LEGAL AND ETHICAL ISSUES *for Health Professionals*

GEORGE D. POZGAR, MBA, CHE, D.LITT.
Consultant
GP Health Care Consulting
Annapolis, Maryland

LEGAL REVIEW
NINA M. SANTUCCI, MSCJ, JD

MEDICAL REVIEW
JOHN W. PINNELLA, MD, DDS, FICS

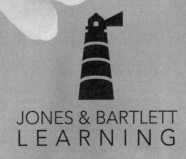

JONES & BARTLETT
LEARNING

World Headquarters
Jones & Bartlett Learning
5 Wall Street
Burlington, MA 01803
978-443-5000
info@jblearning.com
www.jblearning.com

Jones & Bartlett Learning books and products are available through most bookstores and online booksellers. To contact Jones & Bartlett Learning directly, call 800-832-0034, fax 978-443-8000, or visit our website, www.jblearning.com.

Substantial discounts on bulk quantities of Jones & Bartlett Learning publications are available to corporations, professional associations, and other qualified organizations. For details and specific discount information, contact the special sales department at Jones & Bartlett Learning via the above contact information or send an email to specialsales@jblearning.com.

06976-1

Production Credits

VP, Executive Publisher: David D. Cella
Publisher: Cathy L. Esperti
Associate Editor: Sean Fabery
Associate Director of Production: Julie C. Bolduc
Marketing Manager: Grace Richards
Art Development Editor: Joanna Lundeen
Art Development Assistant: Shannon Sheehan
VP, Manufacturing and Inventory Control: Therese Connell
Composition: Cenveo Publisher Services
Cover Design: Kristin E. Parker
Cover Image: © wavebreakmedia/Shutterstock, Inc.
Printing and Binding: Edwards Brothers Malloy

Library of Congress Cataloging-in-Publication Data
Pozgar, George D., author.
  Legal and ethical issues for health professionals / George D. Pozgar.—Fourth edition.
      p. ; cm.
  Includes bibliographical references and index.
  ISBN 978-1-284-03679-4 (alk. paper)
  I. Title.
  [DNLM: 1. Ethics—United States. 2. Legislation, Medical—United States. 3. Ethics, Clinical—United States. 4. Patient Rights—United States. W 32.5 AA1]
  KF3821
  174.2—dc23
                          2014041415

6048

Printed in the United States of America
18 17 16 15 14   10 9 8 7 6 5 4 3 2 1

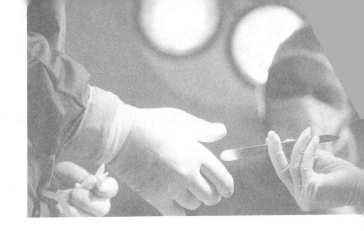

He has achieved success who has lived well, laughed often, and loved much; who has gained the respect of intelligent men and the love of little children; who has filled his niche and accomplished his task; who has left the world better than he found it, whether by an improved poppy, a perfect poem, or a rescued soul; who has never lacked appreciation of earth's beauty or failed to express it; who has always looked for the best in others and given them the best he [or she] had; whose life was an inspiration; whose memory a benediction.

—Bessie Anderson Stanley

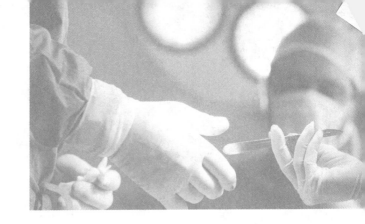

BRIEF CONTENTS

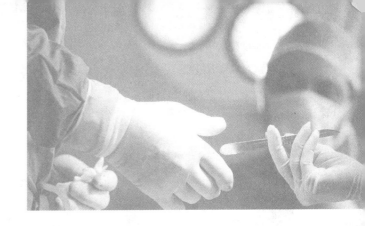

CONTENTS

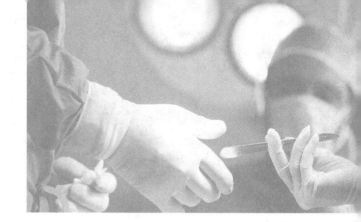

FOREWORD

Good health is an essential and fundamental value that arguably supersedes everything else in our human existence. Thus it is critical to administer it in an ethical, legal, scientifically valid, and efficient manner. This is inherently complicated. Laws are subject to changes. There may even be contradictions among federal, state, and local laws and regulations. Codes of ethics vary among professional organizations, hospitals, and religions. Scientific advances can bring hope for a healthier, longer life but can pose ethical and logistical issues of availability and cost. The pace of change is faster than ever now because of the digital information explosion and promising new avenues of research in such areas as stem cell biology, genetics, nanotechnology, and so much more. It is an exciting time that offers humanity a happier, more optimistic future. The purpose of this *Fourth Edition* is to provide the reader with a reference tool, a framework of fundamentals, and a coherent starting point from which to advance into the future.

Health care is personal. It is perhaps the most personal of any service any of us will receive in our lifetime. We all need it and recognize its importance, and we need to know that our health care delivery system has ethical and legal integrity as well as scientific validity. Sometimes correct choices are not always obvious. There are gray areas. That is why health care administrators and providers need a resource such as this book to help clarify their responsibilities and to help guide them through the tough choices that inevitably occur. Intuition and good intentions are laudable but are not enough when it comes to health care. There are specific criteria that our society requires in this very sensitive area. Awareness of those criteria is crucial. That information, however, comes from a variety of sources that are not always readily accessible. This book concentrates much of that information into one convenient volume. It provides the reader with the proper foundation to make good decisions in the delivery of patient care. That is the ultimate goal of this book.

—John W. Pinnella, MD, DDS, FICS

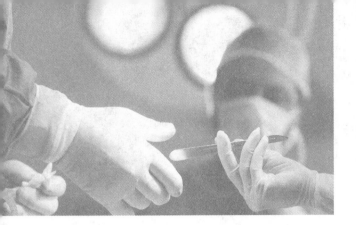

PREFACE

How far you go in life depends on your being tender with the young, compassionate with the aged, sympathetic with the striving, and tolerant of the weak and strong. Because someday in life you will have been all of these.

—GEORGE WASHINGTON CARVER

NEWS

What's the One Thing You Would Invent If You Could?

A "decision-making" machine. You input your life dilemmas, and just like that, the right decision is displayed on a screen. The invention would save me so much time in torment.

Caitlin Ghilarducci, O, The Oprah Magazine, *August 2013*

Legal and Ethical Issues for Health Professionals, Fourth Edition, has been designed to assist the reader in a more comfortable transition from the didactics of the classroom to the practical application in the workplace. The *Fourth Edition* provides the reader with a clearer understanding of how the law and ethics are intertwined as they relate to health care dilemmas. The practical application of ethics in the health care setting is accomplished by interspersing the thoughts of great minds through *Quotes*; current health care events through *News Clippings*; patient, personal, provider, and organizational experiences through *Reality Checks*; and legal rulings and summaries through legal *Cases*. The book concludes with a *closet drama* that illustrates the real world of human behavior and ties together its contents in one case.

The reader will learn how to evaluate and distinguish between the rightness and wrongness of alternative courses of action when faced with complex ethical dilemmas. Ethics in the health care setting focuses on doing the right thing for both patients and caregivers. When people consider matters of ethics they often involve matters of freedom in regard to one's personal choices, judgments about human character, and obligations to others.

This book, as with the first three editions, starts with the premise that to act in an ethical manner means to engage in conduct according to accepted principles of right and wrong. The author's objective is to provide the reader with the background knowledge necessary to understand that ethical behavior begins with understanding that we have alternatives and choices to make about how we treat ourselves and how we treat others. To make good decisions, we must first understand that they will be only as good as our knowledge of what is "right" and what is "wrong."

A study titled "Does Ethics Education Influence the Moral Action of Practicing Nurses and Social Workers?," published in the *American Journal of Bioethics* in July 2008, showed that "ethics education has a significant positive influence on moral confidence, moral action, and use of ethics resources."[1]

This *Fourth Edition* is not an indictment of any profession or organization. It does, however, illustrate how a minority of people can often cast a dark shadow on all the good that is done by so many for so many. It is about learning how the system can fail and how we can so easily fix it simply through good people doing good things. The book is a call to arms to do good things, to stand out from the crowd, because acts of caring, compassion, and kindness often go unnoticed.

The *Fourth Edition*, as with previous editions, has been designed to introduce the reader to various ethical–legal issues and should not be considered an in-depth or comprehensive review of a particular ethical–legal issue. We study ethics because we need to know right from wrong and maintain order in a society that would otherwise be lawless. Ethics distinguishes good from evil. Ethics and the law are inseparable, for it is ethics that describes our values and morality. An unethical person helps create a world of fear, distrust, and tyranny. It is the law that describes our commonly accepted principles of good behavior and provides punishment for those who fail to adhere to the laws of the land.

Cases containing a multitude of legal and ethical issues are included throughout the book. The reader will be asked a series of questions after each case, requiring legal and ethical logic in order to answer them. Caregivers who have a clear grasp of the ethical and legal concepts discussed in this book will be better prepared to make health care decisions that are ethically sound and legally correct. Presented here is a sampling of the wide range of questions that can be asked and discussed when analyzing an ethical dilemma.

1. What are the relevant ethical and legal issues in the case?
2. What could have been done to bring more clarity to the ethical dilemma?
3. How should the legal issues of the case be addressed?
4. How might one's professional code of ethics be violated in the case?
5. How might the principles of patient autonomy, beneficence, nonmaleficence, and justice affect the decision-making process when faced with an ethical dilemma with legal implications?
6. What are the issues that could affect those involved in the resolution of an ethical dilemma (e.g., family members, physicians, other caregivers including nurses, chaplains, and/or ethics committee members)?
7. If you were friendly with the patient, would it affect your ability to give an objective opinion?

---

[1] Grady C., Danis M, Soeken KL, O'Donnell P., Taylor C., Farrar A., and Ulrich C. M. Does ethics education influence the moral action of practicing nurses and social workers? *American Journal of Bioethics*, 2008 Apr; 8(4): 4–11. http://www.ncbi.nlm.nih.gov/pubmed/18576241.

8. How can moral values, religious beliefs, education, and life experiences of both caregivers and patients complicate the resolution of health care dilemmas?
9. How can financial concerns affect the decision-making process?
10. How can corporate culture affect the decision-making process?

One of the most difficult things to come to terms with in the decision-making process is to know when the endless loop of asking questions must end and a decision has to be made.

 Each life is like a novel. Filled with moments of happiness, sadness, crisis, defeat, and triumph. When the last page has been written, will you be happy or saddened by what you read?

—AUTHOR UNKNOWN

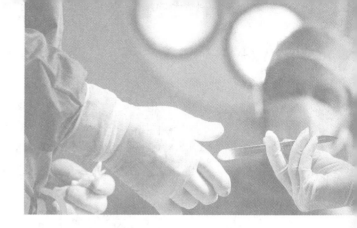

NEW TO THE *FOURTH EDITION*

The fourth edition of *Legal and Ethical Issues for Health Professionals* has been updated to expand discussion on difficult topics and includes a wide variety of current *News Clippings* and *Reality Checks*, which are real life events experienced by both patients and health care professionals in leadership positions in the health care industry. These experiences include those of the author, incorporating his observations from a unique background as a hospital administrator in a multihospital system, instructor, author, consultant, and joint commission surveyor who conducted surveys of more than 1,000 hospitals and outpatient facilities from Alaska to Puerto Rico.

In crafting this edition, some material has been relocated from one chapter to another in order to provide an improved learning experience. In some cases, materials that appear to be duplicative have been removed. As in any update, some sections have been updated to improve understanding and the flow of the text.

The author has made every attempt in this *Fourth Edition* to provide the student with the tools necessary for applying the law and ethics in the health care setting with the end goal of improving the professional's skills, performance, and decision-making processes.

The following is a summary of changes that have been made to improve the readability of the law and ethics content, which can be difficult topics for the reader to grasp owing to the need to learn new terminology, theories, and concepts that have substantial impact on each health care professional's daily tasks.

Changes to all chapters include revisions of the following features:

- Learning Objectives
- Chapter Reviews
- Review Questions

Chapter-specific changes are outlined in the following pages.

CHAPTER 1: INTRODUCTION TO ETHICS

New or expanded topics include the following:

- Morality and moral dilemmas
- Normative ethics
- CPR and paternalism in nursing homes
- Employment-related paternalism
- Nonmaleficence

- Autonomy
- Pillars of moral strength
- Fairness
- Cooperation and teamwork

The following *Reality Checks* have been added:

- "No Good Deed Goes Unpunished"
- "Maximizing Happiness and Reducing Suffering"
- "Duty Compromises Patient Care"
- "Bad Outcome, Good Intentions"
- "Spouse's Grief Leads to Withholding the Truth"
- "Patient Questions Physical Exam"
- "My Journey: How Lucky Am I?"
- "Community Hospital v. Respected Medical Center"

The following *Reality Check* has been revised or expanded:

- "Kill the Messenger"

The following *News Clippings* have been added:

- "Peninsula Child Psychiatrist William Ayres Sentenced to Eight Years for Molesting Patients"
- "The Fear Factor and Patient Satisfaction"
- "Health Costs Cut by Limiting Choices"
- "Cancer Doctor Allegedly Prescribed $35 Million Worth of Totally Unnecessary Chemotherapy"
- "Brooke Greenberg: 20-Year-Old 'Toddler's' Legacy of Hope and Love"
- "Syrian Rebels Combat al-Qaeda Force"
- "Surgeon Uses Ministry in Medical Practice"

CHAPTER 2: CONTEMPORARY ETHICAL DILEMMAS

New or expanded topics include the following:

- Noteworthy historical events
- Informed consent
- Artificial insemination
- Organ donations

The following *News Clippings* have been added:

- "Philadelphia Abortion Doctor Guilty of Murder in Late-Term Procedures"
- "PA Abortion Provider Convicted of Murder"
- "Moral Persuasion on Abortion"
- "Facebook Launches Organ Donation Campaign"

CHAPTER 3: END-OF-LIFE DILEMMAS

New or expanded topics include the following:

- Physician-assisted suicide
- Withholding and withdrawal of treatment
- Do-not-resuscitate orders

The following *News Clippings* have been added:

- "Brain-Dead Girl Jahi McMath Released from California Hospital"
- "Belgium Considering New Euthanasia Law for Kids"
- "California Gov. Signs Assisted Suicide Information Bill into Law"
- "Mass. Doctor-Assisted Suicide Measure Fails"

CHAPTER 4: HEALTH CARE ETHICS COMMITTEE

New or expanded topics include the following:

- Committee structure
- Policy and procedure development
- Consultation and conflict resolution

CHAPTER 5: DEVELOPMENT OF LAW

New or expanded topics include:

- Conflict of laws
- Department of Health and Human Services and Its structure

CHAPTER 6: INTRODUCTION TO LAW

New or expanded topics include the following:

- Duty to care
- Standard of care
- Breach of duty
- Injury/causation
- Causation/proximate cause
- Criminal law
- Grand jury indictment
- Health care fraud
- Investigation and prosecution of fraud
- Schemes to defraud
- Murder
- Contracts

The following *News Clippings* have been added:

- "$12 Million in Medicaid Funds Went to Deceased in Illinois"
- "Renewed Criticism for Google Over Drug Sites"
- "Mother With Terminal Cancer Can Retain Child Custody, Judge Holds"

CHAPTER 7: GOVERNMENT ETHICS AND THE LAW

New or expanded topics include the following:

- House of Representatives Committee on Ethics
- Senate Select Committee on Ethics
- Office of Congressional Ethics
- U.S. Judicial Code of Conduct
- Veterans Administration

The following *Reality Check* has been added:

- VA Hospital

The following *News Clippings* have been added:

- "VA, Heal Thyself, Agency Is Told at Hearing Filled with Pained Testimony"
- "Atlanta VA Exec Scores Bonuses While Audits Found Lapses"
- "Too trapped in a war to be at peace"

CHAPTER 8: ORGANIZATIONAL ETHICS AND THE LAW

New or expanded topics include:

- Implied corporate authority
- Code of ethics for organizations
- Trust and integrity
- Concealing mistakes
- Doctrine of *respondeat superior*
- Independent contractor
- Applicant job screening
- Credentialing, appointment, and privileging
- Complying with accreditation standards
- Accreditation and conflicts of interest
- Financial incentive schemes
- Effective communications builds trust

The following *Reality Checks* have been added:

- "Advertising Unintentionally Misleading"
- "Hospital's Challenge to Survive"
- "One Family's Experience"
- "Veterans' Care Unconscionably Delayed"

The following *Reality Checks* have been revised or expanded:

- "Discrimination: Behind Closed Doors"
- "Accreditation Is Serious Business"

The following *Cases* have been added:

- "Wrong Surgical Procedure Cover-Up"
- "Monitor Alarm Disconnected"

CHAPTER 9: HEALTH CARE PROFESSIONALS LEGAL-ETHICAL ISSUES

New, revised, or expanded topics include the following:

- Ethical and legal issues for nurses
- Float nurses
- Failure to follow instructions
- Diet orders
- Incidence and recognition of malnutrition
- Ethics and inaccurate lab results
- Expanding role of the pharmacist

- Billing fraud
- Resident neglect
- Ethical and legal issues affecting physician assistants
- Sexual harassment by psychologists
- Ethical and legal issues affecting radiology technologists
- Ethical and legal issues affecting respiratory therapists
- Ethical and legal issues affecting social workers

The following *Reality Checks* have been added:

- "Patient's Diet Order Inappropriate"
- "Patient's Nutritional Status Not Addressed"

The following *Case* has been revised:

- "Refusal to Perform HIV Testing"

CHAPTER 10: PHYSICIAN ETHICAL AND LEGAL ISSUES

New, revised, or expanded topics include the following:

- How the law and ethics intertwine in patient care
- Violations of the AMA Code of Ethics
- Compassion
- Trust and breaches of trust
- Justice
- Physician negligence
- Patient assessments
- Failure to respond to emergency call
- Family medical history
- Medical misdiagnosis
- Treatment
- Surgery
- Patient infections

The following *News Clippings* have been added:

- "Suddenly, unexpectedly, he grabs my shirt"
- "Bonded by Blood"
- "As Hands-On Doctoring Fades Away, Patients Lose"
- "Her Doctor Dismissed the Lump in Her Breast"
- "Joint Commission Alert: Preventing Retained Surgical Items"
- "Pregnant Woman Dies After Horrifying Medical Mixup"

CHAPTER 11: EMPLOYEE RIGHTS AND RESPONSIBILITIES

New, revised, or expanded topics include the following:

- Freedom from discrimination
- Equal Employment Opportunity Commission
- Refusal to Participate in Therapeutic Abortion Insubordinate
- Whistleblowing
- Safe environment
- Unemployment compensation
- Complying with hospital policy

- Sexual harassment
- Maintain professional competencies

The following *Reality Checks* have been added:

- "O.R. Becomes an Abusive Environment"
- "My Surgical Journey"
- "Failure to Comply with Hand Hygiene Guidelines"

The following *News Clippings* have been added:

- "Hospitals Crack Down on Tirades by Angry Doctors"
- "Drug Firm to Pay $2.2 Billion in Fraud Settlement"
- "Physician Whistle-Blowers Can Sue Hospitals Without Delay, Appeals Court Rules"
- "Whistleblower Lawsuit Alleges Florida Hospital Filed Millions in False Claims"
- "The Price Whistle-Blowers Pay for Secrets"
- "U.S. Cancer-Care Delivery is 'in Crisis': Report"

CHAPTER 12: PATIENT CONSENT

New, revised, or expanded topics include the following:

- Codes of ethics
- Parental consent
- Right to refuse treatment
- Refusal of treatment based on religious beliefs

The following *News Clippings* have been added:

- "Unreported Robot Surgery Injuries Open New Questions for FDA"
- "Are Teens Old Enough for Life/Death Decisions?"

CHAPTER 13: PATIENT ABUSE

New, revised, or expanded topics include the following:

- Child abuse
- Reporting abuse
- Senior abuse
- Reporting senior abuse

The following *Reality Check* has been added:

- "Child Abuse Can Be Elusive"

CHAPTER 14: PATIENT RIGHTS AND RESPONSIBILITIES

New, revised, or expanded topics include the following:

- Patient rights
- Right to know one's rights
- The Health Insurance Portability and Accountability Act (HIPAA)
- Right to ask questions
- Right to examination and treatment

- Right to emergency care
- Execute advance directives
- Right to trust caregivers
- Right to chaplaincy services
- Right to ethics consultation
- Right to informed consent
- Right to receive quality care
- Right to compassionate care
- Discharge orders
- Right to access lab reports
- Right to know hospital charges
- Maintain healthy lifestyle
- Provide full disclosure of medical history
- Report unexpected changes in health status
- Adhere to the agreed upon treatment plan
- Seek a second opinion
- Stay informed

The following *Reality Checks* have been added:

- "Accreditation Standards and Patient Right to Ask Questions"
- "My Question Disregarded"
- "Hospital Charges Not So Transparent"

The following *Case* has been added:

- "Release from Hospital Contraindicated"

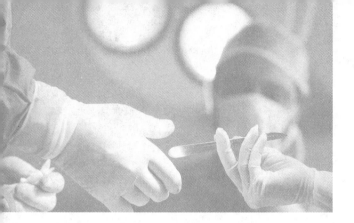

ACKNOWLEDGMENTS

The author especially acknowledges the staff at Jones & Bartlett Learning whose guidance and assistance were so important in making this fourth edition of *Legal and Ethical Issues for Health Professionals* a reality. Special thanks to Katey Bircher and Teresa Reilly during the signing stage of the *Fourth Edition*; Rhonda Dearborn and Sean Fabery, who worked tirelessly during the editorial stages; the production editors, Lou Bruno and Julie Bolduc; and the all-important Grace Richards in marketing. As with the publication of any book, there are numerous people behind the scenes with whom I have not dealt with directly. Please know that your hard work is much appreciated. Thanks to all for allowing me to leave behind this legacy of writing.

I am grateful to the very special people in the more than 1,000 hospitals and ambulatory sites from Alaska to Puerto Rico with whom I have consulted, surveyed, and provided education over many years. Their shared experiences have served to remind me of the importance of making this book valuable in the classroom as well as useful as a reference for practicing health care professionals.

To my students in health care law and ethics classes at the New School for Social Research, Molloy College, Long Island University–C.W. Post Campus, Saint Francis College, and Saint Joseph's College; my intern from Brown University; my resident in hospital administration from The George Washington University; and those I have instructed throughout the years at various seminars, I will always be indebted to you for your inspiration.

Many thanks are also extended to all those special people at the National Library of Medicine and the Library of Congress for their guidance over the years in locating research materials.

CHAPTER 1

ETHICS

INTRODUCTION TO ETHICS

I expect to pass through this world but once. Any good therefore that I can do, or any kindness I can show to any creature, let me do it now. Let me not defer it, for I shall not pass this way again.

—STEPHEN GRELLET

LEARNING OBJECTIVES

Upon completion of this chapter, the reader will be able to:

- Explain what ethics is, its importance, and its application to ethical dilemmas.
- Describe the concepts of morality, codes of conduct, and moral judgments.
- Understand relevant ethical theories and principles.
- Describe virtue ethics and values and how they more clearly describe one's moral character.

- Understand how religious ethics can affect one's moral character.
- Explain the concept of situational ethics and how changes in circumstances can alter one's behavior.
- Understand the importance of reasoning in the decision-making process.

INTRODUCTION

Good can triumph over evil.

—AUTHOR UNKNOWN

This chapter provides the reader with an overview of ethics, moral principles, virtues, and values. The intent here is not to burden the reader with the philosophical arguments surrounding ethical theories, morals, and principles; however, as with the study of any new subject, "words are the tools of thought." The reader who thoroughly absorbs and applies the content of the theories and principles of ethics discussed herein will have the tools necessary to empathize with and guide patients through the conflicts they will face when making difficult care decisions. Therefore, some new vocabulary is a necessary tool, as a building block for the reader to establish a foundation for applying the abstract theories and principles of ethics in order to make practical use of them.

Theories, principles, virtues, and values are a necessary beginning point for the study of ethics. Words are merely labels for ideas and best used for helping the reader to wire his or her mind to think through difficult dilemmas more easily. The directions on a map are of little value until we make the journey. So it is with ethics; we must begin to make the journey inward with a lot of hard mind work so that we can more easily make the right decisions when faced with ethical dilemmas. The learning process for ethics becomes a more enjoyable and rewarding journey as we grasp the ideas, build upon them, and practice all the good we learn by helping all the people we can as long as we can.

ETHICS

How we perceive right and wrong is influenced by what we feed on.

—AUTHOR UNKNOWN

Ethics is the branch of philosophy that seeks to understand the nature, purposes, justification, and founding principles of moral rules and the systems they comprise. Ethics and morals are derivatives from the Greek and Latin terms (roots) for custom. The etymology of the words "ethics" and "morality" are derived from the roots "ethos" and "mos," which both convey a meaning describing customs or habits. This etymology supports the claims of anthropologist Ruth Benedict that all values are rooted in customs and habits of a culture because the words moral and ethics themselves were essentially created to describe these topics.[1]

Ethics deals with values relating to human conduct. It focuses on the rightness and wrongness of actions, as well as the goodness and badness of motives and ends. Ethics encompasses the decision-making process of determining ultimate actions—what should I do and is it the right thing to do. It involves how individuals decide to live with one another within accepted boundaries and how they live in harmony with the environment as well as one another. Ethics is concerned with human conduct as it ought to be, as opposed to what it actually is.

Microethics involves an individual's view of what is right and wrong based on one's personal life teachings, tradition, and experiences. *Macroethics* involves a more global view of right and wrong. Although no person lives in a vacuum, solving ethical dilemmas involves consideration of ethical issues from both a micro and macro perspective.

Man's duty is to improve himself; to cultivate his mind; and, when he finds himself going astray, to bring the moral law to bear upon himself.

–IMMANUEL KANT

The term *ethics* is used in three distinct but related ways, signifying (1) *philosophical ethics*, which involves inquiry about ways of life and rules of conduct; (2) a *general pattern or way of life*, such as religious ethics (e.g., Judeo-Christian ethics); and (3) a *set of rules* of conduct or "moral code" (e.g., professional codes for ethical behavior).

The scope of health care ethics encompasses numerous issues, including the right to choose or refuse treatment and the right to limit the suffering one will endure. Incredible advances in technology and the resulting capability to extend life beyond what would be considered a reasonable quality of life have complicated the process of health care decision making. The scope of health care ethics is not limited to philosophical issues but embraces economic, medical, political, social, and legal dilemmas.

Bioethics addresses such difficult issues as the nature of life, the nature of death, what sort of life is worth living, what constitutes murder, how we should treat people who are especially vulnerable, and the responsibilities that we have to other human beings. It is about making better decisions when faced with diverse and complex circumstances.

WHY STUDY ETHICS?

We study ethics to help us make sound judgments, good decisions, and right choices; if not right choices, then better choices. To those in the health care industry, it is about anticipating and recognizing health care dilemmas and making good judgments and decisions based on universal values that work in unison with the laws of the land and our constitution. Where the law remains silent, we rely on the ability of caregivers to make sound judgments, guided by the Wisdom of Solomon to do good. Doing the right thing by applying the universal morals and values described in this text (e.g., the 10 Commandments) will help shield and protect all from harm.

MORALITY

The three hardest tasks in the world are neither physical feats nor intellectual achievements, but moral acts: to return love for hate, to include the excluded, and to say, "I was wrong."

–SYDNEY J. HARRIS

The following news clippings portray how a deficiency in the morality of society can lead to a betrayal of humanity. Lawlessness and heartless actions run rampant in a land void of courage and compassion. The reader who thoroughly absorbs, understands, and practices the virtues and values discussed in the pages that follow will spring forth hope in what often seems a desperate and hopeless world.

Vietnam—Terror of War

Fire rained down on civilians. Women and children ran screaming. Ut snapped pictures. A little girl ran toward him, arms outstretched, eyes shut in pain, clothes burned off by Napalm. She said, "Too hot, please help me!"

1973 Spot News, Newseum, *Washington, DC*

Ethiopian Famine (1985 Feature)

People searched everywhere for food. Some 30,000 tons of it, from the United States, had been held up by an Ethiopian government determined to starve the countryside into submission. And starve the people it did—half a million Ethiopians, many of them children so hungry their bodies actually consumed themselves.

I'll never forget the sounds of kids dying of starvation.

Newseum, *Washington, DC*

Waiting Game for Sudanese Child . . .

Carter's winning photo shows a heartbreaking scene of a starving child collapsed on the ground, struggling to get to a food center during a famine in the Sudan in 1993. In the background, a vulture stalks the emaciated child.

Carter was part of a group of four fearless photojournalists known as the "Bang Bang Club" who traveled throughout South Africa capturing the atrocities committed during apartheid.

Haunted by the horrific images from Sudan, Carter committed suicide in 1994 soon after receiving the award.

A Pulitzer-Winning Photographer's Suicide, National Public Radio, (NPR), *March 2, 2006*

Trek of tears describes many horrible historic events, from broken treaties with American Indians to an African Journey of horror, where people would flee together as a village to escape the barbaric slaughter of men, women, and children as the remainder of the world stood cowardly by watching the death and starvation of hundreds of thousands of people. Human atrocities committed by humans. Is it not time to stand up and be counted on to do what is right and leave all excuses behind for our complacency toward the genocide that continues throughout the world?

–GP

There are those who have been brainwashed into believing, in the name of religion, that if they blow themselves up in public places, killing innocent people, that they will be rewarded in the afterlife. This is not religion and it is not culture; it is evil people brainwashing young minds to do evil things.

–GP

Aim above morality. Be not simply good; be good for something.

–Henry David Thoreau

Morality describes a class of rules held by society to govern the conduct of its individual members. It implies the quality of being in accord with standards of right and good conduct. Morality is a code of conduct. It is a guide to behavior that all rational persons should put forward for governing their behavior. Morality requires us to reach a decision as to the rightness or wrongness of an action. *Morals* are ideas about what is right and what is wrong; for example, killing is wrong, whereas helping the poor is right, and causing pain is wrong, whereas easing pain is right. Morals are deeply ingrained in culture and religion and are often part of its identity. Morals should not be confused with religious or cultural habits or customs, such as wearing a religious garment (e.g., veil, turban). That which is considered morally right can vary from nation to nation, culture to culture, and religion to religion. In other words, there is no universal morality that is recognized by all people in all cultures at all times.

CODE OF CONDUCT

A *code of conduct* generally prescribes standards of conduct, states principles expressing responsibilities, and defines the rules expressing duties of professionals to whom they apply. Most members of a profession subscribe to certain "values" and moral standards written into a formal document called a code of ethics. Codes of conduct often require interpretation by caregivers as they apply to the specific circumstances surrounding each dilemma.

Michael D. Bayles, a famous author and teacher, describes the differences between standards, principles, and rules:

- *Standards* (e.g., honesty, respect for others, conscientiousness) are used to guide human conduct by stating desirable traits to be exhibited and undesirable ones (dishonesty, deceitfulness, self-interest) to be avoided.
- *Principles* describe responsibilities that do not specify what the required conduct should be. Professionals need to make a judgment about what is desirable in a particular situation based on accepted principles.
- *Rules* specify specific conduct; they do not allow for individual professional judgment.

MORAL JUDGMENTS

Moral judgments are those judgments concerned with what an individual or group believes to be the right or proper behavior in a given situation. Making a moral judgment is being able to choose an option from among choices. It involves assessing another person's moral character based on how he or she conforms to the moral convictions established by the individual and/or group. A lack of conformity can result in moral disapproval and possibly ridicule of one's character.

MORALITY LEGISLATED

When it is important that disagreements be settled, morality is often legislated. Law is distinguished from morality by having explicit rules and penalties, as well as officials who interpret the laws and apply penalties when laws are broken. There is often considerable overlap in the conduct governed by morality and that governed by law. Laws are created to set boundaries for societal behavior. They are enforced to ensure that the expected behavior happens.

MORAL DILEMMAS

Moral dilemmas in the health care setting often arise when values, rights, duties, and loyalties conflict. Caregivers often find that there appears to be no right or wrong answer when faced with the daunting task of deciding which decision path to follow. The best answer when attempting to resolve an ethical dilemma includes the known wishes of the patient and other pertinent information, such as a living will, that might be available when the patient is considered incompetent to make his or her own choices. The right answer is often elusive when the patient is in a coma and there are no known documents as to a patient's wishes and there are no living relatives. However, an understanding of the concepts presented here will help the caregiver in resolving complex ethical dilemmas.

ETHICAL THEORIES

Ethics, too, are nothing but reverence for life. This is what gives me the fundamental principle of morality, namely, that good consists in maintaining, promoting, and enhancing life, and that destroying, injuring, and limiting life are evil.

—ALBERT SCHWEITZER

Ethics seeks to understand and to determine how human actions can be judged as right or wrong. Ethical judgments can be made based on our own experiences or based upon the nature of or principles of reason.

Ethical theories and principles introduce order into the way people think about life. They are the foundations of ethical analysis and provide guidance in the decision-making process. Various theories present varying viewpoints that assist caregivers in making difficult decisions when faced with ethical dilemmas that affect the lives of others. The more commonly discussed ethical theories are presented here.

Metaethics is the study of the origin and meaning of ethical concepts. Metaethics seeks to understand ethical terms and theories and their application. "Metaethics explores as well the connection between values, reasons for action, and human motivation, asking how it is that moral standards might provide us with reasons to do or refrain from doing as it demands, and it addresses many of the issues commonly bound up with the nature of freedom and its significance (or not) for moral responsibility."[2]

NORMATIVE ETHICS

Normative ethics is prescriptive in that it attempts to determine what moral standards should be followed so that human behavior and conduct may be morally right. Normative ethics is primarily concerned with establishing standards or norms for conduct and is commonly associated with investigating how one ought to act. It involves the critical study of major moral precepts, such as what things are right, what things are good, and what things are genuine. One of the central questions of modern normative ethics is whether human actions are to be judged right or wrong solely according to their consequences.

The determination of a universal moral principle for all humanity is a formidable task and most likely not feasible due to the diversity of people and their cultures. However, there is a need to have a commonly held consensus as to right and wrong to avoid chaos. Thus, there are generally accepted moral standards around which laws are drafted.

Normative Ethics and Assisted Suicide

Oregon's Death with Dignity Act of 1997 allows terminally ill state residents to end their lives through the voluntary self-administration of a lethal dose of medications prescribed by a physician.[3] Although this act was voted upon by the Oregon state legislature and agreed upon by referendum, there are those who disagree with the law from a religious or moral standpoint. The Oregon act is controversial at best and has placed morality and the law in conflict. In the middle of the continuing controversy is the terminally ill patient who must make the ultimate decision of life versus death. It could be argued that it is morally wrong to take one's own life regardless of the law or it can be argued that ending one's life is a morally permissible right because the law provides the opportunity for terminally ill patients to make end-of-life decisions that include the right to self-administer a lethal dose of medications.

As there is a diversity of cultures, there is diversity of opinions as to the rightness and wrongness of the Oregon act. From a microethics point of view as it relates to the Oregon law, each individual must decide what is the right thing to do.

Normative ethics prescribes how people should act and descriptive ethics describes how people act. Both theories have application in the Oregon act. The controversial nature of physician-assisted suicide in the various states is but one of many health care dilemmas caregivers will experience during their careers (e.g., abortion, euthanasia).

DESCRIPTIVE ETHICS

Descriptive ethics, also known as comparative ethics, is the study of what people believe to be right and wrong and why they believe it. Descriptive ethics describes how people act, whereas normative ethics prescribes how people ought to act.

APPLIED ETHICS

Applied ethics is "the philosophical search (within western philosophy) for right and wrong within controversial scenarios."[4] *Applied ethics* is the application of normative theories to practical moral problems, such as abortion, euthanasia, and assisted suicide.

Consequential Ethics

The end excuses any evil.

—Sophocles, *Electra* (c. 409 B.C.)

The *consequential theory* of ethics emphasizes that the morally right action is whatever action leads to the maximum balance of good over evil. From a contemporary standpoint, theories that judge actions by their consequences have been referred to as consequential ethics. Consequential ethical theories revolve around the premise that the rightness or wrongness of an action depends on the consequences or effects of an action. The theory of consequential ethics is based on the view that the value of an action derives solely from the value of its consequences. The consequentialist considers the morally right act or failure to act is one that will produce a good outcome. The goal of a consequentialist is to achieve the greatest good for the greatest number. It involves asking such questions as:

- What will be the effects of each course of action?
- Who will benefit?
- What action will cause the least harm?
- What action will lead to the greatest good?

These questions should be applied when answering the questions in the following *reality check*.

No Good Deed Goes Unpunished

Matt was assigned to survey "Community Medical Center" (CMC) in Minnesota with a team of three surveyors and one observer. He related to me his experience of surveying the children's dental clinic.

Following his tour of CMC's dental clinic, Matt reviewed with the clinic's staff the dental program, which served the city's underserved children. He also reviewed the care rendered several patients based on common and complex diagnoses, as well as the clinic's performance improvement activities. During the survey Dr. Seiden, the clinic director asked, "Are surveyors trained about the importance of dental care in disease prevention? As you know, dentistry is often a stepchild when it comes to allocation of scarce resources. Departments like surgery and radiology often receive the lion's share of funds." Matt responded by describing a film sponsored by the American Dental Association that was shown when he was in training to become a surveyor. The film presented a man whose dental care had been sorely neglected throughout his life and not been addressed prior to replacement of a heart valve. The patient developed a systemic infection following surgery, which led to deterioration of the heart valve and the patient's ultimate death. The film described the lessons learned and opportunities for performance improvement that included the need for a dental evaluation by a dentist prior to valve replacement. Dr. Seiden was pleased to learn that the importance of dentistry is included in surveyor training.

Following Matt's survey of the dental clinic, the staff relayed to him their concern that the clinic was going to be closed for lack of funds. Cheryl, the clinic manager, explained, "I sometimes feel the importance of the dental clinic to the underserved population is not well-understood." A bit emotional, Cheryl said, "Matt, have you surveyed other dental clinics?" Matt replied, "Yes, several well-funded clinics that come to mind were in Philadelphia and New York." Cheryl then asked, "Matt, do you have any ideas as to how we can save our clinic from closing?" Matt replied, "I have some time before lunch and I can share a few ideas with you." Cheryl replied, "The staff will be eager to listen." The staff proceeded to place several chairs in a semicircle and brainstormed with Matt a variety of ideas for saving the clinic. The staff discussed several fund-raising activities including a car wash by children to bring awareness to Any Town's dental clinic." Matt looked at his watch and said, "I need to get back to my survey team, but I want to leave you with one other thought to ponder that could be applicable to any department in the hospital. I was surveying a veteran's hospital physical therapy department and noticed on their bulletin board the staff's dream plan for renovation of their department. I asked the physical therapy staff about the plan. They related how their vision of a new physical therapy department had been sketched out and placed on their bulletin board. Several weeks later, a veteran who had been sitting in the waiting area became curious about their dream. After studying the board during his visits for therapy, he walked to the reception desk on his last visit and asked about their vision for physical therapy. They explained it was a $200,000 dream. Gary looked at the staff at the reception desk and said, "It is no longer a dream. I don't have much, but what I do have is enough to make your dream come true." And, so he did. Matt continued, "You see, if people know your dreams, something as small as a bulletin board can make all the difference." Dr. Seiden smiled and said, "I see where this is going, community awareness as to the need to fund the clinic. It's really not merely about a car wash, it's about a concept of how the hospital can save not only the dental clinic but other programs earmarked for closing." Matt smiled, as the staff regained hope. Dr. Seiden, seeing that Matt had little time for lunch, stood up, extended his hand and said, "Matt, you gave us hope when we believed there was none. Thank you so much. I will be sure to discuss this with administration."

Matt presented his observations the following morning to the organization's leadership, which included his round table discussion with the staff. He was however cut short in his presentation by the surveyor team leader, Brad, who later reported to Victor, Matt's manager, that Matt should not be discussing how to save a dental clinic by opening a car wash. Matt received a reprimand from Victor and was removed at the end of day 4 of a 5-day survey without explanation.

Anonymous

Discussion

1. Discuss Matt's approach to addressing the staff's concerns for saving the children's dental clinic.
2. If Matt's round table session led to saving the clinic, was Matt's reprimand worth the risk if he could have foreseen the resulting reprimand?
3. The goal of a consequentialist is to achieve the greatest good for the greatest number. Discuss how this applies in this *reality check*.

Utilitarian Ethics

Happiness often sneaks in a door you did not think was open.

—AUTHOR UNKNOWN

The utilitarian theory of ethics involves the concept that the moral worth of an action is determined solely by its contribution to overall usefulness. It describes doing the greatest good for the most people. It is thus a form of consequential ethics, meaning that the moral worth of an action is determined by its outcome, and, thus, the ends justify the means. The utilitarian commonly holds that the proper course of an action is one that maximizes utility, commonly defined as maximizing happiness and reducing suffering, as noted in the following *reality check*.

Maximizing Happiness and Reducing Suffering

Daniel was the last of five interviews for the CEO's position at Anytown Medical Center. During the interview, a member of the finance committee asked, "Daniel, how would maximize an allocation of $100,000 to spend as you wished for improving patient care, aside from capital budget and construction projects?" Bishop Paul, the board chairman added, "Daniel, think about the question. I will give you five minutes to form an answer." Daniel responded, "Bishop Paul, I am ready now to answer your question." The trustees looked somewhat surprised, as Bishop Paul with a smile quickly responded, "You may proceed with your answer." Daniel replied, "An old Chinese proverb came to mind as quickly as the question was asked: 'Give a man a fish and you feed him for a day. Teach a man to fish and you feed him for a lifetime.' You are interviewing me as CEO of your hospital. I see my job as assuring you that employees are thoroughly trained to care for the patients the hospital serves. I will maximize the value of each and every dollar by determining the staff skill sets that are lacking and retrain staff in the areas deficiencies are noted." Bishop Paul looked around the long oval table at the trustees, "This has been a long day and a grueling interview process for Daniel. Are there any other questions you would like to ask him." There was silence, as the trustees nodded their heads no. Bishop Paul looked at Daniel and thanked him for his interest in becoming the hospital's next CEO.

As Daniel began to leave the boardroom, Bishop Paul smiled and turned his swivel chair around as Daniel was walking towards the exit and asked, "Daniel, could you not leave the building just yet. If you could, just wait outside the room and have a seat in the doctors' lounge area." After about 20 minutes, a trustee went into the lounge where Daniel was sitting and asked him to return to the boardroom. As he entered the room, Bishop Paul stood up and looked at Daniel straight in his eyes and said, "Daniel, you were the last to be interviewed because you were on the 'short list' of candidates selected to be interviewed. Speaking for the board, your response to the last question was merely icing on the cake confirming our interest in you joining our staff. Both the Board of Trustees and members of the Medical Executive Committee unanimously have recommended you as our CEO, with which I unconditionally concur! Welcome to Anytown hospital." The trustees stood and clapped their hands. The bishop turned to the trustees and said, "Wow, that's a first."

Anonymous

Discussion

1. Discuss how Daniel's response to the trustee's question of how he would spend the $100,000 fits the utilitarian theory of ethics.
2. Did Daniel, metaphorically speaking, succeed in maximizing happiness in the eyes of the board? Discuss your answer.

DEONTOLOGICAL ETHICS

Act in such a way that you always treat humanity, whether in your own person or in the person of any other, never simply as a means, but always at the same time as an end.

—IMMANUEL KANT

Deontological ethics is commonly attributed to the German philosopher Immanuel Kant (1724–1804). Kant believed that although doing the right thing is good, it might not always lead to or increase the good and right thing sought after. It focuses on one's duties to others and others' rights. It includes telling the truth and keeping your promises. Deontology ethics is often referred to as duty-based ethics. It involves ethical analysis according to a moral code or rules, religious or secular. *Deon* is derived from the Greek word meaning "duty." Kant's theory differs from consequentialism in that consequences are not the determinant of what is right; therefore, doing the right thing may not always lead to an increase in what is good.

> Duty-based approaches are heavy on obligation, in the sense that a person who follows this ethical paradigm believes that the highest virtue comes from doing what you are supposed to do—either because you have to, e.g., following the law, or because you agreed to, e.g., following an employer's policies. It matters little whether the act leads to good consequences; what matters is "doing your duty."[5]

The following *reality check* illustrates how duty-based ethics focuses on the act and not the consequences of an act.

Duty Compromises Patient Care

At 33 years of age, I was the youngest administrator in New York State and was about to learn that adhering to company policy sometimes conflicts with the needs of the patient. In this case it was a 38-year-old employee who had been diagnosed with cancer. I remember the day well, even though it was more than 30 years ago. My secretary alerted me that Carol, a practical nurse and employee, had been admitted to the 3-North medical-surgical unit, where she worked. Without delay, I left my office and went to the nursing unit and inquired as to what room Carol was in. Beth, the unit's nurse manager, overheard my question. She walked up to me and asked, "Daniel, could I please talk to you for a moment before you visit with Carol?" I looked at her and nodded my head yes and without thought we both walked to her office. She closed the door and said, "As you know, we are self-insured and the health insurance program we have does not cover Carol's chemotherapy treatments. She cannot bear the cost. Is there anything you can do to help her?" I replied that I would make an inquiry with our human resources director to see what could be done.

Beth asked, "Would you mind if I went with you to Carol's room for a few minutes." Daniel compassionately replied, "Of course you can."

They walked to Carol's room. Her husband and children had just left. Beth stayed for a few minutes while Daniel remained behind chatting with Carol for a few moments and said he would be back to talk with her more.

Daniel went to speak with Christine, the human resources director for his hospital. There were two other hospitals in the multihospital system. He explained Carol's financial situation and her lack of funds for chemotherapy treatment. Christine replied, "Daniel, this is corporate policy that is applicable to all three hospitals with which we must comply." Following much discussion, Daniel said, "Christine, Carol is an employee and I realize there are conflicting duties here. One is to follow corporate policy or choose to do, as I see it, what is right for Carol. If you prefer, I can request an exception to the rule. To me, right trumps duty." Christine looked at Daniel and said, "Daniel, I will see what I can do. I have a good relationship with the corporate vice president for human resources. If anyone can make an exception, he can make it happen. I know you would do the same for me and any other employee."

Anonymous

Discussion

1. Discuss the potential long-term effect of granting an exception for Carol.
2. Do you believe that duty should be trumped by good? Discuss your answer.
3. Would you describe Daniel as consequentialist because he favors evaluating the outcome of an act rather than the act itself? Discuss your answer.
4. Discuss how deontological ethics in this case is in conflict with consequential thinking.

NONCONSEQUENTIAL ETHICS

The *nonconsequential ethical theory* denies that the consequences of an action are the only criteria for determining the morality of an action. In this theory, the rightness or wrongness of an action is based on properties intrinsic to the action, not on its consequences. In other words, the nonconsequentialist believes right or wrong depends on the intention not the outcome.

Bad Outcome, Good Intentions

Chelsea was preparing to drape Mr. Smith's leg in OR 6 for surgery, when she was approached by Nicole, the nurse manager, asked, "Chelsea, please come to OR 3. We have an emergency there and urgently need your skills to assist the surgeon." Chelsea turned to Daniel, the surgical technician, and asked him to continue prepping Mr. Smith's leg for surgery. Daniel prepped the leg prior to the surgeon entering the room. The surgeon entered the room a few minutes later and asked, "Where is Chelsea?" Daniel replied, "She was called away for an emergency in OR 3. Karen will be in shortly to assist us."

Following surgery, Mr. Smith was transferred to the recovery room. While he was in the recovery room a nurse was looking at the patient's medical record as to the notes regarding the patient's procedure during surgery. She noticed that surgery was conducted on the wrong leg.

Although there was heated discussion between the surgeon and nursing staff, each member of the staff had good intentions but the outcome was not so good. Nonconsequentialists believe that right or wrong depends on the intention. They generally focus more on deeds and whether those deeds are good or bad. In this case the intentions were good but the outcome was bad. It should be noted that nonconsequentialists do not always ignore the consequences. They accept the fact that sometimes good intentions can lead to bad outcomes. In summary nonconsequentialists focus more on character as to whether someone is a good person or not. Nonconsequentialists believe that right or wrong depends on the intention. Generally, the consequentialist will focus more on outcomes as to whether or not they are good or bad.

Discussion

1. Describe how the nonconsequential theory of ethics applies in this case.
2. What questions might the consequentialist raise after reviewing the facts of this case?

ETHICAL RELATIVISM

The theory of *ethical relativism* holds that morality is relative to the norms of the culture in which an individual lives. In other words, right or wrong depends on the moral norms of the society in which it is practiced. A particular action by an individual may be morally right in one society or culture and wrong in another. What is acceptable in one society may not be considered as such in another. Slavery may be considered an acceptable practice in one society and unacceptable and unconscionable in another. The administration of blood may be acceptable as to one's religious beliefs and not acceptable to another within the same society. The legal rights of patients vary from state to state, as is well borne out, for example, by Oregon's Death with Dignity Act. Caregivers must be aware of cultural, religious, and legal issues that can affect the boundaries of what is acceptable and what is unacceptable practice, especially when delivering health care to persons with beliefs different from their own. As the various cultures of the world merge together in communities, the education and training of caregivers become more complex. The caregiver must not only grasp the clinical skills of his or her profession but also have a basic understanding of what is right and what is wrong from both a legal and ethical point of view. Although decision making is not always perfect, the knowledge gained from this text will aid the reader in making better decisions.

PRINCIPLES OF ETHICS

You cannot by tying an opinion to a man's tongue, make him the representative of that opinion; and at the close of any battle for principles, his name will be found neither among the dead, nor the wounded, but the missing.

—E.P. WHIPPLE (1819–1886)

An army of principles can penetrate where an army of soldiers cannot.

—THOMAS JEFFERSON

Ethical principles are universal rules of conduct, derived from ethical theories that provide a practical basis for identifying what kinds of actions, intentions, and motives are valued. Ethical principles assist caregivers in making choices based on moral principles that have been identified as standards considered worthwhile in addressing health care–related ethical dilemmas. As noted by the principles discussed in the following sections, caregivers, in the study of ethics, will find that difficult decisions often involve choices between conflicting ethical principles.

AUTONOMY

No right is held more sacred, or is more carefully guarded, by the common law, than the right of every individual to the possession and control of his own person, free from all restraint or interference of others, unless by clear and unquestioned authority of law.

—UNION PACIFIC RY. CO. V. BOTSFORD [141 U.S. 250, 251 (1891)]

The principle of *autonomy* involves recognizing the right of a person to make one's own decisions. "Auto" comes from a Greek word meaning "self" or the "individual." In this context, it means recognizing an individual's right to make his or her own decisions about what is best for him or herself. Autonomy is not an absolute principle. The autonomous actions of one person must not infringe upon the rights of another. The eminent Justice Benjamin Cardozo, in *Schloendorff v. Society of New York Hospital*, stated:

> Every human being of adult years and sound mind has a right to determine what shall be done with his own body and a surgeon who performs an operation without his patient's consent commits an assault, for which he is liable in damages, except in cases of emergency where the patient is unconscious and where it is necessary to operate before consent can be obtained.[6]

Each person has a right to make his or her own decisions about health care. A patient has the right to refuse to receive health care even if it is beneficial to saving his or her life. Patients can refuse treatment, refuse to take medications, and refuse invasive procedures regardless of the benefits that may be derived from them. They have a right to have their decisions adhered to by family members who may disagree simply because they are unable to let go. Although patients have a right to make their own choices, they also have a concomitant right to know the risks, benefits, and alternatives to recommended procedures.

Autonomous decision making can be affected by one's disabilities, mental status, maturity, or incapacity to make decisions. Although the principle of autonomy may be inapplicable in certain cases, one's autonomous wishes may be carried out through an advance directive and/or an appointed health care agent in the event of one's inability to make decisions.

What happens when the right to autonomy conflicts with other moral principles, such as beneficence and justice? Conflict can arise, for example, when a patient refuses a blood transfusion considered necessary to save his or her life whereas the caregiver's principal obligation is to do no harm. What is the right thing to do when the spouse decides to have the physician withhold from his wife her true diagnosis?

Spouse's Grief Leads to Withholding the Truth

Annie, a 27-year-old woman with one child, began experiencing severe pain in her abdomen while visiting her family in May. After describing the excruciating pain to her husband Daniel, he scheduled Annie for an appointment with Dr. Sokol, a gastroenterologist, who ordered a series of tests. While conducting a barium scan, a radiologist at Community Hospital noted a small bowel obstruction. Dr. Sokol recommended surgery to which both Annie and Daniel agreed.

After the surgery, on July 7, Dr. Brown, the operating surgeon, paged Daniel over the hospital intercom as he walked down a corridor on the ground floor. Daniel, hearing the page, picked up a house phone and dialed zero for an operator. The operator inquired, "May I help you?" "Yes," Daniel replied. "I was just paged." The operator replied, "Oh, yes. Dr. Brown would like to talk to you. I will connect you with him. Hang on. Don't hang up." (Daniel's heart began to pound.) Dr. Brown asked, "Is this you, Daniel?" Daniel replied, "Yes, it is." Dr. Brown replied, "Well, surgery is over. Your wife is recovering nicely in the recovery room." Daniel was relieved but for a moment. "That's good." Daniel sensed Dr. Brown had more to say. Dr. Brown continued, "I am sorry to say that she has carcinoma of the colon." Daniel replied, "Did you get it all?" Dr. Brown reluctantly replied, "I am sorry, but the cancer has spread to her lymph nodes and surrounding organs." Daniel, with the tears in his eyes, asked, "Can I see her?" Dr. Brown replied, "She is in the recovery room." Before hanging up, Daniel told Dr. Brown, "Please do not tell Annie that she has cancer. I want her to always have hope." Dr. Brown agreed, "Don't worry, I won't tell her. You can tell her that she had a narrowing of the colon."

Daniel hung up the phone and proceeded to the recovery room. After entering the recovery room, he spotted his wife. His heart sank. Tubes seemed to be running out of every part of her body. He walked to her bedside. His immediate concern was to see her wake up and have the tubes pulled out so that he could take her home.

Later, in a hospital room, Annie asked Daniel, "What did the doctor find?" Daniel replied, "He found a narrowing of the colon." "Am I going to be okay?" "Yes, but it will take a while to recover." "Oh, that's good. I was so worried," said Annie. "You go home and get some rest." Daniel said, "I'll be back later," as Annie fell back to sleep.

Daniel left the hospital and went to see his friends, Jerry and Helen, who had invited him for dinner. As Daniel pulled up to Jerry and Helen's home, he got out of his car and just stood there, looking up a long stairway leading to Jerry and Helen's home. They were standing there looking down at Daniel. It was early evening. The sun was setting. A warm breeze was blowing, and Helen's eyes were watering. Those few moments seemed like a lifetime. Daniel discovered a new emotion, as he stood there speechless. He knew then that he was losing a part of himself. Things would never be the same.

Annie had one more surgery 2 months later in a futile attempt to extend her life. In November 2002, Annie was admitted to the hospital for the last time. Annie was so ill that even during her last moments she was unaware that she was dying. Dr. Brown entered the room and asked Daniel, "Can I see you for a few moments?" "Yes," Daniel replied. He followed Dr. Brown into the hallway. "Daniel, I can keep Annie alive for a few more days, or we can let her go." Daniel, not responding, went back into the room. He was now alone with Annie. Shortly thereafter, a nurse walked into the room and gave Annie an injection. Daniel asked, "What did you give her?" The nurse replied, "Something to make her more comfortable." Annie had been asleep; she awoke, looked at Daniel, and said, "Could you please cancel my appointment to be sworn in as a citizen? I will have to reschedule. I don't think I will be well enough to go." Daniel replied, "Okay, try to get some rest." Annie closed her eyes, never to open them again.

Discussion

1. Do you agree with Daniel's decision not to tell Annie about the seriousness of her illness? Explain your answer.
2. Should the physician have spoken to Annie as to the seriousness of her illness regardless of Daniel's desire to give Annie hope and not a death sentence? Explain your answer.
3. Describe the ethical dilemmas in this case (e.g., how Annie's rights were violated).
4. Place yourself in Annie's shoes, the physician's shoes, and Daniel's shoes, and then discuss how the lives of each may have been different if the physician had informed Annie as to the seriousness of her illness.

This true life case raises numerous questions, often resulting in conflicts among ethics, the law, patient rights, and family wishes. From a professional ethics point of view, the American Medical Association provides in its *Principles of Medical Ethics* that:

> IV. A physician shall respect the rights of patients, colleagues, and other health professionals, and shall safeguard patient confidences and privacy within the constraints of the law.[7]

Legally, pursuant to the Patient Self-Determination Act of 1990, patients have a right to make their own health care decisions, to accept or refuse medical treatment, and to execute an advance health care directive. Practically speaking, as discussion of this case illustrates, one shoe does not fit all. Both legal and ethical edicts have often served to raise an unending stream of questions that involve both the law and ethics. Although discussed later, a case here has been made for the need of a well-balanced ethics committee to help caregivers, patients, and family come to a consensus in the decision-making process.

Life or Death: The Right to Choose

A Jehovah's Witness executed a release requesting that no blood or its derivatives be administered during hospitalization. The Connecticut Superior Court determined that the hospital had no common law right or obligation to thrust unwanted medical care on the patient because she had been sufficiently informed of the consequences of the refusal to accept blood transfusions. She had competently and clearly declined that care. The hospital's interests were sufficiently protected by her informed choice, and neither it nor the trial court in this case was entitled to override that choice.

BENEFICENCE

Beneficence describes the principle of doing good, demonstrating kindness, showing compassion, and helping others. In the health care setting, caregivers demonstrate beneficence by providing benefits and balancing benefits against risks. Beneficence requires one to do good. Doing good requires knowledge of the beliefs, culture, values, and preferences of the patient—what one person may believe to be good for a patient may in reality be harmful. For example, a caregiver may decide to tell a patient frankly, "There is nothing else that I can do for you." This could be injurious to the patient if the patient really wants encouragement and information about care options from the caregiver. Compassion here requires the caregiver to tell the patient, "I am not aware of new treatments for your illness; however, I have some ideas about how I can help treat your symptoms and make you more comfortable. In addition, I will keep you informed as to any significant research that may be helpful in treating your disease processes."

Paternalism

Paternalism is a form of beneficence. People sometimes believe that they know what is best for another and make decisions that they believe are in that person's best interest. It may involve, for example, withholding information, believing that the person would be better off that way. Paternalism can occur due to one's age, cognitive ability, and level of dependency.

CPR and Paternalism in Nursing Homes

Some nursing homes have implemented facilitywide no CPR policies, as noted in the following Centers for Medicare and Medicaid Services Memorandum. Nursing home patients have a right to make their own care decisions. To eliminate that option in the nursing home sitting by having a policy of no resuscitation measures is a paternalistic approach to patient care and is a clear violation of patient rights and autonomous decision making. Such policies are unconditionally morally and legally wrong.

Memorandum Summary

- **Initiation of CPR**—Prior to the arrival of emergency medical services (EMS), nursing homes must provide basic life support, including initiation of CPR, to a resident who experiences cardiac arrest (cessation of respirations and/or pulse) in accordance with that resident's advance directives or in the absence of advance directives or a Do Not Resuscitate (DNR) order. CPR-certified staff must be available at all times.
- **Facility CPR Policy**—Some nursing homes have implemented facilitywide no CPR policies. Facilities must not establish and implement facilitywide no CPR policies.
- **Surveyor Implications**—Surveyors should ascertain that facility policies related to emergency response require staff to initiate CPR as appropriate and that records do not reflect instances where CPR was not initiated by staff even though the resident requested CPR or had not formulated advance directives.[8]

Physicians and Paternalism

Medical paternalism involves making decisions for patients who are capable of making their own choices. Physicians often find themselves in situations where they can influence a patient's health care decision simply by selectively telling the patient what he or she prefers based on personal beliefs. This directly violates patient autonomy. The problem of paternalism involves a conflict between the principles of autonomy and beneficence, each of which may be viewed and weighed differently, for example, by the physician and patient, physician and family member, or even the patient and a family member.

Employment-Related Paternalism

Employment-related paternalism at its best is a shared and cooperative style of management in which the employer recognizes and considers employee rights when making decisions in the workplace. Paternalism at its worst occurs when the employer's style of management becomes more authoritarian, sometimes arbitrary, and unpredictable, as noted in the *reality check* presented next. In this scenario the employer has complete discretion in making workplace decisions and the individual employee's freedom is subordinate to the employer's authority. Here the employer requires strict obedience to follow orders without question. The employer in this case lacks respect and consideration for the employee.

Paternalism and Breach of Confidentiality

Nina traveled with her husband, Dan, to a work assignment in Michigan. While visiting with her brother in Michigan, Nina believed that her potassium was low, which was a frequent occurrence with her for many years. Nina's brother suggested she could have her blood tested at a local blood drawing station. Dan later learned Nina's potassium was low.

Later that morning, while at work, Joan, Dan's colleague, called Bill, Dan's supervisor, to discuss Nina's health. Bill, however, had overslept and had not yet arrived at work. Joan decided to speak to the supervisor on call. After that conversation, Joan, being led by three staff members from the organization, tracked Dan down on several occasions that morning. On the first occasion, at approximately 10:15 A.M., Dan was surveying the organization's family practice center when Joan arrived. She rudely called Dan aside, excusing the organization's staff from the immediate area. Joan said, with surprise, "Dan, you are working?" Dan, even more surprised at the question, "Yes, I have been working." Joan replied, "Well, anyway, the corporate office wants to speak to you." Dan said he would call during lunch hour. Joan, somewhat agitated, walked away.

Joan again tracked Dan down with an entourage of the organization's staff at 11:30 A.M. She located Dan while he was in the organization's transfusion center. Again she rudely entered the conference room where Dan was discussing the care being rendered to a cancer patient. She once again asked in a stern tone of voice, "Could everyone please leave the room. I need to talk to Dan." The organization's staff left the room and the nurse said, "I finally reached Bill and he wants you to call him." Dan inquired, "Is he pulling me off this assignment?" The nurse replied, "Yes, he is. I spoke to Bill, and he has decided that out of concern for Nina you should be removed from this particular assignment. He wants you to call him." Dan replied, "I don't understand why you did this, calling Bill and continuously interrupting my work and sharing with others confidential information about my wife. I will wrap up with the staff my review of this patient and call Bill." As Joan left the conference room Dan said, "I trusted you and you shared confidential information about my wife?" Joan, realizing that she had no right to share the information, quickly walked away.

Dan called Bill during his lunch break. During that call Bill said, "I am going to remove you from your assignment because I think your wife's health needs should be addressed, and this could be disruptive to the survey." Dan replied, "The only disruption has been the nurse tracking me down with staff from the organization and not conducting her work activities." Bill said, "My decision stands. You can opt to take vacation time for the remainder of the week."

Discussion

1. Discuss what examples of paternalism you have gleaned from this case.
2. Do you think Dan was treated fairly? Discuss your answer.
3. Discuss the issues of trust, confidentiality, and fairness as they relate to this case.

At present, our federal employment discrimination laws fail to provide uniform and consistent legal protection when an employer engages in applicant-specific paternalism—the practice of excluding an applicant merely to protect that person from job-related safety and/or health risks uniquely attributable to his or her federally protected characteristic(s). Under Title VII of the Civil Rights Act of 1964, the courts and the Equal Employment Opportunity Commission (EEOC) reject such paternalism, demanding that the applicant alone decide whether to pursue (and accept) a job that poses risks related to his or her sex, race, color, religion, or national origin.[9]

CAN A PHYSICIAN "CHANGE HIS OR HER MIND"?

Walls had a condition that caused his left eye to be out of alignment with his right eye. Walls discussed with Shreck, his physician, the possibility of surgery on his left eye to bring both eyes into alignment. Walls and Shreck agreed that the best approach to treating Walls was to attempt surgery on the left eye. Before surgery, Walls signed an authorization and consent form that included the following language:

- I hereby authorize Dr. Shreck . . . to perform the following procedure and/or alternative procedure necessary to treat my condition . . . of the left eye.
- I understand the reason for the procedure is to straighten my left eye to keep it from going to the left.
- It has been explained to me that conditions may arise during this procedure whereby a different procedure or an additional procedure may need to be performed, and I authorize my physician and his assistants to do what they feel is needed and necessary.

During surgery, Shreck encountered excessive scar tissue on the muscles of Walls's left eye and elected to adjust the muscles of the right eye instead. When Walls awoke from the anesthesia, he expressed anger at the fact that both of his eyes were bandaged. The next day,

Walls went to Shreck's office for a follow-up visit and adjustment of his sutures. Walls asked Shreck why he had operated on the right eye, and Shreck responded that "he reserved the right to change his mind" during surgery.

Walls filed a lawsuit. The trial court concluded that Walls had failed to establish that Shreck had violated any standard of care. It sustained Shreck's motion for directed verdict, and Walls appealed. The court stated that the consent form that had been signed indicated that there can be extenuating circumstances when the surgeon exceeds the scope of what was discussed presurgery. Walls claimed that it was his impression that Shreck was talking about surgeries in general.

Roussel, an ophthalmologist, had testified on behalf of Walls. Roussel stated that it was customary to discuss with patients the potential risks of a surgery, benefits, and the alternatives to surgery. Roussel testified that medical ethics requires informed consent.

Shreck claimed that he had obtained the patient's informed consent not from the form but from what he discussed with the patient in his office. The court found that the form itself does not give or deny permission for anything. Rather, it is evidence of the discussions that occurred and during which informed consent was obtained. Shreck therefore asserted that he obtained informed consent to operate on both eyes based on his office discussions with Walls.

Ordinarily, in a medical malpractice case, the plaintiff must prove the physician's negligence by expert testimony. One of the exceptions to the requirement of expert testimony is the situation whereby the evidence and the circumstances are such that the recognition of the alleged negligence may be presumed to be within the comprehension of laypersons. This exception is referred to as the "common knowledge exception."

The evidence showed that Shreck did not discuss with Walls that surgery might be required on both eyes during the same operation. There was evidence that Walls specifically told Shreck he did not want surgery performed on the right eye.

Expert testimony was not required to establish that Walls did not give express or implied consent for Shreck to operate on his right eye. Absent an emergency, it is common knowledge that a reasonably prudent health care provider would not operate on part of a patient's body if the patient told the health care provider not to do so.

On appeal, the trial court was found to have erred in directing a verdict in favor of Shreck. The evidence presented established that the standard of care in similar communities requires health care providers to obtain informed consent before performing surgery. In this case, the applicable standard of care required Shreck to obtain Walls's express or implied consent to perform surgery on his right eye.

[*Walls v. Shreck*, 658 N.W.2d 686 (2003)]

Ethical and Legal Issues

1. Discuss the conflicting ethical principles in this case.
2. Did the physician's actions in this case involve medical paternalism? Explain your answer.

NONMALEFICENCE

Nonmaleficence is an ethical principle that requires caregivers to avoid causing patients harm. It derives from the ancient maxim *primum non nocere*, translated from the Latin, "first, do no harm." Physicians today still swear by the code of Hippocrates, pledging to do no harm. Medical ethics require health care providers to "first, do no harm." A New Jersey court in *In re Conroy*,[10] found that "the physician's primary obligation is . . . First do no harm." Telling the truth, for example, can sometimes cause harm. If there is no cure for a patient's disease, you may have a dilemma. Do I tell the patient and possibly cause serious psychological harm, or do I give the patient what I consider to be false hopes? Is there a middle ground? If so, what is it? To avoid causing harm, alternatives may need to be considered in solving the ethical dilemma.

The caregiver, realizing that he or she cannot help a particular patient, attempts to avoid harming the patient. This is done as a caution against taking a serious risk with the patient or doing something that has no immediate or long-term benefits.

Law and Ethics Intersect

Peninsula Child Psychiatrist William Ayres Sentenced to Eight Years for Molesting Patients

REDWOOD CITY—As one victim after another testified, calling William Ayres a monster and a serial child-abuser who robbed them of their innocence, the once-renowned child psychiatrist sat stoically Monday as a judge sentenced him to eight years in prison for molesting his former patients.

• • •

Ayres used his work with boys having trouble at school, at home or with the law as a setting to abuse them, the victims said. His position of authority allowed him to deflect suspicions about his sexual interest in boys and keep parents from believing their sons' complaints, victims said.

Joshua Melvin, San Jose Mercury News, *August 27, 2013*[11]

The patients described in the news clipping were harmed because the physician who was trained to do good did wrong by taking advantage of the patients' weaknesses. The beneficent person does good and not harm (nonmaleficence). The law in the news clipping is clear. If a person with intent and action causes harm to the patient, that person will be punished.

One of the many lessons in the next *reality check* teaches the reader that one may have good intent but that intent can lead to a perceived wrong and thus be damaging to one's good character and possibly his or her career path.

Patient Questions Physical Exam

Dear Sir:

I was a patient on your short-term acute-care psychiatric unit. It was a voluntary admission as is with all patients on that unit. Dr. X was my psychiatrist. Although he was very good as a psychiatrist, I was somewhat disturbed in the way he conducted my physical examination. He had come to my room on the day of my admission and said that he needed to perform a physical exam. He had already conducted a thorough history of my physical ailments and thoroughly reviewed my family history as far back as I could remember.

We were in the room alone when he entered. He had a gown in his hand and asked me to put it on. He then walked out of the room and said he would be back in a few minutes, as soon as I was gowned. When he returned he began his physical examination. Early on in the exam he asked when I had my last breast examination. I told him that I was 28 and never had one. He said, "Well, I better do one." I thought it was a bit odd that he conducted the exam without a female nurse present. I became more concerned when he touched my breasts in what I considered a sensual manner. It was uncanny. It seemed to be a bit more than what I would've expected during a breast examination. He seemed to be caressing my breasts, as opposed to examining them. I don't know if this is a routine procedure, but I was very uncomfortable in the situation. I think it would be better if you considered having a female nurse present when conducting female examinations in a patient room on a psychiatric unit or on any other unit for that matter.

Thanks for listening to my concerns.

Anonymous

Administrator

I called Dr. X into my office and discussed the patient's concerns with him. He said this is what physicians are trained to do. "We are trained to conduct both history and physical examinations." He had brought with him a letter from one of his professional associations that stated psychiatrists are permitted to perform physical examinations on their patients. I asked him why he did not have someone in the room with him when he examined the patient. He stated, "I generally do but I was extremely busy and the staff was swamped with other patients. It was just a hectic day."

Discussion

1. Discuss how you would respond to the patient.
2. Describe how you would resolve this issue with the physician; assuming this was the first complaint that you had received regarding his care.
3. Explain what policy decisions you would implement.
4. Knowing that the physician is in a position of trust with his patient, discuss what action the physician should take to prevent complaints of this nature from recurring.

The intersection of "law" and "ethics" is clear. Deviation from either can lead to unsatisfactory outcomes for both physicians and patients. Although a caregiver may be trained to conduct a physical examination, the question may not be "can I do it" but "should I do it."

Nonmaleficence and Ending Life

The principle of nonmaleficence is defeated when a physician is placed in the position of ending life by removing respirators, giving lethal injections, or writing prescriptions for lethal doses of medication. Helping patients die violates the physician's duty to save lives. In the final analysis, there needs to be a distinction between killing patients and letting them die. It is clear that killing a patient is never justified.

JUSTICE

Justice is the obligation to be fair in the distribution of benefits and risks. Justice demands that persons in similar circumstances be treated similarly. A person is treated justly when he or she receives what is due, is deserved, or can legitimately be claimed. Justice involves how people are treated when their interests compete with one another.

Distributive justice is a principle requiring that all persons be treated equally and fairly. No one person, for example, should get a disproportional share of society's resources or benefits. There are many ethical issues involved in the rationing of health care. This is often a result of limited or scarce resources, limited access as a result of geographic remoteness, or a patient's inability to pay for services combined with many physicians who are unwilling to accept patients who are perceived as "no-pays" with high risks for legal suits.

Senator Edward M. Kennedy, speaking on health care at the John F. Kennedy Presidential Library in Boston, Massachusetts on April 28, 2002, stated:

> It will be no surprise to this audience that I believe securing quality, affordable health insurance for every American is a matter of simple justice. Health care is not just another commodity. Good health is not a gift to be rationed based on ability to pay. The time is long overdue for America to join the rest of the industrialized world in recognizing this fundamental need.

Later, speaking at the Democratic National Convention on August 25, 2008, Kennedy said:

> And this is the cause of my life—new hope that we will break the old gridlock and guarantee that every American—North, South, East, West, young, old—will have decent, quality health care as a fundamental right and not a privilege.

Although Kennedy did not live to see the day his dream would come true, President Barack Obama signed into law the final piece of his administration's historic health care bill on March 23, 2010.

The costs of health care have bankrupted many, and research dollars have proven to be inadequate, yet many members of Congress elected to address the needs of the country have elected to continue their bipartisan bickering while they "enjoy" the lowest acceptance ratings in the nation's history. They have, however, ensured that their health care needs are met with the best of care in the best facilities with the best doctors. They have taken care of themselves. Their pensions are intact, whereas many Americans have to face such dilemmas as which medications they will take and which they cannot afford. Many often have to decide between food and medications. Is this justice or theft of the nation's resources by the few incompetents who have been elected to protect the American people? Unfortunately, these problems continue to this day as Congress continues to wrangle over national health insurance.

Justice and Government Spending

He Won His Battle With Cancer. Thus, Why Are Millions of Americans Still Losing Theirs?

For an increasing number of cancer activists, researchers and patients, there is too much death and too much waiting for new drugs and therapies. They want a greater sense of urgency, a new approach that emphasizes translational research over basic research—turning knowledge into therapies and getting them to patients pronto. The problem is, that's not the way our sclerotic research paradigm—principally administered by the National Institutes of Health and the National Cancer Institute (NIH/NIC)—is set up. "The fact that we jump up and down when cancer deaths go from 562,000 to 561,000, that's ridiculous. That's not enough," says Lance Armstrong, the cyclist and cancer survivor turned activist, through his Lance Armstrong Foundation (LAF).

Time, *September 15, 2008*

Scarce resources are challenging to the principles of justice. Justice involves equality; nevertheless, equal access to health care, for example, across the United States does not exist. How should government allocate a trillion dollars? Consider the following questions:

- Should the money be distributed equally among families?
- Should the money be distributed equally among all citizens?
- Should the money be invested and saved for a rainy day?
- Should the money be used to improve educational programs, build libraries, build state-of-the-art hospitals, or fund afterschool programs for disadvantaged youths?
- Should the money include both savings for that rainy day and funding for the programs described previously?
- What would be the greater good for all?
- Should health care be rationed based on one's ability to pay?
- Should those individuals found to be ethically corrupt be condemned to poverty and stand in the same food lines as the poorest of Americans?

States Have Double Standards

It is no secret that states have had double standards over the years, one for health care organizations and one for physicians and investors, who often duplicated the financially more lucrative hospital services, while referring Medicaid patients and no-pays to hospital programs for care. As administrator of one hospital, allow me to give you a few examples.

1. A radiology group was able to purchase their own Computed Tomography (CT) scanner, while I had to jump through hoops to be able to purchase one.
2. A group of surgeons and private investors established a surgery center in direct competition with my hospital without scrutiny. At the same time, I was required to justify the hospital's proposed surgery center. The hospital was required to complete lengthy questionnaires and gather supporting documentation to justify construction and operation of an outpatient surgery center.
3. The hospital had to justify opening an outpatient rehabilitation program within the hospital in order to provide a continuum of care for patients needing physical therapy services. While I was busy justifying the need for an outpatient rehabilitation program, orthopedic surgeons were busy setting up their own outpatient programs to compete with the hospital.

I remember walking to my car one day after work and one of my orthopedic surgeons caught up to me and said, "You know Dan, I have made enough money in the 3 years that I have been on your staff to buy your hospital."

Discussion

1. Discuss the issues of justice as they apply to this scenario.
2. Discuss the issues of fairness and how physician competition with hospitals can affect the quality of patient care.

Injustice for the Insured

Even if you're insured, getting ill could bankrupt you. Hospitals are garnishing wages, putting liens on homes and having patients who can't pay arrested. It's enough to make you sick. Think You're Covered? Think Again.

—Sara Austin, *Self*, October 2004

Hospitals are receiving between $4 million and $60 million annually in charity funds in New York City alone, according to Elizabeth Benjamin, director of the health law unit of the Legal Aid Society of New York City; however, even the insured face injustice. In 2003, almost 1 million Americans declared bankruptcy because of medical issues, accounting for nearly half of all of the bankruptcies in the country. When an insured patient gets ill and exhausts his or her insurance benefits, should the hospital be able to:

- Withhold the money from the patient's wages?
- Place a lien on the patient's home?
- Arrest the patient?
- Block the patient from applying for the hundreds of millions of dollars in government funds designated to help pay for care for those who need it?

Age and Justice

New Kidney Transplant Rules Would Favor Younger Patients

The nation's organ transplant network is considering giving younger, healthier people preference over older, sicker patients for the best kidneys.

Some also complain that the new system would unfairly penalize middle-aged and elderly patients at a time when the overall population is getting older.

If adopted, the approach could have implications for other decisions about how to allocate scarce resources, such as expensive cancer drugs and ventilators during hurricanes and other emergencies. . . .

Rob Stein, The Washington Post, *February 24, 2011*

- Should an 89-year-old patient get a heart transplant, rather than a 10-year-old girl, just because he or she is higher on the waiting list?
- Should a 39-year-old single patient, rather than a 10-year-old boy, get a heart transplant because he or she is higher on the waiting list?
- Should a 29-year-old mother of three get a heart transplant, rather than a 10-year-old girl, because she is higher on the waiting list?
- Should a 29-year-old pregnant mother with two children, rather than a 10-year-old boy, get a heart transplant because she is higher on the waiting list?

Justice and Emergency Care

When two patients arrive in the emergency department in critical condition, consider who should receive treatment first. Should the caregiver base his or her decision on the:

- First patient who walks through the door?
- Age of the patients?
- Likelihood of survival?
- Ability of the patient to pay for services rendered?
- Condition of the patient?

Patients are to be treated justly, fairly, and equally. What happens, however, when resources are scarce and only one patient can be treated at a time? What happens if caregivers decide that age should be the determining factor as to who is treated first? One patient is saved, and another dies. What happens if the patient saved is terminal and has an advance directive in his wallet requesting no heroic measures to save his life? What are the legal issues intertwined with the ethical issues in this case?

The principle of distributive justice raises numerous issues, including how limited resources should be allocated. For example, when there is a reduction in staff in health care organizations, managers are generally asked to eliminate "nonessential" personnel. In the health care industry, this translates to those individuals not directly involved in patient care (e.g., maintenance and housekeeping employees). Is this fair? Is this just? Is this the right thing to do?

In Search of Economic Justice

Avery Comarow, in his article "Under the Knife in Bangalore" (*U.S. News and World Report*, May 12, 2008), wrote that the high cost of U.S. hospital care is motivating patients to travel to places like India and Thailand for major procedures. There would be no need for uninsured patients to go abroad if the prices they were quoted in the United States were more in line with what insurers and Medicare pay. The uninsured often pay full price for medical procedures in the United States. For example, a self-pay patient will pay between $70,000 and $133,000 for coronary bypass surgery, whereas Medicare will pay between $18,609 and $23,589. Commercial insurance plans often get up to a 60% discount off the list cost of medical procedures. In India, the same surgery will cost the patient $7,000, and in Thailand, it will be $22,000.

To avoid bankruptcy and loss of assets, maybe their homes, Americans risk the unknowns of going abroad for health care.

Boomer Bubble "Bioeconomics"

As baby boomers become Medicare eligible, there is likely to be a huge strain on the federal budget. Is this dramatically increased cost justified, beneficial, and necessary to the country as a whole?

The revenue from working, taxpaying baby boomers over the past 4 decades has fueled unprecedented prosperity. That revenue has made many entitlements possible, but it is going to diminish drastically as boomers retire and become recipients instead of contributors to the revenue base. Advances in medical technology have increased longevity dramatically, and boomers therefore are likely to be on the receiving end of entitlements for a long time. Medical advances, however, also can increase productivity as well as longevity. Boomers with a lifetime of work experience can be a valuable resource if they are kept healthy enough to remain gainfully employed at some level. Maintenance of a skilled American workforce is essential for future prosperity and economic stability. Boomers are a substantial resource of experienced skilled workers. It is a political necessity that they are encouraged to stay productive. The government's subsidizing health care through Medicare and other programs is therefore an investment that can facilitate this worthwhile goal. Additional incentives may even be appropriate. Even on an ethical basis, boomers that fueled our economy for so long deserve to be taken care of in their later years. Hopefully, many of them will be healthy enough and willing enough to continue being productive beyond the usual retirement age. Thus, from a political perspective, the healthful, moral, and ethical choice may also turn out to be the profitable choice for our society.

Physician

VIRTUE ETHICS AND VALUES

Virtue ethics focuses on the inherent character of a person rather than on the specific actions he or she performs. A *virtue* is a positive trait of moral excellence. Virtues are those characteristics that differentiate good people from bad people. Virtues such as courage, honesty, and justice are abstract moral principles. A morally virtuous person is one who does the good and right thing by habit, not merely based on a set of rules of conduct. The character of a virtuous person is naturally good, as exhibited by his or her unswerving good behavior and actions.

Resilience of the Health Caregiver Spirit

I've been in leadership roles for two sister hospitals in southeast Louisiana, with each experiencing the devastation of hurricane damage twice in the past 3 years. The first experience was temporarily suspending normal operations in New Orleans, and recently, history repeated itself at the sister hospital in Houma, Louisiana.

In both instances, I was stunned at the determination and strength of health care teams to rebuild. Both hospitals needed to resort to MASH-type tent hospitals to allow rebuilding of the hospitals. Health care for the communities was not interrupted. Back-to-basics care ensued, but not without close attention to needed regulatory compliance standards. The regulatory agencies were called and involved from the get-go, and the caregiver teams and support service staff flourished with enthusiasm to survive and care for the patients in need. Was this because of the nonprofit nature of our state-sponsored hospitals? I don't think so. The human spirit takes over when it comes to patient care, no matter what.

I am happy to say that both New Orleans and Houma are back on track, with care being provided in top-quality hospitals. This is only due to the diligence of all, including facilities management, housekeeping, and multiple direct and indirect caregiver departments. What is the ethical issue here? There is no issue. Support for the art of care-giving will never be disappointed—at least not in southeast Louisiana. I stand in awe of what I have seen and look forward to growing with this team of devoted professionals.

Nurse

Values are standards of conduct. They are used for judging the goodness or badness of some action. A *moral value* is the relative worth placed on some virtuous behavior.

Values are rooted in customs and habits of a culture because the words moral and ethics themselves were essentially created to describe these topics.[12]

Values are the standards by which we measure the goodness in our lives. *Intrinsic value* is something that has value in and of itself (e.g., happiness). *Instrumental value* is something that helps to give value to something else (e.g., money is valuable for what it can buy).

Values may change as needs change. If one's basic needs for food, water, clothing, and housing have not been met, one's values may change such that a friendship, for example, might be sacrificed if one's basic needs can be better met as a result of the sacrifice. As mom nears the end of her life, a financially well-off family member may want to take more aggressive measures to keep mom alive despite the financial drain on her estate. Another family member, who is struggling financially, may more readily see the futility of expensive medical care and find it easier to let go. Values give purpose to each life. They make up one's moral character.

All people make value judgments and make choices among alternatives. Values are the motivating power of a person's actions and necessary to survival, both psychologically and physically.

The relationship between abstract virtues (principles) and values (practice) is often difficult to grasp. The virtuous person is one who does good, and his or her character is known through the values he or she practices consistently by habit.

We begin our discussion here with an overview of those virtues commonly accepted as having value when addressing difficult health care dilemmas. The reader should not get overly caught up in the philosophical morass of how virtues and values differ but should be aware that virtues and values have been used interchangeably. This text is not about memorizing words; it is about applying what we learn for the good of all whose lives we touch.

Whether we call compassion a virtue or a value or both, the importance for our purposes in this text is to understand what compassion is and how it is applied in the health care setting.

PILLARS OF MORAL STRENGTH

I am part of all I have met.

—ALFRED TENNYSON

There is a deluge of ethical issues in every aspect of human existence. Although cultural differences, politics, and religion influence who we are, it is all of life experiences that affect who we have become. If we have courage to do right, those who have influenced our lives were most likely courageous. If we are compassionate, it is most likely because we have been influenced by the compassionate.

The *Pillars of Moral Strength* illustrated in **Figure 1-1** describes a virtuous person. What is it that sets each person apart? In the final analysis, it is one's virtues and values that build moral character. Look beyond the words and ask, "Do I know their meanings?" "Do I apply their concepts?" "Do I know their value?" "Are they part of me?"

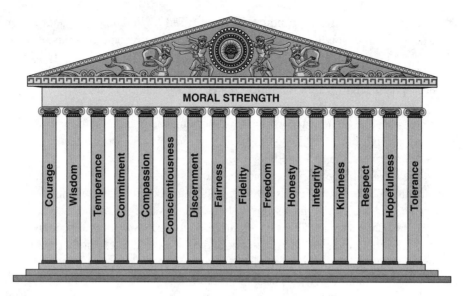

FIGURE 1-1 Pillars of Moral Strength

Courage as a Virtue

Courage is the greatest of all virtues, because if you haven't courage, you may not have an opportunity to use any of the others.

—Samuel Johnson

Courage is the mental or moral strength to persevere and withstand danger. Courage can be characterized as the ladder upon which all the other virtues mount. Courage is the strength of character necessary to continue in the face of fears and the challenges in life. It involves balancing fear, self-confidence, and values. Without courage, we are unable to take the risks necessary to achieve the things most valued. A courageous person has good judgment and a clear sense of his or her strengths, correctly evaluates danger, and perseveres until a decision is made and the right goal that is being sought has been achieved.

My Journey–How Lucky Am I?

No words can be scripted to say what I have been through, so I will just speak from my heart and off the cuff. From the day the Dr. said to me, "Denise, you have a rare cancer and we are sorry there is nothing we can do. I did not waver in my faith in God. He was in me, he was thru me and he was around me. I just asked the Dr., "What Do I Do?" And yet, although he said a whole bunch of words, I wasn't focused so much on what was being said. It's like a calmness was over me, not much worry, just a feeling of I will never be ALONE on this new journey I'm about to experience. I felt calm. Not until I looked at my loved ones FACES did I realize, oh my, this can be bad. But again, a feeling came over me that I will not face this ALONE. God has plans for me and I will surrender in his grace and as time past [sic], I realized how lucky and blessed I am, for most people who may feel that death may be close by, I didn't feel that way. What I felt was WOW!! Everyone gets to show me their love in the NOW and not in the later when I am no longer HERE. How lucky am I.

—Denise

Courage, in differing degrees, helps to define one's character (the essence of one's being) and offers the strength to stand up for what is good and right. It crosses over and unites and affects all other values. Courage must not be exercised to an extreme, causing a person to become so foolish that his or her actions are later regretted.

When the passion to destroy another human being becomes such an obsession that one is willing to sacrifice the lives of others, that person has become a bully and a coward and not a person of courage. History is filled with men and women who have hidden their fears by inciting others to do evil. Such people are not the models of character that we wish to instill thoughts of in the minds of our children.

WISDOM AS A VIRTUE

True wisdom comes to each of us when we realize how little we understand about life, ourselves, and the world around us.

—SOCRATES

We can learn from history how past generations thought and acted, how they responded to the demands of their time and how they solved their problems. We can learn by analogy, not by example, for our circumstances will always be different than theirs were. The main thing history can teach us is that human actions have consequences and that certain choices, once made, cannot be undone. They foreclose the possibility of making other choices and thus they determine future events.

—GERDA LERNER (PIONEER OF WOMEN'S HISTORY)

Wisdom is the judicious application of knowledge. Wisdom begins first by learning from the failures and successes of those who have preceded us. Marcus Tullius Cicero (106–43 BC), a Roman philosopher and politician, is reported to have said, "The function of wisdom is to discriminate between good and evil." In the health care setting, when the patient's wishes and end-of-life preferences are unknown, wisdom with good judgment without bias or prejudice springs forth more easily.

TEMPERANCE AS A VIRTUE

Being forced to work, and forced to do your best, will breed in you temperance and self-control, diligence and strength of will, cheerfulness and content, and a hundred virtues which the idle will never know.

—CHARLES KINGSLEY

Temperance involves self-control and restraint. It embraces moderation in thoughts and actions. Temperance is evidenced by orderliness and moderation in everything one says and does. It involves the ability to control one's actions so as not to go to extremes. The question arises, without the ability to control oneself from substance abuse, for example, how can a person possibly live the life of a virtuous person. The old adage, "the proof is in the pudding" lies in one's actions. A virtuous person stands out from the crowd by actions and deeds.

COMMITMENT

Unless commitment is made; there are only promises and hopes; but no plans.

—PETER F. DRUCKER

I know the price of success: dedication, hard work, and an unremitting devotion to the things you want to see happen.

—FRANK LLOYD WRIGHT

Commitment is the act of binding oneself intellectually or emotionally to a course of action (e.g., pursue a career, adhere to a religious belief) or person (e.g., marriage, family, patient care). It is an agreement or pledge to do something. It can be ongoing, such as in a marriage, or a pledge to do something in the future, such as an engagement as a commitment to marry a particular person.

COMPASSION

Compassion is the basis of morality.

—ARTHUR SCHOPENHAUER

The Fear Factor and Patient Satisfaction

Nurses tend to score highly on measures of empathy, care, and compassion . . . Here is some specific advice about what hospitals can do to help nurses improve at calming their patients' fears.

- Encourage nurses to be sensitive to the level of fear their patients experience when they're admitted to the hospital. Empathy and communication are key . . .
- Set nurses up for success through training and support. In many instances, it is easy to deal with safety concerns by providing detailed protocols, policies, and procedures . . .

Rick Blizzard, D.B.A., Gallup, *August 6, 2013*[13]

Hospital Video Shows No One Helped Dying Woman

A shocking video shows a woman dying on the floor in the psych ward at Kings County Hospital, while people around her, including a security guard, did nothing to help. After an hour, another mental patient finally got the attention of the indifferent hospital workers, according to the tape obtained by the *New York Daily News*.

Worse still, the surveillance tape suggests hospital staff may have falsified medical charts to cover the utter lack of treatment provided to Esmin Green before she died.

John Marzulli, Daily News, *June 30, 2008*

Compassion is the deep awareness of and sympathy for another's suffering. The ability to show compassion is a true mark of moral character. There are those who argue that compassion will blur one's judgment. Caregivers need to show the same compassion for others, as they would expect for themselves or their loved ones.

Elderly Patient Hit by Motorcycle Dies in Japan After Being Rejected by 14 Hospitals

After getting struck by a motorcycle, an elderly Japanese man with head injuries waited in an ambulance as paramedics phoned 14 hospitals, each refusing to treat him.

He died 90 minutes later at the facility that finally relented—one of thousands of victims repeatedly turned away in recent years by understaffed and overcrowded hospitals in Japan.

Maria Yamaguchi, Associated Press, *February 5, 2009*

Compassion is a moral value expected of all caregivers. Those who lack compassion have a weakness in their moral character. In 1996, Dr. Linda Peeno, featured in Michael Moore's 2007 film *Sicko*, testified before Congress (Important issue facing House-Senate conference on health care reform, House of Representatives—March 28, 2000—Page: H1465) to discuss her prior work for Humana, where she worked as a claims reviewer for several health maintenance organizations (HMOs). Dr. Peeno showed compassion as she testified before the Committee on Commerce on May 30, 1996. Here is her story in part:

> I wish to begin by making a public confession. In the spring of 1987, I caused the death of a man. Although this was known to many people, I have not been taken before any court of law or called to account for this in any professional or public forum. In fact, just the opposite occurred. I was rewarded for this. It brought me an improved reputation in my job and contributed to my advancement afterwards. Not only did I demonstrate that I could do what was asked, expected of me, I exemplified the good company employee. I saved a half a million dollars.

Since that day, I have lived with this act and many others eating into my heart and soul. The primary ethical norm is do no harm. I did worse, I caused death. Instead of using a clumsy bloody weapon, I used the simplest, cleanest of tools: my words. This man died because I denied him a necessary operation to save his heart. I felt little pain or remorse at the time. The man's faceless distance soothed my conscience. Like a skilled soldier, I was trained for the moment. When any moral qualms arose, I was to remember, "I am not denying care; I am only denying payment."

Duty-based ethics required Dr. Peeno to follow the rules of her job. In so doing, a life was lost. Although Dr. Peeno eventually came forward with her story, the irony here lies in the fact that Dr. Peeno lacked the courage, integrity, and compassion to report her story sooner. The lack of compassion for others plagues the health care industry in a variety of settings.

Teaching Doctors to Care

At Harvard and other medical schools across the country, educators are beginning to realize that empathy is as valuable to a doctor as any clinical skill . . . doctors who try to understand their patients may be the best antidote for the widespread dissatisfaction with today's health care system.

Nathan Thornburgh, Time magazine, *March 29, 2006*

Detachment

Detachment, or lack of concern for the patient's needs, often translates into mistakes that result in patient injuries. Those who have excessive emotional involvement in a patient's care may be best suited to work in those settings where patients are most likely to recover and have good outcomes (e.g., maternity units). As with all things in life, there needs to be a comfortable balance between compassion and detachment.

Never apologize for showing feeling. When you do so, you apologize for the truth.

—BENJAMIN DISRAELI

Policy Ruled—Compassion Missing

Mr. Jones was trying to get home from a long trip to see his ailing wife. Mrs. Jones had been ill for several years, suffering a great deal of pain. His flight was to leave at 7:00 PM. Upon arrival at the airport in New York at 4:30 pm, he inquired at the ticket counter, "Is there an earlier flight that I can take to Washington?" The counter agent responded, "There is plenty of room on the 5:00 pm flight, but you will have pay a $200 change fee." The passenger inquired, "Could you please waive the change fee? I need to get home to my ailing wife." The ticket agent responded, "Sorry, your ticket does not allow me to make the change. You can, however, try at the gate."

The passenger made a second attempt at the gate to get on an earlier flight, but the manager at the gate was unwilling to authorize the change, saying, "I don't make the rules." Mr. Jones decided to give it one more try. He called the airline's customer service center. The customer service agent responded to Mr. Jones's plea: "We cannot overrule the agent at the gate. Sorry, you just got the wrong supervisor. He is going by the book."

Anonymous

Discussion

1. Should rules be broken for a higher good? Discuss your answer.
2. Do the rules seem to be consistently or inconsistently applied in this *reality check*? Discuss your answer.

CONSCIENTIOUS

The most infectiously joyous men and women are those who forget themselves in thinking about and serving others.

–ROBERT J. MCCRACKEN

A *conscientious* person is one who has moral integrity and a strict regard for doing what is considered the right thing to do. An individual acts conscientiously if he or she is motivated to do what is right, believing it is the right thing to do. Conscience is a form of self-reflection on and judgment about whether one's actions are right or wrong, good or bad. It is an internal sanction that comes into play through critical reflection. This sanction often appears as a bad conscience in the form of painful feelings of remorse, guilt, shame, disunity, or disharmony as the individual recognizes that his or her acts were wrong.

Kill the Messenger

Frank, working as a hospital inspector, found a number of things wrong in his recent building inspection. At first glance the building looked clean and polished—Frank was amazed by how the floors sparkled in the old building. But then, as Frank always does, he asked to look behind a corridor door. Behind the door, Frank found a small storage closet with medical records strewn on the floor and others stored in cardboard boxes. The records had been soaked by water and floor wax that had seeped under the door when the corridors where cleaned. Entries on the records were blurred, making them difficult to read, and the records appeared to have black mold growing on them.

Behind another door was a medical equipment repair room. Dust balls floated on the floor as the door was opened. There was food on the floor, and a can of soda had been spilled and allowed to dry. Equipment parts were also scattered on the floor.

The staff complained about Frank's findings. Before he left, the staff corrected the issues he had noted and asked, "Frank, could you remove these comments from your report.

We cleaned the room and it is spotless. In addition, we stored the records in the medical records department." Frank replied, "I could not in good conscience remove my findings. Yes, the room may be clean but what about the information that had been recorded on the medical records that is not readable. Further, our process for inspecting your facility is a sampling process. I did not look behind every door and I am not sure what we would find if we did. I would suggest, as we discussed earlier, that a written plan of action be prepared and implemented to address the issues I identified. More important, your action plan should be implemented facilitywide. For example, no boxes should be stored on the floors, including medical supplies, as well as medical records."

Anonymous

Discussion

1. Should Frank have overlooked his findings, as the staff pressed him not to report them? Discuss your answer.
2. Assuming you were Frank, would you have deleted the findings from your report? Explain your answer.

DISCERNMENT

Get to know two things about a man—how he earns his money and how he spends it—and you have the clue to his character, for you have a searchlight that shows up the innermost recesses of his soul. You know all you need to know about his standards, his motives, his driving desires, and his real religion.

—ROBERT J. MCCRACKEN

Discernment is the ability to make a good decision without personal biases, fears, and undue influences from others. A person who has discernment has the wisdom to decide the best course of action when there are many possible actions to choose from.

9/11 Value Judgment

James had been scheduled to fly Monday evening, September 10, 2001, from Ronald Reagan Washington National Airport to New York LaGuardia Airport, and then rent a car and drive to Greenwich, Connecticut, where he was assigned to inspect a hospital. As luck would have it, there was one flight cancellation after another. After the last flight to LaGuardia was canceled, he went to the ticket counter and scheduled the first flight out Tuesday morning, September 11, 2001, at 6:00 AM.

The following morning James flew into LaGuardia, picked up his car, and drove to Connecticut to work with an assigned team led by Dr. Matthews. Not long after he arrived at the hospital, the first plane hit the World Trade Center. Shortly after the second plane crashed into the World Trade Center, the corporate office called and asked if the hospital wanted to reschedule the survey. The hospital opted to continue the survey.

On Thursday, the last day of the survey, a hospital staff member approached Dr. Matthews and asked if he and his survey team would like to attend a short memorial service in the lobby at noon for the victims and workers of 9/11. Without hesitation, Dr. Matthews replied, "No, we really have to finish our reports."

Anonymous

Discussion

1. Did the team leader make an appropriate decision? Discuss your answer.
2. Describe the various virtues and values that come into play in this case.
3. Discuss how you would have addressed the hospital's request to attend the memorial service.
4. Realizing that hindsight is 20/20, could you defend the decision not to attend the ceremony? Explain your answer.

FAIRNESS

Do all the good you can, By all the means you can, In all the ways you can, In all the places you can, At all the times you can, To all the people you can, As long as you ever can.

—JOHN WESLEY

In ethics, *fairness* requires each person to be objective, unbiased, dispassionate, impartial, and consistent with the principles of ethics. Fairness is the ability to make judgments free from discrimination, dishonesty, or one's own bias. It is the ability to be objective without prejudice or bias. We often tolerate mediocrity. We sometimes forget to thank those who just do their jobs, and we often praise the extraordinary, sometimes despite questionable faults. To be fair, it is important to see the good in all and to reward that good.

Questions of fairness in the Affordable Care Act have led to lawsuits in a number of the nation's top hospitals including the Mayo Clinic in Minnesota and Cedars-Sinai in Los Angeles because they are cut out of most insurance plans sold on the exchange.

Health Costs Cut by Limiting Choice

"Exchanges exclude, doctors, hospitals; in backlash, some providers file lawsuits"

The result, some argue, is a two-tiered system of health care: Many of the people who buy health plans on the exchanges have fewer hospitals and doctors to choose from than those with coverage through their employers.

• • •

Insurers "looked at the people expected to go on the exchanges and thought: 'these are people coming out of the ranks of the uninsured. They don't care about the Mayo Clinic or the Cleveland Clinic. They will go to community providers,'" explained Robert Laszewski, a consultant to the health-care industry.

Sandhya Somashekhar and Ariana Eunjung Cha, The Washington Post, *August 21, 2013*

Although care is generally cheaper at community-based hospitals than academic medical centers, the quality of that care often comes into question, as noted in the following *reality check*.

Community Hospital v. Respected Medical Center

My closest friend Nick was admitted to a small community hospital for what was described as a minor surgical procedure. During surgery, the surgeon unknowingly nicked the large bowel, which went unknown for several days. Nick, as a result, developed a methicillin-resistant staphylococcus aureus (MRSA) infection. Further surgeries were conducted, complicating an already botched surgery. One evening a nurse called his family aside and said, although I am jeopardizing my job, "I would get Nick out of here if I was you." The family decided to move Nick to a major teaching medical center several hours away from his hometown. Following an extended stay at the medical center and discharged home under hospice care, I visited Nick at his home. He looked intensely straight at me with deep sadness and said, "they took my life from me." He told another friend, "My life is over."

Anonymous

So where are we as it relates to fairness in the delivery of health care? Is it true that people coming out of the ranks of the uninsured don't care about the Mayo Clinic, Cleveland Clinic, the Lahey Hospital and Medical Center, or the Massachusetts General Hospital, to name but a few? Or do they care but just don't know the quality differences from one hospital to the next. Or is it a question of accessibility in remote areas of the country. Do we need hospital selection exchanges more then we need insurance exchanges? If one has money or connections is he or she more likely to get a higher quality of medical care than a poorer patient? Who determines what routine care is? Is routine care based on each patient's needs and comorbidities? Should those who have a financial interest in where a patient is treated be excluded from the decision-making process? Cheaper is not always better and providing care very well may not be enough. Although fairness in the delivery of health is a laudable value, it is most likely unachievable. The disparity as to who holds the nation's wealth continues to widen, as noted in the news clippings that follow. With so much wealth in the hands of the few, fairness in the delivery of high-quality health care for all is unlikely. However, the human race must continue to strive to meet the needs of all.

Of the 1%, by the 1%, for the 1%

Americans have been watching protests against oppressive regimes that concentrate massive wealth in the hands of an elite few. Yet in our own democracy, 1 percent of the people take nearly a quarter of the nation's income—an inequality even the wealthy will come to regret.

Joseph E. Stiglitz, Vanity Fair, *May 2011*

World's Richest 1% Own 40% of All Wealth, UN Report Discovers

The richest 1% of adults in the world own 40% of the planet's wealth, according to the largest study yet of wealth distribution. The report also finds that those in financial services and the internet sectors predominate among the super rich.

Europe, the US and some Asia Pacific nations account for most of the extremely wealthy. More than a third live in the US. Japan accounts for 27% of the total, the UK for 6% and France for 5%.

James Randerson, The Guardian, *December 2006*

FIDELITY

Nothing is more noble, nothing more venerable, than fidelity. Faithfulness and truth are the most sacred excellences and endowments of the human mind.

—CICERO

Fidelity is the virtue of faithfulness, being true to our commitments and obligations to others. A component of fidelity, veracity, implies that we will be truthful and honest in all our endeavors. It involves being faithful and loyal to obligations, duties, or observances. The opposite of fidelity is infidelity, meaning unfaithfulness.

FREEDOM

You can only protect your liberties in this world by protecting the other man's freedom. You can only be free if I am free.

—DOROTHY THOMPSON

Freedom is the quality of being free to make choices for oneself within the boundaries of law. Freedoms enjoyed by citizens of the United States include the freedom of speech, freedom of religion, freedom from want, and freedom from physical aggression.

HONESTY/TRUSTWORTHINESS/TRUTH TELLING

A lie can travel halfway around the world while the truth is still putting on its shoes.
—MARK TWAIN (AMERICAN HUMORIST, WRITER, AND LECTURER, 1835–1910)

Honesty and trust involve confidence that a person will act with the right motives. It is the assured reliance on the character, ability, strength, or truth of someone or something. To tell the truth, to have integrity, and to be honest are most honorable virtues. *Veracity* is devotion to and conformity with what is truthful. It involves an obligation to be truthful.

Truth telling involves providing enough information so that a patient can make an informed decision about his or her health care. Intentionally misleading a patient to believe something that the caregiver knows to be untrue may give the patient false hopes. There is

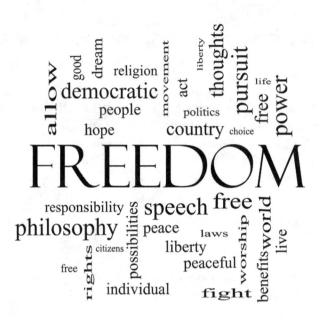

FIGURE 1-2   Freedom Speaks (© Keith Bell/Shutterstock, Inc.)

always apprehension when one must share bad news; the temptation is to play down the truth for fear of being the bearer of bad news. To lessen the pain and the hurt is only human, but in the end, truth must win over fear.

Speaking the truth in times of universal deceit is a revolutionary act.

—GEORGE ORWELL

36,000 Feet over Texas

A few weeks before Frank was to travel to Dodge City, Texas, for a work assignment, he received a call from Dr. Layblame: "Hi Frank. This is Dr. Layblame. Can you be ready for an early afternoon departure from Dodge City on Friday?" Frank replied, "Well you know we have been instructed not to leave early, and the last flight leaves at 4:30 P.M. Anyway, I don't mind flying out Saturday morning." Dr. Layblame replied, "Well, it's only an hour early. If you write most of your report the night before and during lunch on Friday, we should be able to finish up work by 2:30 P.M. The airport is small and close to the hospital. Besides, my team has to drive to Louisiana and we would like to get there so we can go out to dinner and enjoy evening. I am the tour leader, so it should not be a problem." Frank said OK and scheduled a 4:30 P.M. return flight.

While Frank was in a flight to Washington, DC following his work assignment, Ronald, Frank's supervisor was dictating a voicemail message to him. When Frank returned home at about 10:30 that evening, he retrieved his voicemail messages. Ronald had left Frank a message at 4:30 P.M. earlier that day asking Frank, "Call me as soon as you get this message. I will be in my office until about 5:30 P.M. If you miss me, you can reach me over the weekend. My cell phone number is xxx/xxx-xxxx."

Frank called Ronald that evening and the next morning; however, Ronald never answered, nor did he return his call. Frank called Ronald Monday morning. As luck would have it, Ronald was out of the office for the day. Frank called Ronald again on Tuesday morning and Ronald answered. Frank asked, "Ronald, you called?" He replied, "Yes, I did. How were you able to get to the airport on Friday and catch a 4:30 P.M. flight without leaving your job early? I had your flight schedule and you left the survey early. You could not possibly have traveled to the airport in time to catch your flight without leaving early."

Frank replied, "I did not schedule the exit time from the survey. The physician team leader determined the time of the exit. He said that he was conducting a system tour and would like to get the exit briefing started as soon as possible. He asked for everybody to be ready to exit by having draft reports ready the night before." Ronald replied, "Dr. Layblame told me the team had to exit early because you scheduled an early flight."

Frank asked, "Just one question, Ronald. Why would you leave a message for me at 4:30 P.M. to call you by 5:30 P.M. when you knew I was 36,000 feet high in the sky? And why didn't you call the team leader at the beginning of the assignment and not after it was completed? Since you know flight schedules, why would you wait until the assignment was completed to raise this issue? Sounds a bit peculiar, don't you think? Sort of like observing a protocol not being followed in the OR and then chastising the OR team after the surgery is completed for not following protocol. This is a serious business we are in. You need to ask yourself why you would allow an event to occur if you believed it to be wrong."

Discussion

1. Discuss the ethical issues involved in this case.
2. Discuss what you would do if you found yourself in Frank's situation.
3. What should Frank have said if his manager said, "You should have reported Dr. Layblame"?
4. How would you describe Ronald's management style?

Declining Trust in the Health Care System

The declining trust in the nation's ability to deliver high-quality health care is evidenced by a system caught up in the quagmire of managed care companies, which have in some instances inappropriately devised ways to deny health care benefits to their constituency. In addition, the continuing reporting of numerous medical errors serves only to escalate distrust in the nation's political leadership and the providers of health care.

Physicians find themselves vulnerable to lawsuits, often because of misdiagnosis. As a result, patients are passed from specialist to specialist in an effort to leave no stone unturned. Fearful to step outside the boundaries of their own specialties, physicians escalate the problem by ineffectively communicating with the primary care physician responsible for managing the patient's overall health care needs. This can also be problematic if no one physician has taken overall responsibility to coordinate and manage a patient's care.

Cancer Doctor Allegedly Prescribed $35 Million Worth of Totally Unnecessary Chemotherapy

A Michigan oncologist has been charged with giving $35 million in needless chemotherapy to patients—some of whom didn't even have cancer, The Today Show reported.

Popular physician Farid Fata, who had more than 1,000 patients, allegedly misdiagnosed people with cancer just so he could bill Medicare.

He's also accused of giving chemo to "end-of-life" patients who wouldn't benefit and had to endure the treatment's nasty side effects during their final days.

Christina Sterbenz, Business Insider, *August 15, 2013*

Politics and Distrust

Lies or the appearance of lies are not what the writers of our Constitution intended for our country—it's not the America we salute every Fourth of July, it's not the America we learned about in school, and it is not the America represented in the flag that rises above our land.

—ANONYMOUS

Truthfulness is just one measure of one's moral character. Unfortunately, politicians do not always set good examples for the people they serve. The following news clipping is an example of how political decisions can lead to distrust in government.

Cheney's Staff Cut Testimony on Warming

In a letter to Sen. Barbara Boxer (D-Calif.), former EPA deputy associate administrator Jason K. Burnett said an official from Cheney's office ordered last October that six pages be edited out of the testimony of Julie L. Gerberding, director of the Centers for Disease Control and Prevention. Gerberding had planned to say that the "CDC considers climate change a serious public health concern."

Juliet Eilperin, The Washington Post, *July 9, 2008*

Discussion

1. Discuss how headlines such as this affect your opinion of politicians.
2. Assuming a cover-up, discuss how the principles of beneficence and nonmaleficence apply.
3. At the end of our days, the most basic principles of life—trust and survival—are on trial. What is your verdict, if indeed there was a cover-up?

INTEGRITY

Nearly all men can stand adversity, but if you want to test a man's character, give him power.
—ABRAHAM LINCOLN

Wrong-Operation Doctor

Hospitals find it hard to protect patients from wrong-site surgery

Last year a jury returned a $20 million negligence verdict against Arkansas Children's Hospital for surgery on the wrong side of the brain of a 15-year-old boy who was left psychotic and severely brain damaged. Testimony showed that the error was not disclosed to his parents for more than a year. The hospital issued a statement saying it deeply regretted the error and had "redoubled our efforts to prevent" a recurrence.

"Healthcare has far too little accountability for results . . . . All the pressures are on the side of production; that's how you get paid," said Peter Pronovost, a prominent safety expert and medical director of the Johns Hopkins Center for Innovation in Quality Patient Care, who added that increased pressure to turn over operating rooms quickly has trumped patient safety, increasing the chance of error.

Sandra G. Boodman, Kaiser Health News, The Washington Post, *June 20, 2011*

Discussion

1. Discuss the issues of integrity in this case.
2. Should criminal charges be a consideration in this case, if accurately reported? Discuss your answer.

Integrity involves a steadfast adherence to a strict moral or ethical code and a commitment not to compromise this code. A person with integrity has a staunch belief in and faithfulness to, for example, his or her religious beliefs. Patients and professionals alike often make health care decisions based on their integrity and their strict moral beliefs. For example, Jehovah's Witnesses generally refuse blood transfusions because it is contrary to their religious beliefs, even if such refusal may result in death. A provider of health care may refuse to participate in an abortion because it is against the provider's moral beliefs. A person without personal integrity lacks sincerity and moral conviction and may fail to act on professed moral beliefs.

Behind the Smiles

Jeff well remembers what happened after Bill left the hospital boardroom. He, however, remembers more clearly how Bill, a consultant, was treated while he was in the room after presenting his organizational improvement report to the hospital's leadership. Bill was treated with kindness and assurances as to how well he took an educational approach to his audit findings with the staff and how employees appreciated his suggestions for improvement.

Prior to exiting the conference room, Bill asked whether there were any questions about his report. No questions, just smiles, accolades, and goodbyes. Jeff thought to himself, wow, it is good to see good people take suggestions and be so willing to make the changes that Bill suggested.

Oops, hold on, it turns out Bill wasn't as wonderful as the leadership described. The organization's leadership was now disgruntled about Bill's report. Bill was gone and now vilified. Jeff, a consultant not scheduled to finish his assignment for another 2 weeks, asked, "Why didn't you ask questions while Bill was here?" Carol, the finance director replied, "I spent 2 weeks with Bill. He just made up his mind. There was just no changing his mind." Jim said, "Are you saying that you disagree with Bill's report?" Carol, replied, "Yes, I do disagree with it." Jeff continued, "But you did not state that while he was here. You told him you liked his suggestions and that you were already in the process of implementing them." Carol replied, "That's true, but since we made the suggested changes while he was here, he did not have to include them in his written report." Bill replied, "It speaks well of leadership that you have done so; however, it is the hospital board that asked for the audit. We must report what we found." Carol, disgruntled, remained silent. Jim thought to himself, integrity includes being honest and truthful and surely not criticizing a person after leaving the conference room.

Anonymous

Discussion

1. Should Bill have left his findings off the report? Explain your answer.
2. Discuss why Bill's integrity in reporting the deficiencies he found and reported were important to both ABC consulting and the hospital board, which had contracted with ABC to conduct the audit.

Employee Satisfaction Survey

The human resources department manager was reporting on an employee satisfaction survey at a leadership roundtable session with the organization's employees. To maintain employee confidentiality, a third-party consulting firm had conducted the survey. Approximately 49% of employees had responded to the survey, compared with 47% 3 years earlier. The HR manager commented that it is was the first satisfaction survey conducted in 3 years and that the results were excellent, with a 4.2% rise in overall employee satisfaction. Management was all smiles as they sat listening to the report. The HR manager had actually briefed the organization's leadership prior to the roundtable session. Following the report, she asked if there were any questions. The silence was deadly—no one responded. Finally, one employee, Richard, placed his hands on the table to stand up, but he felt a nudge on his right shoulder from Phil, a physician friend. Phil whispered, "Richard, are you sure you want to ask any questions? There is nothing to gain here." Richard, looking down with a smile, said, "I agree, but I can't help myself." Richard then stood up and asked the HR manager, "Do you know what the employee turnover rate has been during the past 3 years?" She responded, "Well, ugh, yes, it was about 30%." Richard replied, "So, then, does this report reflect that we have had a 30% turnover?" The manager replied, "Good point, I will have to get back to you on that."When he returned to his seat, Phil said, "Do you really think you will ever hear back an answer to your question?" Richard smiled and replied, "Not really." Richard was right; she never did get back to him.

Discussion

1. Discuss why employees are often reluctant to ask questions when their questions are solicited by leadership.
2. Knowing that the HR manager never followed up with Richard, should he have followed up with the manager as to the validity of the survey data? Explain your answer.

Medical Integrity and Patient Autonomy

The integrity of the medical profession is not threatened by allowing competent patients to decide for themselves whether a particular medical treatment is in their best interests. Patient autonomy sets the foundation of one's right to bodily integrity, including the right to accept or refuse treatment. Those rights are superior to the institutional considerations of hospitals and their medical staffs. A state's interest in maintaining the ethical integrity of a profession does not outweigh, for example, a patient's right to refuse blood transfusions.

KINDNESS

When you carry out acts of kindness, you get a wonderful feeling inside. It is as though something inside your body responds and says, yes, this is how I ought to feel.

—HAROLD KUSHNER

Kindness involves the quality of being considerate and sympathetic to another's needs. Some people are takers, and others are givers. If you go through life giving without the anticipation of receiving, you will be a kinder and happier person.

Kindness Is Not Always Returned

The widely known saying "actions speak louder than words" is well demonstrated in this *reality check*. Joe was a health care consultant. He had collected thousands of documents of helpful information to share with health care organizations with which he had worked. His thinking was this: Why should hospitals have to reinvent the wheel? If organizations are willing to share with others, why not disseminate such information for the benefit of other hospitals? His hopes were that larger trade organizations would eventually collect the information and freely share with their constituents. After all, the goal was better care for all wherever they lived. Joe would provide copies of his CD to fellow consultants and encourage them to share the information with others. One day upon arriving at work he noticed that one of the consultants to whom he had given a copy of the CD had four or five newspaper clippings about hospitals spread out on a conference room table. Joe thought they looked interesting and asked, "Could I have a copy of your clippings?" The consultant said, "No, these are proprietary information."

On another occasion, after sharing his CD with an organization, he asked, "Would you be willing to share your '12 Step Addiction Program' with other health care organizations?" A representative from the organization said, "We will share it with you but not others." Joe kindly said, "That's okay. I can accept only what you are willing to share with others."

Anonymous

Discussion

1. Should Joe have asked for his CD back from the consultant and organization? Discuss your answer.
2. Discuss why an organization might not be willing to share program information.

RESPECT

Respect for ourselves guides our morals; respect for others guides our manners.

　　　　　　　　　　　　　　　　　　　　　　　　　　　　　　　—LAURENCE STERNE

Respect is an attitude of admiration or esteem. Kant was the first major Western philosopher to put respect for persons, including oneself as a person, at the center of moral theory. He believed that persons are ends in themselves with an absolute dignity, which must always be respected. In contemporary thinking, respect has become a core ideal extending moral respect to things other than persons, including all things in nature.

Caregivers who demonstrate respect for one another and their patients will be more effective in helping them cope with the anxiety of their illness. Respect helps to develop trust between the patient and caregiver and improve healing processes. If caregivers respect the family of a patient, cooperation and understanding will be the positive result, encouraging a team effort to improve patient care.

HOPEFULNESS

Hope is the last thing that dies in man; and though it be exceedingly deceitful, yet it is of this good use to us, that while we are traveling through life, it conducts us in an easier and more pleasant way to our journey's end.

　　　　　　　　　　　　　　　　　　　　　　　　　—FRANCOIS DE LA ROCHEFOUCAULD

Brooke Greenberg: 20-Year-Old "Toddler's" Legacy of Hope and Love

The baffling case of Brooke Greenberg, a 20-year-old who never developed beyond the toddler stage, may provide clues to help scientists unlock the secrets of longevity and fight age-related disorders, such as Alzheimer's, Parkinson's, and heart disease. Brooke, who passed away last Thursday, had the body and cognitive function of a 1-year-old. She didn't grow after the age of 5—and basically, she stopped aging entirely.

Brooke may have been the only person in the world suffering from a mysterious genetic disease that her doctors called Syndrome X. "Finding out that her DNA makeup is completely different than anyone else brought to our attention that we could help," her father, Howard Greenberg, told Yahoo Shine in a previous interview. "So eventually, at the end of the rainbow, there will be something that comes out of all this. I believe everyone is here for a reason."

Sarah B. Weir, Healthy Living, *October 29, 2013*[14]

Hopefulness in the patient care setting involves looking forward to something with the confidence of success. Caregivers have a responsibility to balance truthfulness while promoting hope. The caregiver must be sensitive to each patient's needs and provide hope. As noted by Brooke's father, we can pass on hope and love to others.

TOLERANCE

There is a criterion by which you can judge whether the thoughts you are thinking and the things you are doing are right for you. The criterion is: Have they brought you inner peace? If they have not, there is something wrong with them—so keep seeking! If what you do has brought you inner peace, stay with what you believe is right.

—PEACE PILGRIM

Tolerance can be viewed in two ways, positive or negative. *Positive tolerance* implies that a person accepts differences in others and that one does not expect others to believe, think, speak, or act as he or she does. Tolerant people are generally free of prejudice and discrimination. Recognizing this fact, Thomas Jefferson incorporated theories of tolerance into the U.S. Constitution. *Negative tolerance* implies that one will reluctantly put up with another's beliefs. In other words, he or she merely tolerates the views of others.

Although tolerance can be viewed as a virtue, however, not all tolerance is virtuous nor is all intolerance necessarily wrong. An exaggerated tolerance may amount to a vice, whereas intolerance may sometimes be a virtue. For example, tolerating everything regardless of its repugnance (e.g., persecution for religious beliefs) is no virtue, and having intolerance for that which should not be tolerated and is evil is no vice (e.g., mass executions).

COOPERATION AND TEAMWORK

If we do not hang together, we will all hang separately.

—BENJAMIN FRANKLIN (1706–1790)

Cooperation is the process of working with others. In the health care setting, caregivers must work together to improve patient outcomes. The health care worker today works in an environment where change is the norm. Those unwilling to accept change and work in unity will eventually be working alone. Change is the only constant in today's workplace and society in general. Technological change is occurring at a pace faster than the human mind can absorb, thus requiring teamwork between individuals with a wide variety of skills sets. Congress, as noted in the following news clipping, is an example of how little can be accomplished when its members are dysfunctional and unwilling to cooperate and work together towards common goals.

Congress Gets Stuck Again—Over FAA

Parties Blame Each Other in Funding Dispute and Partial Shutdown

A dispute over funding for the Federal Aviation Administration has left an estimated 74,000 people out of work for a dozen days and tossed Congress into the throes of yet another interparty battle.

Now, with lawmakers leaving town or already on recess, there seems to be little hope of a resolution on the horizon.

Ashley Halsey III, The Washington Post, *August 4, 2011*

Failure to cooperate has a rippling effect in any setting. The failure of Congress to cooperate and resolve funding issues for the Federal Aviation Administration (FAA) before taking its summer recess in 2011 left 74,000 people out of work, costing the nation nearly a billion dollars for the month of August. Failure of the few to cooperate and act responsibly not only affected employees placed on a leave of absence but also placed a financial hardship on their families, not to mention the effect it has had on the communities where they live. In addition, passenger safety on airline flights was placed in jeopardy. If hospitals operated in this manner, there would be even more recorded bad outcomes. Teamwork is effective only as long as each member of the team cooperates and fulfills the duties assigned. High-quality patient care is more likely to be better in those organizations where respect and cooperation abounds.

Tying together the Patient Protection and Portable Care Act, commonly referred to as Obamacare, as a prerequisite to approving the national budget has merely resulted in name-calling by government officials, which has stirred bitterness between citizens of varying beliefs. Pundits and politicians alike fill the airways with contemptuous remarks that stoke the flames of division. The need to win one's point of view has selfishly become the norm and more important than the nation itself. Pride and self-appointed power brokers are the hallmarks of those responsible for crisis after crisis. Change comes when the players learn to cooperate for the common good.

FORGIVENESS

Forgiveness is a virtue of the brave.

–INDIRA GANDHI

Forbearing one another, and forgiving one another, if any man have a quarrel against any: even as Christ forgave you, so also do ye.

–COLOSSIANS 3:13 KJV

Forgiveness is a virtue and a value. It is the willingness to pardon someone who has wronged you in some way. It is also a form of mercy. Forgiveness is to forgive and let lose the bonds of blame. It is a form of cleansing souls of both those who forgive and those who accept the forgiveness offered.

The following *reality check* is an excerpt of a Facebook discussion between two friends involving courage and forgiveness by two very special people.

Courage and Forgiveness

7:38 am

Scotty: Did you see this link http://www.josieking.org/page.cfm?pageID=10 on the internet?

7:38 am

Diane: Reading it now

[Josie was 18 months old.... In January of 2001 Josie was admitted . . . after suffering first and second degree burns from climbing into a hot bath. She healed well and within weeks was scheduled for release. Two days before she was to return home she died of severe dehydration and misused narcotics ...

Josie spent 10 days in the PICU. I [Josie's mother] was by her side every day and night. I paid attention to every minute detail of the doctors' and nurses' care, and I was quick to ask questions. I bonded with them and was in constant awe of the medical attention she received . . . . She was sent down to the intermediate care floor with expectations of being sent home in a few days. Her three older siblings prepared for her welcome home celebration . . .

The following week her central line had been taken out. I began noticing that every time she saw a drink she would scream for it, and I thought this was strange. I was told not to let her drink. While a nurse and I gave her a bath, she sucked furiously on a washcloth. As I put her to bed, I noticed that her eyes were rolling back in her head. Although I asked the nurse to call the doctor, she reassured me that oftentimes children did this and her vitals were fine. I told her Josie had never done this and perhaps another nurse could look at her. After yet another reassurance from another nurse that everything was fine, I was told that it was okay for me to sleep at home. I called to check in two times during the night and returned to the hospital at 5:30 am. I took one look at Josie and demanded that a doctor come at once. She was not fine. Josie's medical team arrived and administered two shots of Narcan. I asked if she could have something to drink. The request was approved, and Josie gulped down nearly a liter of juice. Verbal orders were issued for there to be no narcotics given. As I sat with Josie, I noticed that the nurse on morning duty was acting very strangely. She seemed nervous, overly demonstrative and in a hurry. Uneasy, I asked the other nurses about her and they said she had been a nurse for a long time. Still worried, I expressed my concern to one of the doctors, and he agreed that she was acting a bit odd. Meanwhile, Josie started perking up. She was more alert and had kept all liquids down. I was still scared and asked her doctors to please stay close by. At 1:00 the nurse walked over with a syringe of methadone. Alarmed, I told her that there had been an order for no narcotics. She said the orders had been changed and administered the drug.

Josie's heart stopped as I was rubbing her feet. Her eyes were fixed, and I screamed for help. I stood helpless as a crowd of doctors and nurses came running into her room. I was ushered into a small room with a chaplain.

The next time I saw Josie she had been moved back up to the PICU. Doctors and nurses were standing around her bed. No one seemed to want to look at me. She was hooked up to many machines, and her leg was black and blue. I looked into their faces, and said to them, You did this to her now YOU must fix her. I was told to pray. Two days later Jack, Relly and Eva were brought to the hospital to kiss their beloved Josie goodbye. Josie was taken off of life support. She died in our arms on a snowy night in what's considered to be one of the best hospitals in the world. Our lives were shattered and changed forever.

Josie died from severe dehydration and misused narcotics. Careless human errors. On top of our overwhelming sorrow and intense grief we were consumed by anger. They say anger can do one of two things to you. It can cause you to rot away or it can propel you forward. There were days when all I wanted was to destroy the hospital and then put an end to my own pain. My three remaining children were my only reason for getting out of bed and functioning. One day I will tell them how they saved my life. My husband Tony and I decided that we had to let the anger move us forward. We would do something good that would help prevent this from ever happening to a child again.

7:43 am

Diane: I've experience first hand human error in the hospital. I was told by my Dr. it could have been critical and I would have died.

7:45 am

Diane: The nurses don't like him and he told me to write a letter to file a complaint, but the thing is, the nursing staff was so good to me before and after that incident. Evidently when it was happening he yelled at the staff without me knowing. I had no clue what had happened till days later the nurse involved apologized to me profusely.

7:46 am

Diane: But I was so ill I didn't give it much thought you ever heard of tpn? Its a sugar mixture via iv cuz i couldn't eat. Supposedly it was supposed to be infused in me I think over a 12 hr period?

7:47 am

Diane: But the nurse put it for 4 hrs. I could have gone into diabetic shock. I do remember trying to wake up but I couldn't open my eyes and I heard a lot of movement in my room with the nurses. I yelled out. I can't open my eyes and I'm dretched in sweat. I had no idea wat was happening. I was then put on insulin.

7:50 am

Scotty: I must say you are an amazing young lady.

Anonymous Patient

Discussion

1. This young lady forgave the nurse and suggested that when the nurse was setting the timing for the TPN, she may have distracted the nurse, and she blamed herself for the wrong setting. Discuss how courage and forgiveness were displayed in this case.
2. Discuss the similarities in values that Josie's mother and the young lady on the Internet have in common.
3. Discuss your thoughts as to how human errors can be prevented; including what roles patients, families, caregivers, hospitals, and regulatory agencies should play in preventing similar errors.

RELIGIOUS ETHICS

The Great Physician: Dear Lord, You are the great physician. I turn to you in my sickness, asking you for help. I place myself under Your loving care, praying that I may know Your healing grace and wholeness. Help me to find love in this strange world and to feel your presence by my bed both day and night. Give my doctors and nurses wisdom, that they may understand my illness. Steady and guide them with your strong hand. Reach out Your hand to me and touch my life with Your peace. Amen.

—University of Pennsylvania Health System

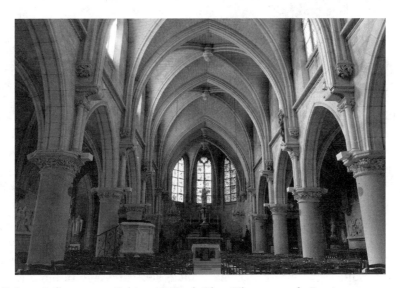

FIGURE 1-3 Religious Influence on Ethics (© Pack-Shot/Shutterstock, Inc.)

Religious ethics serve a moral purpose by providing codes of conduct for appropriate behavior through revelations from a divine source. These codes of conduct are enforced through fear of pain and suffering in the next life and/or reward in the next life for adhering to religious codes and beliefs. The prospect of divine justice helps us to tolerate the injustices in this life, where goodness is no guarantee of peace, happiness, wellness, or prosperity.

Many Think God's Intervention Can Revive the Dying

When it comes to saving lives, God trumps doctors for many Americans. An eye-opening survey reveals widespread belief that divine intervention can revive dying patients. And, researchers said, doctors "need to be prepared to deal with families who are waiting for a miracle."

Lindsey Tanner, USA Today, *August 18, 2008*

Religion should be a component of the education, policy development, and consultative functions of ethics committees. There is a need to know, for example, how to respond to Jehovah's Witnesses who refuse blood transfusions. Some hospitals provide staff with materials that describe various religious beliefs and how those beliefs might affect the patient's course of care while in the hospital.

Religion is often used as a reason to justify what otherwise could be considered unjustifiable behavior. Political leaders often use religion to legitimize and consolidate their power. Leaders in democratic societies speak of the necessity to respect the right to "freedom of religion."

Political leaders often use religion to further their political aspirations. They have often used religion to justify their actions. Religious persecution has plagued humanity from the beginning of time.

Syrian Rebels Combat al-Qaeda Force

The ISIS extremists "have not the support of the people because they treated them badly. They were cutting off people's heads all of the time to scare them in the name of religion," said Col. Qassim Saadeddine, spokesman for the Revolutionary Front.

Liz Sly, The Washington Post, *January 6, 2013*

The world today, with the aid of the news media, is able to see firsthand the results of what can happen to innocent people in the name of religion. The atrocities of evil people strapping bombs to the mentally deficient with the purpose of blowing themselves up in public places, killing and maiming men, women, and children, are but a few of the numerous atrocities of what has occurred throughout the ages.

Spirituality implies that there is purpose and meaning to life; spirituality generally refers to faith in a higher being. For a patient, injury and sickness are frightening experiences. This fear is often heightened when the patient is admitted to a hospital or nursing facility. Health care organizations can help reduce patient fears by making available to them appropriate emotional and spiritual support and coping resources. It is a well-proven fact that patients who are able to draw on their spirituality and religious beliefs tend to have a more comfortable and often improved healing experience. To assist both patients and caregivers in addressing spiritual needs, patients should be provided with information as to how their spiritual needs can be addressed.

Surgeon Uses Ministry in Medical Practice

DALLAS–At 83, Carl Smith found himself facing quadruple bypass surgery and the real possibility that he might not survive.

Within hours on this spring morning, Dr. Daniel Pool would temporarily bring Smith's heart to a stop in an attempt to circumvent its blocked passages.

And to help his patient confront the uncertainty, Pool did something unusual in his profession: He prayed with him.

The power of healing: Medicine and religion have had their day, and they haven't always been able to coexist. But as today's medical treatment becomes more holistic, doctors are increasingly taking spirituality into account.

Marc Ramirez, Altoona Mirror, *August 9, 2013*

Discussion

1. Discuss the pressure, if any, placed on the patient in responding to the suggestion of prayer prior to surgery.
2. Describe how you, as the surgeon, would address a patient's religious or spiritual needs if the risks of a complex surgical procedure appear to be threatening.

Difficult questions regarding a patient's spiritual needs and how to meet those needs are best addressed on admission by first collecting information about the patient's religious or spiritual preferences. Caregivers often find it difficult to discuss spiritual issues for fear of offending a patient who may have beliefs different from their own. If caregivers know from admission records a patient's religious beliefs, the caregiver can share with the patient those religious and spiritual resources available in the hospital and community.

A variety of religions are described next for the purpose of understanding some of the basic tenets of these religions. They are presented here to note the importance of better understanding why patients differ in decision-making processes and how religion affects their beliefs and to encourage further study of how each religion affects the decision-making process. Hospitals should maintain a directory of the various religions that includes contacts for referral and consultation purposes.

Judaism

Jewish Law refers to the unchangeable 613 mitzvot (commandments) that God gave to the Jews. Halakhah (Jewish Law) comes from three sources: (1) the Torah (the first five books of the Bible); (2) laws instituted by the rabbis; and (3) longstanding customs. The Jewish People is another name for the Children of Israel, referring to the Jews as a nation in the classical sense, meaning a group of people with a shared history and a sense of a group identity rather than a specific place or political persuasion.[15]

Judaism is a monotheistic religion based on principles and ethics embodied in the Hebrew Bible (Old Testament). The notion of right and wrong is not so much an object of philosophical inquiry as an acceptance of divine revelation. Moses, for example, received a list of 10 laws directly from God. These laws were known as the 10 Commandments. Some of the 10 Commandments are related to the basic principles of justice that have been adhered to by society since they were first proclaimed and published. For some societies, the 10 Commandments were a turning point, where essential commands such as "thou shalt not kill" or "thou shalt not commit adultery" were accepted as law. The 10 Commandments (King James Version of the Bible) are as follows:

1. Thou shalt have no other gods before me.
2. Thou shalt not make unto thee any graven image, or any likeness of anything that is in heaven above, or that is in the earth beneath, or that is in the water under the earth. Thou shalt not bow down thyself to them, nor serve them.
3. Thou shalt not take the name of the Lord thy God in vain.
4. Remember the Sabbath day, to keep it holy.
5. Honor thy father and thy mother: that thy days may be long upon the land which the Lord thy God giveth thee.
6. Thou shalt not kill.
7. Thou shalt not commit adultery.
8. Thou shalt not steal.
9. Thou shalt not bear false witness against thy neighbor.
10. Thou shalt not covet thy neighbor's house, thou shalt not covet thy neighbor's wife, nor his manservant, nor his maidservant, nor his ox, nor his ass, nor anything that is thy neighbor's.

When caring for the dying, family members will normally want to be present and prayers spoken. If a rabbi is requested, the patient's own rabbi should be contacted first.

Hinduism

Hinduism is a polytheistic religion with many gods and goddesses. Hindus believe that God is everything and is infinite. The earliest known Hindu Scriptures were recorded around 1200 BC. Hindus believe in reincarnation and that one's present condition is a reflection of one's virtuous behavior or lack thereof in a previous lifetime.

When caring for the dying, relatives may wish to perform rituals at this time. In death, jewelry, sacred threads, or other religious objects should not be removed from the body. Washing the body is part of the funeral rites and should be carried out by the relatives.[16]

BUDDHISM

Buddhism is a religion and philosophy encompassing a variety of traditions, beliefs, and practices, based largely on teachings attributed to Prince Siddhartha Gautama (563–483 BC), son of King Suddhodana and Queen Mayadevi, who lived in the present-day border area between India and Nepal. He had gone on a spiritual quest and eventually became enlightened at the age of 35, and from then on, he took the name Buddha. Simply defined, Buddhism is a religion to some and a philosophy to others that encourages one "to do good, avoid evil, and purify the mind."

When caring for the dying, Buddhists like to be informed about their health status in order to prepare themselves spiritually. A side room with privacy is preferred.[17]

Falun Gong

Falun Gong, also referred to as *Falun Dafa*, is a traditional Chinese spiritual discipline belonging to the Buddhist school of thought. It consists of moral teachings, a meditation, and four exercises that resemble tai chi and are known in Chinese culture as *qigong*. Falun Gong does not involve physical places of worship, formal hierarchies, rituals, or membership and is taught without charge. The three principles practiced by the followers are truthfulness, compassion, and forbearance/tolerance toward others. The followers of Falun Gong claim a following in 100 countries.

Zen

Zen evolved from Buddhism in Tibet. It emphasizes dharma practice (from the master to the disciple) and experiential wisdom based on learning through the reflection on doing, going beyond scriptural readings. In Zen, Buddhism learning comes through a form of seated meditation known as *zazen*, where practitioners perform meditation to calm the body and the mind and experience insight into the nature of existence and thereby gain enlightenment.

TAOISM

Taoists believe that ultimate reality is unknowable and unperceivable. The founder of Taoism is believed to be Lao Tzu (6 BC). Taoist doctrine includes the belief that the proper way of living involves being in tune with nature. Everything is ultimately interblended and interacts.

CHRISTIANITY

Christianity is based on the Bible's New Testament teachings. Christians accept both the Old and New Testament as being the word of God. The New Testament describes Jesus as being God, taking the form of man. He was born of the Virgin Mary, sacrificed his life by suffering crucifixion, and after being raised from the dead on the third day, he ascended into Heaven from which he will return to raise the dead, at which time the spiritual body will be united with the physical body. His death, burial, and resurrection provide a way of salvation through belief in Him for the forgiveness of sin. God is believed to be manifest in three persons: the Father, Son, and Holy Spirit.

The primary and final authority for Christian ethics is found in the life, teachings, ministry, death, and resurrection of Jesus Christ. He clarified the ethical demands of a God-centered life by applying the obedient love that was required of Peter. The 10 Commandments are accepted and practiced by both Christians and Jews.

Christians, when determining what is the right thing to do, often refer to the Golden Rule, which teaches us to "do unto others as you would have them do unto you," a common principle in many moral codes and religions.

There have been and continue to be numerous interpretations of the meaning of the scriptures and their different passages by Christians over the centuries. This has resulted in a plethora of churches with varying beliefs. As noted later, such beliefs can affect a patient's wishes for health care. However, the heart of Christian beliefs is found in the book of John:

For God so loved the world, that he gave his only begotten Son, that whoever believeth in him should not perish, but have everlasting life.

— King James Version, John 3:16

The Apostle Paul proclaimed that salvation cannot be gained through good works but through faith in Jesus Christ as savior. He recognized the importance of faith in Christ over good works in the pursuit of salvation.

That if thou shalt confess with thy mouth the Lord Jesus, and shalt believe in thine heart that God hath raised him from the dead, thou shalt be saved.

— King James Version, Romans 10:9

The Apostle Paul, however, did not dismiss the importance of good works. Works are the fruit of one's faith. In other words, good works follows faith.

Anointing of the Sick

When caring for the dying, services of the in-house chaplain and/or one's religious minister should be offered the patient. A Catholic priest should be offered when last rites need to be administered to those of the Catholic faith.

Islam

The Islamic religion believes there is one God: Allah. Muhammad (570–632 AD) is considered to be a prophet/messenger of God. He is believed to have received revelations from God. These revelations were recorded in the Qur'an, the Muslim Holy Book. Muslims accept Moses and Jesus as prophets of God. The Qur'an is believed to supersede that of the Torah and the Bible. Muslims believe that there is no need for God's grace and that their own actions can merit God's mercy and goodness. Humans are believed to have a moral responsibility to submit to God's will and to follow Islam as demonstrated in the Qur'an. The five pillars of the practice of Islam are believing the creed, performing five prayers daily, giving alms, fasting during Ramadan, and making a pilgrimage to Mecca at least once in a lifetime.

When caring for the dying, patients may want to die facing Mecca (toward the southeast) and be with relatives. In death, many Muslims follow strict rules in respect of the body after death.

RELIGIOUS BELIEFS AND DUTY CONFLICT

Religious beliefs and codes of conduct sometimes conflict with the ethical duty of caregivers to save lives. For example, Jehovah's Witnesses, believe that it is a sin to accept a blood transfusion because the Bible states that we must "abstain from blood" (Acts 15:29). Current Jehovah's Witness doctrine, in part, states that blood must not be transfused. In order to respect this belief, bloodless surgery is available in a number of hospitals to patients who find it against their religious beliefs to receive a blood transfusion.

Every attempt should be made to resolve blood transfusion issues prior to any elective surgery. The transfusion of blood to an emergent unconscious patient may be necessary to save the patient's life. Because some Jehovah's Witnesses would accept blood in such situations, most courts would most likely find such a transfusion acceptable. When transfusion of a minor becomes necessary and parental consent is refused, it may be necessary to seek a court order to allow for such transfusions. Because time is of the essence in many cases, it is important for hospitals to work out such issues in advance with legislative bodies and the judicial system in order to provide legal protection for caregivers who find it necessary to transfuse blood in order to save a life. In those instances in which the patient has a right to refuse a blood transfusion, the hospital should seek a formal signed release from the patient.

SECULAR ETHICS

Unlike religious ethics, *secular ethics* is based on codes developed by societies that have relied on customs to formulate their codes. The Code of Hammurabi, for example, carved on a black Babylonian column 8 feet high, now located in the Louvre in Paris, depicts a mythical sun god presenting a code of laws to Hammurabi, a great military leader and ruler of Babylon (1795–1750 BC). Hammurabi's code of laws is an early example of a ruler proclaiming to his people an entire body of laws. The following excerpts are from the Code of Hammurabi.

Code of Hammurabi

5

If a judge try a case, reach a decision, and present his judgment in writing; if later error shall appear in his decision, and it be through his own fault, then he shall pay twelve times the fine set by him in the case, and he shall be publicly removed from the judge's bench, and never again shall he sit there to render judgment.

194

If a man give his child to a nurse and the child die in her hands, but the nurse unbeknown to the father and mother nurse another child, then they shall convict her of having nursed another child without the knowledge of the father and mother and her breasts shall be cut off.

215

If a physician make a large incision with an operating knife and cure it, or if he open a tumor (over the eye) with an operating knife, and saves the eye, he shall receive ten shekels in money.

> ### 217
>
> *If he be the slave of some one, his owner shall give the physician two shekels.*
>
> ### 218
>
> *If a physician make a large incision with the operating knife, and kill him, or open a tumor with the operating knife, and cut out the eye, his hands shall be cut off.*
>
> ### 219
>
> *If a physician make a large incision in the slave of a freed man, and kill him, he shall replace the slave with another slave.*
>
> ### 221
>
> *If a physician heal the broken bone or diseased soft part of a man, the patient shall pay the physician five shekels in money.*

ATHEISM

Atheism is the rejection of belief in any god, generally because atheists believe there is no scientific evidence that can prove God exists. They argue that there is no objective moral standard for right and wrong and that ethics and morality are the products of culture and politics, subject to individual convictions.

Those of various religious faiths, however, believe there is overwhelming evidence that there is reason to believe that God does exist and that the evidence through historical documents, archeological finds, and the vastness of space and time clearly supports and confirms the existence of God. Christians often refer to the Old Testament and cite the book of Isaiah:

It is He that sitteth upon the circle of the earth . . .

—ISAIAH 40:22 (KING JAMES VERSION)

Christians argue when citing this verse that Isaiah could not possibly know that the earth is the shape of a circle. He presents no magical formula or scientific argument in his writings as to why the earth is round. Furthermore, Isaiah does not belabor the fact that the earth is round. The argument continues in the book of Job:

He stretcheth out the north over the empty place, and hangeth the earth upon nothing.

—JOB 26:7 (KING JAMES VERSION)

The obvious question then arises, how did Job know, 3,000 years before it became a scientific, verifiable fact, the earth hangs upon nothing?

SITUATIONAL ETHICS

Be careful how you judge others. . . . As Scottish author J.M. Barrie said, "Never ascribe to an opponent motives meaner than your own." We tend to judge others based on their behavior, and ours based on our intent. In almost all situations, we would do well to recognize the possibility— even probability—of good intent in others . . . sometimes despite their observable behavior.

—STEPHEN M. R. COVEY, *THE SPEED OF TRUST* (FREE PRESS)

Situational ethics is concerned with the outcome or consequences of an action in which the ends can justify the means. It refers to those times when a person's beliefs and values can change as circumstances change. Why do good people behave differently in similar situations? Why do good people sometimes do bad things? The answer is fairly simple: One's moral character can sometimes change as circumstances change; thus the term situational ethics. A person, therefore, may contradict what he believes is the right thing to do and do what he morally considers wrong. For example, a decision not to use extraordinary means to sustain the life of an unknown 84-year-old may result in a different decision if the 84-year-old is one's mother.

The news clipping that follows illustrates how far society can regress when there are no common rules, values, or boundaries to guide us.

Viet Cong Execution

"And out of nowhere came this guy who we didn't know." Gen. Nguyen Ngoc Loan, chief of South Viet Nam's national police, walked up and shot the prisoner in the head. His reason: The prisoner, a Viet Cong lieutenant, had just murdered a South Vietnamese colonel, his wife, and their six children.

The peace movement adopted the photo as a symbol of the war's brutality. But Adams, who stayed in touch with Loan, said the photo wrongly stereotyped the man. "If you're this general and you caught this guy after he killed some of your people . . . how do you know you wouldn't have pulled that trigger yourself? You have to put yourself in that situation. . . . It's a war."

1969 Spot News, Newseum, *Washington, DC*

Have we lost our way? Have we lost our sense as to what is right and what is wrong? We say we have become a melting pot with some common themes but uncommon beliefs. In religion, there are those who sometimes seek a place of worship not always because one seeks what is right but because unconsciously it supports an individual's beliefs of what is right and wrong. Sometimes one's ever-changing choice of lifestyle contradicts earlier beliefs and can often result in a change in place of worship.

The values held ever so strongly in one situation may conflict with the same values given a different fact pattern. To better understand the concept of situational ethics, consider the desire to live and the extreme measures one will take in order to do so, remembering that ethical decision making is the process of determining the right thing to do when faced with moral dilemmas.

Consider the account of the plane crash on October 13, 1972, high in the Andes Mountains. The survivors of the crash, until the day they were rescued, were faced with difficult decisions in order to survive. Of the original 40 passengers and 5 crewmembers, 16 emerged alive 72 days later to tell the story of the difficult ethical dilemmas and survival decisions they had to make.

Those who wished to survive had to eat the flesh of those who did not. They realized that to survive, they would have to deviate from their beliefs that teach it is morally wrong to eat the flesh of another human being. Given a different fact pattern, where there would have been an abundance of food at the site of the plane crash, the survivors would have found it reprehensible to eat human flesh. This is a gruesome story indeed, but it illustrates how there are no effective hard and fast rules or guidelines to govern ethical behavior when faced with life or death decisions. The reader here should consider here how one's beliefs, decisions, and or actions can change as circumstances change. Such is the case in the patient care setting where individual differences emerge based on needs, beliefs, and values.

ABSENCE OF A MORAL COMPASS

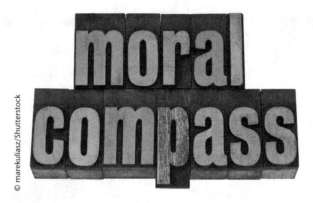

© marekuliasz/Shutterstock

The world is a dangerous place. Not because of the people who are evil; but because of the people who don't do anything about it.

—ALBERT EINSTEIN

The nation's health care system is off course as noted by the absence of a moral compass. Trust in the health care system continues to decline when those who are entrusted with providing health care prescribe unnecessary procedures (e.g., cardiac catheterizations, hysterectomies, tonsillectomies), molest our children, secretly record photographic pictures of patients while they are receiving physical examinations, numerous fraudulent billing scams costing the nation billions of dollars annually, tampering with chemotherapy agents by diluting them (unbeknown by patients who trust they are being treated by caregivers with integrity), unwarranted high-risk life-saving treatment delays for our veterans and falsification of records, and the list of unethical behavior continues to grow, seemingly unabated. The failure of government and those in leadership roles have failed to reset the nation's moral compass. The present path to better health care for all continues on an unacceptable course of corruption and is increasingly becoming a disturbing public concern.

Political corruption, antisocial behavior, declining civility, and rampant unethical conduct have heightened discussions over the nation's moral decline and decaying value systems in the delivery of health care. The numerous instances of questionable political decisions; numbers-cooking executives with exorbitant salaries, including health care executives working for both profit and nonprofit organizations, have all contributed to the nation's moral decline.

The continuing trend of consumer awareness of declining value systems mandates that the readers of this book understand ethics and the law and how they intertwine. Applying the generally accepted ethical principles (e.g., do good and not harm) and the moral values (e.g., respect, trust, integrity, compassion) described in this chapter will help sit a better course for those who are guided by a moral compass. It is the responsibility of every person to participate in resetting the moral compass, in our nation and in the world at large.

SUMMARY THOUGHTS

Be careful of your thoughts, for your thoughts inspire your words. Be careful of your words, for your words precede your actions. Be careful of your actions, for your actions become your habits. Be careful of your habits, for your habits build your character. Be careful of your character, for your character decides your destiny.

—Chinese Proverb

Although you cannot control the amount of time you have in this lifetime, you can control your behavior by adopting the virtues and values that will define who you are and what you will become and how you will be remembered or forgotten.

Become who you want to be and behave how you want to be remembered. The formula is easy and well described previously in what has been claimed to be a Chinese proverb. Read it. Reread it. Write it. Memorize it. Display it in your home, at work, and in your car, and most of all, practice it, always remembering that it all begins with thoughts.

Control your thoughts, and do not let them control you. As to words, they are the tools of thought. They can be sharper than any double-edged sword and hurt, or they can do good and heal.

It is never too late to change your thoughts, as long as you have air to breathe. Your legacy may be short, but it can be powerful. Remember the Gettysburg address. In the final analysis:

People are often unreasonable, illogical and self-centered; forgive them anyway. If you are kind, people may accuse you of selfish, ulterior motives; be kind anyway. If you are successful, you will win some false friends and some true enemies; succeed anyway. What you spend years building, someone may destroy overnight; build anyway. The good you do today, people will often forget tomorrow; do good anyway. Give the world the best you have, and it may never be enough; give the world the best you have anyway. You see, in the final analysis, it is between you and God; It was never between you and them anyway.

—Author Unknown

CHAPTER REVIEW

1. *Ethics* is the branch of philosophy that seeks to understand the nature, purposes, justification, and founding principles of moral rules and the systems they compose.
   * *Microethics* involves an individual's view of what is right and wrong based on his or her life experiences.
   * *Macroethics* involves a more generalized view of right and wrong.
2. *Bioethics* addresses such difficult issues as the nature of life, the nature of death, what sort of life is worth living, what constitutes murder, how we should treat people who are especially vulnerable, and the responsibilities we have to other human beings.
3. We study ethics to aid us in making sound judgments, good decisions, and right choices.
4. Ethics signifies a general pattern or way of life, such as religious ethics; a set of rules of conduct or "moral code," which involves professional ethics; or philosophical ethics, which involves inquiry about ways of life and rules of conduct.
5. *Morality* is a code of conduct. It is a guide to behavior that all rational persons would put forward for governing the behavior of all moral agents.
6. There is no "universal morality." Whatever guide to behavior that an individual regards as overriding and wants to be universally adopted is considered that individual's morality.
7. *Moral judgments* are those judgments concerned with what an individual or group believes to be the right or proper behavior in a given situation.
8. Morality is often legislated when differences cannot be resolved because of conflicting moral codes with varying opinions as to what is right and what is wrong (e.g., abortion). Laws are created to set boundaries for societal behavior, and they are enforced to ensure that the expected behavior is followed.
9. *Ethical theories* and principles introduce order into the way people think about life. *Metaethics* seeks to understand ethical terms and theories and their application. The following are ethical theories:
   * *Normative ethics* is the attempt to determine what moral standards should be followed so that human behavior and conduct may be morally right.
   * *Descriptive ethics*, also known as comparative ethics, deals with what people believe to be right and wrong.
   * *Applied ethics* is the application of normative theories to practical moral problems. It is the attempt to explain and justify specific moral problems such as abortion, euthanasia, and assisted suicide.
   * The *consequential theory* emphasizes that the morally right action is whatever action leads to the maximum balance of good over evil. The consequential theory is based on the view that the value of an action derives solely from the value of its consequences.
   * *Utilitarian ethics* involves the concept that the moral worth of an action is determined solely by its contribution to overall utility, that is, its contribution to happiness or pleasure as summed among all persons.

- *Deontological ethics* focuses on one's duties to others. It includes telling the truth and keeping your promises. Deontology is an ethical analysis according to a moral code or rules.
- The *nonconsequential ethical theory* denies that the consequences of an action or rule are the only criteria for determining the morality of an action or rule.
- *Ethical relativism* is the theory that holds that morality is relative to the norms of one's culture.

10. Common principles of ethics include:
    - *Autonomy* involves recognizing the right of a person to make his or her own decisions.
    - *Beneficence* describes the principle of doing good, demonstrating kindness, showing compassion, and helping others.
      - *Paternalism* is a form of beneficence. It may involve withholding information from a person because of the belief that doing so is in the best interest of that person.
      - *Medical paternalism* involves making choices for (or forcing choices on) patients who are capable of choosing for themselves. It directly violates patient autonomy.
    - *Nonmaleficence* is an ethical principle that requires caregivers to avoid causing harm to patients.
    - *Justice* is the obligation to be fair in the distribution of benefits and risks.
      - *Distributive justice* is a principle that requires treatment of all persons equally and fairly.

11. *Virtue ethics and values*
    - *Virtue* is normally defined as some sort of moral excellence or beneficial quality. In traditional ethics, virtues are characteristics that differentiate good people from bad people.
    - *Virtue ethics* focuses on the inherent character of a person rather than on the specific actions he or she performs.
    - *Value* is something that has worth. Values are used for judging the goodness or badness of some action.
      - *Ethical values* imply standards of worth.
      - *Intrinsic value* is something that has value in and of itself.
      - *Instrumental value* is something that helps to give value to something else (e.g., money is valuable for what it can buy).
      - Values may change as needs change.

12. *Religious ethics* serves a moral purpose by providing codes of conduct for appropriate behavior through revelations from a divine source.

13. *Secular ethics* is based on codes developed by societies that have relied on customs to formulate their codes.

14. *Situational ethics* describes how a particular situation may influence how one's reaction and values may change in order to cope with changing circumstances.

15. The acceptance, understanding, and application of the ethical and moral concepts learned in this chapter will provide a *Moral Compass* to guide the reader through life's journey.

TEST YOUR UNDERSTANDING

TERMINOLOGY

applied ethics
autonomy
beneficence
bioethics
code of ethics
commitment
compassion
conscientiousness
consequential theory
cooperation
courage
deontological ethics
descriptive ethics
detachment
distributive justice
discernment
employment-related
   paternalism
ethical principles

ethical relativism
ethical theories
ethics
fairness
fidelity
freedom
honesty
hopefulness
instrumental value
integrity
intrinsic value
justice
kindness
macroethics
medical paternalism
metaethics
microethics
moral dilemmas
moral judgments

morality
moral values
nonconsequential ethics
nonmaleficence
normative ethics
paternalism
religious ethics
respect
secular ethics
situational ethics
spirituality
tolerance
truth telling
values
veracity
virtue ethics
virtues

REVIEW QUESTIONS

1. What is ethics?

2. Why should one study ethics?

3. What is morality?

4. Describe the ethical theories presented in this chapter.

5. What is ethical relativism? What is the relevance of this concept to individuals of various cultures living in the same society?

6. Describe the various ethical principles reviewed and how they might be helpful in resolving health care ethical dilemmas.

7. Describe virtue ethics and values. How do virtues and values differ?

8. Discuss why "courage" could be considered as the greatest of all virtues.

9. Discuss how religion can affect one's character.

10. Describe the principle of justice and how it can affect the decision-making process.

11. Explain how you would allocate scarce resources in the provision of health care?

12. What is "situational ethics"? Why do people behave differently in different situations?

NOTES

1. http://www.bukisa.com/articles/15091_the-root-of-ethics-and-morality.
2. Ayer, A. J., 1946. "A Critique of Ethics," in *Language, Truth and Logic*, London: Gollanz, pp. 102–114.
3. http://public.health.oregon.gov/ProviderPartnerResources/EvaluationResearch/DeathwithDignityAct/Pages/index.aspx.
4. http://www.ethicsmorals.com/ethicsapplied.html.
5. http://smallbusiness.chron.com/workplace-example-duty-based-ethics-11972.html
6. 105 N.E. 92, 93 (N.Y. 1914).
7. http://www.ama-assn.org/ama/pub/physician-resources/medical-ethics/code-medical-ethics/principles-medical-ethics.page
8. http://www.healthlawyers.org/Members/PracticeGroups/PALS/emailalerts/Documents/131111_Surveyand-CertLetter.pdf.
9. Craig Robert Senn, Fixing Inconsistent Paternalism Under Federal Employment Discrimination Law 58 UCLA L. Rev. 947. http://uclalawreview.org/?p=1679.
10. 464 A.2d 303, 314 (N.J. Super. Ct. App. Div. 1983).
11. http://www.mercurynews.com/san-mateo-county-times/ci_23948856/peninsula-child-psychiatrist-william-ayres-sentenced-eight-years?source=rss&cid=dlvr.it.
12. http://www.bukisa.com/articles/15091_the-root-of-ethics-and-morality.
13. http://www.gallup.com/poll/7288/Fear-Factor-Patient-Satisfaction.aspx.
14. http://shine.yahoo.com/healthy-living/brooke-greenberg-20-old-8220-toddler-8217-8221-185100345.html.
15. Tracey R. Rich, "Halakhah: Jewish Law," http://www.jewfaq.org/halakhah.htm (accessed October 13, 2010).
16. *Id.*
17. *Id.*

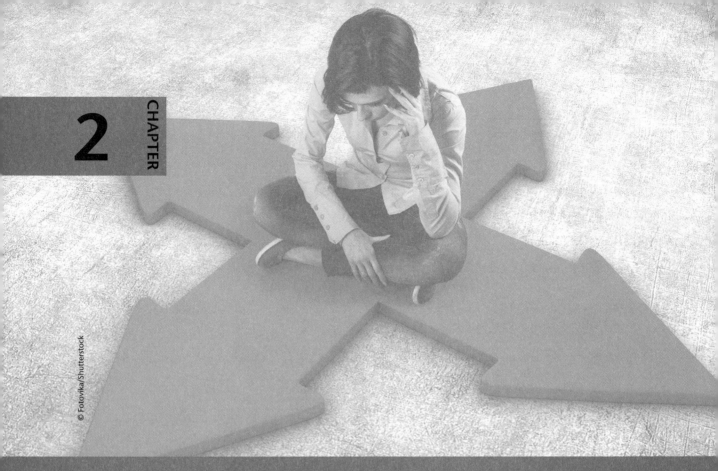

CHAPTER

2

© Fotovika/Shutterstock

CONTEMPORARY ETHICAL DILEMMAS

No right is held more sacred, or is more carefully guarded, by the common law, than the right of every individual to the possession and control of his own person, free from all restraint or interference of others, unless by clear and unquestioned authority of law.

—UNION PAC. RY. CO. V. BOTSFORD[1]

LEARNING OBJECTIVES

Upon completion of this chapter, the reader will be able to:

- Describe various historical events that have had an impact on the resolution of ethical dilemmas.

- Describe common ethical dilemmas and the various ethical issues that have in many instances divided many segments of the population. Topics include abortion; sterilization; artificial insemination; surrogacy; organ donations; research, experimentation, and clinical trials; human genetics, stem cell research; and, AIDS.

INTRODUCTION

An *ethical dilemma* arises in situations where a choice must be made between unpleasant alternatives. It can occur whenever a choice involves giving up something good and suffering something bad, no matter what course of action is taken. Ethical dilemmas often require caregivers to make decisions that may break some ethical norm or contradict some ethical value. For example, should I choose life knowing that an unborn child will be born with severe disabilities, or should I choose abortion and thus prevent pain for both parent and child? Should I adhere to my spouse's wishes not to be placed on a respirator, or should I choose life over death, disregarding her wishes and right to self-determination? Should I encourage my daughter—the victim of a gang rape—to have an abortion or should I choose life and "do no harm" to the unborn child? Such dilemmas give rise to conflicting answers.

There is a wide range of ethical and legal issues impacting the health care system. This chapter focuses on some of the more common ethical and legal dilemmas facing the providers of health care. In reviewing this chapter, the reader should apply court decisions and the ethical theories, principles, and values previously discussed.

NOTEWORTHY HISTORICAL EVENTS

I was created at the end of the Renaissance, watched pirates rule the oceans as Ivan the Terrible ruled Russia, and witnessed the arrest of Galileo for believing the earth revolved around the sun.

—I AM HISTORY

The historical events presented in this section describe some of the many milestones that have had a significant impact on health care ethics.

58,000–68,000 BC

Neanderthal Burial Sites

Evidence of belief in an afterlife was found in Neanderthal burial sites, where various implements and supplies were buried with the deceased.

> According to anthropologist F. Clark Howell the flexed position of the body, and discoveries of other sites where stone slabs were placed over the Neanderthal graves, along with food and tools, suggests that Neanderthal man believed in life after death. Their concept of the afterlife must not have been that much different than the life they experienced on earth; they provided the dead with food, tools, and other everyday items, much like the Egyptians did for their journey to the next life.[2]

1932–1972

Tuskegee Study of Syphilis

The Tuskegee Study of Syphilis, involving African American men, was designed to analyze the natural progression of untreated syphilis. The study was conducted from 1932 through the early 1970s. The participants were not told during the study that there was a cure for syphilis (e.g., penicillin). They believed that they were receiving adequate care and unknowingly suffered unnecessarily. The Tuskegee syphilis study used disadvantaged, rural black men to investigate the untreated course of a disease, one that is by no means confined to that population. We know now that the selection of research subjects must be closely monitored to ensure that specific classes of individuals (e.g., terminally ill patients, welfare patients, racial and ethnic minorities, or persons confined to institutions) are not selected for research studies because of their easy availability, compromised position, or manipulability. Rather, they must be selected for reasons directly related to the research being conducted.

1933–1945

The Holocaust

The Holocaust was one of the most violent events in human history. Over 6 million Jews were murdered as well as millions of people from other cultural groups, including Slavs, homosexuals, and Gypsies.

> Doctors have always been thought of as the saviors of mankind, the healers, and caretakers of our utter existence. Even ancient civilizations revered the medicine men as having special power to protect life. The trust of a physician is sacred. This is why the practice of medicine by the doctors of the Third Reich is egregious, outrageous, and shocking. The Nazi doctors violated the trust placed in them by humanity. The most painful truth is for the most part the doctors escaped their crimes against Humanity and lived a life, unlike their victims.[3]

1946

Military Tribunal for War Crimes

In 1946, the Military Tribunal for War Crimes began criminal proceedings against 23 German physicians and administrators for war crimes and crimes against humanity. As a direct result of these proceedings, the Nuremberg Code was established, which made it clear that the voluntary and informed consent of human subjects is essential to research and that benefits of research must outweigh risks to human subjects involved.[4]

1949

WMA International Code of Medical Ethics

The World Medical Association International Code of Medical Ethics was adopted in October 1949 after it was learned that the Nazis conducted numerous inhumane experiments on prisoners in concentration camps. Prisoners were exposed to cholera, diphtheria, malaria, mustard gas, yellow fever, and typhus and forced to participate in other horrendous experiments, ultimately claiming thousands of lives. This exploitation of unwilling prisoners as research subjects was condemned as a particularly flagrant injustice. The code was amended at the 57th WMA General Assembly, Pilanesberg, South Africa, October 2006.[5]

1954

Guidelines on Human Experimentation

The National Institutes of Health published guidelines on human experimentation following the first kidney transplant[6] conducted in 1954. The transplantation of human organs has generated numerous ethical issues (e.g., the harvesting and selling of organs, who should have first access to freely donated human organs, how death is defined).

1960s

Cardiopulmonary Resuscitation Raises Ethical Dilemmas

Cardiopulmonary resuscitation was developed, leading to numerous ongoing ethical dilemmas because it involves the prolonging of life beyond what would reasonably be expected. Should limited resources, for example, be spent on those who have been determined to be in a comatose vegetative state without hope of recovery? Or, should limited resources be spent on preventative medicine, aimed at improving the quality of life?

1964

WHO Guidelines for Conducting Biomedical Research

The World Medical Association[7] established guidelines for medical doctors conducting biomedical research involving human subjects. The Declaration of Helsinki is the basis for advanced clinical practices today.[8]

1968

Harvard Ad Hoc Committee on Brain Death

The Harvard Ad Hoc Committee on Brain Death published the following criteria to aid in determining a permanently nonfunctioning brain, a condition it referred to as "irreversible coma," now known as brain death:

1. Patient shows total unawareness to external stimuli and unresponsiveness to painful stimuli.
2. No movements or breathing: All spontaneous muscular movement, spontaneous respiration, and response to stimuli are absent.
3. No reflexes: Fixed, dilated pupils; no eye movement even when hit or turned, or when ice water is placed in the ear; no response to noxious stimuli; no tendon reflexes.

In addition to these criteria, the report recommended adding the presence of a flat electroencephalogram.[9]

1970

Patient as a Person

The Patient as a Person by Paul Ramsey discusses the question of *paternalism*. As physicians are faced with many options for saving lives, transplanting organs, and furthering research, they also must wrestle with new and troubling choices, for example, who should receive scarce resources (e.g.., organ transplants), how to determine when life ends, and what limits should be placed on care for the dying.

1971

Kennedy Institute of Ethics

The Joseph P. and Rose F. Kennedy Institute of Ethics was established at Georgetown University in 1971 by a generous grant from the Joseph P. Kennedy, Jr., Foundation. Today it is the world's oldest and most comprehensive academic bioethics center. The institute and its library serve as an unequaled resource for those who research and study ethics, as well as those who debate and make public policy. The Kennedy Institute is home to scholars who engage in research, teaching, and public service on issues that include protection of research subjects, reproductive and feminist bioethics, end-of-life care, health care justice, intellectual disability, cloning, gene therapy, eugenics, and other major bioethical issues. Institute scholars figure prominently among the pioneers of the discipline. They are extending the boundaries of the field to incorporate emerging issues of racial and gender equality, international justice and peace, and other policies affecting the world's most vulnerable populations.[10]

1972

Informed Consent

Informed consent in the *Canterbury v. Spence*[11] case set the *reasonable man standard*, requiring informed consent for treatment. Patients must be informed of the risks, benefits, and alternatives associated with recommended treatments. The court found that Dr. Spence negligently failed to disclose a risk of serious disability inherent in the operation and that the Washington Hospital Center provided negligent postoperative care.[12]

1973

Women's Right to Abortion

The *Roe v. Wade*[13] abortion case gave strength to a woman's right to privacy in the context of matters relating to her own body, including how a pregnancy would end.

1974

National Research Act (NRA) of 1974

Because of publicity from the Tuskegee Syphilis Study, the National Research Act (NRA) of 1974 was passed. The NRA created the National Commission for the Protection of Human Subjects of Biomedical and Behavioral Research. One of the commission's charges was to identify the basic ethical principles that should underlie the conduct of biomedical and behavioral research involving human subjects and to develop guidelines to ensure that such research is conducted in accordance with those principles.[14]

The commission was directed to consider the following:[15]

1. The boundaries between biomedical and behavioral research and the accepted and routine practice of medicine
2. The role of assessment of risk-benefit criteria in determining the appropriateness of research involving human subjects
3. Appropriate guidelines for the selection of human subjects for participation in such research
4. The nature and definition of informed consent in various research settings

1976

Substitute Judgment—Karen Ann Quinlan

The New Jersey Supreme Court in the *Matter of Karen Ann Quinlan*[16] rendered a unanimous decision providing for the appointment of Joseph Quinlan as personal guardian of his daughter, Karen Ann Quinlan. The record was remanded to the trial court to implement without further testimonial hearing:

> To appoint Joseph Quinlan as guardian of the person of Karen Quinlan with full power to make decisions with regard to the identity of her treating physicians.
>
> We repeat for the sake of emphasis and clarity that upon the concurrence of the guardian and family of Karen, should the responsible attending physicians conclude that there is no reasonable possibility of Karen's ever emerging from her present comatose condition to a cognitive, sapient state and that the life-support apparatus now being administered to Karen should be discontinued, they shall consult with the hospital "Ethics Committee" or like body of the institution in which Karen is then hospitalized. If that consultative body agrees that there is no reasonable possibility of Karen's ever emerging from her present comatose condition to a cognitive, sapient state, the present life-support system may be withdrawn and said action shall be without any civil or criminal liability therefor, on the part of any participant, whether guardian, physician, hospital or others.
>
> By the above ruling we do not intend to be understood as implying that a proceeding for judicial declaratory relief is necessarily required for the implementation of comparable decisions in the field of medical practice.

First Living Will Legislation Enacted

In California, the first living will legislation was enacted, permitting a person to sign a declaration stating that if there is no hope of recovery, no heroic measures need to be taken to prolong life. This provision is now available in every state.

1978

Commission for the Study of Ethical Problems

The President's Commission for the Study of Ethical Problems in Medicine includes studies regarding the ethical and legal issues of informed consent for research participants;

the matter of defining death, including the advisability of developing a uniform definition of death; the voluntary testing, counseling, and information and education programs with respect to genetic diseases and conditions, taking into account the essential equality of all human beings, born and unborn; the differences in the availability of health services, as determined by the income or residence of the persons receiving the services; current procedures and mechanisms designed to safeguard the privacy of human subjects of behavioral and biomedical research, to ensure the confidentiality of individually identifiable patient records and to ensure appropriate access of patients to information; and such other matters relating to medicine or biomedical or behavioral research as the president may designate for study by the commission.[17]

1980

Hemlock Society

The Hemlock Society was an organization formed to advocate for physician-assisted dying for the terminally ill, mentally competent patient suffering with incurable illnesses.

> Controversial in death as in life, the Hemlock Society USA as a name died suddenly on June 13, 2003, in a boardroom in Denver, Colorado. It was 23 years old. Public relations experts and political strategists—leaning heavily on focus groups—were on hand to usher in the death knell. Months of agonizing debate had preceded the decision because no one could think of a better name![18]

1983

First Durable Power of Attorney Legislation

California enacted the first durable power of attorney legislation permitting an advance directive to be made describing the kind of health care that one would desire when facing death by designating an agent to act on the patient's behalf. Currently the California Health Care Directive form in part reads:

> You have the right to give instructions about your own health care. You also have the right to name someone else to make health care decisions for you. This form lets you do either or both of these things. It also lets you express your wishes regarding donation of organs and the designation of your primary physician. If you use this form, you may complete or modify all or any part of it. You are free to use a different form. [CALIFORNIA PROBATE CODE SECTION 4700-4701][19]

Compassion and Choices

The Hemlock Society evolved into "End-of-Life Choices, which in 2005 merged with Compassion in Dying to form Compassion & Choices."[20]

> Compassion & Choices is the leading nonprofit organization committed to helping everyone have the best death possible. We offer free counseling, planning resources, referrals and guidance, and across the nation we work to protect and expand options at the end of life.

For over thirty years we have reduced people's suffering and given them some control in their final days—even when injury or illness takes their voice. We are experts in what it takes to die well.[21]

1990

Patient Self-Determination Act

The Patient Self-Determination Act of 1990[22] was enacted to ensure that patients are informed of their rights to execute advance directives and accept or refuse medical care. The act was intended to reinforce a person's constitutional right to make his or her own health care decisions. The act requires that federally funded health care organizations explain to patients their right to complete an advance directive.

Nancy Cruzan Feeding Tube Removed

The Supreme Court ruled that the parents of Nancy Cruzan, a 32-year old woman who had been unconscious since a 1983 car accident, could have her feeding tube removed.[23] The court determined the Missouri Department of Health was permitted to require clear and convincing evidence of the wishes of a patient regarding provision of artificial nutrition and hydration.[24] Thus affirming the right of Americans to refuse unwanted medical treatment and their right to appoint a healthcare proxy.

Kevorkian Illegally Assists Terminally Ill Patients in Suicide

Dr. Jack Kevorkian assisted terminally ill patients in suicide outside the boundaries of law. He used a suicide machine to assist Janet Adkins, a 54-year-old woman with Alzheimer's disease, in ending her life at her request.

Timothy Quill and Prescription for Death

Timothy Quill, a primary care physician, published an article describing how he had prescribed a lethal dose of sedatives to end the life of a young woman whose suffering from leukemia had become unbearable.

Final Exit and Freedom of Speech

Derek Humphry's popular text, *Final Exit: The Practicalities of Self-Deliverance and Assisted Suicide for the Dying,* was published. Although there were calls for it to be banned, it was not possible under the First Amendment to the U.S. Constitution.

Congress shall make no law respecting an establishment of religion, or prohibiting the free exercise thereof; or abridging the freedom of speech, or of the press; or the right of the people peaceably to assemble, and to petition the Government for a redress of grievances.[25]

1993

Patient's Wishes Honored

In the case of *DeGrella v. Elston,* the Kentucky Supreme Court ruled on an incompetent's right to die. The decision determined that a patient's wishes will be honored if the attending physician, the hospital, or nursing home ethics committee where a patient resides and the legal guardian or next of kin all agree upon and document the patient's wishes and the patient's condition. If no one disputes their decision, no court order is required to proceed to carry out the patient's wishes. Future criminal sanctions or civil liability turn not on the existence or absence of a court order, but on the facts of the case. No liability attaches to a decision to refuse or withdraw treatment if the necessary facts are established and carefully documented by the parties involved. In contrast, the court cannot absolve the parties from liability where the facts do not exist to support the action taken.[26]

1994

Oregon—Physician Assisted Suicide Legal

Oregon's Death with Dignity Act, involving physician-assisted suicide, became a legal medical option for terminally ill patients in Oregon. The Oregon Death with Dignity Act allows terminally ill Oregon residents to obtain from their physicians and use prescriptions for self-administered, lethal medications.

Michigan—Physician Assisted Suicide Illegal

The Supreme Court of Michigan ruled on December 13, 1994, that assisted suicide is illegal in the state of Michigan. The ruling overturned several lower court decisions. The court determined that there is no constitutional right to aid in carrying out a suicide in Michigan. Jack Kevorkian, a physician, assisted terminally ill patients in suicide outside the boundaries of the law. He claims to have assisted 130 patients.

1996

Health Insurance Portability and Accountability Act

The Health Insurance Portability and Accountability Act (Public Law 104191) was enacted to protect the privacy, confidentiality, and security of patient information.

Dolly the Sheep Cloned

Ian Wilmut Keith Campbell and colleagues at the Roslin Institute, University of Edinburgh and the biotechnology company PPL Therapeutics near Edinburgh in Scotland successfully cloned Dolly, the Sheep.

> Several clones had been produced in the lab before Dolly, including frogs, mice, and cows, which had all been cloned from the DNA from embryos. Dolly was remarkable in being the first mammal to be cloned from an adult cell. This was a major scientific achievement as it demonstrated that the DNA from adult cells, despite having specialised as one particular type of cell, can be used to create an entire organism.[27]

Fourteenth Amendment and Terminally Ill

The Second and Ninth U.S. Circuit Courts of Appeals ruled that there is a constitutional right under the Fourteenth Amendment for a terminally ill person to receive help from a physician when dying.

1997

Physician-Assisted Suicide

Physician-assisted suicide, through referendum, became a legal medical option within narrowly prescribed circumstances for terminally ill Oregon residents.

Kevorkian Charged with Murder

Kevorkian was charged with murder in five cases of physician-assisted suicide and was acquitted.

Supreme Court—States May Enact Assisted Suicide Laws

The Supreme Court ruled that it is up to the individual states to enact laws regarding medically assisted death.

1998

Oregon Voters Reaffirm Death with Dignity Act

Oregon voters reaffirm their support for the Death with Dignity Act by a 60% majority.

Kevorkian Administers Lethal Injection

Kevorkian administered a lethal injection to Thomas Youk, a 52-year-old man with Lou Gehrig's disease, on national television.

Ballot Physician-Assisted Suicide Defeated

Michigan voters defeated a ballot measure that would legalize physician-assisted suicide.

1999

Kevorkian Convicted of Second-Degree Murder

Kevorkian was convicted of second-degree murder for Youk's death and sentenced 10 to 20 years in prison.

Patients Receive Lethal Doses of Medication

Twenty-three terminally ill patients were reported as having received lethal doses of medication since passage of Oregon's Death with Dignity Act.

2000

Seven Myths About End-of-Life Care

Legal myths about end-of-life care may prevent doctors and patients and families from providing adequate comfort measures to dying patients, according to an article published in the November 15 issue of the *Journal of the American Medical Association* (AMA).[28]

2001

President's Council on Bioethics

President George W. Bush created the President's Council on Bioethics. The council was charged with advising the president on bioethical issues that may emerge as a consequence of advances in biomedical science and technology.

Assisted Suicide Act Challenged

U.S. Attorney General John Ashcroft abrogated former Attorney General Janet Reno's mandate allowing physician-assisted suicide. Instead, he decided that physician-assisted suicide was a violation of the federal Controlled Substance Act. In *State of Oregon v. Ashcroft*, CV01-1647 (D-Oregon), the judge allowed Oregon's law to remain in effect.

Oregon—Assisted Suicide Cases

Since 1991, the total number of physician-assisted suicide cases totaled 129. On April 17, U.S. District Court Judge Robert Jones upheld Oregon's Death with Dignity Act.

2002

Attorney General Appeals District Court's Ruling

Attorney General John Ashcroft filed an appeal, asking the Ninth U.S. Circuit Court of Appeals to lift the District Court's ruling.

2003

Human Genome System Fully Sequenced

The human genome system became fully sequenced, allowing molecular genetics and medical research to accelerate at an unprecedented rate. The ethical implications of human genome research are as immense as the undertaking of the totality of the research that was conducted to map the human genome system (e.g., cloning of humans).[29]

Oregon—Assisted Suicide Cases

Forty-two residents of the State of Oregon ingested medications under provisions of the Death with Dignity Act.

2004

Death with Dignity Act Upheld

The U.S. Circuit Court of Appeals upheld Oregon's Death with Dignity Act, blocking the attempt by the U.S. Justice Department, under Attorney General Ashcroft, to use the federal Controlled Substances Act to prevent doctors in the state from prescribing drugs to assist the suicide of their patients. The Ashcroft directive interfered with Oregon's authority to regulate medical care within its borders and therefore altered the usual constitutional balance between state and the federal governments.[30]

2005

The United Nations Educational, Scientific, and Cultural Organization released the second edition to the 2005 *Human Cloning, Ethical Issues* publication.[31]

2006

U.S. Supreme Court Upholds Death with Dignity Act

On January 17, 2006, the U.S. Supreme Court voted six to three to uphold an Oregon physician-assisted suicide law in the case *Gonzales v. Oregon*,[32] ruling that former Attorney General John Ashcroft overstepped his authority in seeking to punish doctors who prescribed drugs to help terminally ill patients end their lives. In the decision, the Supreme Court said that the Oregon law supersedes federal authority to regulate physicians and that the Bush administration improperly attempted to use the Controlled Substances Act to prosecute Oregon physicians who assist in patient suicides.

Supreme Court Blocks Bush's Attempt to Punish Doctors

The Supreme Court blocks the Bush administration's attempt to punish doctors who help terminally ill patients die, protecting Oregon's one-of-a-kind assisted-suicide law.[33]

Morning-after Pill

The Food and Drug Administration approved the morning-after pill to prevent contraception for use without a prescription. This decision has added another dimension to the ongoing controversy between right-to-life and pro-choice advocates. Opponents claim that it is just another way to end human life.

2009

Right to Know End-of-Life Options

On January 1, the Terminal Patients' Right to Know End-of-Life Options Act, AB 2747, goes into effect in California.

2010

California—Living Donor Registry

Legislation was introduced in California that would make it the first state in the country to build a living donor registry. Under Senate Bill 1395, people could declare their wishes regarding organ donation by checking a box when obtaining or renewing their driver's license.

2013

Information and Referral Service for Kidney Donors

California launched a state-authorized information and referral service to inspire and inform people to be altruistic living kidney donors. Through its website, www.LivingDonationCalifornia.org, the free service provides information about living kidney donation and refers potentially eligible individuals for evaluation at a transplant center.[34]

NEWS

Vermont Set to Become Third U.S. State to Allow Assisted Suicide

Vermont is poised to become the third U.S. state to allow doctor-assisted suicide, after its legislature passed a bill allowing physicians to prescribe lethal drugs to terminally ill patients.

The bill passed late on Monday, and the governor has pledged to sign it into law.

Oregon and Washington state have legalized doctor-assisted suicide in voter referendums.

Scott Malone, Reuters, *May 14, 2013*

ABORTION

We shall have to fight the politician, who remembers only that the unborn have no votes and that since posterity has done nothing for us we need do nothing for posterity.
—William Ralph Inge (1860–1954)[35]

An *abortion* is the termination of pregnancy by removal or expulsion from the uterus of a fetus or embryo before it is viable. The question of viability has been strongly debated between pro-life (the right to life) and pro-choice (the right to choose) advocates. An abortion can be a spontaneous abortion, often referred to as a miscarriage, or it can be an elective abortion, meaning purposely induced, which continues to be a hotly debated controversial issue nationwide. The controversy in its simplest form involves the question of the rights of the fetus to be born and the rights of the mother to make decisions regarding her body.

A consensus as to when life begins has not been reached. There has been no final determination as to the proper interplay among a mother's liberty, the interests of an unborn child, and the state's interests in protecting life. In abortion cases, the law presupposes a theory of ethics and morality, which in turn presupposes deeply personal ideas about being and existence. Answers to such questions as when life begins define ethical beliefs, and these ethical beliefs should determine how we govern ourselves. Abortion in this context is less a question about constitutional law and more about who we are as a people. This is a decision the Supreme Court cannot make. Taking these issues out of the public discourse threatens to foment hostility, stifle the search for answers, distance people from the Constitution, and undermine the credibility of that document.[36]

With more than 1 million abortions performed annually in the United States, it is certain that the conflict between pro-choice and pro-life advocates will continue to pervade America's landscape. The issues are numerous and emotions run high. Common ethical dilemmas include:

- When does life begin?
- Who decides?
- Who protects the unborn fetus?
- What are the rights of the child or woman who has been raped?
- What are the rights of the spouse?
- What are the rights of the father of an unwed child or woman?
- What are the rights of society and the state to interfere with another's rights?
- Should the principles of autonomy and right to self-determination prevail?
- Should an abortion be considered murder?
- Can the use of contraception be considered a form of killing by preventing a birth that might have otherwise occurred?
- What are the religious implications of a woman who is Catholic, for example, who chooses to undergo an abortion?
- Is it morally acceptable to save the life of the mother by aborting the fetus?
- Is an abortion for mere convenience morally wrong?
- What role should education play in the woman's decision to undergo an abortion?
- What alternatives should the woman be educated about (e.g., the choice of adoption) before undergoing an abortion?
- At what age should the decision to abort be that of the mother?
- Should the feelings of guilt that may accompany an abortion and how those feelings may haunt the mother through the years be explained?
- Should the feelings that might occur after giving birth be explained to the victim of a rape (e.g., anger and resentment)?
- When does control over one's body begin, and when does it end?

These are but a few of the many questions that need to be addressed in the pursuit of doing the right thing. As the following pages point out, for each new issue decided in the courts, numerous new issues arise, all of which seem to involve both legal and moral questions as to what is acceptable behavior. In addition to having substantial ethical, moral, and religious implications, abortion has proven to be a major political issue and will continue as such in the future. As the following court decisions illustrate, new laws will be enacted by the various states and challenged, often winding their way up to the Supreme Court for decision.

Right to Abortion

The *Roe v. Wade* 1973 landmark case gave strength to a woman's right to privacy in the context of matters relating to her own body, including how a pregnancy would end.[37] The U.S. Supreme Court has also recognized the interest of the states in protecting potential life and has attempted to spell out the extent to which the states may regulate and even prohibit abortions. The Supreme Court in this case found the Texas penal abortion law unconstitutional, stating, "State criminal abortion statutes . . . that except from criminality only a lifesaving procedure on behalf of the mother, without regard to the stage of her pregnancy and other interests involved, is violating the Due Process Clause of the Fourteenth Amendment."[38] The court then went on to delineate what regulatory measures a state lawfully may enact during the three stages of pregnancy.

First Trimester

During the first trimester of pregnancy, the decision to undergo an abortion procedure is between the woman and her physician. A state may require that abortions be performed by a licensed physician pursuant to law; however, a woman's right to an abortion is not unqualified because the decision to perform the procedure must be left to the medical judgment of her attending physician. "For the stage prior to approximately the end of the first trimester, the abortion decision and its effectuation must be left to the medical judgment of the pregnant woman's attending physician."[39]

Second Trimester

In *Roe v. Wade*, the Supreme Court stated, "For the stage subsequent to approximately the end of the first trimester, the State, in promoting its interest in the health of the mother, may, if it chooses, regulate the abortion procedure in ways that are reasonably related to maternal health."[40] Thus, during approximately the fourth to sixth months of pregnancy, the state may regulate the medical conditions under which the procedure is performed. The constitutional test of any legislation concerning abortion during this period would be its relevance to the objective of protecting maternal health.

Third Trimester

The Supreme Court reasoned that by the time the final stage of pregnancy has been reached the state has acquired a compelling interest in the product of conception, which would override the woman's right to privacy and justify stringent regulation even to the extent of prohibiting abortions. In the *Roe v. Wade* case, the court formulated its ruling as to the last trimester in the following words: "For the stage subsequent to viability, the State in promoting its interest in the potentiality of human life, may, if it chooses, regulate, and even proscribe, abortion except where it is necessary, in appropriate medical judgment, for the preservation of the life or health of the mother."[41]

Thus, during the final stage of pregnancy, a state may prohibit all abortions except those deemed necessary to protect maternal life or health. The state's legislative powers over the performance of abortions increase as the pregnancy progresses toward term.

ABORTION RESTRICTIONS UNCONSTITUTIONAL

Abortion Committee Review

In a 1973 companion decision, the U.S. Supreme Court ruled in *Doe v. Bolton*,[42] that Georgia's abortion statute requiring residency requirements for women seeking an abortion and calling for the procedure to be performed in a hospital accredited by the Joint Commission is constitutionally invalid. Further, the court found there was no constitutionally justifiable rationale for a statutory requirement necessitating advance approval by the abortion committee of the hospital's medical staff prior to abortion. The court ruled that "interposition of the hospital abortion committee is unduly restrictive of the patient's rights and needs that . . . have already been medically delineated and substantiated by her personal physician. To ask more serves neither the hospital nor the State."[43] Insofar as statutory consultation requirements are concerned, the court reasoned that the acquiescence of two copractitioners has no rational connection with a patient's needs and, further, unduly infringes on the physician's right to practice.

Abortion Counseling

The U.S. Supreme Court in 1983 in *City of Akron v. Akron Center for Reproductive Health*[44] decided that the different states cannot (1) mandate what information physicians give abortion patients or (2) require that abortions for women more than 3 months pregnant be performed in a hospital. With respect to a requirement that the attending physician must inform the woman of specified information concerning her proposed abortion, it was found unreasonable for a state to insist that only a physician is competent to provide information and counseling relative to informed consent. A state may not adopt regulations to influence a woman's informed choice between abortion and childbirth.

With regard to a second-trimester hospital requirement, this could significantly limit a woman's ability to obtain an abortion. This is especially so in view of the evidence that a second-trimester abortion may cost more than twice as much in a hospital as in a clinic.

Undue Burden Rule

In *Planned Parenthood v. Casey*,[45] the U.S. Supreme Court ruling, as enunciated in *Roe v. Wade*, reaffirmed:

- The constitutional right of women to have an abortion before viability of the fetus, as first enunciated in *Roe v. Wade*
- The state's power to restrict abortions after fetal viability, so long as the law contains exceptions for pregnancies that endanger a woman's life or health
- The principle that the state has legitimate interests from the outset of the pregnancy in protecting the health of the woman and the life of the fetus

The U.S. Supreme Court rejected the trimester approach in *Roe v. Wade*, which limited the regulations states could issue on abortion depending on the development stage of the fetus. In place of the trimester approach, the court will evaluate the permissibility of state abortion rules based on whether they unduly burden a woman's ability to obtain an abortion. A rule is an *"undue burden"* if its purpose or effect is to place a substantial obstacle in the path of a woman seeking an abortion before the fetus attains viability. The Supreme Court ruled that it is "not an undue burden" to require that a woman be informed of the nature of the abortion procedure and the risks involved, be offered information on the fetus and alternatives to abortion, and be given informed consent before the abortion procedure. In addition, it is not an undue burden to require parental consent for a minor seeking an abortion, providing for a judicial bypass option if a minor does not wish to or cannot obtain parental consent, and requiring a 24-hour waiting period before any abortion can be performed.

FUNDING

Some states have placed an indirect restriction on abortion through the elimination of funding. Under the Hyde Amendment, the U.S. Congress, through appropriations legislation, has limited the types of medically necessary abortions for which federal funds may be spent under the Medicaid program. Although the Hyde Amendment does not prohibit states from funding nontherapeutic abortions, this action by the federal government opened the door to state statutory provisions limiting the funding of abortions.

Denial of Financial Assistance for Elective Abortions

In *Beal v. Doe*[46] in 1977, the Pennsylvania Medicaid plan was challenged based on denial of financial assistance for nontherapeutic abortions. The U.S. Supreme Court held that Title XIX of the Social Security Act (the Medicaid program) does not require the funding of nontherapeutic abortions as a condition of state participation in the program. The state has a strong interest in encouraging normal childbirth, and nothing in Title XIX suggests that it is unreasonable for the state to further that interest. The court ruled that it is not inconsistent with the Medicaid portion of the Social Security Act to refuse to fund unnecessary (although perhaps desirable) medical services.

In *Maher v. Roe*[47] in 1977, the U.S. Supreme Court considered the Connecticut statute that denied Medicaid benefits for first-trimester abortions that were not medically necessary. The court rejected the argument that the state's subsidy of medical expenses incident to pregnancy and childbirth created an obligation on the part of the state to subsidize the expenses incident to nontherapeutic abortions. The Supreme Court voted six to three that states may refuse to spend public funds to provide nontherapeutic abortions for women.

Funding Not Required for Therapeutic Abortions

The U.S. Supreme Court in 1980 in *Harris v. McRae*,[48] upheld in a five-to-four vote the Hyde Amendment, which restricts the use of federal funds for Medicaid abortions. Under this case, the different states are not compelled to fund Medicaid recipients' medically necessary abortions for which federal reimbursement is unavailable but may choose to do so.

Funding Bans Unconstitutional in California

The California Supreme Court in 1981 held that funding bans were unconstitutional; the court asked rhetorically:

> If the state cannot directly prohibit a woman's right to obtain an abortion, may the state by discriminatory financing indirectly nullify that constitutional right? Can the state tell an indigent person that the state will provide him with welfare benefits only

upon the condition that he join a designated political party or subscribe to a particular newspaper that is favored by the government? Can the state tell a poor woman that it will pay for her needed medical care but only if she gives up her constitutional right to choose whether or not to have a child?[49]

Funding Discrimination Prohibited in Arizona

The Arizona Supreme Court, in 2002 in *Simat Corp. v. Arizona Health Care Cost Containment Sys.*,[50] found that the state's constitution does not permit the state and the Arizona Health Care Cost Containment System (AHCCCS) to refuse to fund medically necessary abortion procedures for pregnant women suffering from serious illness while funding such procedures for victims of rape or incest or when the abortion was necessary to save the woman's life (A.R.S. § 35-196.02. AHCCCS). After the state has chosen to fund abortions for one group of indigent, pregnant women for whom abortions are medically necessary to save their lives, the state may not deny the same option to another group of women for whom the procedure is also medically necessary to save their health. An example is cancer, for which chemotherapy or radiation therapy ordinarily cannot be provided if the patient is pregnant, making an abortion necessary before proceeding with the recognized medical treatment. Other therapy regimens that must at times be suspended during pregnancy include those for heart disease, diabetes, kidney disease, liver disease, chronic renal failure, inflammatory bowel disease, and lupus. In many of the women suffering from these diseases, suspension of recognized therapy during pregnancy will have serious and permanent adverse effects on their health and lessen their life span. In such a situation, the state is not simply influencing a woman's choice but is actually conferring the privilege of treatment on one class and withholding it from another.

A woman's right to choose preservation and protection of her health and, therefore, in many cases, her life is at least as compelling as the state's interest in promoting childbirth. The court's protection of the fetus and promotion of childbirth cannot be considered so compelling as to outweigh a woman's fundamental right to choose and the state's obligation to be evenhanded in the design and application of its health care policies. The majority of states that have examined similar Medicaid funding restrictions have determined that their state statutes or constitutions offer broader protection of individual rights than does the U.S. Constitution, and they have found that medically necessary abortions should be funded if the state also funds medically necessary expenses related to childbirth. The case was remanded to the trial court for further proceedings consistent with this opinion.

Refusal to Fund Abortion Counseling Not Unconstitutional

Federal regulations that prohibit abortion counseling and referral by family planning clinics that receive funds under Title X of the Public Health Service Act were found not to violate the constitutional rights of pregnant women or Title X grantees in a five-to-four decision by the Supreme Court in *Rust v. Sullivan*.[51] Proponents of abortion counseling argued (1) that the regulations impermissibly burden a woman's privacy right to abortion and (2) that by prohibiting the delivery of abortion information, even as to where such information could be obtained, the regulations deny a woman her constitutionally protected right to choose under the First Amendment. The question arises: How can a woman make an informed choice between two options when she cannot obtain information as to one of them? The plaintiff had argued that the government may not condition receipt of a benefit on the relinquishment of constitutional rights. In *Sullivan*, however, the Supreme Court found that there was no violation of a woman's or provider's First Amendment rights to freedom of speech. The court extended the doctrine that government need not subsidize the exercise of the fundamental rights to free speech.

SPOUSAL CONSENT

Husband's Interest Insufficient

Provisions of the Florida Therapeutic Abortion Act, which required a married woman to obtain the husband's consent before abortion, were found to be unconstitutional in *Poe v. Gerstein*.[52] The state's interest was found not to be sufficiently compelling to limit a woman's right to abortion. The husband's interest in the baby was held to be insufficient to force his wife to face the mental and physical risks of pregnancy and childbirth.

Husband's Required Consent Unconstitutional

In *Doe v. Zimmerman* (1975),[53] the court declared unconstitutional the provisions of the Pennsylvania Abortion Control Act, which required that the written consent of the husband of a married woman be secured before performing an abortion. The court found that these provisions impermissibly permitted the husband to withhold his consent either because of his interest in the potential life of the fetus or for capricious reasons. The natural father of an unborn fetus in *Doe v. Smith* (1988)[54] was not entitled to an injunction to prevent the mother from submitting to an abortion. Although the father's interest in the fetus was legitimate, it did not outweigh the mother's constitutionally protected right to an abortion, particularly in light of evidence that the mother and father had never married.

In the 1992 decision of *Planned Parenthood v. Casey*, the Supreme Court ruled that spousal consent would be an undue burden on the woman.

PARENTAL CONSENT

Competent Persons Under 18

The U.S. Supreme Court ruled in 1973 in *Danforth v. Planned Parenthood*[55] that it is unconstitutional to require all women younger than the age of 18 years to obtain parental consent in writing prior to obtaining an abortion. The court, however, failed to provide any definitive guidelines as to when and how parental consent may be required if the minor is too immature to comprehend fully the nature of the procedure.

The U.S. Supreme Court in 1979 in *Bellotti v. Baird*[56] ruled eight to one that a Massachusetts statute requiring parental consent before an abortion could be performed on an unmarried woman younger than the age of 18 years was unconstitutional. Justice John P. Stevens, joined by Justices William J. Brennan, Jr., Thurgood Marshall, and Harry Blackmun, concluded that the Massachusetts statute was unconstitutional because under that statute as written and construed by the Massachusetts Supreme Judicial Court, no minor, no matter how mature and capable of informed decision making, could receive an abortion without the consent of either both parents or a superior court judge, thus making the minor's abortion subject in every instance to an absolute third-party veto.

Incompetent Persons

Abortion was found to be proper by a family court in *In re Doe* (1987)[57] for a profoundly retarded woman. She had become pregnant during her residence in a group home as a result of a sexual attack by an unknown person. The record had supported a finding that if the woman had been able to do so she would have requested the abortion. The court properly chose welfare agencies and the woman's guardian ad litem (a guardian appointed to prosecute or defend a suit on behalf of a party incapacitated by infancy, mental incompetence, etc.) as the surrogate decision makers.

Parental Notification Permitted

The U.S. Supreme Court in 1981 in *H. L. v. Matheson*,[58] by a six-to-three vote, upheld a Utah statute that required a physician to "notify, if possible" the parents or guardian of a minor on whom an abortion is to be performed. In this case, the physician advised the patient that an abortion would be in her best medical interest but, because of the statute, refused to perform the abortion without notifying her parents. The Supreme Court ruled that although a state may not constitutionally legislate a blanket, unreviewable power of parents to veto their daughter's abortion, a statute setting out a mere requirement of parental notice when possible does not violate the constitutional rights of an immature, dependent minor.

Emancipated Minor

The trial court in 1987 *In re Anonymous*[59] was found to have abused its discretion when it refused a minor's request for waiver of parental consent to obtain an abortion. The record indicated that the minor lived alone, was within 1 month of her 18th birthday, lived by herself most of the time, and was employed full time.

Parental Notification Not Required

The issue in 2000 in *Planned Parenthood v. Owens*[60] was whether the Colorado Parental Notification Act (Colorado Revised Statute §§ 12-37.5-101, et seq. [1998]), which requires a physician to notify the parents of a minor prior to performing an abortion upon her, violates the minor's rights protected by the U.S. Constitution. The act, a citizen-initiated measure, was approved at Colorado's general election. The act generally prohibits physicians from performing abortions on an unemancipated minor until at least 48 hours after written notice has been delivered to the minor's parent, guardian, or foster parent.

The U.S. District Court decided that the act violated the rights of minor women protected by the Fourteenth Amendment. The Supreme Court, for more than a quarter of a century, has required that any abortion regulation except from its reach an abortion medically necessary for the preservation of the mother's health. The act fails to provide such a health exception.

INFORMED CONSENT

The Fifth U.S. Circuit Court of Appeals determined that a Texas law requiring a pregnant mother to undergo an ultrasound prior abortion is constitutional. Although a pregnant woman cannot be compelled to view the ultrasound image, the physician is required to describe what the image shows. The pregnant woman, however, has a concomitant right to refuse to listen to any detailed explanation. Chapter 171 of the Texas Health and Safety Code requires the following as prerequisites for a woman's informed and voluntary consent to an abortion:

> (1) the physician who is to perform the abortion, or a certified sonographer agent thereof, must perform a sonogram on the pregnant woman;

> (2) the physician must display the sonogram images "in a quality consistent with current medical practice" such that the pregnant woman may view them;

> (3) the physician must provide, "in a manner understandable to a layperson," a verbal explanation of the results of the sonogram images, including a variety of detailed descriptions of the fetus or embryo; and

> (4) the physician or certified sonographer agent must "make . . . audible the heart auscultation for the pregnant woman to hear, if present, in a quality consistent with current medical practice and provide . . . , in a manner understandable to a layperson, a simultaneous verbal explanation of the heart auscultation," H.B. 15, Sec. 2 (amending TEX. HEALTH & SAFETY CODE ANN. Ann. § 171.012).

STATES MAY PROTECT FETUS

The U.S. Supreme Court in 1979 in *Colautti v. Franklin*[61] voted six to three that states can seek to protect a fetus that a physician has determined could survive outside the womb. Determination of whether a particular fetus is viable is, and must be, a matter for judgment of the responsible attending physician. State abortion regulations that impinge on this determination, if they are to be constitutional, must allow the attending physician the room that he or she needs to make the best medical judgment.

ABORTION RIGHTS NARROWED

Webster v. Reproductive Health Services[62] began the U.S. Supreme Court's narrowing of abortion rights by upholding a Missouri statute providing that no public facilities or employees should be used to perform abortions and physicians should conduct viability tests before performing abortions.

PARTIAL BIRTH ABORTION

The Supreme Court in 1998 in *Women's Medical Professional Corp. v. Voinovich*[63] involved an Ohio statute that banned the use of the intact dilation and extraction (D&X) procedure in the performance of any previability or postviability abortion. The Sixth Circuit Court of Appeals held that the statute banning any use of the D&X procedure was unconstitutionally vague. It is likely that a properly drafted statute will eventually be judged constitutionally sound.

Partial Birth Abortion Ban Struck Down

On June 28, 2002, the U.S. Supreme Court struck down a Nebraska ban on "partial-birth abortion," finding it an unconstitutional violation of *Roe v. Wade*. The court found these types of bans to be extreme descriptive attempts to outlaw abortion—even early in pregnancy—that jeopardizes women's health [192 F.3d 1142 (8th Cir. 1999), 120 S. Ct. 2597 (2000)].

Partial Birth Abortion Ban Made Law

President Bush, on November 6, 2003, signed the first federal restrictions banning late-term partial-birth abortions. (The *partial birth abortion,* also referred to as the D&X procedure, is a late-term abortion involving partial delivery of the baby before its being aborted.) Both houses of Congress passed the ban. The ban permits no exceptions when a woman's health is at risk or the fetus has life-threatening disabilities. A U.S. District Court in Nebraska issued a restraining order on the ban.

Partial-Birth Abortion Ban Unconstitutional

The Partial-Birth Abortion Ban Act, 18 U.S.C. Section 1531, in *National Abortion Fed'n v. Gonzages,*[64] was found to be unconstitutional because it lacked any exception to preserve the health of the mother, where such exception was constitutionally required. Also, the act was unconstitutional because it imposed an undue burden on a woman's right to choose previability abortion and was constitutionally vague.

STATE ABORTION STATUTES

The effect of the Supreme Court's 1973 decisions in *Roe* and *Doe* was to invalidate all or part of almost every state abortion statute then in force. The responses of state legislatures to these decisions were varied, but it is clear that many state laws had been enacted to restrict the performance of abortions as much as possible. Although *Planned Parenthood v. Casey* was expected to clear up some issues, it is evident that the states have been given more power to regulate the performance of abortions.

24-Hour Waiting Period Not Burdensome

In 1992, the U.S. Supreme Court in *Planned Parenthood of Southeastern Pennsylvania v. Casey*[65] determined that in asserting an interest in protecting fetal life, a state may place some restrictions on previability abortions, so long as those restrictions do not impose an "undue burden" on the woman's right to an abortion. The court determined that the 24-hour waiting period, the informed consent requirement, and the medical emergency definitions did not unduly burden the right to an abortion and were therefore constitutional.

The 1993 Utah Abortion Act Revision, Senate Bill 60, provides for informed consent by requiring that certain information be given to the pregnant woman at least 24 hours before performing an abortion. The law allows for exceptions to this requirement in the event of a medical emergency. The Utah Women's Clinic, in *Utah Women's Clinic, Inc. v. Leavitt,*[66] filed a 106-page complaint challenging the constitutionality of the new Utah law. It was determined that the 24-hour waiting period did not impose an undue burden on the right to an abortion. On appeal, a U.S. District Court held that the Utah abortion statute's 24-hour waiting period and informed consent requirements do not render the statute unconstitutionally vague.

LAW AND MORALITY OF ABORTION—CONFLICTING BELIEFS

The abortion issue is obviously one that invokes strong feelings on both sides. Individuals are free to urge support for their cause through debate, advocacy, and participation in the political process. The subject also might be addressed in the courts so long as there are valid legal issues in dispute. Where, however, a case presents no legitimate legal arguments, the courthouse is not the proper forum. Litigation, or the threat of litigation, should not be used as economic blackmail to strengthen one's hand in the political battle.[67]

The morality of abortion involves philosophy, ethics, and theology. It is a subject wherein reasonable people adhere to vastly divergent convictions and principles. The obligation of society is to define the liberties of all and not to mandate one's own moral code.[68]

Two or more ethical principles in conflict with one another are considered "ethical dilemmas," such as in the case of abortion. Further complication of ethical dilemmas occurs when laws and regulations affect the decision-making process and, further, when the courts enter the melting pot by interpreting laws and regulations while recognizing the rights of individuals as provided under the Constitution.

Pro-life advocates argue on constitutional, ethical, and religious grounds that the unborn child has a right to life and that right must be protected. Pro-choice advocates argue that a woman has a right to choose preservation and protection of her health, and therefore, in many cases, her life is at least as compelling as the state's interest in promoting childbirth. Two viewpoints, as different as day and night, opposite opinions surrounded by highly charged emotional and religious beliefs as to what is right and what is wrong.

Dr. Gosnell, a Philadelphia physician, was found guilty of murder in some instances by severing the spinal cord of a fetus during late-term abortions. As illustrated in the following news headlines, there is a stream of court cases that continue to stoke the flames of the abortion controversy.

Philadelphia Abortion Doctor Guilty of Murder in Late-Term Procedures

While abortion rights groups argued that Dr. Gosnell operated far outside the legalities and norms of women's health care, abortion opponents seized on the case to raise questions about the ethics of late-term abortions. Put simply, they asked why a procedure done to a living baby outside the womb is murder, but destroying a fetus of similar gestation before delivery can be legal.

John Hurdle and Trip Gabriel, The New York Times, *May 13, 2013*

Pa. Abortion Provider Convicted of Murder

. . . "Some abortionists may have cleaner sheets than Gosnell, and better sterilized equipment and better trained accomplices, but what they do—what Gosnell did—kill babies and hurt women is the same," Rep. Christopher H Smith (R-NJ) said in a statement.

Meanwhile, abortion-rights groups insisted that Gosnell's crimes are an anomaly and that the abysmal conditions inside his clinic persisted only because numerous regulators ignored red flags for years.

Brady Dennis, The Washington Post, *May 14, 2013*

To make the right choices in the resolution of ethical dilemmas, it is often necessary to value one ethical principle more than another. The difficulty in the abortion dilemma arises because beliefs, religion, culture, education, and life experiences can differ from person to person. Good people cannot be considered bad people merely because their beliefs differ from another's beliefs. Values differ, and, therefore, determinations of morality may differ. It is certain that the controversies and ethical dilemmas surrounding abortion will continue for many years to come.

Common ground must be the beginning point for resolving this emotionally charged dilemma.

Moral Persuasion on Abortion

If you wish to persuade someone to adopt your viewpoint on any issue, it is usually counter-productive to begin by insulting that person. The reason is simple: Your target is likely to want to defend himself or herself from the insult, and consequently will not be in a position to hear your argument.

Joseph B. Kadane, Huffington Post, *September 27, 2013*[69]

STERILIZATION

Sterilization is the termination of the ability to produce offspring. Sterilization often is accomplished by either a *vasectomy* for men or a tubal ligation for women. A vasectomy is a surgical procedure in which the vas deferens is severed and tied to prevent the flow of the seminal fluid into the urinary canal. A *tubal ligation* is a surgical procedure in which the fallopian tubes are cut and tied, preventing passage of the ovum from the ovary to the uterus. Sterilizations are often pursued for such reasons as:

- Birth control
- Economic necessity
- Therapeutic necessity (e.g., prevent harm to a woman's health)
- Genetic concerns (e.g., prevent birth defects)

ELECTIVE STERILIZATION

Voluntary or *elective sterilizations* on competent individuals present few legal problems, so long as proper consent has been obtained from the patient and the procedure is performed properly. Civil liability for performing a sterilization of convenience may be imposed if the procedure is performed in a negligent manner. Like abortion, voluntary sterilization is the subject of a variety of debates concerning its moral and ethical propriety.

THERAPEUTIC STERILIZATION

If the life or health of a woman may be jeopardized by pregnancy, the danger may be avoided by terminating: (1) her ability to conceive or (2) her husband's ability to impregnate. Such an operation is a *therapeutic sterilization*—one performed to preserve life or health. The medical necessity for sterilization renders the procedure therapeutic. Sometimes a diseased reproductive organ has to be removed to preserve the life or health of the individual. The operation results in sterility, although this was not the primary reason for the procedure. Such an operation technically should not be classified as sterilization because it is incidental to the medical purpose.

EUGENIC STERILIZATION

The term *eugenic sterilization* refers to the involuntary sterilization of certain categories of persons described in statutes, without the need for consent by, or on behalf of, those subject to the procedures. Persons classified as mentally deficient, feebleminded, and, in some instances, epileptic are included within the scope of the statutes. Several states also have included certain sexual deviants and persons classified as habitual criminals. Such statutes ordinarily are designed to prevent the transmission of hereditary defects to succeeding generations, but several statutes also have recognized the purpose of preventing procreation by individuals who would not be able to care for their offspring.

Although there have been judicial decisions to the contrary, the United States Supreme Court in *Buck v. Bell*[70] specifically upheld the validity of such eugenic sterilization statutes, provided that certain procedural safeguards are observed. Several states have laws authorizing eugenic sterilization. The decision in *Wade v. Bethesda Hospital*[71] strongly suggests that in the absence of statutory authority the state cannot order sterilization for eugenic purposes. Eugenic sterilization statutes provide the following: a grant of authority to public officials supervising state institutions for the mentally ill or prisons and to certain public health officials to conduct sterilizations; a requirement of personal notice to the person subject to sterilization and, if that person is unable to comprehend what is involved, notice to the person's legal representative, guardian, or nearest relative; a hearing by the board designated in the particular statute to determine the propriety of the prospective sterilization; at the hearing, evidence that may be presented, and the patient, who must be present or represented by counsel or the nearest relative or guardian; and an opportunity to appeal the board's ruling to a court.

The procedural safeguards of notice, hearing, and the right to appeal must be present in sterilization statutes to fulfill the minimum constitutional requirements of due process. An Arkansas statute was found to be unconstitutional in that it did not provide for notice to the incompetent patient and opportunity to be heard or for the patient's entitlement to legal counsel.[72]

NEGLIGENT STERILIZATION

The improper performance of sterilization can result in lawsuits based on such theories as *wrongful birth*, *wrongful life*, and *wrongful conception*. Wrongful life suits are generally unsuccessful, primarily because of the court's unwillingness, for public policy reasons, to permit financial recovery for the "injury" of being born into the world.

Some success, however, has been achieved in litigation by the patient (and his or her spouse) who allegedly was sterilized and subsequently proved fertile. Damages have been awarded for the cost of the unsuccessful procedure; pain and suffering as a result of the pregnancy; the medical expense of the pregnancy; and the loss of comfort, companionship services, and consortium of the spouse. Again, as a matter of public policy, the courts have indicated that the joys and benefits of having the child outweigh the cost incurred in the rearing process.

There have been many cases in recent years involving actions for wrongful birth, wrongful life, and wrongful conception. Litigation originated with the California case in which a court found that a genetic testing laboratory could be held liable for damages from incorrectly reporting genetic tests, leading to the birth of a child with defects.[73] Injury caused by birth had not been previously actionable by law. The court of appeals held that medical laboratories engaged in genetic testing owe a duty to parents and their unborn child to use ordinary care in administering available tests for the purpose of providing information concerning potential genetic defects in the unborn. Damages in this case were awarded on the basis of the child's shortened life span.

Wrongful Birth

In a wrongful birth action, the plaintiffs claim that but for a breach of duty by the defendant(s) (e.g., improper sterilization), the child would not have been born. A wrongful birth claim can be brought by the parent(s) of a child born with genetic defects against a physician who or a laboratory that negligently fails to inform them, in a timely fashion, of an increased possibility that the mother will give birth to such a child, therefore precluding an informed decision as to whether to have the child.

NEGLIGENT STERILIZATION

Chaffee performed a partial salpingectomy on Seslar. The purpose of the procedure was to sterilize Seslar, who had already borne four children, so that she could not become pregnant again. After undergoing the surgery, however, Seslar conceived and delivered a healthy baby. Seslar sued Chaffee.

The Court of Appeals held that damages for the alleged negligent sterilization procedure could not include the costs of raising a normal healthy child. Although raising an unplanned child is costly, all human life is presumptively invaluable. A child, regardless of the circumstances of birth, does not constitute harm to the parents so as to permit recovery for the costs associated with raising and educating the child. As with a majority of jurisdictions, the court held that the value of a child's life to the parents outweighs the associated pecuniary burdens as a matter of law. Recoverable damages may include pregnancy and childbearing expenses but not the ordinary costs of raising and educating a normal, healthy child conceived after an allegedly negligent sterilization procedure.[74]

Ethical and Legal Issues

1. Do you agree with the court's decision?
2. Under what circumstances would you not agree with the court's decision?
3. Describe the ethical issues in this case.

In a New Jersey case, *Canesi ex rel. Canesi v. Wilson*,[75] the New Jersey Supreme Court reviewed the dismissal of an action for wrongful birth on the claim of the parents that had the mother been informed of the risk that a drug, Provera, which she had been taking before she learned that she was pregnant, might cause the fetus to be born with congenital anomalies, such as limb reduction, she would have decided to abort the fetus. It was alleged that the physicians failed to disclose the risks associated with the drug. The physicians argued that the informed consent doctrine requires that the plaintiffs establish that the drug in fact caused the birth anomalies. The court rejected the argument and distinguished the wrongful birth action from one based on informed consent:[76]

> In sum, the informed consent and wrongful birth causes of action are similar in that both require the physician to disclose those medically accepted risks that a reasonably prudent patient in the plaintiff's position would deem material to her decision. What is or is not a medically acceptable risk is informed by what the physician knows or ought to know of the patient's history and condition. These causes of action, however, have important differences. They encompass different compensable harms and measures of damages. In both causes of action, the plaintiff must prove not only that a reasonably prudent patient in her position, if apprised of all material risks, would have elected a different course of treatment or care. In an informed consent case, the plaintiff must additionally meet a two-pronged test for proximate causation: She must prove that the undisclosed risk actually materialized and that it was medically caused by the treatment. In a wrongful birth case, on the other hand, a plaintiff need not prove that the doctor's negligence was the medical cause of her child's birth defect. Rather, the test of proximate causation is satisfied by showing that an undisclosed fetal risk was material to a woman in her position; the risk materialized was reasonably foreseeable and not remote in relation to the doctor's negligence; and had plaintiff known of that risk, she would have terminated her pregnancy. The emotional distress and economic loss resulting from this lost opportunity to decide for herself whether or not to terminate the pregnancy constitute plaintiff's damages.

With the increasing consolidation of hospital services and physician practices, a case could be made for finding a hospital liable for the physician's failure to obtain informed consent where the hospital actually owns or controls the physician's practice or where both the hospital and the physician's practice are owned or controlled by another corporation that sets policy for both the hospital and the physician's practice.

Wrongful Life

Wrongful life claims are initiated by the parent(s) or child based on harm suffered as a result of being born. The plaintiffs generally contend that the physician or laboratory negligently failed to inform the child's parents of the risk of bearing a genetically defective infant and hence prevented the parents' right to choose to avoid the birth.[77] Because there is no recognized legal right not to be born, wrongful life cases are generally not successful.

> [L]egal recognition that a disabled life is an injury would harm the interests of those most directly concerned, the handicapped. Disabled persons face obvious physical difficulties in conducting their lives. They also face subtle yet equally devastating

handicaps in the attitudes and behavior of society, the law, and their own families and friends. Furthermore, society often views disabled persons as burdensome misfits. Recent legislation concerning employment, education, and building access reflects a slow change in these attitudes. This change evidences a growing public awareness that the handicapped can be valuable and productive members of society. To characterize the life of a disabled person as an injury would denigrate both this new awareness and the handicapped themselves.[78]

A cause of action for wrongful life was not cognizable under Kansas law in *Bruggeman v. Schimke*.[79] Human life is valuable, precious, and worthy of protection. Not to be born rather than to be alive with deformities cannot be recognized. The Kansas Supreme Court held that there was no recognized cause for wrongful life.

In *Kassama v. Magat*,[80] Kassama alleged that Dr. Magat failed to advise her of the results of an alpha-fetoprotein blood test that indicated a heightened possibility that her child, Ibrion, might be afflicted with Down syndrome. Had she received that information, Kassama contends, she would have undergone amniocentesis, which would have confirmed that prospect. Kassama claims that if that had occurred she would have chosen to terminate the pregnancy through an abortion.

The Supreme Court of Maryland decided that for purposes of tort law, an impaired life was not worse than nonlife, and, for that reason, life itself was not and could not be considered an injury. There was no evidence that Ibrion was not deeply loved and cared for by her parents or that she did not return that love. Studies have shown that people afflicted with Down syndrome can lead productive and meaningful lives. They can be educated and employed, form friendships, and get along in society. Allowing a recovery of extraordinary life expenses on some theory of fairness—that the physician or his or her insurance company should pay not because the physician was negligent causing the injury or impairment but because the child was born—ignores that fundamental issue.

Wrongful birth is based on the premise that being born and having to live with the affliction are disadvantages and thus cognizable injuries. The injury sued upon was the fact that Ibrion was born; she bears the disability and will bear the expenses only because, due to the alleged negligence of Magat, her mother was unable to terminate the pregnancy and avert her birth. The issue here is whether Maryland law is prepared to recognize that kind of injury—the injury of life itself.

The child has not suffered any damage cognizable at law by being brought into existence. One of the most deeply held beliefs of our society is that life, whether experienced with or without a major physical handicap, is more precious than nonlife. No one is perfect, and each person suffers from some ailments or defects (whether major or minor) that make impossible participation in all of the activities life has to offer. Our lives are not thereby rendered less precious than those of others whose defects are less pervasive or less severe. Despite their handicaps, Down syndrome children are able to love and be loved and to experience happiness and pleasure—emotions that are truly the essence of life and that are far more valuable than the suffering that may be endured.

The right to life and the principle that all are equal under the law are basic to our constitutional order. To presume to decide that a child's life is not worth living would be to forsake these ideals. To characterize the life of a disabled person as an injury would denigrate the handicapped themselves. Measuring the value of an impaired life as compared with nonexistence is a task that is beyond mortals.

Unless a judgment can be made on the basis of reason rather than the emotion of any given case, that nonlife is preferable to impaired life—that the child–plaintiff would, in fact, have been better off had he or she never been born—there can be no injury, and if there can be no injury, whether damages can or cannot be calculated becomes irrelevant.

The crucial question, a value judgment about life itself, is too deeply immersed in each person's own individual philosophy or theology to be subject to a reasoned and consistent community response in the form of a jury verdict.

Wrongful Conception

Wrongful conception refers to a claim for damages sustained by the parents of an unexpected child based on an allegation that conception of the child resulted from negligent sterilization procedures or a defective contraceptive device.[81] Damages sought for a negligently performed sterilization might include:

- Pain and suffering associated with pregnancy and birth
- Expenses of delivery
- Lost wages
- Father's loss of consortium
- Damages for emotional or psychological pain
- Suffering resulting from the presence of an additional family member in the household
- The cost and pain and suffering of a subsequent sterilization
- Damages suffered by a child born with genetic defects

The most controversial item of damages claimed is that of raising a normal healthy child to adulthood. The mother in *Hartke v. McKelway*[82] had undergone sterilization for therapeutic reasons to avoid endangering her health from pregnancy. The woman became pregnant as a result of a failed sterilization. She delivered a healthy child without injury to herself. It was determined that "the jury could not rationally have found that the birth of this child was an injury to this plaintiff. Awarding child-rearing expense would only give Hartke a windfall."[83]

The cost of raising a healthy newborn child to adulthood was recoverable by the parents of the child conceived as a result of an unsuccessful sterilization by a physician employee at Lovelace Medical Center. The physician in *Lovelace Medical Center v. Mendez*[84] found and ligated only one of the patient's two fallopian tubes and then failed to inform the patient of the unsuccessful operation. The court held that:[85]

> the Mendezes' interest in the financial security of their family was a legally protected interest which was invaded by Lovelace's negligent failure properly to perform Maria's sterilization operation (if proved at trial), and that this invasion was an injury entitling them to recover damages in the form of the reasonable expenses to raise Joseph to maturity.

Some states bar damage claims for emotional distress and the costs associated with the raising of healthy children but will permit recovery for damages related to negligent sterilizations. In *Butler v. Rolling Hill Hospital*,[86] the Pennsylvania Superior Court held that the patient stated a cause of action for the negligent performance of a laparoscopic tubal ligation. The patient was not, however, entitled to compensation for the costs of raising a normal, healthy child. "In light of this Commonwealth's public policy, which recognizes the paramount importance of the family to society, we conclude that the benefits of joy, companionship, and affection which a normal, healthy child can provide must be deemed as a matter of law to outweigh the costs of raising that child."[87]

As the Court of Common Pleas of Lycoming County, Pennsylvania, in *Shaheen v. Knight*, stated:[88]

> Many people would be willing to support this child were they given the right of custody and adoption, but according to plaintiff's statement, plaintiff does not want such. He wants to have the child and wants the doctor to support it. In our opinion, to allow such damages would be against public policy.

ARTIFICIAL INSEMINATION

Artificial insemination is the process by which sperm is placed into the reproductive tract of a female, for the purpose of impregnating the female by using means other than sexual intercourse. There are two sources of the sperm for impregnation of a female: (1) homologous artificial insemination involves the use of the husband's semen to impregnate the female; and heterologous artificial insemination (HAI) involves the use of semen from a donor other than a woman's husband. The absence of answers to many questions concerning HAI may discourage couples from seeking to use the procedure and physicians from performing it. Some of the questions concern the procedure itself; others concern the status of the offspring, the effect of the procedure on the marital relationship, and the risk of multiple births that can be financially challenging. Further worrying is the potential for legal actions for multiple births and even lead to the loss of a physician's license to practice medicine such as occurred when the Medical Board of California revoked Dr. Michael Kamrava medical license. Dr. Kamrava had transplanted multiple embryos that resulted in the birth of octuplets. The Medical Board determined that Dr. Kamrava had acted beyond the reasonable judgment of a physician by implanting a number of embryos that exceeded existing guidelines. "The Board subsequently found Kamrava guilty of gross negligence, repeated negligent acts, and inadequate medical records in the first case. In the additional two cases, Kamrava was found guilty of gross negligence and repeated negligent acts in one case and guilty of repeated negligent acts in the other case."[89]

CONSENT

The Oklahoma HAI statute specifies that husband and wife must consent to the procedure.[90] It is clear that the wife's consent must be obtained; without it, the touching involved in the artificial insemination would constitute a battery. Besides the wife's consent, it is important to obtain the husband's consent to ensure against liability accruing if a court adopted the view that without the consent of the husband, HAI was a wrong to the husband's interest, for which he could sustain a suit for damages.

The Oklahoma statute also deals with establishing proof of consent. It requires the consent to be in writing, and it must be executed and acknowledged by the physician performing the procedure and by the local judge who has jurisdiction over the adoption of children, as well as by the husband and wife.

In states without specific statutory requirements, medical personnel should attempt to avoid such potential liability by establishing the practice of obtaining the written consent of the couple requesting the HAI procedure.

CONFIDENTIALITY

Another problem that directly concerns medical personnel involved in heterologous artificial insemination birth is preserving confidentiality. This problem is met in the Oklahoma HAI statute, which requires that the original copy of the consent be filed pursuant to the rules for filing adoption papers and is not to be made a matter of public record.[91]

SURROGACY

Surrogacy is a method of reproduction whereby a woman agrees to give birth to a child she will not raise but hand over to a contracted party, who is often unable to conceive a natural child of her or his own. A surrogate "may be the child's genetic mother (the more traditional form of surrogacy), or she may as a gestational carrier, carry the pregnancy to delivery after having been implanted with an embryo. In some cases surrogacy is the only available option for parents who wish to have a child that is biologically related to them."[92]

Surrogacy raises a variety of ethical and legal issues that should be considered before searching for a surrogate mother. For example, is it ethical to enter a contract with a woman by offering her money in exchange for bearing a child and then transferring all parental rights and physical custody of the child to the "commissioning couple"? Although the long-term effects of surrogacy contracts are not known, the adverse psychological impact could be detrimental to the child who learns that he or she is the offspring of someone who gave birth only to obtain money. Would the child want to search for his or her gestational mother? Should records be kept, and should the child have access to the records? After the child is taken, the surrogate mother may be negatively affected as her feeling of isolation is felt along with the reality of the sale of her body.

Although there are arguments offered for and against surrogacy contracts, there are many parents who have experienced the joy of raising happy, psychologically well-balanced, and career-successful surrogate children. Those who have done their research and understand the issues live as happy together as those in any other family relationship.

ORGAN DONATIONS

Becoming a Donor

Organ and tissue donation and transplantation provide a second chance at life for thousands of people each year. You have the opportunity to be one of the individuals who make these miracles happen.

By deciding to be a donor, you give the gift of hope ... hope for the thousands of individuals awaiting organ transplants and hope for the millions of individuals whose lives could be enhanced through tissue transplants. [organdonor.gov.]

U.S. Department of Health and Human Services[93]

Federal regulations require that hospitals have and implement written protocols regarding their organ procurement responsibilities. The regulations impose specific notification duties, as well as other requirements concerning informing families of potential donors. It encourages discretion and sensitivity in dealing with the families and in educating hospital staff on a variety of issues involved with donation matters in order to facilitate timely donation and transplantation.

Organ transplantations are performed to treat patients with end-stage organ disease who face organ failure. Developments in medical science have enabled physicians to take tissue from persons immediately after death for use in replacing or rehabilitating diseased or damaged organs or other parts of living persons. Interest in organ transplantation increased in 1954 when the Herrick twins became the first successful kidney transplant.[94] The success rates of organ transplants have improved because of advances in the patient selection process, improved clinical and operative management and skills, and immunosuppressant drugs that aid in decreasing the incidence of tissue rejection (e.g., cyclosporin A, which acts to suppress the production of antibodies that attack transplanted tissue); nevertheless, this progress has created the problem of obtaining a sufficient supply of replacement body parts. There is a corresponding cry for more organs as the success rate in organ transplantation increases. Because of the fear of people buying and selling organs, the National Organ Procurement Act was enacted in 1984, making it illegal to buy or sell organs. Throughout the country, there are tissue banks and other facilities that store and preserve organs and tissue that can be used for transplantation and other therapeutic services.

The ever-increasing success of organ transplants and the demand for organ tissue require the close scrutiny of each case, to make sure that established procedures have been followed in the care and disposal of all body parts. Section 1138, Title XI, of the Omnibus Budget Reconciliation Act of 1986 requires hospitals to establish organ procurement protocols or face a loss of Medicare and Medicaid funding. Physicians, nurses, and other paramedical personnel assigned this responsibility often are confronted with several legal issues. Liability can be limited by complying with applicable regulations. Organs and tissues to be stored and preserved for future use must be removed almost immediately after death; therefore, it is imperative that an agreement or arrangement for obtaining organs and tissue from a body be completed before death, or very soon after death, to enable physicians to remove and store the tissue promptly.

There is a shortage of cadavers needed for medical education and transplantation. Mark Zuckerburg, chairman and chief executive officer of Facebook, aware of the severe shortage, launched an organ donation campaign in 2012.

Facebook Launches Organ Donation Campaign

May 1 (Reuters)—Facebook on Tuesday launched an organ donation tool aimed at encouraging the 900 million users of the social networking site to help combat a shortage of organs needed for life-saving transplants.

"What we hope will happen is that by just having a simple tool, we think that people can really help spread awareness of organ donation and that they want to participate in this to their friends, and we think that can be a big part in helping to solve the crisis," chief executive Mark Zuckerberg said on ABC-TV's "Good Morning America" program on Tuesday.

Nicola Leske, Jill Serjeant, Patricia Reaney, Chicago Tribune, *May 1, 2012*

Some people may wish to make arrangements for the use of their bodies after death for such purposes. A surviving spouse may, however, object to such disposition. In such cases, the interest of the surviving spouse or other family member could supersede that of the deceased.

Who Lives? Who Dies? Who Decides?

Who lives? Who dies? Who decides? These are but a few of the ethical questions that arise when deciding to whom an organ shall be given. The answers are not easy. The decision makers, even with guidelines to follow, often become the judge and jury and often find that the answers to who lives and dies are not always easy decisions. If there were unlimited sources of organs, there would be no supply-and-demand issues. Because supply is limited, numerous ethical principles come into play. In the case of a 70-year-old patient with multiple life-threatening health problems, the patient may not be considered a suitable candidate for a transplant, whereas a 15-year-old patient with few health issues would be considered a more appropriate candidate.

Uniform Anatomical Gift Act

The American Bar Association endorsed a *Uniform Anatomical Gift Act* drafted by the Commission on Uniform State Laws. This statute has been enacted by all 50 states and has many detailed provisions that apply to the wide variety of issues raised in connection with the making, acceptance, and use of anatomical gifts. The act allows a person to make a decision to donate organs at the time of death and allows potential donors to carry an anatomical donor card. State statutes regarding donation usually permit the donor to execute the gift during his or her lifetime.

The right to privacy of the donor and his or her family must be respected. Information should not be publicized regarding transplant procedures as well as the names the donor or donee without consent.

States have enacted legislation to facilitate donation of bodies and body parts for medical uses. Virtually all of the states have based their enactments on the Uniform Anatomical Gift Act, but it should be recognized that in some states there are deviations from this act or additional laws dealing with donation.

Individuals who are of sound mind and 18 years of age or older are permitted to dispose of their own bodies or body parts by will or other written instrument for medical or dental education, research, advancement of medical or dental science, therapy, or transplantation. Among those eligible to receive such donations are any licensed, accredited, or approved hospitals; accredited medical or dental schools; surgeons or physicians; tissue banks; or specified individuals who need the donation for therapy or transplantation. The statute provides that when only a part of the body is donated, custody of the remaining parts of the body shall be transferred to the next of kin promptly after removal of the donated part.

A donation by will becomes effective immediately on the death of the testator, without probate, and the gift is valid and effective to the extent that it has been acted on in good faith. This is true even if the will is not probated or is declared invalid for testimonial purposes.

Failure to Obtain Consent

Although failure to obtain consent for removal of body tissue can give rise to a lawsuit, not all such claims are successful. In *Nicoletta v. Rochester Eye & Human Parts Bank*,[95] emotional injuries resulted from the removal of the eyes of Nicoletta's son for donation after a fatal motorcycle accident. The hospital was immune from liability under the provisions of the Uniform Anatomical Gift Act because the hospital had neither actual nor constructive knowledge that the woman who had authorized the donation was not the decedent's wife. The hospital was entitled to the immunity afforded by the "good faith" provisions of Section 4306(3) of the act, under which its agents had made reasonable inquiry as to the status of the purported wife, who had resided with the decedent for 10 years and was the mother of their two children. The hospital had no reason to believe that any irregularity existed. The father, who was present at the time his son was brought to the emergency department, failed to object to any organ donation and failed to challenge the authority of the purported wife to sign the emergency department authorization. There are several methods by which a donation may be revoked. If the document has been delivered to a named donee, it may be revoked by:

- A written revocation signed by the donor and delivered to the donee
- An oral revocation witnessed by two persons and communicated to the donee
- A statement to the attending physician during a terminal illness that has been communicated to the donee
- A written statement that has been signed and is on the donor's person or in the donor's immediate effects

If the written instrument of donation has not been delivered to the donee, it may be revoked by destruction, cancellation, or mutilation of the instrument. If the donation is made by a will, it may be revoked in the manner provided for revocation or amendment of wills. Any person acting in good-faith reliance on the terms of an instrument of donation will not be subject to civil or criminal liability unless there is actual notice of the revocation of the donation.

RESEARCH, EXPERIMENTATION, AND CLINICAL TRIALS

Medical progress and improved patient care are dependent on advances in medicine made through research. Research studies are designed to answer specific questions, including a drug or device's safety and effectiveness. Ethical considerations, to name but a few, that should be addressed when conducting research on human subjects include honesty, integrity, autonomy; self-determination; the Hippocratic maxim of do no harm; the application of justice; and, how to fairly conduct blind trials. The basic principle of research is honesty, which must be ensured through institutional protocols. Honesty and integrity must govern all stages of research.

The science of medicine, which by its very nature studies the human body, is prevented from making progress through direct experimentation. A necessary part of research is to conduct laboratory tests on animals and observe their effects prior to testing them on humans. Advances in research occurs by observation and study of how a normal healthy body functions and when the body malfunctions, studying the cause of those changes that occur and finding a way to slow and possibly reverse the progression of a disease.

Federal regulations control federal grants that apply to experiments involving new drugs, new medical devices, or new medical procedures. Generally, a combination of federal and state guidelines and regulations ensures proper supervision and control over experimentation that involves human subjects. For example, federal regulations require hospital-based researchers to obtain the approval of an *institutional review board.*

OFFICE OF RESEARCH INTEGRITY

The Office of Research Integrity (ORI) oversees and directs Public Health Service (PHS) research integrity activities on behalf of the Secretary of Health and Human Services with the exception of the research integrity activities of the Food and Drug Administration. The ORI carries out its responsibility by developing policies, procedures, and regulations related to the detection, investigation, and prevention of research misconduct and the responsible conduct of research. The ORI is responsible for implementing activities and programs to teach the responsible conduct of research, promote research integrity, prevent research misconduct, and improve the handling of allegations of research misconduct. The ORI administers programs for: maintaining institutional assurances, responding to allegations of retaliation against whistleblowers, approving intramural and extramural policies and procedures, and responding to Freedom of Information Act and Privacy Act requests.

FOOD AND DRUG ADMINISTRATION

The Food and Drug Administration (FDA) regulates the conduct of clinical trials. A variety of regulations that describe good clinical practices for studies with both human and nonhuman animal subjects are listed next. More detail on these and other research-related regulations can be found at the FDA website.[96]

- Electronic Records
- Protection of Human Subjects
- Informed Consent Elements
- Financial Disclosure by Investigators
- Institutional Review Boards
- Investigational Drug New Application
- Investigational Device Exemptions
- Good Laboratory Practice for Nonclinical Laboratory Studies
- Expanded Access to Investigational Drugs for Treatment

The FDA—after much criticism over the years because of the red tape involved in the approval of new drugs—issued new rules to speed up the approval process. The rules permit the use of experimental drugs outside a controlled clinical trial if the drugs are used to treat a life-threatening condition. In *Abigail Alliance for Better Access to Developmental Drugs v. Eschenbach,* [33] the U.S. Court of Appeals for the District of Columbia ruled that terminally ill patients have a "fundamental right" protected by the U.S. Constitution to access to experimental drugs that have not yet been fully approved by the FDA. The appeals court ruled that once the FDA has determined, after Phase I trials, that a potentially lifesaving new drug is sufficiently safe for expanded human trials, terminally ill patients have a constitutional right to seek treatment with the drug if no other FDA-approved drugs are available. The court said that if the FDA wishes to prevent such patients from gaining access to investigational drugs that have completed Phase I trials, it bears the burden of demonstrating that its restrictions are "narrowly tailored" to serve a compelling governmental interest.

Patients participating in research studies should fully understand the implications of their participation. Health care organizations involved in research studies should have appropriate protocols in place that protect the rights of patients. Consent forms should describe both the risks and benefits involved in the research activity.

INSTITUTIONAL REVIEW BOARD

Health care organizations conducting medical research must have a mechanism in place for approving and overseeing the use of investigational protocols. This is accomplished through the establishment of an institutional review board (IRB). An IRB is a committee designated by organizations (e.g., hospitals) conducting clinical trials to provide initial approval and periodic monitoring of biomedical research studies. The primary responsibilities of an IRB include:

- Protecting the rights and welfare of human subjects
- Ensuring protocols are presented by the sponsor(s)
- Ensuring sponsor(s) of a protocol discloses
  - Areas of concern that might give the impression of a conflict of interest in the outcome of the clinical research
  - Financial interests that might occur should the clinical trials prove to be successful or give the impression of success, including stock options and cash payouts
  - Reviewing, monitoring, and approving clinical protocols for investigations of drugs and medical devices involving human subjects
  - Ensuring that the rights, including the privacy and confidentiality, of each individual are protected
  - Ensuring that all research is conducted within appropriate state and federal guidelines (e.g., FDA guidelines)

INFORMED CONSENT

My husband . . . participated in a clinical trial involving both an autologous (self) and allogeneic (donor) transplant for a hopeful cure of the disease. We both understood the risks involved and the no-promise guarantee, as such is the nature of a clinical trial. The ultimate responsibility for whatever the outcome rested with us, as we were the ones who voluntarily entered into the program. Three years later, we have just learned of the disease's progression, but we continue to look forward, remain optimistic, and support those who dedicate their lives for the betterment of those afflicted with these cursed cancers.

The reality is that someday, probably sooner than later, my husband will lose the battle with this tenacious enemy, but we are still thankful for the compassionate and learned members of the Fred Hutchinson Cancer Research Center who helped and are still helping us to navigate a most challenging road.[97]

Mary Ellen Stokes and Bill Stokes, "Relentless Assault on a Research Hospital," *Wall Street Journal*, *March 15, 2004*

Health care organizations involved in research studies should have appropriate protocols in place that protect the rights of patients. Patients participating in research studies should fully understand the implications of their participation. Physicians have a clear duty to warn patients as to the risks, benefits, and alternatives of an experimental procedure. Written consent should be obtained from each patient who participates in a clinical trial. The consent form must not contain any coercive or exculpatory language through which the patient is forced to waive his or her legal rights, including the release of the investigator, sponsor, or organization from liability for negligent conduct.

Organizations conducting clinical trials on human subjects, at the very least, must:

- Fully disclose to the patient the inherent risks, benefits, and treatment alternatives to the proposed research protocol(s)
- Determine the competency of the patient to consent
- Obtain written consent from the patient
- Educate the staff as to the potential side effects, implementation of, and ongoing monitoring of protocols
- Require financial disclosure issues associated with the protocols
  - Promote awareness of ethical issues
  - Promote education in regard to ethical decision making
  - Increase nurse participation in ethical decision making
  - Have ongoing monitoring of approved protocols

The Centers for Medicare and Medicaid Services accreditation survey process for nursing facilities includes a review of the rights of nursing facility residents participating in experimental research. Surveyors will review the records of residents identified as participating in a clinical research study. They will determine whether informed consent forms have been executed properly. The form will be reviewed to determine whether all known risks have been identified. Appropriate questions may be directed to both the staff and residents or the residents' guardians.

Possible questions to ask staff include:[98]

- Is the facility participating in any experimental research?
- If yes, what residents are involved? (Interview a sample of these residents.)[99]
- Residents or guardians may be asked questions, such as:
  - Are you participating in the study?
  - Was this explained to you well enough so that you understand what the study is about and any risks that might be involved?

EXPERIMENTAL SUBJECT'S BILL OF RIGHTS

The following is a bill of rights developed by the Veterans Administration system for patients involved in research studies. Human subjects have the following rights. These rights include, but are not limited to, the subject's right to:[100]

- Be informed of the nature and purpose of the experiment
- Be given an explanation of the procedures to be followed in the medical experiment and any drug or device to be used
- Be given a description of any attendant discomforts and risks reasonably to be expected
- Be given an explanation of any benefits to the subject reasonably to be expected, if applicable
- Be given a disclosure of any appropriate alternatives, drugs, or devices that might be advantageous to the subject, their relative risks, and benefits
- Be informed of the avenues of medical treatment, if any, available to the subject after the experiment if complications should arise
- Be given an opportunity to ask questions concerning the experiment or the procedures involved
- Be instructed that consent to participate in the medical experiment may be withdrawn at any time and the subject may discontinue participation without prejudice
- Be given a copy of the signed and dated consent form
- Be given the opportunity to decide to consent or not to consent to a medical experiment without the intervention of any element of force, fraud, deceit, duress, coercion, or undue influence on the subject's decision

CASE: MEDICAL RESEARCH AND DUTY TO WARN

About 5,000 patients at Michael Reese Hospital and Medical Center, located in Chicago, Illinois, were treated with X-ray therapy for some benign conditions of the head and neck from 1930 to 1960. Among them was Joel Blaz, now a citizen of Florida, who received this treatment for infected tonsils and adenoids while a child in Illinois from 1947 through 1948. He has suffered various tumors, which he now attributes to this treatment. Blaz was diagnosed with a neural tumor in 1987.

In 1974, Michael Reese set up the Thyroid Follow-Up Project to gather data and conduct research among the people who had been subjected to the X-ray therapy. In 1975, the program notified Blaz by mail that he was at increased risk of developing thyroid tumors because of the treatment. In 1976, someone associated with the program gave him similar information by phone and invited him to return to Michael Reese for evaluation and treatment at his own expense, which he declined to do.

Dr. Arthur Schneider was placed in charge of the program in 1977. In 1979, Schneider and Michael Reese submitted a research proposal to the National Institutes of Health stating that a study based on the program showed "strong evidence" of a connection between X-ray treatments of the sort administered to Blaz and various sorts of tumors: thyroid, neural, and others. In 1981, Blaz received but did not complete or return a questionnaire attached to a letter from Schneider in connection with the program. The letter stated that the purpose of the questionnaire was to "investigate the long-term health implications" of childhood radiation treatments and to "determine the possible associated risks." It did not say anything about "strong evidence" of a connection between the treatments and any tumors.

In 1996, after developing neural tumors, Blaz sued Michael Reese's successor, Galen Hospital in Illinois, and Dr. Schneider, alleging, among other things, that they failed to notify and warn him of their findings that he might be at greater risk of neural tumors in a way that might have permitted their earlier detection and removal or other treatment. There is a clear duty to warn the subject of previously administered radiation treatments when there is a strong connection between those treatments and certain kinds of tumors. The harm alleged, neural and other tumors would here be reasonably foreseeable as a likely consequence of a failure to warn and was in fact foreseen by Schneider. A reasonable physician, indeed any reasonable person, could foresee that if someone were warned of "strong evidence" of a connection between treatments to which he had been subjected and tumors, he would probably seek diagnosis or treatment and perhaps avoid these tumors, and if he were not warned he probably would not seek diagnosis or treatment, increasing the likelihood that he would suffer from such tumors. Other things being equal, therefore, a reasonable physician would warn the subject of the treatments.[101]

Ethical and Legal Issues

1. Discuss the ethical and legal principles violated in this case.
2. What preventative measures should be taken to prevent recurrence of cases such as this?

PATIENT RESPONSIBILITIES

Patients in National Institutes of Health (NIH) clinical trials have responsibilities, as well as rights. The following describes the responsibilities of NIH patients.

> In the spirit of working together toward a common goal, our patients (and their parents, guardians, and surrogates) have responsibilities as partners in medical research and as patients at the Clinical Center.
> You have the responsibility:
>
> 1. To provide, to the best of your knowledge, complete information about your current medical condition and past medical history, including current illness, prior hospitalizations, current medications, allergies, and all other health-related matters;
> 2. To discuss your protocol (study or treatment plan) with the research staff before indicating agreement to take part in it by signing a consent;
> 3. To inform the medical staff about your wishes regarding treatment plans. You may provide for a duly authorized family member or spokesperson to make medical decisions on your behalf in the event that you become unable to communicate;
> 4. To comply with your protocol, to cooperate with hospital staff, to ask questions if directions or procedures are not clear, and to participate in your health care decisions. You may withdraw from the study for any reason, but it is desirable to discuss your concerns with the attending physician before taking that action.

Parents of pediatric patients have the responsibility to indicate if and how they want to be involved in their child's plan of care;

5. To refrain from taking any medications, drugs, or alcoholic beverages while participating in the protocol, except those approved by an NIH physician;

6. To adhere to the no-smoking policy of the NIH;

7. To report on time for scheduled procedures and to keep all clinic appointments. If unable to do so, you have the responsibility of notifying the protocol physician and canceling and rescheduling the appointment;

8. To report promptly to the medical or nursing staff any unexpected problems or changes in your medical condition;

9. To inform the appropriate staff or the patient representative of any concerns or problems with the care and treatment that you feel are not being adequately addressed;

10. To respect the property of the U.S. government, fellow patients, and others; to follow NIH rules and regulations affecting patient care and treatment; to respect the rights of other patients and hospital staff. This includes the responsibility of respecting the privacy of other patients and treating information concerning them as confidential;

11. To pay all medical or laboratory expenses incurred outside the Clinical Center, except when you have received written authorization on the appropriate NIH form to have such expenses billed to the NIH;

12. To obtain medical care and medications from your own health care provider for all conditions unrelated to the protocol in which you are participating, except while being treated as an inpatient at the Clinical Center;

13. To provide your own transportation to and from the Clinical Center and to pay living expenses except when all or part of these expenses are covered by the protocol or authorized by the responsible NIH physician; to advise accompanying escorts or others who travel to and remain in the Bethesda area that they must pay for their travel and living expenses except when designated by NIH as a guardian for you when your expenses are covered;

14. To provide complete information, so that contacts and communications to schedule visits and monitor health status can be maintained. This information should include (1) your current address and phone number; (2) the names, addresses, and phone numbers of next of kin or persons to be notified in the event of an emergency; and (3) the names, addresses, and phone numbers of physicians responsible for your ongoing care, including your family physician and the physician(s) who referred you to the NIH;

15. To return to the care of your own health-care provider when participation in the protocol is completed or stopped and your medical condition permits.[102]

If you have questions about your rights, you may contact the Clinical Center Patient Representative.

PATENTS DELAY RESEARCH

The legal system—caught up in the rights of patent holders—has resulted in delayed cures. What happens to the rights of those who would have benefited from the cures? The rights of the few, those who could be viewed as seeing money as the ultimate good, hold hostage the rights of many. That is, until they need the cure. The legal system is so ruled by rules that it cannot get out of its own harmful way.

Where Are the Cures? How Patent Gridlock Is Blocking the Development of Lifesaving Drugs

A curious thing happened on the way to the biotech revolution. While investment in biotech research and development has increased over the last three decades, new drugs that improve human health have not been forthcoming at the same rate.

What explains this drug discovery gap? Patent gridlock plays a large role. Since a 1980 Supreme Court decision allowing patents on living organisms, 40,000 DNA-related patents have been granted. Now picture a drug developer walking into an auditorium filled with dozens of owners of the biotech patents needed to create a potential lifesaving cure. Unless the drug maker can strike a deal with every person in the room, the new drug won't be developed.

Peter Ringrose, former chief science officer at Bristol-Myers Squibb, told the *New York Times* that the company would not investigate some 50 proteins that could be cancer-causing, because patent holders would either decline to cooperate or demand big royalties.

Michael Heller, Forbes, *August 11, 2008*

Discussion

- Discuss the ethical principles (e.g., beneficence [doing good] and nonmaleficence [avoiding causing harm]) and issues of morality of a legal system that delays research because of the legal rights of patent holders.
- Discuss what steps could be taken to right the wrongs of patents that delay and often discourage research.

HUMAN GENETICS

The most promising frontier of the future of medical practice is in the area of human genetics, which describes the study of inheritance as it occurs in human beings. It includes such areas as stem cell research, clinical genetics (e.g., genetic disease markers), and molecular genetics. Inevitably there will be ethical issues that will become manifest in these new areas. We have already had a preview of this in the controversy regarding the use of fetal stem cells versus adult stem cells for research and therapy.

The ethics of modern science is a challenging and evolving area, but it is nothing new. In ancient China, for instance, physician Sun Simiao (580–682 AD) had a difficult medical ethical dilemma. In his book *Qianjinfang (Prescriptions Worth a Thousand Pieces of Gold),* he is credited with formulating the first ethical basis for the practice of medicine in China. The ethical conundrum he faced was the clash between Confucian and Buddhist ethics. The relatively new religion of Buddhism had taboos against using any animal-derived product for the treatment of disease, as this violated the principle of respect for all life. The more ancient Confucian idea of compassion and kindness could be interpreted to overrule this, however.

Sun Simiao dealt with this conflict by prohibiting a "standard physician" from using any medication derived from an animal source. He then included many prescriptions in his book that did have animal-sourced remedies. In other words, he seems to have artfully navigated an ethical gray zone between the two philosophies but with a less than clear distinction between right and wrong. Now in modern times we are still faced with continuing and evolving issues of ethics in the practice of medicine.[103]

GENETIC MARKERS

Genetic markers are genes or DNA sequences with a known location on a chromosome that can be used to identify specific cells and diseases, as well as individuals and species. They are often used to study the relationship between an inherited disease and its genetic cause in order to determine an individual's predisposition/proclivity to a specific disease. Genetic markers show observable information in DNA sequence variation, which may arise as a result of mutation of a specific gene. There are companies that will evaluate a person's DNA for these markers and provide a person with a report of his or her potential health risks. Health insurers, life insurers, employers, and others could potentially use this information to determine one's insurance premiums and even one's job future and so forth. There is going to be ethical issues that will arise. For instance, suppose a woman has a family history of breast cancer and has a genetic marker for it, but she is young (e.g., 30 years old) and free of any evidence of cancer. If a physician recommends prophylactic mastectomy or if the patient wants a prophylactic mastectomy, should this be covered by insurance? Should this same logic be extended to other body organs?

GENETIC INFORMATION NONDISCRIMINATION ACT OF 2008 (HR493)

On May 21, 2008, President George W. Bush signed into law the Genetic Information Nondiscrimination Act (GINA), which resulted largely from the efforts of Senator Ted Kennedy. The law prohibits discrimination on the basis of genetic information with respect to the availability of health insurance and employment. The GINA prohibits group health plans and insurers from denying coverage to a healthy individual or charging that person higher premiums based solely on a genetic predisposition to developing a specific disease (e.g., cancer or heart disease) at some future time. The GINA also prohibits employers from using an individual's genetic information when making hiring, firing, job placement, or promotion decisions.

The relatively recent mapping of the human genome and the likelihood of increasing clinical application of advances in genetic disease markers make this an issue of potential increasing importance in the practice of medicine. Most states also have legislation that addresses this issue. Unfortunately, there remains, no federal legislation that protects the individual from discrimination in the availability of life insurance, disability insurance coverage, or long-term care insurance. Because of this loophole, patients and their doctors need to consider the potential downside of ordering prognostic genetic tests.[104]

STEM CELL RESEARCH

Stem cell research involves the use of embryonic stem cells to create organs and various body tissues. It continues to be a highly controversial issue generally involving religious beliefs and fears as to how far scientists might go in their attempt to create, for example, another human being. Researchers must be free to unlock the secrets that stem cells hold and learn from them with the hope to develop effective therapies.

Some opponents of stem cell research argue that this practice is a slippery slope to reproductive cloning and fundamentally devalues the worth of a human being. Contrarily, some medical researchers in the field argue that it is necessary to pursue embryonic stem cell research because the resultant technologies could have significant medical potential and that excess embryos created for in vitro fertilization could be donated with consent and used for the research. This, in turn, conflicts with opponents in the pro-life movement, who advocate for the protection of human embryos. The ensuing debate has prompted authorities around the world to seek regulatory frameworks and highlighted the fact that embryonic stem cell research represents a social and ethical challenge that includes concern for the natural order of the ecosystem and, ultimately, the survival of the human race.

ACQUIRED IMMUNE DEFICIENCY SYNDROME

NEWS

WHO Issues New HIV Recommendations Calling for Earlier Treatment

GENEVA—New HIV treatment guidelines by WHO recommend offering antiretroviral therapy (ART) earlier. Recent evidence indicates that earlier ART will help people with HIV to live longer, healthier lives, and substantially reduce the risk of transmitting HIV to others. The move could avert an additional 3 million deaths and prevent 3.5 million more new HIV infections between now and 2025.

News Release, World Health Organization, *June 30, 2013*

The epidemic of *acquired immune deficiency syndrome (AIDS)* is considered to be the deadliest epidemic in human history. The first case appeared in the literature in 1981.[105] It has been estimated that more than 35 million people have died of AIDS.

> **Global situation and trends:** Since the beginning of the epidemic, almost 70 million people have been infected with the HIV virus and about 35 million people have died of AIDS. Globally, 34.0 million (31.4–35.9 million) people were living with HIV at the end of 2011. An estimated 0.8% of adults aged 15–49 years worldwide are living with HIV, although the burden of the epidemic continues to vary considerably between countries and regions. Sub-Saharan Africa remains most severely affected, with nearly 1 in every 20 adults (4.9%) living with HIV and accounting for 69% of the people living with HIV worldwide.[106]

AIDS, generally, is accepted as a syndrome—a collection of specific, life-threatening, opportunistic infections and manifestations that are the result of an underlying immune deficiency. AIDS is caused by the human immunodeficiency virus (HIV) and is the most severe form of HIV, a highly contagious blood-borne virus. It is a fatal disease that destroys the body's capacity to ward off bacteria and viruses that ordinarily would be fought off by a properly functioning immune system. Although there is no effective long-term treatment of the disease, indications are that proper management of the disease can improve the quality of life and delay progression of the disease. Internationally, AIDS is posing serious social, ethical, economic, and health problems.

SPREAD OF AIDS

AIDS is spread by direct contact with infected blood or body fluids, such as vaginal secretions, semen, and breast milk. Currently, there is no evidence that the virus can be transmitted through food, water, or casual body contact. HIV does not survive well outside the body. Although there is currently no cure for AIDS, early diagnosis and treatment with new medications can help HIV-infected persons remain healthy for longer periods. High-risk groups include those who have had unprotected sexual encounters, intravenous drug users, and those who require transfusions of blood and blood products, such as hemophiliacs.

Blood Transfusions

The administration of blood is considered to be a medical procedure. It results from the exercise of professional medical judgment that is composed of two parts: (1) diagnosis, deciding the need for blood, and (2) therapy, the actual administration of blood.

Lawsuits often arise as a result of a person with AIDS claiming that he or she contracted the disease as a result of a transfusion of contaminated blood or blood products. In blood transfusion cases, the standards most commonly identified as having been violated concern blood testing and donor screening. An injured party generally must prove that a standard of care existed, that the defendant's conduct fell below the standard, and that this conduct was the proximate cause of the plaintiff's injury.

The most common occurrences that lead to lawsuits in the administration of blood involve:

- Transfusion of mismatched blood
- Improper screening and transfusion of contaminated blood
- Unnecessary administration of blood
- Improper handling procedures (e.g., inadequate refrigeration and storage procedures)

The risk of HIV infection and AIDS through a blood transfusion has been reduced significantly through health history screening and blood donations testing. Since May 1985, all blood donated in the United States has been tested for HIV antibodies. Blood units that do test positive for HIV are removed from the blood transfusion pool.

ADMINISTRATION OF THE WRONG BLOOD

The patient-plaintiff in *Bordelon v. St. Francis Cabrini Hospital* (1994)[107] was admitted to the hospital to undergo a hysterectomy. Before surgery, she provided the hospital with her own blood in case it was needed during surgery. During surgery, the patient did indeed need blood but was administered donor blood other than her own. The patient filed a lawsuit claiming that the hospital's failure to provide her with her own blood resulted in her suffering mental distress.

The court of appeals held that the plaintiff stated a cause of action for mental distress. It is well established in law that a claim for negligent infliction of emotional distress unaccompanied by physical injury is a viable claim of action. It is indisputable that HIV can be transmitted through blood transfusions even when the standard procedure for screening for the virus is in place. The plaintiff's fear was easily associated with receiving someone else's blood and therefore a conceivable consequence of the defendant's negligent act. The hospital had a "duty" to administer the plaintiff's own blood. The hospital breached that duty by administering the wrong blood.

Ethical and Legal Issues

1. Do you agree with the court's decision? Explain your answer.
2. In cases such as this, do you believe that financial awards are effective in preventing future incidents? Explain your answer.

Health Care Workers

HIV test urged for 7,000 Oklahoma dental patients

Health officials are urging 7,000 patients of an Oklahoma dentist to be tested for potential exposure to HIV, hepatitis B and hepatitis C.

• • •

Harrington, an oral surgeon who has been licensed since the 1970s, surrendered his credentials March 20 and discontinued his practice after investigators discovered alleged health and safety violations. Authorities say he is cooperating.

Katharine Lackey and Michael Winter, USA Today, *March 28, 2013*[108]

Although transmission of HIV from an infected dentist, physician, or other caregiver to his or her patient during invasive procedures is not a common occurrence, there is a foreseeable risk. Because of the potentially deadly consequence of such transmission, physicians should not engage in any activity that creates a risk of transmission.

The ever-increasing likelihood that health care workers will come into contact with persons carrying the AIDS virus demands that health care workers comply with approved safety procedures. This is especially important for those who come into contact with blood and body fluids of HIV-infected persons.

An AIDS-infected surgeon in New Jersey was unable to recover on a discrimination claim when the hospital restricted his surgical privileges. In *Estate of Behringer v. Medical Center at Princeton* (1991),[109] the New Jersey Superior Court held that the hospital acted properly in initially suspending a surgeon's surgical privileges, thereafter imposing a requirement of informed consent and ultimately barring the surgeon from performing surgery. The court held that in the context of informed consent, the risk of a surgical accident involving an AIDS-positive surgeon and implications thereof would be a legitimate concern to a surgical patient that would warrant disclosure of the risk. "The 'risk of harm' to the patient includes not only the actual transmission of HIV from the surgeon to patient but the risk of a surgical accident (e.g.., a scalpel cut or needle stick), which may subject the patient to post-surgery HIV testing."[110]

CONFIDENTIALITY

Guidelines drafted by the Centers for Disease Control and Prevention call on health care workers who perform "exposure-prone" procedures to undergo tests voluntarily to determine whether they are infected. The guidelines also recommend that patients be informed. Both health care workers and patients claim that mandatory HIV testing violates their Fourth Amendment right to privacy. The dilemma is how to balance these rights against the rights of the public in general to be protected from a deadly disease.

State laws have been developed that protect the confidentiality of HIV related information. Some states have developed informational brochures and consent, release, and partner notification forms. The unauthorized disclosure of confidential HIV-related information can subject an individual to civil and/or criminal penalties. Information regarding a patient's diagnosis as being HIV positive must be kept confidential and should be shared with other health care professionals only on a need-to-know basis. Each person has a right to privacy as to his or her personal affairs. The plaintiff surgeon in *Estate of Behringer v. Medical Center at Princeton* (1991)[111] was entitled to recover damages from the hospital and its laboratory director for the unauthorized disclosure of his condition during his stay at the hospital. The hospital and the director had breached their duty to maintain confidentiality of the surgeon's medical records by allowing placement of the patient's test results in his medical chart without limiting access to the chart, which they knew was available to the entire hospital community. "The medical center breached its duty of confidentiality to the plaintiff, as a patient, when it failed to take reasonable precautions regarding the plaintiff's medical records to prevent the patient's AIDS diagnosis from becoming a matter of public knowledge."[112]

The hospital in *Tarrant County Hospital District v. Hughes* (1987)[113] was found to have properly disclosed the names and addresses of blood donors in a wrongful death action alleging that a patient contracted AIDS from a blood transfusion administered in the hospital. The physician–patient privilege expressed in the Texas Rules of Evidence did not apply to preclude such disclosure because the record did not reflect that any such relationship had been established. The disclosure was not an impermissible violation of the donors' right of privacy. The societal interest in maintaining an effective blood donor program did not override the plaintiff's right to receive such information. The order prohibited disclosure of the donors' names to third parties.

In *Doe v. University of Cincinnati* (1988),[114] a patient who was infected with HIV-contaminated blood during surgery brought an action against a hospital and a blood bank. The trial court granted the patient's request to discover the identity of the blood donor, and the defendants appealed. The court of appeals held that the potential injury to a donor in revealing his identity outweighed the plaintiff's modest interest in learning of the donor's identity. A blood donor has a constitutional right to privacy not to be identified as a donor of blood that contains HIV. At the time of the plaintiff's blood transfusion in July 1984, no test had been developed to determine the existence of AIDS antibodies. By May 27, 1986, all donors donating blood through the defendant blood bank were tested for the presence of HIV antibodies. Patients who had received blood from donors who tested positive were to be notified through their physicians. In this case, the plaintiff's family was notified because of the plaintiff's age and other disability.

HIV-related regulations must continue to address the rights and responsibilities of both patients and health care workers. Although this will always be a delicate balancing act, it must be handled with privacy, safety, and compassion in mind.

DISCLOSURE OF PHYSICIAN'S HIV STATUS

The physician, Doe, was a resident in obstetrics and gynecology at a medical center. In 1991, he cut his hand with a scalpel while he was assisting another physician. Because of the uncertainty that blood had been transferred from Doe's hand wound to the patient through an open surgical incision, he agreed to have a blood test for HIV. His blood tested positive for HIV, and he withdrew himself from participation in further surgical procedures. The medical center and Harrisburg Hospital, where Doe also participated in surgery, identified those patients who could be at risk. The medical center identified 279 patients, and Harrisburg identified 168 patients, who fell into this category. Because hospital records did not identify those surgeries in which physicians may have accidentally cut themselves, the hospitals filed petitions in the Court of Common Pleas, alleging that there was, under the Confidentiality of HIV-Related Information Act [35 P.S. § 7608(a)(2)], a "compelling need" to disclose information regarding Doe's condition to those patients who conceivably could have been exposed to HIV. Doe argued that there was no compelling need to disclose the information and that he was entitled to confidentiality under the act.

The Pennsylvania Supreme Court held that a compelling need existed for at least a partial disclosure of the physician's HIV status.

The medical experts who testified agreed that there was some risk of exposure and that some form of notice should be given to the patients at risk. Even the expert witness presented by Doe agreed that there was at least some conceivable risk of exposure and that giving a very limited form of notice would not be unreasonable. Failure to notify the patients at risk could result in the spread of the disease to other noninfected individuals through sexual contact and through exposure to other body fluids. Doe's name was not revealed to the patients, only the fact that a resident physician who had participated in their care had tested HIV positive. "No principle is more deeply embedded in the law than that expressed in the maxim Salus populi suprema lex . . . (The welfare of the people is the supreme law), and a more compelling and consistent application of that principle than the one presented would be quite difficult to conceive."[115]

Ethical and Legal Issues

1. Do you agree that there was a need for a partial disclosure of the physician's HIV status?
2. If "the welfare of the people is the supreme law," did the court fall short of its responsibility by not allowing disclosure of the physician's name? Discuss your answer.

News Media and Confidentiality

The Pennsylvania Superior Court in *Stenger v. Lehigh Valley Hospital Center*[116] upheld the Court of Common Pleas' order denying the petition of The Morning Call, Inc., which challenged a court order closing judicial proceedings to the press and public in a civil action against a hospital and physicians. A patient and her family had all contracted AIDS after the patient received a blood transfusion. The access of the media to pretrial discovery proceedings in a civil action is subject to reasonable control by the court in which the action is pending. The protective order limiting public access to pretrial discovery material did not violate the newspaper's First Amendment rights. The discovery documents were not judicial records to which the newspaper had a common-law right of access. Good cause existed for nondisclosure of information about the intimate personal details of the plaintiffs' lives, disclosure of which would cause undue humiliation.

HIV AUTONOMY AND CONFIDENTIALITY

Jones, a divorcee with two children, was sentenced to 10 years in prison for repeated robberies of three banks. He was in prison for 8 years. His wife, Nora, disappeared shortly after he was sentenced. Five of his close inmate friends at Sing Prison had tested positive for the HIV virus and had since passed away. Prison officials wanted to test Jones for the HIV virus. He objected and sought legal counsel. Local school officials were informed of the deaths of Mr. Jones's friends and his refusal to be tested for the HIV virus. Strangely, the community at large became aware of Jones's situation and the fact that his children were attending school with their children. The parents insisted that the Jones kids be removed from school or else they would remove their children from class. Meanwhile, Nora showed up at a local navy recruiting station posing as a single woman with no children. She admitted to being bisexual several years earlier but claimed that she was now straight. The navy learned of this situation and required her to undergo HIV testing. She objected and sought legal counsel.

Ethical and Legal Issues

1. What are Mr. Jones's rights?
2. What are the rights of other prisoners?
3. Is there a legitimate need for a physician to disclose otherwise confidential testing data to the spouse and other intimate sexual partners of an HIV-infected patient?

THE RIGHT TO TREATMENT

A variety of health care organizations have included in their ethics statements that HIV-infected patients have a right not to be discriminated against in the provision of treatment. The Ethics Committee of the American Academy of Dermatology, for example, states "it is unethical for a physician to discriminate against a class or category of patients and to refuse the management of a patient because of medical risk, real or imagined."[117] Patients with HIV infection, therefore, should receive the same compassionate and competent care provided to other patients.

Basketball Camp's Exclusion of HIV-Positive Boy Ruled Discrimination

An HIV-positive 10-year-old boy was discriminated against when he was denied admission to a New York basketball camp, a federal judge has ruled. Judge Donald C. Pogue granted a motion for declaratory relief, finding the camp had violated the Americans with Disabilities Act. "The court agrees that defendants were obligated to protect other campers from a very serious, life-threatening viral infection," Pogue said. "But this obligation does not excuse defendants' actions when based on unsubstantiated fears."

Mark Hamblet, New York Law Journal, *January 22, 2010*

DISCRIMINATION IN THE COMMUNITY

The plaintiff Adam Doe claimed that the defendants, Deer Mountain Day Camp, Inc. (DMDC) and Deer Mountain Basketball Academy (DMBA), discriminated against him by denying him admission to a basketball camp on the basis of his disability, an HIV infection, in violation of the Americans with Disabilities Act (ADA), 42 U.S.C. §§ 12101-213 (2000) (ADA) and the New York State Human Rights Law (NYHRL), N.Y. Exec. Law §§ 290301 (2004) (NYHRL).

Adam had contracted HIV at birth due to a perinatal infection. He took antiretroviral medications to treat his condition, and his syndrome has been undetectable for years. On the advice of Dr. Neu, Adam's HIV specialist, Adam and his mother had kept and continued to keep Adam's HIVseropositivity confidential. Adam liked to play basketball, and in 2004, his HIV clinic recommended that he attend a basketball camp.

Mrs. Doe had been notified that the camp was unable to make reasonable accommodations for Adam and, as a consequence, they could not allow him to attend DMBA. According to Mrs. Doe, she was told that Adam could potentially transmit HIV through blood in his urine or in his stool. Mrs. Doe denied that Adam had problems with bloody stool or urine. Mrs. Doe, however, was told that DMBA could not accept Adam. She later received a refund of Adam's admission fees.

The plaintiff brings this action for violations of Title III of the ADA and the NYHRL, arguing that the defendants unlawfully discriminated against him on the basis of his disability, e.g., his HIV-seropositivity, by excluding him from participation in the basketball camp. To redress his injuries, including emotional and psychological harm, Adam requested declaratory, compensatory, and injunctive relief, as well as attorney's fees and costs.

Both parties made motions for summary judgment. The defendants failed to present any evidence of the objective reasonableness of their determination that the plaintiff's condition posed a threat to other campers.

In their cross motions for summary judgment, the parties placed before the court the issues of whether HIV-seropositivity qualifies as a "disability" and whether defendants' denial of admission constitutes discrimination "on the basis of" that disability. The plaintiff's motion argued that the defendants conclusively qualify as "public accommodations," thus prohibiting them from engaging in such discrimination.

The United States District Court, S.D. of New York, granted the plaintiff's motion for Summary Judgment of ADA and NYHRL declaratory relief, as to DMDC's discrimination "on the basis of" Adam's disability, and denied the defendants' motion for summary judgment in its entirety.[118]

Ethical and Legal Issues

1. Since Adam's HIV syndrome has been undetectable for years, discuss why you agree or disagree with the basketball camp's decision to revoke Adam's registration.
2. Do you agree with the court's ruling? Discuss your answer.

AIDS Education

The ever-increasing likelihood that health care workers will come into contact with persons carrying HIV demands continuing development of and compliance with approved safety procedures. This is especially important for those who come into contact with blood and body fluids of HIV-infected persons. The Centers for Disease Control and Prevention (CDC) expanded its infection control guidelines and has urged hospitals to adopt universal precautions to protect their workers from exposure to patients' blood and other body fluids. Hospitals are following universal precautions in the handling of body fluids, which is the accepted standard for employee protection.

A wide variety of AIDS-related educational materials are available on the market. One of the most important sources of AIDS information is the CDC. The process of staff education in preparing to care for patients with AIDS is extremely important and must include a training program on prevention and transmission in the work setting. Educational requirements specified by the Occupational Safety and Health Administration (OSHA) for health care employees include epidemiology, modes of transmission, preventive practices, and universal precautions. See the following websites for some helpful information: www.aids.gov. and http://www.caps.ucsf.edu/.

CHAPTER REVIEW

1. Ethical dilemmas arises whenever a choice has to be made in which something good has to be given up or something bad has to be suffered no matter what is chosen.
2. Noteworthy historical events (see text at the beginning of the chapter).
3. *Abortion* is the premature termination of a pregnancy, either spontaneous or induced.
   - The morality of abortion is not a legal or constitutional issue; it is a matter of philosophy, ethics, and theology. It is a subject where reasonable people can and do adhere to vastly divergent convictions and principles.
   - *Partial birth abortion* is a late-term abortion that involves partial delivery of the baby prior to its being aborted.
4. *Sterilization* is defined as the termination of the ability to produce offspring.
   - *Therapeutic sterilization* is performed to preserve life or health.

- *Eugenic sterilization* refers to the involuntary sterilization of certain categories of persons described in statutes, without the need for consent by, or on behalf of, those subject to the procedures.
- *Wrongful birth* actions claim that, but for breach of duty by the defendant, a child would not have been born.
- *Wrongful life* suits—those in which a parent or child claims to have suffered harm as a result of being born—are generally unsuccessful.
- *Wrongful conception*/pregnancy actions claim that damages were sustained by the parents of an unexpected child based on the allegation that the child's conception was the result of negligent sterilization procedures or a defective contraceptive device.

5. *Artificial insemination* most often takes the form of the injection of seminal fluid into a woman to induce pregnancy.
   - *Homologous artificial insemination* is when the husband's semen is used in the procedure.
   - *Heterologous artificial insemination* is when the semen is from a donor other than the husband.

6. Surrogacy refers to a method of reproduction whereby a woman agrees to become pregnant for the purpose of gestating and giving birth to a child she will not raise but hand over to a contracted party.

7. Organ donations: Federal regulations require that hospitals have and implement written protocols regarding the organization's organ procurement responsibilities.
   - Organ transplantation is the result of the need for treating patients with end-stage organ disease facing organ failure.
   - Uniform Anatomical Gift Act has many provisions that apply to the wide variety of issues raised in connection with the making, acceptance, and use of anatomical gifts.
     ○ Act allows a person to make a decision to donate organs at the time of death.
     ○ Allows potential donors to carry an anatomical donor card.

8. Research, experimentation, and clinical trials.
   - Ethical principles that are relevant to the ethics of research involving human subjects include respect for person, beneficence, and justice. These principles cannot always be applied to resolve ethical problems beyond dispute. The objective in applying ethical principles is to provide an analytical framework that will guide the resolution of ethical problems arising from research involving human subjects.

9. Human genetics describes the study of inheritance as it occurs in human beings.
   - The Genetic Information Nondiscrimination Act (GINA) prohibits discrimination on the basis of genetic information with respect to the availability of health insurance and employment.

10. Stem cell research is being conducted to create tissues and organs that can be matched to patients for transplant.
    - Genetic markers are genes or DNA sequences that have a known location on chromosomes and can be associated with particular genes or traits.

11. *Acquired immune deficiency syndrome* is a fatal disease that destroys the body's ability to fight bacteria and viruses.
    - Concerns involve the spread of AIDS, issues of confidentiality, discrimination, and AIDS education.

TEST YOUR UNDERSTANDING

TERMINOLOGY

abortion	institutional review board	surrogacy
AIDS	partial birth abortion	therapeutic sterilization
artificial insemination	paternalism	undue burden
elective sterilization	reasonable man standard	Uniform Anatomical Gift Act
ethical dilemma	*Roe v. Wade*	wrongful birth
eugenic sterilization	stem cell research	wrongful conception
genetic marker	sterilization	wrongful life

REVIEW QUESTIONS

1. Discuss under what circumstances ethical dilemmas arise.

2. Discuss the controversy over the Supreme Court decision in *Roe v. Wade*.

3. What ethical principles surround the abortion issue? Discuss these principles.

4. Do you agree that individual states should be able to impose reasonable restrictions or waiting periods on women seeking abortions? Who should determine what is reasonable?

5. Should a married woman be allowed to abort without her husband's consent?

6. Discuss the arguments for and against partial birth abortions.

7. Why is the medical issue of abortion an example of legislating morality?

8. What is artificial insemination? What questions should be asked when considering artificial insemination?

9. Discuss the importance of organ donations.

10. Describe the ethical considerations that should be addressed before conducting research on human subjects.

11. Why is it important that written consent be obtained from each patient who participates in a clinical trial?

12. What is sterilization, as discussed in this chapter? Do you agree that eugenic sterilization should be allowed? Explain your answer.

13. Describe the distinctions among wrongful birth, wrongful life, and wrongful conception. Discuss the moral dilemmas of these concepts.

14. Describe the controversy over surrogacy.

15. Discuss why there is controversy over genetic markers and stem cell research.

16. What is AIDS, and how is it spread?

17. Discuss the controversy that can occur when considering a patient's right to know whether a caregiver has AIDS and the caregiver's right to privacy and confidentiality.

NOTES

1. *Union Pac. Ry. Co. v. Botsford,* 141 U.S. 250, 251 (1891).
2. http://www.encyclopedia.com/doc/1G2-3406300011.html/
3. http://www.remember.org/educate/medexp.html/
4. http://www.ushmm.org/wlc/en/article.php?ModuleId=10007069.
5. http://www.wma.net/en/30publications/10policies/c8/.
6. "First Successful Kidney Transplant Performed," PBS.org, http://www.pbs.org/wgbh/aso/databank/entries/dm54ki.html.
7. http://www.ncbi.nlm.nih.gov/pmc/articles/PMC1154799/.
8. "Protection and Use of Human Subjects," Eastern Michigan University,
9. "Issues and Concepts," Ascension Health, http://www.ascensionhealth.org/ethics/public/ issues/harvard.asp.
10. https://kennedyinstitute.georgetown.edu/.
11. 464 F.2d 772 (D.C. Cir. 1972).
12. http://www.lawandbioethics.com/demo/Main/LegalResources/C5/Canterbury.htm.
13. http://caselaw.lp.findlaw.com/scripts/getcase.pl?court=us&vol=410&invol=113.
14. http://www.hhs.gov/ohrp/humansubjects/guidance/belmont.html.
15. *Id.*
16. *In re Quinlan,* 70 N.J.10, 355 A.2d 647 (N.J. 1976).
17. United States Code, Title 42—The Public Health and Welfare, Chapter 6A—Public Health Service, Subchapter XVI—President's Commission for the Study of Ethical Problems in Medicine and Biomedical and Behavior Research, Section 300v-1, http://caselaw.lp.findlaw.com/casecode/uscodes/42/chapters/6a/subchapters/xvi/sections/section_300v-1.html.
18. http://assistedsuicide.org/farewell-to-hemlock.html.
19. http://ag.ca.gov/consumers/pdf/ProbateCodeAdvancedHealthCareDirectiveForm-fillable.pdf.
20. http://www.compassionandchoices.org/who-we-are/timeline/.
21. http://www.compassionandchoices.org/who-we-are/about/.
22. 42 U.S.C. 1395cc(a)(1).
23. *Cruzan v. Director of the Mo. Dep't of Health,* 497 U.S. 261 (1990).
24. *Id.*
25. http://www.usconstitution.net/xconst_Am1.html
26. *DeGrella v. Elston,* 858 S.W.2d 698 (1993).
27. http://www.animalresearch.info/en/medical-advances/151/cloning-dolly-the-sheep/.
28. http://jama.jamanetwork.com/article.aspx?articleid=193273.
29. "Biological Sciences," Intute, http://bioresearch.ac.uk/browse/mesh/C0020125L0020125.html.
30. State of Oregon v. Ashcroft, No. 02-35587 (C.A. 9, Ore. 2004).
31. http://unesdoc.unesco.org/images/0013/001359/135928e.pdf.
32. Gonzales v. Oregon, 04-623.
33. Death with Dignity National Center, "Legal and Political Timeline in Oregon,"http://www.deathwithdignity.org/in-oregon.
34. http://donatelifecalifornia.org/livingdonationcalifornia/.

35. English Clergy, Dean of Westminster.

36. *Causeway Medical Suite v. Ieyoub,* 109 F.3d 1096 (1997).

37. 410 U.S. 113 (1973).

38. *Id.* at 164.

39. *Id.*

40. *Id.*

41. *Id.*

42. 410 U.S. 179 (1973).

43. *Id.* at 198.

44. 103 S. Ct. 2481 (1983).

45. *Planned Parenthood v. Casey,* 112 S. Ct. 2792 (1992).

46. 432 U.S. 438 (1977).

47. 432 U.S. 464 (1977).

48. 448 U.S. 297 (1980).

49. *Committee to Defend Reproductive Rights v. Myers,* 625 P.2d 779, 798 (Cal. 1981).

50. 56 P.3d 28 (Ariz. 2002).

51. 111 S. Ct. 1759 (1991).

52. Poe v. Gerstein, 517 F.2d 787 (5th Cir. 1975).

53. 405 F. Supp. 534 (M.D. Pa. 1975).

54. 486 U.S. 1308 (1988).

55. 428 U.S. 52 (1976).

56. 443 U.S. 622 (1979).

57. 533 A.2d 523 (R.I. 1987).

58. 101 S. Ct. 1164 (1981).

59. 515 So. 2d 1254 (Ala. Civ. App. 1987).

60. 107 F. Supp. 1254 (Ala. Civ. App. 1987).

61. 99 S. Ct. 675 (1979).

62. 492 U.S. 490 (1989).

63. 118 S. Ct. 1347 (1998).

64. 437 F.3d. 278 (C.A. N.Y. 2006).

65. 112 S. Ct. 2791 (1992).

66. 844 F. Supp. 1482 (D. Utah 1994).

67. 844 F. Supp. 1482 (D. Utah 1994) at 1494.

68. *American Acad. of Pediatrics v. Lungren,* 940 P.2d 797 (1997).

69. http://www.huffingtonpost.com/joseph-b-kadane/moral-persuasion-on-abortion_b_4004735.html

70. 224 U.S. 200 (1927).

71. 337 F. Supp. 671 (E.D. Ohio 1971).

72. *McKinney v. McKinney,* 805 S.W.2d 66 (Ark. 1991).

73. 165 Cal. Rptr. 477 (Cal. Ct. App. 1980).

74. *Chaffee v. Seslar,* 786 N.E.2d 705 (2003).

75. 730 A.2d 806 (N.J. 1999).

76. *Id.* at 18.

77. *Smith v. Cote,* 513 A.2d 344 (N.H. 1986).

78. *Id.* at 353.

79. 718 P.2d 635 (Kan. 1986).

80. 136 Md. App. 38 (2002).

81. *Cowe v. Forum Group, Inc.,* 575 N.E.2d 630, 631 (Ind. 1991).

82. 707 F.2d 1544 (D.C. Cir. 1983).

83. *Id.* at 1557.
84. 805 P.2d 603 (N.M. 1991).
85. *Id.* at 612.
86. 582 A.2d 1384 (Pa. Super. Ct. 1990).
87. *Id.* at 1385.
88. 11 Pa. D. & C.2d 41, 46 (Lycoming Co. Ct. Com. Pl. 1957).
89. http://www.mbc.ca.gov/About_Us/Media_Room/2011/news_releases_2011.pdf
90. Okla. Stat. Ann. 10, §§ 551–553.
91. *Id.*
92. *Id.*
93. http://www.organdonor.gov/becomingdonor/index.html?utm_source=bing&utm_medium=cpc&utm_camp.aign=2013+Sign+Up
94. U.S. Dept. of Health & Human Services, Task Force on Organ Donation and Transplantation (1986). http://www.pbs.org/wgbh/aso/databank/entries/dm54ki.html
95. 519 N.Y.S.2d 928 (N.Y. Sup. Ct. 1987).
96. http://www.fda.gov/ScienceResearch/SpecialTopics/RunningClinicalTrials/ucm155713.htm#FDARegulations.
97. Mary Ellen Stokes and Bill Stokes, "Relentless Assault on a Research Hospital," Wall Street Journal, March 15, 2004, at A17.
98. 2 C.F.R. § 488.115 (1989).
99. *Id.*
100. *Id.*
101. *Blaz v. Michael Reese Hosp. Found,* 74 F. Supp. 2d 803 (D.C. Ill. 1999).
102. http://www.cc.nih.gov/participate/patientinfo/legal/responsibilities.shtml.
103. Yuanyi S. Chun, *History of Medicine* (Wuhan, China, 1988).
104. National Human Genome Research Institute, http://www.genome.gov.
105. Cantwell, *AIDS: The Mystery and the Solution* (Los Angeles: Aries Rising Press, 1986), at 54.
106. http://www.who.int/gho/hiv/en/index.html.
107. 640 So. 2d 476 (La. App. 3d Cir. 1994).
108. http://www.usatoday.com/story/news/nation/2013/03/28/hiv-oklahoma-dentist/2028865/.
109. 592 A.2d 1251 (N.J. Super. Ct. Law Div. 1991).
110. *Id.* at 1255.
111. 592 A.2d 1251 (N.J. Super. Ct. Law Div. 1991).
112. *Id.* at 1255.
113. 734 S.W.2d 675 (Tex. Ct. App. 1987).
114. 538 N.E.2d 419 (Ohio Ct. App. 1988).
115. Application of Milton S. Hershey Med. Ctr., 639 A.2d 159, 163 (Pa. 1993).
116. 554 A.2d 954 (Pa. Super. Ct. 1989).
117. Ethics Committee of the American Academy of Dermatology, Ethics in Medical Practice, 1992, at 6.
118. *Doe v. Deer Mountain Day Camp, Inc.; Deer Mountain Basketball Academy* 682 F. Supp. 2d 324 (2010).

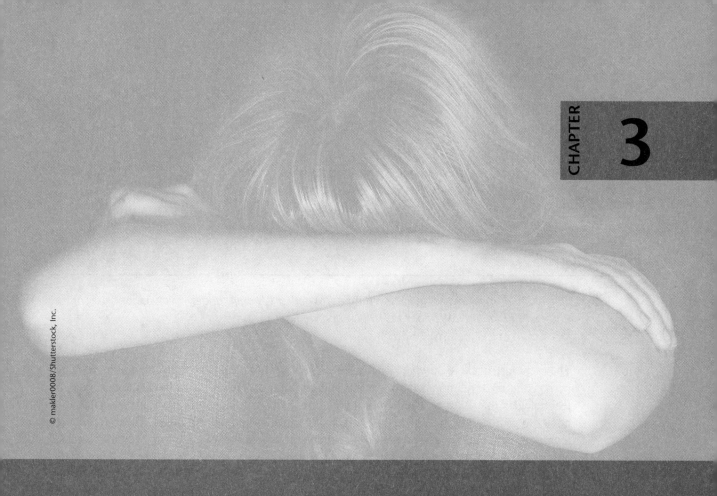

END-OF-LIFE DILEMMAS

When we finally know we are dying, and all other sentient beings are dying with us, we start to have a burning, almost heartbreaking sense of the fragility and preciousness of each moment and each being, and from this can grow a deep, clear, limitless compassion for all beings.

—SOGYAL RINPOCHE

LEARNING OBJECTIVES

Upon completion of this chapter, the reader will be able to:

- Describe the human struggle to survive.
- Discuss end-of-life issues, including:
  - Euthanasia
  - Right to self-determination
  - Defining death

- Legislative response
- Assisted suicide
- Patient Self-Determination Act of 1990
- Advance directives (e.g., living will, durable power of attorney)
- Futility of treatment
- Withholding and withdrawal of treatment

INTRODUCTION

One of the hardest lessons in life is letting go. Whether it's guilt, anger, love, loss or betrayal. Change is never easy. We fight to hold on and we fight to let go.

— SHERRY JONES

The human struggle to survive and dreams of immortality have been instrumental in pushing humankind to develop means to prevent and cure illness. Advances in medicine and related technologies that have resulted from human creativity and ingenuity have given society the power to prolong life; however, the process of dying also can be prolonged. Those victims of long-term pain and suffering, as well as patients in vegetative states and irreversible comas, are the most directly affected.

The struggle to survive and a family's inability to let go is as real today as when Methuselah, a descendant of Adam, passed away at the age of 969 (Genesis 5:27). Most likely Methuselah's family had a great deal of pain as they observed his passing. At the time of this writing, the family of 13-year-old Jahi McMath's continues their struggle to hold on, as she lapsed into a coma following a tonsillectomy and physicians determined she was brain dead.

Brain-Dead Girl Jahi McMath Released from California Hospital

Jahi McMath is no longer inside the hospital where doctors declared her brain-dead after tonsil surgery last month.

• • •

"We're very relieved that she got safely to where she needed to be, because we were all very afraid, given the fragile condition as she wasted away at Children's, that she might not make it," attorney Chris Dolan told reporters Monday.

The move ends one chapter of a weeks-long struggle between the hospital, which sought to remove Jahi from a ventilator after doctors and a judge concluded she was brain-dead, and her relatives, who fought in court to keep her on the ventilator and contended she showed signs of life.

Ed Payne. Catherine E. Shoichet, and Jason Hanna, CNN Health, *January 7, 2014*[1]

Rather than watching hopelessly as a disease destroys a person or as a body part malfunctions, causing death to a patient, physicians now can implant artificial body organs. Exotic machines (e.g., ventilators) and antibiotics are weapons in a physician's arsenal to help extend a patient's life. Such situations have generated vigorous debate. This chapter reviews many of the issues that inevitably arise as one approaches the end of life.

End of Life or Beginning of Life?

My mother is 92 years old, and she is more active and is enjoying life more than when she was much younger. Her advanced age has actually proven to be something of an advantage, as it has given her the time and freedom to do some of the things she couldn't do while she was raising a family. It has been a joy to me, as her son, and to the rest of the family to witness her joy and vigor. Even strangers have found her stamina to be an inspiration as to the value of the end years of life. Three years ago, however, it wasn't so. Mother was critically ill, comatose on a respirator in an intensive care unit. Survival was not considered likely. I am embarrassed to say that I was making arrangements for a funeral. I am even more embarrassed because I am a physician and did not see how she could survive for long except as a vegetable. Then the unlikely occurred. She recovered! Her condition, including both physical and mental status, rapidly and surprisingly improved dramatically and she promptly resumed a life even more active than before. It would have been a tragedy to deprive her of these joyous years of her life after she worked and sacrificed so much for others most of her life. I had thought it would be an act of mercy to disconnect the respirator when her condition had looked so hopeless. I was so wrong. I learned that we must not make life and death decisions casually. Life is a beautiful mystery with many wonderful surprises if we will let them happen.

Advances in medical technology have made it possible to survive to an older age. That longer survival inevitably involves considerable cost and can therefore be a substantial financial burden to the family and the government. Is it worth it? How do we make a judgment about quality of life? What is the financial value of another day, week, or year of life? Should we assume that younger years are better than older years? Although our bodies may physically decline over time, our treasure trove of life experiences accrues over time. Our knowledge and judgment may often be better than when we were younger. Furthermore, the aged may be a source of comfort and joy to their children, grandchildren, and even great-grandchildren. As long as we are alive, we have value.

Physician

EUTHANASIA

There is nothing more sacred than life and there is nothing more natural in life to wish to cling on to it for those you love! And nothing more cruel than to play god by artificially holding onto that which god wants to bring home.

–Author Unknown

When patients and their families perceive a deterioration of the quality of life with no end in sight, conflict often arises between health care professionals, who are trained to save lives, and patients and their families, who wish to hold on to their loved ones. This conflict centers on the concept of euthanasia and its place in the modern world. There seems to be an absence of controversy only when a patient who is kept alive by modern technology is still able to appreciate and maintain control over his or her life.

Any discussion of euthanasia obliges a person to confront humanity's greatest fear—death. The courts and legislatures have faced it and have made advances in setting forth some guidelines to assist decision makers in this arena; however, much more must be accomplished. Society must be protected from the risks associated with permitting the removal of life-support systems. Society cannot allow the complex issues associated with this topic to be simplified to the point where it is accepted that life can be terminated based on subjective quality-of-life considerations. The legal system must ensure that the constitutional rights of the patient are maintained, while protecting society's interests in preserving life, preventing suicide, and maintaining the integrity of the medical profession. For example, can competent adult patients who ask that no extraordinary lifesaving measures be taken recover damages for finding themselves alive after unwanted resuscitative measures? During a medical emergency, it seems unrealistic to ask a caregiver to first look in a patient's medical record for an advance directive before tending to the immediate needs of the patient. In the final analysis, the boundaries of patient rights often remain uncertain.

From its inception, euthanasia has evolved into an issue with competing legal, medical, and moral implications that continues to generate debate, confusion, and conflict. Currently, there is a strong movement advocating death with dignity, which excludes machines, monitors, and tubes.

Even the connotation of the word "euthanasia" has changed with time depending on who is attempting to define it. Euthanasia originated from the Greek word *euthanatos*, meaning "good death" or "easy death," was accepted in situations where people had what was considered to be incurable diseases. *Euthanasia* is defined broadly as "the mercy killing of the hopelessly ill, injured, or incapacitated."[2]

In the Confucian and Buddhist religions, suicide was an acceptable answer to unendurable pain and incurable disease. The Celtics went a step further, believing that those who chose to die of disease or senility, rather than committing suicide, would be condemned to Hell. Such acceptance began to change during the 1800s when Western physicians refused to lessen suffering by shortening a dying patient's life. Napoleon's physician, for example, rejected Napoleon's plea to kill plague-stricken soldiers, insisting that his obligation was to cure rather than kill people.

In the late 1870s, writings on euthanasia began to appear, mainly in England and the United States. Although such works were written, for the most part, by lay authors, the public and the medical community began to consider the issues raised by euthanasia. Then defined as "the act or practice of painlessly putting to death persons suffering from incurable conditions or diseases," it was considered to be a merciful release from incurable suffering. By the beginning of the 20th century, however, there were still no clear answers or guidelines regarding the use of euthanasia. Unlike in prior centuries when society as a whole supported or rejected euthanasia, different segments of today's society apply distinct connotations to the word, generating further confusion. Some believe euthanasia is meant to allow a painless death when one suffers from an incurable disease yet is not dying. Others, who remain in the majority, perceive euthanasia as an instrument to aid only dying people in ending their lives with as little suffering as possible.

It has been estimated that of the 2 million Americans who die each year, 80% die in hospitals or nursing homes, and 70% of those die after a decision to forgo life-sustaining treatment has been made. Although such decisions are personal in nature and based on individual moral values, they must comply with the laws applicable to the prolonging of the dying process. Courts have outlined the ways in which the government is allowed to participate in the decision-making process. Yet the misconceptions and lack of clear direction regarding the policies and procedures have resulted in wide disparity among jurisdictions, both in legislation and in judicial decisions. As a result, the American Medical Association, the American Bar Association, legislators, and judges are actively attempting to formulate and legislate clear guidelines in this sensitive, profound, and not yet fully understood area. To ensure compliance with the law while serving the needs of their patients, it is incumbent on health care providers to keep themselves informed of regulatory requirements in this ever-changing field.

ACTIVE OR PASSIVE EUTHANASIA

Active euthanasia is commonly understood to be the intentional commission of an act, such as providing a patient a lethal dose of a medication that results in death. The act, if committed by the patient, is thought of as suicide. Moreover, because in most states the patient cannot take his or her own life, any person who assists in the causing of the death could be subject to criminal sanction for aiding and abetting suicide.

Passive euthanasia occurs when lifesaving treatment (such as a respirator) is withdrawn or withheld, allowing the terminally ill patient to die a natural death. Passive euthanasia is generally accepted pursuant to legislative acts and judicial decisions. These decisions, however, generally are based on the facts of a particular case.

The distinctions are important when considering the duty and liability of a physician who must decide whether to continue or initiate treatment of a comatose or terminally ill patient. Physicians are obligated to use reasonable care to preserve health and to save lives, and, thus, unless fully protected by the law, they will be reluctant, for example, to abide by a patient's or family's wishes to terminate life-support devices.

Although there may be a duty to provide life-sustaining equipment in the immediate aftermath of cardiopulmonary arrest, there is no duty to continue its use after it has become futile and ineffective to do so in the opinion of qualified medical personnel. An example is a patient who suffered severe brain damage, placing him in a comatose and vegetative state, from which, according to tests and examinations by other specialists, he was unlikely to recover. The patient, on the written request of his family, was taken off life-support equipment. The patient's family (his wife and eight children) made the decision together after consultation with the physicians. Evidence had been presented that the patient, before his incapacitation, had expressed to his wife that he would not want to be kept alive by a machine. Decisions by family members are based on love and concern for the dignity of their loved one [*Barber v. Superior Court*, 147 Cal. App. 3d 1006 (Cal. Ct. App. 1983)].

The controversy over euthanasia is a common issue throughout the world. Belgium, for example, legalized the practice of euthanasia for adults in 2002 and is at this writing considering legalizing euthanasia for children.

Belgium Considering New Euthanasia Law for Kids

Should children have the right to ask for their own deaths?

In Belgium, where euthanasia is now legal for people over the age of 18, the government is considering extending it to children—something that no other country has done. The same bill would offer the right to die to adults with early dementia.

Advocates argue that euthanasia for children, with the consent of their parents, is necessary to give families an option in a desperately painful situation. But opponents have questioned whether children can reasonably decide to end their own lives.

Maria Cheng, News Daily, *October 31, 2013*[3]

VOLUNTARY OR INVOLUNTARY EUTHANASIA

Both active and passive euthanasia may be either voluntary or involuntary. *Voluntary euthanasia* occurs when a person suffering an incurable illness makes the decision to die. To be considered voluntary, the request or consent must be made by a legally competent adult and be based on material information concerning the possible ramifications and alternatives available.

Involuntary euthanasia, however, occurs when the decision to terminate the life of an incurable person (e.g., an incompetent or nonconsenting competent person) is made by someone other than that incurable person.

A patient's lack of consent can be due to mental impairment or a comatose state. Important value questions face courts struggling with the boundaries for making voluntary euthanasia decisions:

- Who should decide to withhold or withdraw treatment?
- On what factors should the decision be based?
- Are there viable standards to guide the courts?
- Should criminal sanctions be imposed on a person assisting in ending a life?
- When does death occur?

RIGHT TO SELF-DETERMINATION

To analyze the important questions regarding whether life-support treatment can be withheld or withdrawn from an incompetent patient, it is necessary to consider first what rights a competent patient possesses. Both statutory law and case law have presented a diversity of policies and points of view. Some courts point to common law and the early case of *Schloendorff v. Society of New York Hospital*[4] to support their belief in a patient's right to self-determination. The *Schloendorff* court stated:[5]

> Every human being of adult years has a right to determine what shall be done with his own body; and the surgeon who performs an operation without his patient's consent commits an assault for which he is liable for damages.

This right of self-determination was emphasized in *In re Storar*[6] when the court announced that every human being of adult years and sound mind has the right to determine what shall be done with his or her own body. The *Storar* case was a departure from the New Jersey Supreme Court's rationale in the case of *In re Quinlan*.[7] The *Quinlan* case was the first to address significantly the issue of whether euthanasia should be permitted when a patient is terminally ill. The *Quinlan* court, relying on *Roe v. Wade*,[8] announced that the constitutional right to privacy protects a patient's right to self-determination. The court noted that the right to privacy "is broad enough to encompass a patient's decision to decline medical treatment under certain circumstances, in much the same way as it is broad enough to encompass a woman's decision to terminate pregnancy under certain conditions."[9]

The *Quinlan* court, in reaching its decision, applied a test balancing the state's interest in preserving and maintaining the sanctity of human life against Karen Quinlan's privacy interest. It decided that, especially in light of the prognosis (physicians determined that Quinlan was in an irreversible coma), the state's interest did not justify interference with her right to refuse treatment. Thus, Karen Quinlan's father was appointed her legal guardian, and the respirator was shut off.

In the same year as the *Quinlan* decision, the case of *Superintendent of Belchertown State School v. Saikewicz*[10] was decided. There, the court, using the balancing test enunciated in *Quinlan*, approved the recommendation of a court-appointed guardian ad litem that it would be in Saikewicz's best interests to end chemotherapy treatment. Saikewicz was a mentally retarded, 67-year-old patient suffering from leukemia. The court found from the evidence that the prognosis was dim, and even though a "normal person" would probably have chosen chemotherapy, it allowed Saikewicz to die without treatment to spare him the suffering.

Although the court also followed the reasoning of the *Quinlan* opinion in giving the right to an incompetent person to refuse treatment, based on either the objective "best interests" test or the subjective "substituted judgment" test, which it favored because Saikewicz always had been incompetent, the court departed from *Quinlan* in a major way. It rejected the *Quinlan* approach of entrusting a decision concerning the continuance of artificial life support to the patient's guardian, family, attending physicians, and a hospital ethics committee. The *Saikewicz* court asserted that even though a judge might find the opinions of physicians, medical experts, or hospital ethics committees helpful in reaching a decision, there should be no requirement to seek out the advice. The court decided that questions of life and death with regard to an incompetent person should be the responsibility of the courts, which would conduct detached but passionate investigations. The court took a "dim view of any attempt to shift the ultimate decision-making responsibility away from duly established courts of proper jurisdiction to any committee, panel, or group, ad hoc or permanent."[11]

This main point of difference between the *Saikewicz* and *Quinlan* cases marked the emergence of two different policies on the incompetent person's right to refuse treatment. One line of cases has followed *Saikewicz* and supports court approval before physicians are allowed to withhold or withdraw life support. Advocates of this view argue that it makes more sense to leave the decision to an objective tribunal than to extend the right of a patient's privacy to a number of interested parties, as was done in *Quinlan*. They also attack the *Quinlan* method as being a privacy decision effectuated by popular vote.[12]

Six months after *Saikewicz*, the Massachusetts Appeals Court narrowed the need for court intervention in *In re Dinnerstein*[13] by finding that "no code" orders are valid to prevent the use of artificial resuscitative measures on incompetent terminally ill patients. The court was faced with the case of a 67-year-old woman who was suffering from Alzheimer's disease. It was determined that she was permanently comatose at the time of trial. Furthermore, the court decided that *Saikewicz*-type judicial proceedings should take place only when medical treatment could offer a reasonable expectation of effecting a permanent or temporary cure of or relief from the illness.

The Massachusetts Supreme Judicial Court attempted to clarify its *Saikewicz* opinion with regard to court orders in *In re Spring*.[14] The court here held that different factors such as the patient's mental status and his or her medical prognosis with or without treatment must be considered before judicial approval is necessary to withdraw or withhold treatment from an incompetent patient. The problem in all three cases is that there is still no clear guidance as to exactly when the court's approval of the removal of life-support systems would be necessary. *Saikewicz* seemed to demand judicial approval in every case. *Spring*, however, in partially retreating from that view, stated that it did not have to articulate what combination of the factors it discussed, thus making prior court approval necessary.

The inconsistencies presented by the Massachusetts cases led courts since 1977 to follow the parameters set by *Quinlan*, requiring judicial intervention. In cases in which physicians have certified the irreversible nature of a patient's loss of consciousness, an ethics committee (actually a neurologic team) could certify the patient's hopeless neurologic condition. Then a guardian would be free to take the legal steps necessary to remove life-support systems. The main reason for the appointment of a guardian is to ensure that incompetent patients, like all other patients, maintain their right to refuse treatment. Most holdings indicate that because a patient has the constitutional right of self-determination, those acting on the patient's behalf can exercise that right when rendering their best judgment concerning how the patient would assert the right. This substituted judgment doctrine could be argued on standing grounds, whereby a second party has the right to assert the constitutional rights of another when that second party's intervention is necessary to protect the other's constitutional rights. The guardian's decision is sounder if it is based on the known desires of a patient who was competent immediately before becoming comatose.

An advance directive, such as a living will, is persuasive evidence of an incompetent person's wishes. An incompetent patient can act as a guardian and in accordance with the terms of a living will. An agent can substitute his or her judgment for that of the patient.

A court may require the attending physician to certify that a patient is in a permanent vegetative state, with no reasonable chance for recovery, before a family member or guardian can request termination of extraordinary means of medical treatment.

The decision maker would attempt to ascertain the incompetent patient's actual interests and preferences. A court can appoint a guardian if:[15]

- family members disagree as to the incompetent person's wishes.
- physicians disagree on the prognosis.
- the patient's wishes cannot be known because he or she has always been incompetent.
- evidence exists of wrongful motives or malpractice.
- no family member can serve as a guardian.

DEFINING DEATH

When is a patient considered to be legally dead, and what type of treatment can be withheld or withdrawn? Most cases dealing with euthanasia speak of the necessity for a physician to diagnose a patient as being either in a persistent vegetative state or terminally ill.

Traditionally, the definition of death adopted by the courts has been according to *Black's Law Dictionary*: "cessation of respiration, heartbeat, and certain indications of central nervous system activity, such as respiration and pulsation."[16] Currently, however, modern science has the capacity to sustain vegetative functions of those in irreversible comas. Machinery can sustain heartbeat and respiration even in the face of brain death. It is now generally accepted that the irreversible cessation of brain function constitutes death.

Ethicists who advocate the prohibition on taking action to shorten life agree "where death is imminent and inevitable, it is permissible to forgo treatments that would only provide a precarious and painful prolongation of life, as long as the normal care due to the sick person in similar cases is not interrupted."[17]

Relying on the 1968 Harvard Criteria set forth by the Ad Hoc Committee of the Harvard Medical School to Examine the Definition of Brain Death, the American Medical Association in 1974 accepted that death occurs when there is "irreversible cessation of all brain functions including the brain stem."[18] Most states now recognize brain death by statute or judicial decision. New York, for example, in *People v. Eulo*,[19] in rejecting the traditional cardiopulmonary definition of death, announced that the determination of brain death can be made according to acceptable medical standards. The court also repeated its holding in *In re Storar*[20] that clear and convincing evidence of a person's desire to decline extraordinary medical care may be honored and that a third person may not exercise this judgment on behalf of a person who has not expressed or cannot express the desire to decline treatment.

Some courts hold that artificial nutrition can be withheld from a patient who is unable to converse or feed ones-self. Unequivocal proof of a patient's wishes will suffice when the decision to terminate life support is at issue. Factors for determining the existence of clear and convincing evidence of a patient's intention to reject the prolongation of life by artificial means include the:

1. persistence of statements regarding an individual's beliefs.
2. desirability of the commitment to those beliefs.
3. seriousness with which such statements were made.
4. inferences that may be drawn from the surrounding circumstances.

The family of a patient who is in a persistent vegetative state cannot necessarily order physicians to remove artificial nutrition. In 1983, Nancy Cruzan sustained injuries in a car accident in which her car overturned, after which she was found face down in a ditch without respiratory or cardiac function. Although the patient was unconscious, her breathing and heartbeat were restored at the site of the accident. After examining her at the hospital, a neurosurgeon diagnosed her as having suffered cerebral contusions and anoxia. It was estimated that she had been deprived of oxygen for 12 to 14 minutes. After remaining in a coma for 3 weeks, Cruzan went into an unconscious state. At first she was able to ingest some food orally. Thereafter, surgeons implanted a gastrostomy feeding and hydration tube, with the consent of her husband, to facilitate feeding her. She did not improve, and until December 1990, she lay in a Missouri state hospital in a persistent vegetative state that was determined to be irreversible, permanent, progressive, and ongoing. She was not dead, according to the accepted definition of death in Missouri, and physicians estimated that she could live in the vegetative state for an additional 30 years. Because of the prognosis, Cruzan's parents asked the hospital staff to cease all artificial nutrition and hydration procedures. The staff refused to comply with their wishes without court approval. The state trial court granted authorization for termination, finding that Cruzan had a fundamental right—grounded in both the state and federal constitutions—to refuse or direct the withdrawal of death-prolonging procedures. Testimony at trial from a former roommate of Cruzan indicated to the court that she had stated that if she were ever sick or injured she would not want to live unless she could live halfway normally. The court interpreted that conversation, which had taken place when Cruzan was 25 years old, as meaning that she would not want to be forced to take nutrition and hydration while in a persistent vegetative state.

The case was appealed to the Missouri Supreme Court, which reversed the lower court decision. The court not only doubted that the doctrine of informed consent applied to the circumstances of the case, it moreover would not recognize a broad privacy right from the state constitution that would support the right of a person to refuse medical treatment in every circumstance. Because Missouri recognizes living wills, the court held that Cruzan's parents were not entitled to order the termination of her treatment because "no person can assume that choice for an incompetent person in the absence of the formalities required under Missouri's Living Will statutes or the clear and convincing, inherently reliable evidence absent here."[21] The court found that Cruzan's statements to her roommate did not rise to the level of clear and convincing evidence of her desire to end nutrition and hydration.

In June 1990, the U.S. Supreme Court after hearing oral arguments held that:[22]

1. the U.S. Constitution does not forbid Missouri from requiring that there be clear and convincing evidence of an incompetent person's wishes as to the withdrawal of life-sustaining treatment.
2. the Missouri Supreme Court did not commit constitutional error in concluding that evidence adduced at trial did not amount to clear and convincing evidence of Cruzan's desire to cease hydration and nutrition.
3. due process did not require the state to accept the substituted judgment of close family members, absent substantial proof that their views reflected those of the patient.

In delivering the opinion of the court, Justice William Rehnquist noted that although most state courts have applied the common-law right to informed consent or a combination of that right and a privacy right when allowing a right to refuse treatment, the Supreme Court analyzed the issues presented in the *Cruzan* case in terms of a Fourteenth Amendment liberty interest. They found that a competent person has a constitutionally protected right grounded in the due process clause to refuse lifesaving hydration and nutrition. Missouri provided for the incompetent patient by allowing a surrogate to act for the patient in choosing to withdraw hydration and treatment. Moreover, it put into place procedures to ensure that the surrogate's action conforms to the wishes expressed by the patient when he or she was competent. Although recognizing that Missouri had enacted a restrictive law, the Supreme Court held that right-to-die issues should be decided pursuant to state law, subject to a due process liberty interest, and in keeping with state constitutional law. After the Supreme Court rendered its decision, the Cruzans returned to Missouri probate court, where on November 14, 1990,

Judge Charles Teel authorized physicians to remove the feeding tubes from Cruzan. The judge determined that testimony presented to him early in November demonstrated clear and convincing evidence that Nancy would not have wanted to live in a persistent vegetative state. Several of her coworkers had testified that she told them before her accident that she would not want to live "like a vegetable." On December 26, 1990, 2 weeks after her feeding tubes were removed, Nancy Cruzan died.

LEGISLATIVE RESPONSE

After the Cruzan decision, states began to draft new legislation in the areas of living wills, durable powers of attorney, health care proxies, and surrogate decision making. Pennsylvania and Florida were two of the first states to react to the *Cruzan* decision. Pennsylvania law is applied to terminally ill or permanently unconscious patients. The statute, the Advance Directive for Health Care Act,[23] deals mainly with individuals who have prepared living wills. It includes in its definition of life-sustaining treatment the administration of hydration and nutrition by any means if it is stated in the individual's living will. The statute mandates that a copy of the living will must be provided to the patient's physician in order to be effective. Furthermore, the patient must be incompetent or permanently unconscious. If there is no evidence of the presence of a living will, the Pennsylvania probate codes allow an attorney-in-fact who is designated in a properly executed durable-power-of-attorney document to give permission for "medical and surgical procedures to be utilized on an incompetent patient."[24] States subsequently have been addressing the problem of surrogate decision making for those who are incompetent. Evidence of an incompetent person's wishes that had been expressed when he or she was competent is required by the courts.

Unless there is some national uniformity in the legislation, some patients and their families will shop for states that will allow them to have medical treatment terminated or withdrawn with fewer legal hassles. For example, on January 18, 1991, a Missouri probate court judge authorized a father to take his 20-year-old brain-damaged daughter, Christine Busalacchi, from the Missouri Rehabilitation Center to Minnesota for testing by a proeuthanasia physician, Dr. Ronald Cranford. Cranford, who practiced at the Hennepin County Medical Center, had been at the center of controversy in Minnesota. In January 1991, Pro Life Action Ministries demanded Cranford's resignation, claiming that he "desires to make Minnesota the killing fields for the disabled."[25] He, however, viewed himself as an advocate of patients' rights. It is clear that the main reason Busalacchi sought authorization to take his daughter to Minnesota is that he believed he would have to deal with fewer legal impediments there to allow his daughter to die.

Because of continuing litigation involving the right to die, it is clear that the public must be educated as to the importance of expressing their wishes concerning medical treatment while they are competent. Uniformity with regard to the legal instruments available for demonstrating what a patient wants should be a common goal of legislators, courts, and the medical profession. If living wills, surrogates, and durable powers of attorney were to be enacted pursuant to national rather than individual state guidelines, the process of resolving end-of-life issues might be less complicated. Some states have addressed the problem by statutorily providing for these instruments, thereby enabling individuals to have a say in the medical care they would like to receive should they become unable to speak for themselves.

Chief Justice Fred Dore of the Washington Supreme Court voiced his opinion that a legislative response to right-to-die issues could be better addressed by the legislature.

The United States Supreme Court, in *Cruzan*, questioned whether a federally protected right to forgo nutrition and hydration existed. The *Cruzan* Court confronted the same philosophical issues that we face today and wisely recognized and deferred to the Legislature's superior policy-making abilities. As was the case in *Cruzan*, our legislature is far better equipped to evaluate this complex issue and should not have its power usurped by this court.[26]

ASSISTED SUICIDE

Assisted suicide presents profound questions of ethics, religious beliefs, and public policy issues. These are precisely the kinds of issues in which public input is vital, and courts are simply not equipped to conduct the type of comprehensive review required. The legislative and executive branches of government are uniquely well equipped to pursue these issues. Courts have before them only the legal arguments and although questions of law are certainly part of the equation, the core issues presented are fundamentally grounded in questions of policy and how we view ourselves as a society. Those who must answer to the people for their policy product and not those who have no accountability to the people are best suited to answer these questions.[27]

Physician-Assisted Suicide

Physician-assisted suicide is an action in which a physician voluntarily aids a patient in bringing about his or her death. Dr. Jack Kevorkian of Michigan announced in October 1989 that he had developed a device that would end one's life quickly, painlessly, and humanely. He chose to assist a 54-year-old Alzheimer's disease patient in committing suicide on June 4, 1990. In December 1990, he was charged with first-degree murder, but the charge was later dismissed because Michigan had no law against assisted suicide. He was however ordered not to assist in a patient's suicide or to give advice about it. On February 6, 1991, he violated the court order by giving advice about the preparation of a drug to a terminally ill cancer patient.[28] Additional murder charges were lodged against Kevorkian in October 1991, when he instructed two Michigan women how to use of his "suicide machine." In dismissing the charges against him, the circuit court judge stated, "Some people with intractable pain cannot benefit from treatment." Although emphasizing that Michigan has no law against assisting suicide, the judge also expressed his belief that physician-assisted suicide remains an alternative for patients experiencing "unmanageable pain."[29]

The Michigan House on November 22, 1992 approved legislation placing a temporary ban on assisted suicide. The Senate approved the temporary ban after Kevorkian helped a sixth terminally ill patient kill herself. On December 15, 1992, Michigan Governor John Engler signed the law just hours after two more women committed suicide with Kevorkian's aid.

The new law, which became effective on April 1, 1993, made assisting suicide a felony punishable by up to 4 years in prison and a $2,000 fine. Under the new law, assisted suicide was banned for 15 months. During this time, a special commission studied assisted suicide and submitted its recommendations to the Michigan legislature for review and action. The new law apparently raised constitutional questions and was challenged by the Civil Liberties Union of Michigan because of the claim that it failed to recognize that the terminally ill have the right to end their lives painlessly and with dignity.

Kevorkian faced prosecution for murdering two people and for assisting in the suicides of three others. As a result, he appealed a Michigan Supreme Court ruling that found there is no right to assisted suicide.[30] The U.S. Supreme Court rejected his argument that assisted suicide is a constitutional right. The high court's decision allowed the State of Michigan to move forward and prosecute Kevorkian on the pending charges. At the time of the high court's ruling, Kevorkian had attended his 22nd suicide, involving a retired clergyman, less than a month after he was left facing murder charges in Michigan.[31] As of March 1998, Kevorkian had aided in or witnessed 100 suicides. Kevorkian was eventually convicted of second-degree murder for physician suicide and sentenced 10 to 25 years in prison. He was released on June 1, 2007, after serving 8 years in prison.

At the time of this writing, Oregon, Washington, and Vermont have legalized physician-assisted suicide. Vermont became the third state to legalize physician-assisted suicide, when Governor Peter Shumlin signed into law a bill allowing physicians to legally prescribe lethal doses of medication for terminally ill patients.[32]

The Montana Supreme Court ruled that state law protects physicians from prosecution for assisting terminally ill patients in committing suicide. The court, however, did not address whether assisted suicide was guaranteed under the state's constitution.[33] Montana Bill "HB 505 which would have explicitly prohibited doctor-prescribed suicide was introduced by Rep. Krayton Kerns. The bill passed in the House and was sent to the Senate, where it failed on April 15, 2013 in a 27–23 vote."[34]

In 1967, the United States Supreme Court, in two unanimous and separate decisions, ruled that state laws prohibiting assisted suicide are constitutional; nevertheless, the U.S. Supreme Court ruled that states can allow physicians to assist in the suicide of terminally ill patients.[35]

The physician-assisted suicide debate, as noted in the following news clippings, continues throughout the nation.

California Gov. Signs Assisted Suicide Information Bill into Law

California Gov. Arnold Schwarzenegger has signed into law a bill that opponents say could open the door to the eventuality of physician-assisted suicide in the nation's most populous state.

AB 2747 mandates that physicians, nurse practitioners and physician assistants provide patients diagnosed with a terminal illness—or who have been given a diagnosis of one year or less to live—with "comprehensive information and counseling regarding legal end-of-life options, as specified."

Matt Hadro, CNSNews.com, *October 3, 2008*[36]

Mass. Doctor-Assisted Suicide Measure Fails

BOSTON (AP)—A Massachusetts ballot question that would have legalized physician-assisted suicide for the terminally ill has been defeated by a narrow margin.

The measure voted on Tuesday was defeated 51 percent to 49 percent with 96 percent of precincts counted, and was the closest of the three questions on the Massachusetts ballot.

"We believe the voters came to see this as a flawed approach to end of life care, lacking in the most basic safeguards," Rosanne Bacon Meade, chairwoman of the Committee Against Assisted Suicide, said in a statement.

Associated Press, Boston.com, *November 7, 2012*[37]

ASSISTED SUICIDE VERSUS REFUSAL OR WITHDRAWAL OF TREATMENT

The Supreme Court in *Quill v. Vacco*[38] found that neither the assisted suicide ban nor the law permitting patients to refuse medical treatment treats anyone differently from anyone else or draws any distinctions between persons. There is a distinction between letting a patient die and making one die. Most legislatures have allowed the former but have prohibited the latter. The Supreme Court disagreed with the respondents' claim that the distinction is arbitrary and irrational.

In its decision, the Supreme Court determined that New York had valid reasons for distinguishing between the refusal of treatment and assisting suicide. Those reasons included prohibiting intentional killing and preserving life, preventing suicide, maintaining the physician's role as his or her patient's healer, and protecting vulnerable people from indifference, prejudice, and psychological and financial pressure to end their lives. All of those reasons, the court decided, constitute valid and important public interests fulfilling the constitutional requirement that a legislative classification bear a rational relation to a legitimate end.

In the Washington case, *Washington v. Glucksberg*,[39] the U.S. Supreme Court held that assisted suicide is not a liberty protected by the Constitution's due process clause. A majority of states now ban assisted suicide. These rulings, however, do not affect the right of patients to refuse treatment. It is clear that this emotionally charged issue is not settled. Legislative, judicial, and public debates continue to rage. Ultimately, the quality of a patient's life must be improved so that physician-assisted suicide does not become the answer for those who are suffering. Society must learn to address more effectively end-of-life issues including pain management, fear of death, self-worth, and hopelessness. Thus far, progress is slow and inadequate.

OREGON'S DEATH WITH DIGNITY ACT (1994)

On October 27, 1997, physician-assisted suicide became a legal medical option for the terminally ill residents of Oregon. The *Oregon Death with Dignity Act* allows a terminally ill

Oregon resident to obtain a lethal dose of medication from his or her physician. The act legalizes physician-assisted suicide but specifically prohibits euthanasia, where a physician or other person directly administers a medication to end another's life. The following are excerpts from the Oregon Death with Dignity Act:

Or. Rev. Stat. Sects. 127.800-.897 Section 1.01. Definitions...

(12) "Terminal disease" means an incurable and irreversible disease that has been medically confirmed and will, within reasonable medical judgment, produce death within (6) months...

Section 2.01. Who may initiate a written request for medication?

An adult who is capable, is a resident of Oregon, and has been determined by the attending physician and consulting physician to be suffering from a terminal disease, and who has voluntarily expressed his or her wish to die, may make a written request for medication for the purpose of ending his or her life in a humane and dignified manner.

Section 2.02. Form of the Written Request.

(1) A valid request for medication . . . shall be in substantially the form described in ORS 127.897, signed and dated by the patient and witnessed by at least two individuals who, in the presence of the patient, attest that to the best of their knowledge and belief the patient is capable, acting voluntarily, and is not being coerced to sign the request . . .

Section 3.01. Attending physician responsibilities. The attending physician shall: and has made the request voluntarily.

(2) Inform the patient of:

(a) His or her medical diagnosis;

(b) His or her prognosis;

(c) The potential risks associated with taking the medication to be prescribed;

(d) The probable result of taking the medication to be prescribed; and

(e) The feasible alternatives, including, but not limited to, comfort care, hospice care, and pain control.

(3) Refer the patient to a consulting physician for medical confirmation of the diagnosis, and for a determination that the patient is capable and acting voluntarily...

Section 3.06. Written and oral requests.

In order to receive a prescription for medication to end his or her life in a humane and dignified manner, a qualified patient shall have made an oral request and a written request, and reiterate the oral request to his or her attending physician no less than (15) days after making the initial oral request. At the time the qualified patient makes his or her second oral request, the attending physician shall offer the patient an opportunity to rescind the request.

Section 3.07. Right to rescind request. A patient may rescind his or her request at any time and in any manner without regard to his or her mental state. . . .

Section 3.08. Waiting periods.

No less than (15) days shall elapse between the patient's initial oral request and the writing of a prescription. . . . No less than 48 hours shall elapse between the patient's written request and the writing of a prescription. . . .

Section 6.01. Form of the request.

A request for a medication . . . shall be in substantially the following form. [**Figure 3-1**.]

Request for Medication to End My Life in a Humane and Dignified Manner

I, _____, am an adult of sound mind.

I am suffering from _____, which my attending physician has determined is a terminal disease and which has been medically confirmed by a consulting physician.

I have been fully informed of my diagnosis, prognosis, the nature of medication to be prescribed and potential associated risks, the expected result, and the feasible alternatives, including comfort care, hospice care, and pain control.

I request that my attending physician prescribe medication that will end my life in a humane and dignified manner.

Initial One:

_____ I have informed my family of my decision and taken their opinions into consideration.

_____ I have decided not to inform my family of my decision.

_____ I have no family to inform of my decision.

I understand that I have the right to rescind this request at any time.

I understand the full import of this request and I expect to die when I take the medication to be prescribed.

I make this request voluntarily and without reservation, and I accept full moral responsibility for my actions.
Signed: _____
Dated: _____

Declaration of Witnesses
We declare that the person signing this request:

(a) Is personally known to us or has provided proof of identity;

(b) Signed the request in our presence;

(c) Appears to be of sound mind and not under duress, fraud or undue influence;

(d) Is not a patient for whom either of us is attending physician.

FIGURE 3-1   Oregon Request Form to End Life

PATIENT SELF-DETERMINATION ACT OF 1990

The *Patient Self-Determination Act of 1990*[40] provides that patients have a right to formulate advance directives and to make decisions regarding their health care. Self-determination includes the right to accept or refuse medical treatment. Health care providers (including hospitals, nursing homes, home health agencies, health maintenance organizations, and hospices) receiving federal funds under Medicare are required to comply with the new regulations. Providers are required to:[41]

1. Provide individuals written information concerning their rights under state law (whether statutory or recognized by courts of the state) to make decisions including the right to accept or refuse medical or surgical treatment and the right to formulate advance directives.
2. Document in the individual's medical record whether the individual has executed an advance directive.
3. Not condition the provision of care or otherwise discriminate against an individual based on whether the individual has executed an advance directive.
4. Ensure compliance with requirements of state law (whether statutory or recognized by the courts of the state) regarding advance directives. The provider must inform individuals that complaints concerning the advance directive requirements may be filed with the state survey and certification agency.
5. Provide education for staff concerning its policies and procedures on advance directives.
6. Provide for community education regarding issues concerning advance directives by defining what constitutes an advance directive, emphasizing that an advance directive is designed to enhance an incapacitated individual's control over medical treatment and describe applicable state law concerning advance directives. A provider must be able to document its community education efforts.

Providers are not entitled to reimbursement under the Medicare program if they fail to meet Patient Self-Determination Act of 1990 requirements.

ADVANCE DIRECTIVES

Patients have a right to make decisions about their health care with their physician. They may agree to a proposed treatment, choose among alternative treatments, or refuse a treatment. Patients have this right even if they become incapacitated and are unable to make decisions regarding their health care. Because of the advances in modern medical technology, everyone should give serious consideration as to their health care wishes, to decide what they would want done should they become incapacitated, to execute advance directives and make their wishes known so that family and health care providers can respect their decision.

Advance directives, in the form of a "living will" or "durable power of attorney," allow the patient to state in advance the kinds of medical care that he or she considers acceptable or not acceptable. The patient can appoint an agent, a *surrogate decision maker*, to make those decisions on his or her behalf. A patient should be asked at the time of admission if he or she has an advance directive. If a patient does not have an advance directive, the health care facility should provide the patient with information about an advance directive and the opportunity to execute a directive. A patient should clearly understand that an advance directive is a guideline for caregivers describing his or her wishes for medical care—what he or she would and would not want—in the event of incapacitation and inability to make decisions. This interaction should be documented in the patient's medical record. If the patient has an advance directive, a copy should be requested for insertion into the patient's record. If the patient does not have a copy of the advance directive with him or her, the substance thereof should be documented and flagged in the patient's medical record. Documentation should include the location of the advance directive, the name and telephone number of the designated health care agent, and any information that might be helpful in the immediate care situation (e.g., patient's desire for food and hydration). The purpose of such documentation should not be considered to be a need to recreate a new directive, but should be considered a desire to adhere to a patient's wishes in the event some untoward event occurs while waiting for a copy of the directive.

The patient can execute a new directive at any time if desired. Patient and family education should be provided regarding the existence of the directive and its contents. The patient should be periodically queried about whether he or she wishes to make any changes with regard to an advance directive.

LIVING WILL

A *living will* is the instrument or legal document that describes those treatments an individual wishes or does not wish to receive should he or she become incapacitated and unable to communicate treatment decisions. Typically, a living will allows a person, when competent, to inform caregivers in writing of his or her wishes with regard to withholding and withdrawing life-supporting treatment, including nutrition and hydration. The living will is helpful to health care professionals because it provides guidance about a patient's wishes for treatment, provides legally valid instructions about treatment, and protects the patient's rights and the provider who honors them.

The Supreme Court of Kentucky's Living Will Directive Act was determined to be constitutional in *T. Bruce Simpson, Jr., v. Commonwealth of Kentucky and Cabinet for Human Resources*, 142 S.W.3d 24 (Ky. 2004). The act allows a judicially appointed guardian or other designated surrogate to remove a ward's life support. After suffering cardiac arrest, it was agreed that the patient, Woods, would never regain consciousness. After a recommendation of the hospital's ethics committee, Wood's guardian asked for the removal of Woods's life support. If there was no legal guardian but the physicians, family, and ethics committee all agree with the surrogate's decision—in this case, the state's—there is no need for judicial approval. The Supreme Court did determine that when there is disagreement in a particular case, withdrawal of life support would be prohibited absent clear and convincing evidence that the patient is permanently unconscious or in a persistent vegetative state and that withdrawal of life support was in the patient's best interest. In support of its holding, the Supreme Court cited the ethical standards of the National Center for State Courts, the Council on Ethical and Judicial Affairs of the American Medical Association, an Address to an International Congress of Anesthesiologists by Pope Pius XII, and the Declaration on Euthanasia by Pope John Paul II:[42]

In determining the patient's best interests, courts may consider, but are not limited to considering: (1) the patient's present level of physical, sensory, emotional, and cognitive functioning and possibility of improvement thereof; (2) any relevant statements or expressions made by the patient, when competent, as to his or her own wishes with a rebuttable presumption attaching to a valid living will or a designation of a health care surrogate; (3) to the extent known, the *patient's own philosophical, religious, and moral views, life goals, values about the purpose of life and the way it should be lived, and attitudes toward sickness, medical procedures, suffering, and death;* (4) the degree of physical pain caused by the patient's condition, treatment, and termination of treatment; (5) the degree of humiliation, dependence, and loss of dignity probably resulting from the condition or treatment; (6) the life expectancy and prognosis for recovery with and without the treatment; (7) the various treatment options and their risks, benefits, and side effects; (8) whether any particular treatment would be proportionate or disproportionate in terms of the benefits gained; and (9) the impact on the patient's family (the assumption being that the patient would be concerned about the well-being and happiness of his or her own family members).

The living will should be signed and dated by two witnesses who are not blood relatives or beneficiaries of property. A living will should be discussed with the patient's physician, and a signed copy should be placed in the patient's medical record. A copy also should be given to the individual designated to make decisions in the event the patient is unable to do so. A person who executes a living will when healthy and mentally competent cannot predict how he or she will feel at the time of a terminal illness; therefore, it should be updated regularly so that it accurately reflects a patient's wishes. The written instructions become effective when a patient is either in a terminal condition, permanently unconscious, or suffering irreversible brain damage. An example of a living will is illustrated in **Figure 3-2**.

Right to Die Without a Living Will

In *San Juan-Torregosa v. Garcia*,[43] the evidence at trial established that Garcia suffered a cardiac arrest. Although she was later resuscitated, she suffered oxygen deprivation to her brain for more than 10 minutes and was in a chronic vegetative state. Medical opinion established that she was breathing reflexively, but there was no evidence that she would be able to recover "cortical functions." Garcia also had metastatic breast cancer. Her treating physician, Dr. Parrish, testified at trial that within a reasonable degree of medical certainty Garcia would not recover and that he had never seen anyone in her condition recover. He stated that Garcia was functioning on a low brain level, whereby the brainstem kept her blood circulating, maintained blood pressure, and maintained respiration, and that she was in a persistent vegetative state with zero chance of recovering any cortex activity. Parrish further stated that he discussed the discontinuation of artificial nutrition and hydration with the family and that they had ultimately decided to continue the fluids but stop the nutrition, which he felt was reasonable.

When asked why Garcia had been given life support in the first place, Parrish explained that although Garcia's injury initially seemed very severe, he could not say from the beginning whether she would recover and wanted to give her every chance to improve if she could.

The trial court ruled that because Garcia, who was in a chronic vegetative state, had not executed a living will, the court had no authority to authorize discontinuance of artificial

My Living Will

To my Family, Doctors, and All Those Concerned with My Care:

I, _____, being of sound mind, make this statement as a directive to be followed if for any reason I become incapacitated and unable to participate in decisions regarding my medical care.

If I should be in an incurable or irreversible mental or physical condition with no reasonable expectation of recovery, I direct my attending physician to withhold or withdraw treatment that merely prolongs my dying. I direct that my treatment in this instance be limited to comfort care and the control of and relief from pain.

Care I Want:

_____

_____

_____

_____

_____

_____

To live as long as possible regardless of the quality of life that I may experience:

- I direct that all appropriate medical/surgical measures be provided to sustain my life regardless of my mental or physical condition.
- Upon my death, I want to donate any parts of my body that may be of benefit to others.

Care I Do Not Want:

_____

_____

_____

_____

_____

- I am permanently unconscious with and permanently connected to a ventilator.
- I am permanently unconscious with a feeding tube and/or intravenous hydration.
- I am on a ventilator when there is little or no chance of recovery.
- I am conscious but unable to communicate, being fed with a feeding tube and/or hydrated.
- I am in the end stage of a fatal irreversible mental or physical illness, disease, or condition.
- I do not want: _____ Mechanical ventilation _____ CPR _____ Dialysis _____ Feeding tubes
- Other exceptions and/or comments:

_____

_____

_____

FIGURE 3-2 Living Will

Additional Comments or Exceptions:
This living will describes my express wishes and legal right to accept or refuse treatment. As I am of sound mind, I expect my family, physician/s, and all those concerned with my care to regard themselves as legally and morally bound to act in accord with my wishes.
Signed _____
Date _____

Witness (Cannot be designated healthcare agent). I declare that the person who signed the document or asked another to sign this document on his/her behalf did so in my presence and that he/she appears to be of sound mind and free of duress or undue influence.

Signed _____
Date _____

Signed _____
Date _____

Note: A copy of the executed living will should be provided to the patient's physician and healthcare agent.

FIGURE 3-2 Living Will (*Continued*)

nutrition. On appeal, the appellants asserted that the trial court erred in refusing to allow Garcia's family to terminate the artificial nutrition and hydration that was keeping her body alive, thereby failing to honor her wishes and denying her constitutional right to bodily integrity.

The United States Supreme Court, in *Cruzan v. Director, Missouri Dept. of Health*, 497 U.S. 261, 110 S. Ct. 2841 (1990), recognized that a competent person had a constitutionally protected liberty interest in refusing unwanted medical treatment. The court stopped short of finding that an incompetent person would have the same right; however, the court said: "An incompetent person is not able to make an informed and voluntary choice to exercise a hypothetical right to refuse treatment, or any other right. Such a 'right' must be exercised for her, if at all, by some sort of surrogate."

Tennessee's public policy on this issue is set forth in the "Legislative intent" section of the Tennessee Right to Natural Death Act, codified at Tenn. Code Ann. §32-11-102. This statute reads:

> The general assembly declares it to be the law of the state of Tennessee that every person has the fundamental and inherent right to die naturally with as much dignity as circumstances permit and to accept, refuse, withdraw from, or otherwise control decisions relating to the rendering of the person's own medical care, specifically including palliative care and the use of extraordinary procedures and treatment.

This policy applies to every person and does not distinguish between those who are competent and those who are not. An individual has a right to refuse treatment so long as that individual is competent. When an individual is incompetent to make such a decision, the state has a duty to become involved by trying to determine what the desires of the patient would have been had he been conscious and competent. The initial assumption would be that the patient desired lifesaving treatment unless that assumption was contradicted by previous statements made when the patient was competent. It is clear from state court decisions that artificial nutrition and hydration are to be included in the realm of medical treatment that a patient has a right to refuse.

The appeals court concurred with the trial court's fact-finding that evidence is clear and convincing that Garcia would not want to be kept alive by artificial means and that her wishes, expressed while she was competent, would be to have these services discontinued. Courts have the duty to protect constitutional rights and when necessary enable individuals to exercise them. The appeals court ordered that a conservator be appointed to carry out Garcia's wishes, including the refusal of medical care.

Durable Power of Attorney

A *durable power of attorney* is a legal device that permits one individual, known as the "principal," to give to another person, called the "attorney-in-fact," the authority to act on his or her behalf. The attorney-in-fact is authorized to handle banking and real estate affairs, incur expenses, pay bills, and handle a wide variety of legal affairs for a specified period of time. The power of attorney may continue indefinitely during the lifetime of the principal so long as that person is competent and capable of granting power of attorney. If the principal becomes comatose or mentally incompetent, the power of attorney automatically expires, just as it would if the principal dies.

Because a power of attorney is limited by the competency of the principal, some states have authorized a special legal device for the principal to express intent concerning the durability of the power of attorney, to allow it to survive disability or incompetency. The durable power of attorney is more general in scope and applies to a wider range of situations than those involving a patient in imminent danger of death, as is necessary for a living will to apply. Although it need not delineate desired medical treatment specifically, it must indicate the identity of the principal's attorney-in-fact and that the principal has communicated his or her health care wishes to the attorney-in-fact. Although the laws vary from state to state, all 50 states and the District of Columbia have durable power of attorney statutes. This legal device is an important alternative to guardianship, conservatorship, or trusteeship. Because a durable power of attorney places a considerable amount of power in the hands of the attorney-in-fact, an attorney in the state where the client resides should draw up the power of attorney. In the health care setting, a *durable power of attorney for health care* (e.g., **Figure 3-3**) is a legal instrument that designates and grants authority to an agent to, for example, make health care decisions for another.

Surrogate Decision Making

A surrogate decision maker is an agent who acts on behalf of a patient who lacks the capacity to participate in a particular decision. A health care agent's rights are no greater than those of a competent patient; however, the agent's rights are limited to any specific instructions included in the proxy document. An agent's decisions take priority over those of any

Durable Power of Attorney for Health Care

I, _____ , appoint:

1. Name _____   Phone _____

   Address _____

as my attorney-in-fact or agent to make my health and personal care decisions for me if I become unable to make my own decisions.

If the person I have named above is unable to act as my agent, I hereby designate the following person to serve as my agent:

2. Name _____   Phone _____

   Address _____

This *durable power of attorney* shall become effective upon my incapacity to make health or personal care decisions. (Please initial the statement/s below that best expresses your wishes.)

_____ I authorize my admission to or discharge from any medical, nursing, residential, or similar facility and to enter into agreements for my care.

_____ I authorize my agent to refuse or withdraw consent to any and all types of treatment, including, but not limited to, nutrition and hydration administered by artificial or invasive means.

I have discussed with my agent my wishes for health care. If my agent is not able to determine what I would want, I trust my agent to make his/her decision based on what he/she believes would be my wishes. This durable power of attorney is meant to replace all others.

Signed _____ Date _____

Witness (Cannot be the principal's designated healthcare agent). I declare that the person who signed this document or asked another to sign this document on his/her behalf did so in my presence and that he/she appears to be of sound mind and free of duress or undue influence.

Signed _____ Date _____

Signed _____ Date _____

Primary Agent

I, _____, have read the above durable power of attorney and am the person identified as the agent for _____. My signature below indicates that I acknowledge and accept responsibility to act as the agent and will exercise the powers herein granted in the best interest of the principal.

Signed _____ Date _____

FIGURE 3-3   Durable Power of Attorney for Health Care

Substitute Agent

I, _____, have read the above durable power of attorney and am the person identified as the agent for _____. My signature below indicates that I acknowledge and accept responsibility to act as the agent and will exercise the powers herein granted in the best interest of the principal.

Signature _____ Date _____

State of _____

County of _____

On this date, the _____ day of, 201_____, before me, the undersigned officer, personally appeared _____, known to me (satisfactorily proven) to be the person whose name is subscribed to the foregoing instrument, and acknowledged that he/she executed it for the purposes therein contained.

Witness my hand and official seal the day and year aforesaid _____.

Notary Public

Note: A copy of the executed durable power of attorney should be provided to the patient's physician and healthcare agent.

FIGURE 3-3   Durable Power of Attorney for Health Care (*Continued*)

other person except the patient. The agent has the right to consent or refuse to consent to any service or treatment, routine or otherwise, to refuse life-sustaining treatment, and to access all of the patient's medical information to make informed decisions. The agent must make decisions based on the patient's moral and religious beliefs. If a patient's wishes are not known, decisions must be based on a good-faith judgment of what the patient would have wanted.

Substituted Judgment

Substituted judgment is a form of surrogate decision making where the surrogate attempts to establish what decision the patient would have made if that patient were competent to do so. This conclusion can be based on the patient's preference expressed in previous statements or the surrogate's knowledge of the patient's beliefs (e.g., religious) and values.[44]

CASE: SPOUSAL RIGHTS IN DECISION MAKING

Mr. Martin sustained debilitating injuries as the result of an automobile accident. He suffered severe subcortical brain damage, significantly impairing his physical and cognitive functioning.[45] His injuries left him totally paralyzed on the left side. He could not speak or eat and had no bladder or bowel control. Martin remained conscious and had some awareness of his surroundings. He could communicate to a very minimal degree through head nods.

The trial court determined that Martin did not have nor would he ever have the ability to have the requisite capacity to make decisions regarding the withdrawal of life-support equipment. The evidence demonstrated that Martin's preference would have been to decline life-support equipment given his medical condition and prognosis. The trial court's decision was based on the following *four-part test* for determining whether a person has the requisite capacity to make a decision: Does the person have sufficient mind to reasonably understand the condition? Is the person capable of understanding the nature and effect of the treatment choices? Is the person aware of the consequences associated with those choices? Is the person able to make an informed choice that is voluntary and not coerced?

The trial court also determined that Mrs. Martin, the patient's spouse, was a suitable guardian for him. She petitioned to withdraw her husband's life support. Martin's mother and sister counter petitioned to have Mrs. Martin removed as the patient's guardian. The Michigan Court of Appeals held that the evidence was sufficient to support a finding that the patient lacked capacity to make decisions regarding the withholding or withdrawal of life-sustaining treatment. As to the patient's desire not to be placed on life-support equipment, there was sufficient evidence to show that the patient had a medical preference to decline treatment under circumstances such as those that occurred. There was also sufficient evidence to show that the patient's spouse was a suitable guardian.

The test for determining whether Martin had the requisite capacity to make a decision regarding the withholding or withdrawal of life-supporting medical treatment was clear and convincing—he did not have sufficient decision-making capacity. The evidence was just as clear that he never would regain sufficient decision-making capacity that would enable him to make such a decision. It was the general consensus of all of the experts that Martin's condition and cognitive level of functioning would not improve in the future.

Testimony from two of Martin's friends described statements made by him that he would never want to be maintained in a coma or in a vegetative state. In addition, Mrs. Martin described numerous statements made to her by Martin prior to the accident that he would not want to be maintained alive, given the circumstances described previously here. The trial court found that Mrs. Martin was credible. The court of appeals found no reason to dispute the trial court's finding as to Mrs. Martin's credibility.

In contrast to allegations made by the patient's mother and sister, the evidence was clear that Mrs. Martin's testimony was credible. There was no evidence that Mrs. Martin had anything but her husband's best interest at heart. There were allegations, but no evidence, that financial considerations or pressure from another individual influenced Mrs. Martin's testimony.

Ethical and Legal Issues

1. Knowing that the patient had some ability to interact with his environment, discuss the four-part test for determining the patient's ability to make a decision.
2. Do you agree with the court's decision? Explain.
3. Should the concern of the mother and sister have carried more weight in removing custody from Mrs. Martin?
4. What influence do you believe the mother and sister might have had on Mrs. Martin?

Guardianship

Guardianship is a legal mechanism by which the court declares a person incompetent and appoints a guardian. The court transfers the responsibility for managing financial affairs, living arrangements, and medical care decisions to the guardian. The right to refuse medical treatment on behalf of an incompetent person is not limited to legally appointed guardians but may be exercised by health care proxies or surrogates, such as close family members or friends. When a patient has not expressed instructions concerning his or her future health care in the event of later incapacity but has merely delegated full responsibility to a proxy, designation of a proxy must have been made in writing.

Health Care Proxy

A *health care proxy* allows a person to appoint a health care agent to make treatment decisions in the event he or she becomes incompetent and is unable to make decisions for him- or herself. The agent must be made aware of the patient's wishes regarding nutrition and hydration in order to be allowed to make a decision concerning withholding or withdrawing them. In contrast to a living will, a health care proxy does not require a person to know about and consider in advance all situations and decisions that could arise. Rather, the appointed agent would know about and interpret the expressed wishes of the patient and then make decisions about the medical care and treatment to be administered or refused. The *Cruzan* decision indicates that the Supreme Court views advance directives as clear and convincing evidence of a patient's wishes regarding life-sustaining treatment.

Although most statutes fail to cover incompetence, cases such as *Quinlan* and *Saikewicz* created a constitutionally protected obligation to terminate the incurable incompetent patient's life when guardians use the doctrine of substituted judgment. Furthermore, some states provide for proxy consent in the form of durable power of attorney statutes. Generally, these involve designation of a proxy to speak on the incurable incompetent person's behalf. They represent a combination of the intimate wishes of the patient and the medical recommendations of the physicians.

Oral declarations are accepted only after the patient has been declared terminally ill. Moreover, the declarant bears the responsibility of informing the physician to ensure that the document becomes a part of the medical record. The California statute provides that the document be reexecuted after 5 years. Other statutes differ in the length of time of effectiveness. Most states allow the document to be effective until revoked by the individual. To revoke, the patient must sign and date a new writing, destroy the first document himself or herself, direct another to destroy the first document in his or her presence, or orally state to the physician an intent to revoke. The effect of the directive varies among jurisdictions; however, there is unanimity in the promulgation of regulations that specifically authorize health care personnel to honor the directives without fear of incurring liability. The highest court of New York in *In re Eichner*[46] complied with the request of a guardian to withdraw life-support systems from an 83-year-old brain-damaged priest. The court reached its result by finding the patient's previously expressed wishes to be determinative.

Before exercising an incompetent patient's right to forgo medical treatment, the surrogate decision maker must satisfy the following conditions:

- The surrogate must be satisfied that the patient executed a document (e.g., Durable Power of Attorney for Health Care and Health Care Proxy) knowingly, willingly, and without undue influence and that the evidence of the patient's oral declaration is reliable.

- The patient must not have reasonable probability of recovering competency so that the patient could exercise the right.
- The surrogate must take care to ensure that any limitations or conditions expressed either orally or in written declarations have been considered carefully and satisfied.

FUTILITY OF TREATMENT

Futility of treatment, as it relates to medical care, occurs when the physician recognizes that the effect of treatment will be of no benefit to the patient. Morally, the physician has a duty to inform the patient when there is little likelihood of success. The determination as to futility of medical care is a scientific decision.

After a diagnosis has been made that a person is terminally ill with no hope of recovery and is in a chronic vegetative state with no possibility of attaining cognitive function, a state generally has no compelling interest in maintaining life. The decision to forgo or terminate life-support measures is, at this point, simply a decision that the dying process will not be artificially extended. Although the state has an interest in the prolongation of life, it has no interest in the prolongation of dying, and although there is a moral and ethical decision to be made to end the process, that decision can be made only by the surrogate. The decision whether to end the dying process is a personal decision for family members or those who bear a legal responsibility for the patient.

A determination as to the futility of medical care is a decision that must be made by a physician. Even if death is not imminent but a patient's coma is irreversible beyond doubt and there are adequate safeguards to confirm the accuracy of the diagnosis with the concurrence of those responsible for the patient's care, it is not unethical to discontinue all means of life-prolonging medical treatment.

WITHHOLDING AND WITHDRAWAL OF TREATMENT

Withholding of treatment is a decision not to initiate treatment or medical intervention for the patient. This is a decision often made when death is imminent and no hope of recovery. *Withdrawal of treatment* is a decision to discontinue treatment or medical interventions for the patient. When death is imminent and cannot be prevented by available treatment. Withholding or withdrawing treatment should be considered when:

- the patient is in a terminal condition and there is a reasonable expectation of imminent death of the patient;
- the patient is in a noncognitive state with no reasonable possibility of regaining cognitive function; and/or
- restoration of cardiac function will last for a brief period.

Theologians and ethicists have long recognized a distinction between ordinary and extraordinary medical care. The theological distinction is based on the belief that life is a gift from God that should not be destroyed deliberately by humans. Therefore, extraordinary therapies that extend life by imposing grave burdens on the patient and family are not required.

Although the courts have accepted decisions to withhold or withdraw extraordinary care, especially the respirator, from those who are comatose or in a persistent vegetative state with no possibility of emerging, they have been unwilling until recent years to discontinue feeding, which they have considered to be ordinary care. For example, the Illinois Supreme Court, in *In re Estate of Longeway*,[47] found that the authorized guardian of a terminally ill patient in an irreversible coma or persistent vegetative state has a common-law right to refuse artificial nutrition and hydration. The court found that there must be clear and convincing evidence that the refusal is consistent with the patient's interest. The court also required the concurrence of the patient's attending physician and two other physicians. Court intervention is also necessary to guard against the possibility that greed may taint the judgment of the surrogate decision maker. Although there may be a duty to provide life-sustaining equipment in the immediate aftermath of cardiopulmonary arrest, there is no duty to continue its use when it has become futile and ineffective to do so in the opinion of qualified medical personnel.

The Texas Natural Death Act provided immunity to caregivers in the following case for what the plaintiffs claimed was a failure of caregivers to withdraw lifesaving treatment.

CASE: FAILURE TO *WITHDRAW* LIFE SAVING TREAMENT

In this medical malpractice suit, the Stolles (appellants) sought damages from physicians and hospitals (appellees) for disregard of their instructions not to use "heroic efforts" or artificial means to prolong the life of their child, Mariel, who was born with brain damage. The Stolles argued that such negligence resulted in further brain damage to Mariel, prolonged her life, and caused them extraordinary costs that will continue as long as the child lives.

The Stolles had executed a written "Directive to Physicians" on behalf of Mariel in which they made known their desire that Mariel's life not be artificially prolonged under the circumstances provided in that directive.

Mariel suffered a medical episode after regurgitating her food. An unnamed, unidentified nurse–clinician administered chest compressions for 30 to 60 seconds, and Mariel survived.

The Stolles sued, alleging the following, among other things: Appropriate medical entries were not made in the medical record to reflect the Stolles' wishes that caregivers refrain from "heroic" life-sustaining measures. Lifesaving measures were initiated in violation of the physician's orders. The hospital did not follow the physician's orders, which were in Mariel's medical chart, when chest compressions and mechanically administered breathing to artificially prolong Mariel's life were applied, and a bioethics committee meeting was not convened to consider the Stolles' wishes and the necessity of a do-not-resuscitate (DNR) order.

The central issue in this case is whether appellees are immune from liability under the Texas Natural Death Act. Section 672.016(b) of the Texas Natural Death Act provides the following: "A physician, or a health professional acting under the direction of a physician, is not civilly or criminally liable for failing to effectuate a qualified patient's directive" [Tex. Health & Safety Code Ann. A4 672.016(b) (Vernon 1992)]. A "qualified patient" is a "patient with a terminal condition that has been diagnosed and certified in writing by the attending physician and one other physician who have personally examined the patient." A "terminal condition" is an "incurable condition caused by injury, disease, or illness that would produce death regardless of the application of life-sustaining procedures, according to reasonable medical judgment, and in which the application of life-sustaining procedures serves only to postpone the moment of the patient's death."

Mariel was not in a terminal condition, as appellees alleged. The Stolles failed to cite any authority that would have allowed the withdrawal of life sustaining procedures in a lawful manner. The Texas Natural Death Act, therefore, provided immunity to the caregivers for their actions in the treatment and care of Mariel.[48]

Ethical and Legal Issues

1. Describe the ethical principles in conflict in this case.
2. Do you agree with the court's decision? Explain your answer.

PATIENT NOT IN A PERSISTENT VEGETATIVE STATE

A guardian may direct the withdrawal of life-sustaining medical treatment, including nutrition and hydration, *only* if the incompetent ward is in a persistent vegetative state and the decision to withdraw is in the best interests of the ward.

In *Spahn v. Eisenberg,* Edna's sister and court-appointed guardian, Spahn, sought permission to direct the withholding of Edna's nutrition, claiming that her sister would not want to live in this condition; however, the only testimony presented at trial regarding Edna's views on the use of life-sustaining medical treatment involved a statement made 30 years earlier. At that time, Spahn and Edna were having a conversation about their mother, who was recovering from depression, and Spahn's mother-in-law, who was dying of cancer. Spahn testified that during this conversation, Edna said to her that she would rather die of cancer than lose her mind. Spahn further testified that this was the only time that she and Edna discussed the subject and that Edna never said anything specifically about withholding or withdrawing life-sustaining medical treatment.

The ethics committee at the nursing facility where Edna lived met to discuss the issue of withholding artificial nutrition from Edna. The committee approved withholding nutrition if no family member objected; however, one of Edna's nieces refused to sign a statement approving the withdrawal of nutrition.

The record spoke very little to what Edna's desires would be, and there was no clear statement of what her desires would be today under the current conditions. Her friends and family never had any conversations or discussions with her regarding her feelings or opinions about withdrawing nutrition or hydration, and she did not execute any advance directives expressing her wishes while she was competent.

Consequently, the court held that a guardian could only direct the withdrawal of life-sustaining medical treatment, including nutrition and hydration, if the incompetent ward is in a persistent vegetative state and the decision to withdraw is in the best interests of the ward. In this case, where the only indication of Edna's desires was made at least 30 years earlier and under different circumstances, there was not a clear statement of intent such that Edna's guardian might authorize the withholding of her nutrition.

The circuit judge concluded his own questioning of one member of the ethics committee, "The way I understand it, what you really have is a liability problem, and that's why you want everybody to consent, is that correct?" Dr. Erickson answered, "That is correct."[49]

Removal of Life-Support Equipment

Although there may be a duty to provide life-sustaining equipment in the immediate aftermath of cardiopulmonary arrest, there is no duty to continue its use after it has become futile and ineffective to do so in the opinion of qualified medical personnel. Two physicians in *Barber v. Superior Court*[50] were charged with the crimes of murder and conspiracy to commit murder. The charges were based on their acceding to requests of the patient's family to discontinue life-support equipment and intravenous tubes. The patient had suffered a cardiopulmonary arrest in the recovery room after surgery. A team of physicians and nurses revived the patient and placed him on life-support equipment. The patient had suffered severe brain damage, placing him in a comatose and vegetative state from which, according to tests and examinations by other specialists, he was unlikely to recover. On the written request of the family, the patient was taken off life-support equipment. The family, his wife and eight children, made the decision together after consultation with the physicians. Evidence had been presented that the patient, before his incapacitation, had expressed to his wife that he would not want to be kept alive by a machine. There was no evidence indicating that the family was motivated in their decision by anything other than love and concern for the dignity of their loved one. The patient continued to breathe on his own. Because the patient showed no signs of improvement, the physicians again discussed the patient's poor prognosis with the family. The intravenous lines were removed, and the patient died sometime thereafter.

A complaint then was filed against the two physicians. The magistrate who heard the evidence determined that the physicians did not kill the deceased because their conduct was not the proximate cause of the patient's death. On motion of the prosecution, the superior court determined as a matter of law that the evidence required the magistrate to hold the physicians to answer and ordered the complaint reinstated. The physicians then filed a writ of prohibition with the court of appeals. The court of appeals held that the physicians' omission to continue treatment, although intentional and with knowledge that the patient would die, was not an unlawful failure to perform a legal duty. The evidence amply supported the magistrate's decision. The superior court erred in determining that, as a matter of law, the evidence required the magistrate to hold the physicians to answer. The preemptory writ of prohibition to restrain the Superior Court of Los Angeles from taking any further action in this matter—other than to vacate its order reinstating the complaint and to enter a new and different order denying the People's motion—was granted.

Feeding Tubes

The New Jersey Supreme Court in 1985 heard the case of *In re Claire C. Conroy*.[51] The case involved an 84-year-old nursing home patient whose nephew petitioned the court for authority to remove the nasogastric tube that was feeding her. The court overturned the appellate division decision and held that life-sustaining treatment, including nasogastric feeding, could be withheld or withdrawn from incompetent nursing home patients who will, according to physicians, die within 1 year, in three specific circumstances. These are as follows:[52]

1. When it is clear that the particular patient would have refused the treatment under the circumstances involved (the subjective test)

2. When there is some indication of the patient's wishes (but he or she has not "unequivocally expressed" his or her desires before becoming incompetent) and the treatment "would only prolong suffering" (the limited objective test)
3. When there is no evidence at all of the patient's wishes, but the treatment "clearly and markedly outweighs the benefits the patient derives from life" (the pure objective test, based on pain)

A procedure involving notification of the state Office of the Ombudsman is required before withdrawing or withholding treatment under any of the three tests. The ombudsman must make a separate recommendation.

The court also found tubal feeding to be a medical treatment, and as such, as intrusive as other life-sustaining measures. The court in its analysis emphasized duty, rather than causation, with the result that medical personnel acting in good faith will be protected from liability. If physicians follow the *Quinlan/Conroy* standards and decide to end medical treatment of a patient, the duty to continue treatment ceases. Thus, the termination of treatment becomes a lawful act.

Although *Conroy* presents case-specific guidelines, there is concern that the opinion will have far-reaching repercussions. There is fear that decisions to discontinue treatment will not be based on the "balancing of interests" test, but rather that a "quality-of-life" test will be used to end the lives of severely senile, old, and economic burdensome people.

Those quality-of-life judgments would be most dangerous for nursing home patients whose age would be a factor in the decision-making process. "Advocates of 'the right to life' fear that the 'right to die' for the elderly and handicapped will become a 'duty to die.'"[53] In both the *Saikewicz* and *Spring* cases, age was a determining factor weighing against life-sustaining treatment. Furthermore, in *In re Hier*,[54] the court found that Mrs. Hier's age of 92 years made the "proposed gastrostomy substantially more onerous or burdensome . . . than it would be for a younger, healthier person." Moreover, a New York Superior Court held that the burdens of an emergency amputation for an elderly patient outweighed the benefit of continued life.[55] Finding that prolonging her life would be cruel, the court stated that life had no meaning for her. Although some courts have recognized the difference, other courts must still address the difference between *Quinlan*-type patients and older, confined, and conscious patients who can interact but whose mental or physical functioning is impaired.

In a New Jersey case, however, the ombudsman denied a request to remove feeding tubes from a comatose nursing home patient.[56] In applying the *Conroy* tests, the ombudsman decided that Hilda Peterson might live more than 1 year, the period that *Conroy* used as a criterion for determining whether life support can be removed.

To complicate this issue further, on March 17, 1986, the American Medical Association (AMA) changed its code of ethics on comas. Now physicians may ethically withhold food, water, and medical treatment from patients in irreversible comas or persistent vegetative states with no hope of recovery— even if death is not imminent.[57] Although physicians can consider the wishes of the patient and family or the legal representatives, they cannot cause death intentionally. The wording is permissive, and, thus, those physicians who feel uncomfortable withdrawing food and water may refrain from doing so. The AMA's decision does not comfort those who fear abuse or mistake in euthanasia decisions, nor does it have any legal value as such. There are physicians, nurses, and families who have their own, and not the patient's, interests in mind. Even with the *Conroy* decision and the AMA's code of ethics change, the feeding tube issue is not settled.

On April 23, 1986, the New Jersey Superior Court ruled that the husband of severely brain-damaged Nancy Jobes could order the removal of her life-sustaining feeding tube, which would ultimately cause the 31-year-old comatose patient, who had been in a vegetative state in a hospice for the past 6 years, to starve to death.[58] Dr. Fred Plum created and defined the term "persistent vegetative state" as one in which:[59]

> The body functions entirely in terms of its internal controls. It maintains temperature. It maintains digestive activity. It maintains heart beat and pulmonary ventilation. It maintains reflex activity of muscles and nerves for low-level conditioned responses. But there is no behavioral evidence of either self-awareness or awareness of the surroundings in a learned manner.

Medical experts testified that the patient could, under optimal conditions, live another 30 years. Relieving the nursing home officials from performing the act on one of its residents, the court ruled that the patient may be taken home to die (with the removal to be supervised by a physician and medical care to be provided to the patient at home).

The nursing home had petitioned the court for the appointment of a "life advocate" to fight for continuation of medical treatment for Jobes, which, it argued, would save her life. The court disallowed the appointment of a life advocate, holding that case law does not support requiring the continuation of life-support systems in all circumstances. Such a requirement, according to the court, would contradict the patient's right of privacy.

The court's decision applied "the principles enunciated in *Quinlan* and . . . *Conroy*" and the "ruling by the AMA's Council on Judicial Affairs that the provision of food and water is, under certain circumstances, a medical treatment like any other and may be discontinued when the physician and family of the patient feel it is no longer benefiting the patient."[60]

An Illinois court found that the authorized guardian of a terminally ill patient in an irreversible coma or persistent vegetative state has a common law right to refuse artificial nutrition and hydration. The court found that there must be clear and convincing evidence that the refusal is consistent with the patient's interest. The court also required the concurrence of the patient's attending physician and two other physicians. "Court intervention is also necessary to guard against the remote, yet real possibility that greed may taint the judgment of the surrogate decision maker."[61] Dissenting, Judge Ward said, "The right to refuse treatment is rooted in and dependent on the patient's capacity for informed decision, which an incompetent patient lacks."[62]

Also, Elizabeth Bouvia, a mentally competent cerebral palsy victim, won her struggle to have feeding tubes removed even though she was not terminally ill.[63] The California Court of Appeals announced on April 16, 1986, that she could go home to die. The court found that Bouvia's decision to "let nature take its course" did not amount to a choice to commit suicide with people aiding and abetting it. The court stated that it is not "illegal or immoral to prefer a natural, albeit sooner, death than a drugged life attached to a mechanical device."[64] The court's finding that it was a moral and philosophical question, not a legal or medical one, leaves one wondering whether the courts are opening the door to permitting "legal starvation" to be used by those who are not terminally ill but who do wish to commit suicide.

Do-Not-Resuscitate Orders

Do-not-resuscitate orders (DNR) are physician orders not to resuscitate a patient in the event of cardiac or respiratory arrest. Determination as to futility of medical care is a medical decision based on scientific evidence that further treatment is futile and one's quality of life has been so diminished that "heroic" rescue methods are no longer in the patient's best interests. DNR orders must be written, signed, and dated by the physician. Appropriate consents must be obtained either from the patient or his or her health care agent. Many states have acknowledged the validity of DNR orders in cases involving terminally ill patients in which the patients' families make no objections to such orders. Such orders are generally written as the result of a patient wishes as a result of an advance directive (e.g., living will). If a patient lacks the ability to make a decision regarding a DNR order, the patient's legally *appointed decision maker* can make such decisions provided it can be demonstrated that the decision maker is following the patient's wishes. Advance directives, such as living wills, are helpful in determining a patient's wishes. DNR orders can also be made at the family's request.

DNR orders must comply with statutory requirements, be of short duration, and be reviewed periodically to determine whether the patient's condition or other circumstances (e.g., change of mind by the patient or family) surrounding the "no code" orders have changed. Currently, it is generally accepted that if a patient is competent, the DNR order is considered to be the same as other medical decisions in which a patient may choose to reject life-sustaining treatment. In the case of an incompetent patient, absent any advance written directives, the best interests of the patient would be considered.

Competent Patients Make Their Own Decisions

Should relatives of a patient agree to a no code order when the patient is competent to make his or her own decision?

In *Payne v. Marion General Hospital*,[65] the Indiana Court of Appeals overturned a lower court decision in favor of the physician. The physician had issued a no code status on Payne despite evidence given by a nurse that up to a few minutes before his death Payne could communicate. The physician had determined that Payne was incompetent, thereby rendering him unable to give informed consent to treatment. Because Payne left no written directives, the physician relied on one of Payne's relatives, who asked for the DNR order. The court found that there was evidence that Payne was not incompetent and should have been consulted before a DNR order was given.

Furthermore, the court reviewed testimony that 1 year earlier Payne had suffered and recovered from the same type of symptoms, leading to the conclusion that there was a possibility that he could have survived if resuscitation had continued. There was no DNR policy in place at the hospital to assist the physician in making his decision. To avoid this type of problem, health care providers should adopt an appropriate process with respect to issuing no code orders.

Help Me Bear the Pain

Some say, "Men don't cry." Not true! You may find yourself crying alone someday. But for now, you have to be strong for Sunshine. Sunshine was her name, as given to her by her grandmother. For purposes of this case, she remains Sunshine. Not Miss or Ms. or Mrs., for Sunshine is her name. If you were to ask Sunshine what she thought about her life, this is what she would tell you.

As a hard-charging former district attorney, Sunshine knows what it's like to be under the constant threat of death. In the notorious 1990 "Angel Gabriel" case, a key witness to a cult leader's rape spree was murdered. As a result, the district attorney ordered that a panic alarm be placed in Sunshine's home.

Still, one enemy has done more damage than all of her former enemies combined. Sunshine has been battling systemic sclerosis for more than 6 years and has beaten the long-shot odds for survival.

Early on, she lost 20 pounds in 3 weeks. One by one, from her esophagus to her bottom, her internal organs came under painful attack. Her skin hardened in patches. Her fingers became discolored and swollen. Fingernails fell off. Calcification set in, and she nearly lost several digits. At the moment, she has a mysterious edema throughout her body.

Maintaining a full-time work schedule, she bounced from physician to physician for 3 years, seeking to find a reason for the sudden illness. The clues were finally put together, and her illness was diagnosed as systemic sclerosis—a degenerative connective tissue disease.

Most people don't know she has an illness. She's always in good spirits. She hides it well. Sunshine admits to putting a mask on in the morning. "When I cannot hide the pain, I disappear—go away or go home. I don't want to be defined by my illness. You go through mourning and anger. You feel tethered by the disease. It's a sadness you have to cope with."

With her mask firmly in place, a smiling Sunshine says she is not bitter. "I had a great life. I had fun. If it ended, I had fun."

Sunshine's Prayer: Strength to Cope
O God, you know my feelings. You know that I want to feel better. I want to be better. I want to have my health restored. But the hours of testing, the days of diagnosis, and the question marks concerning my future seem nearly more than I can bear! Grant me, O God, the strength to face each hour of this and every day. In fact, when it seems that I cannot face even this hour, fill me with strength to face the next five minutes. Amen.

Wherever Sunshine goes, the sun always shines, for she, as always, recognizes the beauty of each day.

–Anonymous

CHAPTER REVIEW

1. Euthanasia
   - *Mercy killing* of the hopelessly ill, injured, or incapacitated.
   - Debate over euthanasia is complex.
     - Legal system must maintain a balance between ensuring the patient's constitutional rights are protected and protecting society's interests in preserving life, preventing suicide, and maintaining the integrity of the medical profession.
   - When there is uncertainty regarding a patient's wishes in an emergency
     - The situation should be resolved in a way that favors the preservation of life.
     - Protect the patient's right to freedom of religion and self-determination.
   - *Active euthanasia* is the intentional commission of an act that will result in death.
   - *Passive euthanasia* is when a potentially lifesaving treatment is withdrawn or withheld.
   - *Voluntary euthanasia*
     - When a competent adult patient with an incurable condition who has been informed of the possible ramifications and alternatives available gives consent.
   - *Involuntary euthanasia*
     - When the decision to terminate the life of an incurable person is made by someone other than the incurable person.
   - Supreme Court ruled there is no constitutional right to assisted suicide.
     - Decision allowed the state of Michigan to prosecute Dr. Jack Kevorkian for assisting patients in committing suicide.
2. Right to self-determination
3. Assisted suicide
   - Oregon legislates physician-assisted suicide.
4. Patient Self-Determination Act of 1990
   - Health care organizations have a responsibility to explain to patients, staff, and families that patients have legal rights to direct their medical and nursing care as it corresponds to existing state law.
5. *Advance directives*, in the form of a "living will" or "durable power of attorney," allow the patient to make end-of-life choices.
   - *Living will* is the instrument or legal document that describes those treatments an individual wishes or does not wish to receive should he or she become incapacitated and unable to communicate treatment decisions.
   - *Durable power of attorney* is a legal device that permits one individual, known as the "principal," to give to another person, called the "attorney-in-fact," the authority to act on his or her behalf.
   - *Guardianship* is a legal mechanism by which the court declares a person incompetent and appoints a guardian. The court transfers the responsibility for managing financial affairs, living arrangements, and medical care decisions to the guardian.
   - *Health care proxy* allows a person to appoint a health care agent to make treatment decisions in the event that he or she becomes incompetent and is unable to make decisions for him- or herself.

- *Surrogate decision maker* is an agent who acts on behalf of a patient who lacks the capacity to participate in a particular decision.
- *Substituted judgment* is a form of surrogate decision making where the surrogate attempts to establish what decision the patient would have made if that patient were competent to do so.

6. Futility of treatment
   - When the physician recognizes further treatment will be of no benefit to the patient.
   - Morally, the physician has a duty to inform the patient when there is little likelihood of success of further treatment.
   - Determination as to futility of medical care is a medical decision based on scientific evidence.

7. Withholding or withdrawal of treatment
   - *Withholding of treatment* is a decision not to initiate treatment or medical intervention for the patient.
   - *Withdrawal of treatment* is a decision to discontinue treatment or medical interventions for the patient.
   - *Do-not-resuscitate orders* are physician orders not to resuscitate a patient in the event of a cardiac or respiratory arrest.
     - Generally written as the result of a patient wishes or at the family's request
     - Orders must be in written form, signed and dated by the physician.

TEST YOUR UNDERSTANDING

TERMINOLOGY

active euthanasia
advance directives
appointed decision makers
do-not-resuscitate (DNR) order
durable power of attorney
durable power of attorney for
 health care
euthanasia

futility of treatment
guardianship
health care proxy
involuntary euthanasia
living will
Oregon Death with Dignity
 Act
passive euthanasia

Patient Self-Determination
 Act
physician-assisted suicide
substituted judgment
surrogate decision maker
voluntary euthanasia
withdrawal of treatment
withholding of treatment

REVIEW QUESTIONS

1. Describe why there is such a struggle when addressing end-of-life issues.

2. Describe the difference between active and passive euthanasia.

3. Describe the difference between voluntary and involuntary euthanasia.

4. What are the differences between allowing a patient to die and physician-assisted suicide?

5. Constitutionally, what gives patients the right to self-determination?

6. Describe Oregon's Death with Dignity Act.

7. What was the purpose of the Patient Self-Determination Act of 1990?

8. What are advance directives?

9. Describe how a living will differs from a durable power of attorney for health care.

NOTES

1. http://www.cnn.com/2014/01/06/health/jahi-mcmath-girl-brain-dead/index.html.
2. J. Podgers, *Matters of Life and Death*, A.B.A.J. May 1992, at 60.
3. http://www.newsdaily.com/article/b177a24caf91af300f25679219db15c1/belgium-considering-new-euthanasia-law-for-kids.
4. 105 N.E. 92 (N.Y. 1914).
5. *Id.* at 93.
6. 438 N.Y.S.2d 266, 272 (N.Y. 1981).
7. *In re Quinlan*, 355 A.2d 647 (N.J. 1976).
8. 410 U.S. 113 (1973).
9. *Quinlan*, 355 A.2d at 663.
10. 370 N.E.2d 417 (Mass. 1977).
11. *Id.* at 434.
12. Gelford, *Euthanasia and the Terminally Ill Patient*, 63 Neb. L. Rev. 741, 747 (1984).
13. 380 N.E.2d 134 (Mass. 1978).
14. 405 N.E.2d 115 (Mass. 1980).
15. *John F. Kennedy Mem'l Hosp. v. Bludworth*, 452 So. 2d 921, 925 (Fla. 1984) (citing *In re Welfare of Colyer*, 660 P.2d 738 (Wash. 1983), in which the court found prior court approval to be "unresponsive and cumbersome").
16. *Schmitt v. Pierce*, 344 S.W.2d 120 (Mo. 1961).
17. Connery, *Prolonging Life: The Duty and Its Limits, Moral Responsibility in Prolonging Life's Decisions*, in To Treat or Not To Treat, 25 (1984).
18. Statement of Medical Opinion Re: "Brain Death," A.M.A. House of Delegates Res. (June 1974).
19. 482 N.Y.S.2d 436 (1984).
20. 438 N.Y.S.2d 266 (1981).
21. *Id.* at 425.
22. *Cruzan v. Director of the Mo. Dep't of Health*, 497 U.S. 261 (1990).
23. Pa. S.646, Amendment A3506, Printer's No. 689, Oct. 1, 1990.
24. 20 Pa. Cons. Stat. Ann. § 5602(a)(9) (1988).
25. "Hospital wants to let wife die," *Newsday*, Jan. 11, 1991, at 13.
26. *Farnam v. Crista Ministries*, 807 P.2d 830, 849 (Wash. 1991).
27. *Kevorkian v. Thompson*, 947 F. Supp. 1152 (1997).
28. "Dr. Death at work," *Newsday*, February 7, 1991, at 12.
29. "Kevorkian charges dropped," *Newsday*, July 22, 1992, at 4.
30. *Hobbins v. Attorney Gen. of Mich.*, No. 94–1473 (Mich. 1994); *Kevorkian v. Michigan*, No. 94–1490 (Mich. 1994).
31. "22nd Death for 'Dr. Death,'" *USA Today*, May 9, 1995, at 2A.

32. http://townhall.com/tipsheet/danieldoherty/2013/05/21/sigh-vermont-legalizes-physicianassisted-suicide-n1602510.
33. *Baxter v. State*, 354 Mont. 234, 224 P.3d 1211 (2009)
34. http://www.patientsrightscouncil.org/site/montana/.
35. http://righttodie.uslegal.com/physician-assisted-suicide/supreme-court-rulings/.
36. http://cnsnews.com/news/article/california-gov-signs-assisted-suicide-information-bill-law.
37. http://www.myfoxboston.com/story/20027701/2012/11/07/backers-of-mass-doctor-assisted-suicide-concede>
38. 117 S. Ct. 2293 (1997).
39. *Washington v. Glucksberg*, 117 S.Ct. 2258 (1997).
40. 42 U.S.C. 1395cc(a)(1).
41. http://www.wsha.org/EOL-FedState.cfm
42. http://www.euthanasia.com/vatican.html.
43. No. E2001-02906-COA-R3-CV (2002).
44. Ascension Health, "Issues and Concepts," http://www.ascensionhealth.org/ethics/public/issues/substituted.asp.
45. *In re Martin*, 517 N.W.2d 749 (Mich. Ct. App. 1994).
46. 420 N.E.2d 64 (N.Y. 1981).
47. 549 N.E.2d 292 (Ill. 1989).
48. *Stolle v. Baylor College of Medicine*, 981 S.W.2d 709 (1998).
49. *Spahn v. Eisenberg*, 563 N.W.2d 485 (1997).
50. 195 Cal. Rptr. 484 (Cal. Ct. App. 1983).
51. 486 A.2d 1209 (N.J. Sup. Ct. 1985).
52. *Id.*
53. U.S. Congress, Off. of Technology Assessment, Pub. No. OTA-BA-306, Life-Sustaining Technologies and the Elderly 48 (1987).
54. 464 N.E.2d 959 (Mass. 1984).
55. *In re Beth Israel Med*. Ctr., 519 N.Y.S.2d 511, 517 (N.Y. Sup. Ct. 1987).
56. Ronald Sullivan, "Ombudsman bars food tube removal," *New York Times*, March 7, 1986, at 82.
57. "AMA changes code of ethics on comas," *Newsday*, March 17, 1986, at 2.
58. *In re Jobes*, 529 A.2d 434 (N.J. 1987).
59. *Id.* at 438.
60. "Man wins right to let wife die," *Newsday*, Apr. 24, 1986, at 3.
61. *Id.* at 790.
62. *Id.* at 793.
63. *Bouvia v. Superior Court (Glenchur)*, 225 Cal. Rptr. 297 (Cal. Ct. App. 1986).
64. *Id.* at 306.
65. 549 N.E.2d 1043 (Ind. Ct. App. 1990).

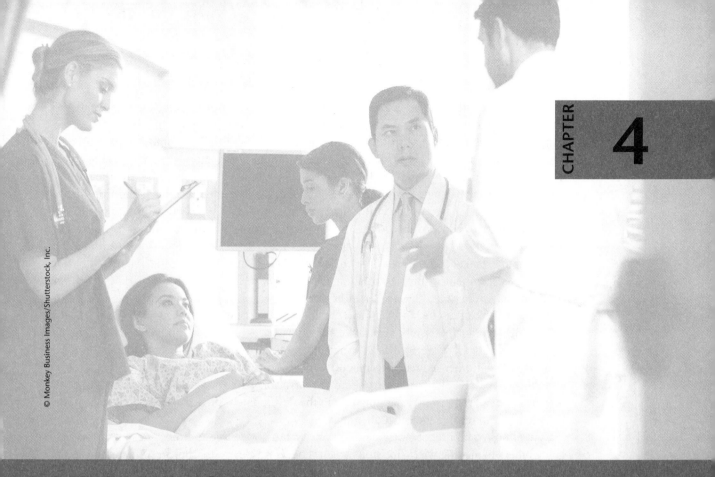
© Monkey Business Images/Shutterstock, Inc.

HEALTH CARE ETHICS COMMITTEE

LEARNING OBJECTIVES

Upon completion of this chapter, the reader will be able to:

- Describe the function and purpose of ethics committees.
- Describe the structure and goals of ethics committees.
- Explain the consultation process of ethics committees.
- Describe the expanding role of ethics committees.
- Discuss why the resolution of ethical dilemmas is no easy task.

INTRODUCTION

A *health care ethics committee* is an advisory body whose purpose is to facilitate discussion and consultation on ethical issues arising in the patient care setting. The goal of the ethics committee is to improve patient care and outcomes through recognition of the needs, interests, and rights of each patient and participants in the delivery of each patient's care. Health care ethics committees address legal–ethical issues that arise during the course of a patient's care and treatment. They serve as a resource for patients, families, and staff. They offer objective counsel when dealing with difficult health care issues. Ethics committees provide both educational and consultative services to patients, families, and caregivers. They enhance but do not replace important patient/family–physician relationships; nevertheless, they afford support for decisions made within those relationships. The numerous ethical questions facing health professionals involve the entire life span from the right to be born to the right to die. Ethics committees concern themselves with issues of morality, patient autonomy, legislation, and states' interests.

Although ethics committees first emerged in the 1960s in the United States, attention was focused on them in the 1976 landmark *Quinlan* case,[1] wherein the parents of Karen Ann Quinlan were granted permission by the New Jersey Supreme Court to remove Karen from a ventilator after she had been in a coma for a year. She died 10 years later at the age of 31, having been in a persistent vegetative state the entire time. The Quinlan court looked to a prognosis committee to verify Karen's medical condition. It then factored in the committee's opinion with all other evidence to reach the decision to allow withdrawing her life-support equipment. To date, ethics committees do not have sole surrogate decision-making authority; however, they play an ever-expanding role in the development of policy and procedural guidelines to assist in resolving ethical dilemmas.

An ethics committee is not a decision maker but a resource that provides advice to help guide others in making wiser decisions when there is no clear best choice. A unanimous opinion is not always possible when an ethics committee convenes to consider the issues of an ethical dilemma; however, consultative advice as to a course of action to follow in resolving the dilemma is a major the role of the ethics committee. Any recommendations for issue resolution reached by the ethics committee need to be communicated to those most closely involved with the patient's care. Being sensitive to each family member's values and assisting them in coping with whatever consensus decision is reached are crucial to the success of the committee. Unresolved issues often need to be addressed and a course of action followed. Each new consultation presents new opportunities for learning and teaching others how to cope with similar issues. Guidelines for resolving ethical issues will always be in a state of flux. Each new case presents new challenges and learning opportunities.

Making a decision, suggesting a course of action, recommending a path to follow, and making a choice require accepting the fact that there will be elements of right and wrong in the final decision. The idea is to cause the least pain and provide the greatest benefit.

COMMITTEE STRUCTURE

A hospital-based ethics committee should be composed of a multidisciplinary group of individuals whose membership includes representatives from the hospital (e.g., administrator, chaplain, nurse, physician, patient advocate) and community (e.g., clergy, legal counsel, ethicist). Members may also include those in positions of corporate and political stature, respect, and diversity. Appointment and rotation of new members to the ethics committee should be staggered in order to maintain continuity and stability.

Ethics committee members should be carefully vetted as to their skills in *conflict resolution*. Members of the ethics committee should complete a mandatory orientation that includes training and coaching. They should participate in continuing education programs. Committee members are expected to be active participants in committee activities. Self-study interest in the law and ethics should prove helpful. Those members of the committee who participate in consultative services involving patient care dilemmas should have appropriate medical, legal, and ethics training.

COMMITTEE GOALS

The goals of ethics committees often include the following:

- Provide a forum for review and discussion of ethical and moral issues relative to patient care.
- Provide information to patients as to the functioning of the ethics committee and how to access the committee at the time of admission. This information is generally provided in patient handbooks and/or informational brochures. The electronic media through patient room TVs is also helpful in educating patients as to their rights and responsibilities including the process for requesting a consultation.
- Serve as support and resource for hospital staff, families, and patients.
- Provide consultation, as requested, when there are conflicts in care options.
- Provide assistance in clarifying situations that are ethical, legal, or religious in nature that extend beyond the scope of daily practice.
- Clarify issues and discuss alternatives to ethical dilemmas.
- Promote patient rights.
- Assist the patient and family in coming to consensus with the options that best meet the patient's care needs.
- Review cases for educational purposes.
- Enhance the ethical tenor of both the hospital and health care professionals.

COMMITTEE FUNCTIONS

The functions of ethics committees are multifaceted and include development of policy and procedure guidelines to assist in resolving ethical dilemmas; staff and community education; conflict resolution; case reviews, support, and consultation; and political advocacy. The degree to which an ethics committee serves each of these functions varies in different health care organizations.

POLICY AND PROCEDURE DEVELOPMENT

The ethics committee is a valuable resource for assisting in the development of hospital policies and procedures pertinent to addressing ethical dilemmas (e.g., consultation procedures, confidentiality of information, staff and community education, annual review of the committee's activities and effectiveness). The following policies are a sampling of those often recommended by ethics committees.

Policy: Staff and Community Education

The director of education collaborates with hospital staff college faculty, when available, and ethicists to teach and train caregivers to resolve ethical issues that occur in the work environment. Programs are also arranged for community members interested in such topics as understanding and executing advance directives. To learn more about the community-sponsored ethics education programs, community members are encouraged to contact the hospital's department of education at xxx-xxx-xxxx.

Policy: Requests for Consultations

Ethics consultations are available to caregivers, patients, or family members who request an ethics consult. Ethics consultations are available 24 hours a day 365 days a year by calling the ethics hotline xxx-xxx-xxxx. Consultations shall be requested on a form prepared by the ethics committee and reviewed and approved by the hospital's administration, legal counsel, and board of directors.

Policy: Confidentiality of Information

Ethics committee information shall be considered confidential and shall not be used in any way except as provided herein or as required by law. Any information or case study developed for use by the committee shall not be required to become part of a patient's medical record. Committee members shall not make entries in a patient's medical record unless required by law and/or hospital policy.

Policy: Annual Review

An overall review of the ethics committee's activities will be conducted on an annual basis to determine the effectiveness of the committee and if it is accomplishing its stated goals. This review may take the form of a self-study or external review, preferably by a qualified ethicist.

EDUCATION

The ethics committee typically provides education on current ethical concepts and issues to committee members, staff, and the community at large. Some community hospitals provide ethics education to the staff at ambulatory care facilities, home health agencies, long-term care facilities, and physicians' offices. Such education helps reduce the need for emergent end-of-life consultations in acute-care settings.

The ethics committee provides resources for educational purposes to support staff in the development of the appropriate competencies for addressing ethical, legal, and spiritual issues, for example, those common to end-of-life issues (e.g., surrogate decision-making, the patient's refusal to accept recommended medical treatment, family conflict). Educational programs on ethical issues are developed for ethics committee members and staff on such topics as moral theories and principals, as well common ethical dilemmas that occur as they relate to such services common to emergency departments and critical care units. Community education often includes such topics as how to prepare and execute an advance directive.

CONSULTATION AND CONFLICT RESOLUTION

Ethics consultations are helpful in resolving uncertainty and disagreements over health care dilemmas. Ethics committees often provide consultation services for patients, families, and caregivers struggling with difficult treatment decisions and end-of-life dilemmas. Always mindful of its basic orientation toward the patient's best interests, the committee provides options and suggestions for resolution of conflict in actual cases. Consultation with an ethics committee is not mandatory but is conducted at the request of a physician, patient, family member, or other caregiver.

The ethics committee strives to provide viable alternatives that will lead to the optimal resolution of dilemmas confronting the continuing care of the patient. It is important to remember that an ethics committee functions in an advisory capacity and should not be considered a substitute proxy for the patient.

A representative of the ethics committee is often able to intervene, when requested, in resolving ethical dilemmas. On occasion it may be necessary to request the assistance of one or more additional members of the ethics committee. An on-call roster is generally helpful when a consultation is necessary during evening, night, and weekend hours. Ethics committee members of the hospital staff generally provide on-call services.

Requests for Committee Consultations

Requests for ethics consultations often involve clarification of issues regarding decision-making capacity, informed consent, advance directives, and withdrawal of treatment. Consultations should be conducted in a timely manner considering the following information:

- Who requested the consultation?
- What are the issues?
- Is there is a problem that needs referral to another service?
- What specifically is being requested of the ethics committee (e.g., clarification of the problem or mediation)?

When conducting a consultation, all patient records must be reviewed and discussed with the attending physician, family members, and other caregivers involved in the patient's treatment. If an issue can be resolved easily, a designated member of the ethics committee should be able to consult on the case without the need for a full committee meeting. If the problem is unusual, problematic, or delicate, or has important legal ramifications, a full committee meeting may be necessary. Others who can be invited to an ethics committee case review, as appropriate, include the patient, if competent; relatives; agent or surrogate decision maker; and caregivers. Evaluation of a case consultation should take the following into consideration:

- Patient's current medical and mental status, diagnosis, and prognosis
- Patient's mental status and ability to make decisions, understand the information that is necessary to make a decision, and clearly understand the consequences of his or her choice
- Benefits and burdens of recommended treatment, or alternative treatments
- Life expectancy, treated and untreated

- Views of caregivers and consultants
- Pain and suffering
- Quality-of-life issues
- Financial burden on family (e.g., if the patient is in a comatose state with no hope of recovery, should the spouse deplete his or her finances to maintain the spouse on a respirator?)

Decisions concerning patient care must take into consideration the patient's:

- Personal assessment of the quality of life
- Current expressed choices
- Advance directives
- Competency to make decisions
- Ability to process information rationally to compare risks, benefits, and alternatives to treatment
- Ability to articulate major factors in decisions and reasons for them and ability to communicate

The patient must have all the information necessary to allow a reasonable person to make a prudent decision on his or her own behalf. The patient's choice must be voluntary and free from coercion by family, physicians, or others.

Family members must be identified and the following questions considered when making decisions:

- Do family members understand the patient's wishes?
- Is the family in agreement with the patient's wishes?
- Does the patient have an advance directive?
- Has the patient appointed an agent?
- Are there any religious proscriptions?
- Are there any financial concerns?
- Are there any legal concerns that need to be addressed (applicable state statutes and case law)?

When an ethics committee is engaged in the consulting process, its recommendations should be offered as suggestions, imposing no obligation for acceptance on the part of the patient, family, surrogate decision maker, organization, its governing body, medical staff, attending physicians, or other persons. **Figure 4-1** presents an ethics consultation form for documenting an ethics committee consultation.

When conducting a formal consultation, ethics committees should:

1. Identify the ethical dilemma (e.g., reasons why the consult was requested).
2. Be sure that the appropriate "Consultation Request" form has been completed.
3. Identify relevant facts.
   a. Diagnosis and prognosis.
   b. Patient goals and wishes.
   c. Regulatory and legal issues.

Ethics Consultation

Date: _____ Time: _____ Caller: _____

Reason for call _____

Action taken: _____

Patient: _____ Age: _____

Record #: _____ Consultation requested by: _____

Relationship (e.g., caregiver, spouse) _____

Attending physician: _____

Other physicians: _____

Will the patient participate in the consultation? ❑ Yes ❑ No

Does the patient have decision-making capacity? ❑ Yes ❑ No Explain _____

Surrogate decision maker? ❑ Yes ❑ No If yes, name: _____

Phone #: _____ Advance directives (e.g., living will)? _____

Availability of advance directive _____

Consultation participants:

❑Family/relationship_____

❑ Physicians _____

❑ Nurses _____

❑ Ethics committee members (e.g., Chaplain, social worker, community representative) _____

_____

_____

_____

Medical Treatment/Care Information

Diagnoses _____ Prognosis _____

Course of illness _____

Treatment options appropriate _____

Treatment options medically beneficial: _____

Treatment options available: _____

Would the patient have wanted the treatment? _____

Ethical issues: _____

Legal issues: _____

Other persons to contact for input, if any. _____

Consultative guidance: _____

Guidance communicated? ❑ Yes ❑ No If yes, to whom? _____

Consultation noted on the medical record ❑ Yes ❑ No

Disposition: _____

_____

Form completed by: _____ Date/Time: _____

FIGURE 4-1 Hospital Consultation Request Form

    d. Professional standards and codes of ethics.

    e. Institutional policies and values.

4. Identify stakeholders.

5. Identify moral issues.

    a. Human dignity.

    b. Common good.

    c. Justice.

    d. Beneficence.

    e. Respect for autonomy.

    f. Informed consent.

    g. Medical futility and so on.

6. Identify legal issues.

7. Consider alternative options.

8. Conduct consultation.

9. Review, discuss, and provide reasoning for recommendations made.

10. Review and follow up.

11. Committee discussion includes family members.

12. Family members are queried as to their hopes and expectations.

13. Consultations are documented.

Case: Ethics Committee Serves as Guardian

The Kentucky Supreme Court ruled in *Woods v. Commonwealth*, 1999-SSC0773 (August 24, 2004) that Kentucky's Living Will Directive, allowing a court-appointed guardian or other designated surrogate to remove a patient's life support systems, is constitutional. The patient in this case, Woods, had been placed on a ventilator after having a heart attack. It was generally agreed that he would never regain consciousness and would die in 2 to 10 years. After a recommendation of the hospital ethics committee, Woods's guardian at the time asked for approval to remove Woods's life support. The Kentucky Supreme Court affirmed an appeals court decision, holding that: (1) "If there is no guardian," but the family, physicians, and ethics committee all agree with the surrogate, there is no need to appoint a guardian; (2) "If there is a guardian" and all parties agree, there is no need for judicial approval; (3) "If there is disagreement," the parties may petition the courts.

    Withdrawal of life support from a patient is prohibited absent clear and convincing evidence that the patient is permanently unconscious or in a persistent vegetative state and that withdrawing life support is in the patient's best interest.

Ethical and Legal Issues

1. Discuss the ethical issues of this case.

2. Discuss under what circumstances an ethics committee should serve as a legal guardian.

3. Discuss the pros and cons of an ethics committee serving as a patient's guardian.

EXPANDING ROLE OF THE ETHICS COMMITTEE

Typically, hospital ethics committees concern themselves with biomedical issues as they relate to end-of-life issues; unfortunately, they often fail to address external decisions that affect internal operations. The role of an organization's ethics committee is evolving into more than a group of individuals who periodically gather together to meet a regulatory requirement and address advance directives and end-of-life issues. The organizational ethics committee has an ever-expanding role. This expanded role involves addressing external issues that affect internal operations (e.g., managed care, malpractice insurance, and complicated Health Insurance Portability and Accountability Act regulations that often increase legal and other financial costs). Ethics committees need to review their functions periodically and redefine themselves.

The ethics committee is health care's sleeping giant. Because of its potential to bring about change, its mission must not be limited to end-of-life issues. Its vision must not be restricted to issues internal to the organization but must include external matters that affect internal operations.

Failure to increase the good of others when one is knowingly in a position to do so is morally wrong. Preventative medicine and active public health interventions exemplify this conviction. After methods of treating yellow fever and smallpox were discovered, for example, it was universally agreed that positive steps ought to be taken to establish programs to protect public health.

The wide variety of ethical issues that an ethics committee can be involved in is somewhat formidable. Although an ethics committee cannot address every issue that one could conceivably imagine, the ethics committee should periodically reevaluate its scope of activities and effectiveness in addressing ethical issues. Some of the internal and external issues facing an organization's ethics committee are listed here.

INTERNAL ETHICAL ISSUES

1. Dilemma of blind trials: Who gets the placebo when the investigational drug looks very promising?
2. Informed consent: Are patients adequately informed as to risks, benefits, and alternative procedures that may be equally effective, knowing that one procedure may be more risky or damaging than another (e.g., lumpectomy versus a radical mastectomy)?
3. What is the physician's responsibility for informing the patient of his or her education, training, qualifications, and skill in treating a medical condition or performing an invasive procedure?
4. What is the role of the ethics committee when the medical staff is reluctant or fails to take timely action, knowing that one of its members practices questionable medicine?
5. Should a hospital's medical staff practice evidence-based medicine or follow its own best judgment?
6. To what extent should the organization participate in and/or support genetic research?
7. How should the ethics committee address confidentiality issues?
8. To what extent should medical information be shared with the patient's family?

9. To what extent should the organization's leadership control the scope of issues that the ethics committee addresses?
10. What are the demarcation lines as to what information should or should not be provided to the patient when mistakes are made relative to his or her care?

EXTERNAL ETHICAL ISSUES

1. Does the ethics committee have a role in addressing questionable reimbursement schemes?
2. Should an ethics committee have its own letterhead? What value would this serve?
3. What role, if any, should an ethics committee play in the following scenario?

CASE: CHOOSING THE RIGHT HOSPITAL

Emergency services ambulance personnel regularly transport suspected stroke patients to Hospital A. This hospital has no neurologists or neurosurgeons on its medical staff but does provide coffee and donuts to transport personnel. Ambulance personnel have an option to take the suspected stroke victim to Hospital B, which is within five blocks of Hospital A. Hospital B has a well-trained stroke team with staff neurologists and neurosurgeons readily available.

Ethical and Legal Issues

1. Describe the ethical issues in this case.
2. Describe the organizational politics that might come into play.
3. Discuss how organizational politics may prevent an ethics committee from becoming involved in many of the issues just described.

Although an ethics committee's serves in an advisory capacity, its value to an organization has yet to be fully realized.

RESOLUTION OF ETHICAL DILEMMAS

The difference between moral dilemmas and ethical ones, philosophers say, is that in moral issues the choice is between right and wrong. In ethics, the choice is between two rights.
—PAMELA WARRICK

The resolution of ethical dilemmas is a perplexing task at best, especially when two opposite answers both have elements of right and wrong—good and bad, regardless of the ultimate decision made. Finding compromise is no easy task when ethical principles, values, and morals are in conflict and vary from individual to individual. This is no easy task for members of an ethics committee, especially when the mix of opinions of caregivers, family members, and the health care entity's mission of healing collide. Although decision-making can be much easier when the patient has executed end-of-life directives, ethics committees often do not have this luxury, thus creating a need for ethics committees to help guide others in making difficult care decisions. With outcomes that often result in the decision-maker reflecting back and doubting his or her own decisions, it is important that each committee member reflect on the following thoughts prior to participating in an ethics consultation:

- I will accept the patient's wishes, if known.
- I will accept the dialogue of committee members with varying beliefs, expectations, and values, knowing some will undoubtedly challenge my own sense of right and wrong.
- I will help the ethics committee seek a morally acceptable resolution to an ethical dilemma.
- I will not be too fearful to seek clarification of issues and ask questions.
- I will contribute to making consultations meaningful and not argumentative.
- My compassion will outweigh my need to be right.
- The ultimate decision is not mine to make.
- I will provide guidance, consultation, and education.

An ethical dilemma can arise when, for example, the principles of autonomy and beneficence conflict with one another. The following cases illustrate how one's right to make his or her decisions can conflict with the principle of doing good and not harm.

CASE: PATIENT REFUSES BLOOD

Mrs. Jones has gangrene of her left leg. Her hemoglobin slipped to 6.4. She has a major infection and is diabetic. There is no spouse and no living will. The patient has decided that she does not want to be resuscitated if she should go into cardiopulmonary arrest. She may need surgery. She has agreed to surgery but refuses a blood transfusion, even though she is not a Jehovah's Witness. The surgeon will not perform the surgery, which is urgent, without Jones agreeing to a blood transfusion, if it becomes necessary. The attending physician questions the patient's capacity to make decisions. Her children have donated blood. She says she is not afraid to die.

Ethical and Legal Issues

1. Should the physician refuse to treat this patient? Explain your answer.
2. Should the family have a right to override the patient's decision to refuse blood? Explain your answer.

CASE: A SON'S GUILT, A FATHER'S WISHES

Following a massive stroke, Mr. Smith was transported from the Rope nursing facility to a local hospital by ambulance on July 4, 2004. Smith, 94 years of age, had been a resident at the Rope nursing facility for the past 12 years. Before being placed in Rope, Smith had been living with Mr. Curry, a close friend, for the previous 8 years. He had an advance directive indicating that he would never want to be placed on a respirator.

Smith's son and only child, Barry, who now lives in Los Angeles and had been estranged from his dad for more than 20 years, was notified by Curry that his dad had been admitted to the hospital in a terminal condition. Smith had mistakenly been placed on a respirator by hospital staff contrary to the directions in his advance directive, which had been placed on the front cover of Smith's medical chart. Curry, who was legally appointed by Smith to act as his health care surrogate decision maker, called Barry and explained that, according to his dad's wishes and advance directives, he was planning to ask hospital staff to have the respirator removed. Barry asked Curry to wait until he flew in from California to see his dad. Curry agreed to wait for Barry's arrival the following day, July 5. After arriving at the hospital, Barry told Curry that he would take responsibility for his dad's care and that Curry's services would no longer be needed. Barry told hospital staff that he objected to the hospital's plan to remove his father from the respirator. He said that he needed time to say goodbye to his dad, which he did by whispering his sorrows in his dad's ears. Smith, however, did not respond. Barry demanded that the hospital do everything that it could to save his dad's life, saying, "I don't know if Dad heard me. We have to wait until he wakes up so that I can tell him how sorry I am for not having stayed in touch with him over the years." Smith's physicians explained to Barry that there was no chance Smith would ever awaken out of his coma. Barry threatened legal action if the hospital did not do everything it could to keep his dad alive. Smith's physician again spoke to Barry about the futility of maintaining his dad on a respirator. Barry remained uncooperative. The hospital chaplain was called to speak to Barry, but had little success. Finally, hospital staff requested an ethics consult.

Ethical and Legal Issues

1. Discuss the ethical dilemmas in this case.
2. Discuss the issues and the role of the ethics committee in this case.

HELPFUL HINTS

The reason for studying ethical and legal issues is to understand and help guide others through the decision-making process as it relates to ethical dilemmas. The following are some helpful guidelines when faced with ethical dilemmas:

- Be aware of how everyday life is full of ethical decisions and that numerous ethical issues can arise when caring for patients.
- Help guide others to make choices.
- Ask your patient how you might help him or her.

- Be aware of why you think the way you do. Do not impose your beliefs on others.
- Ask yourself whether you agree with the things you do. If the answer is no, ask yourself how you should change.
- When you are not sure what to do, the wise thing to do is to talk it over with another person, someone whose opinion you trust.
- Do not sacrifice happiness for devotion to others.
- Do not lie to avoid hurting someone's feelings.

CHAPTER REVIEW

1. Ethics committee serves as a resource for patients, families, and staff, offering an objective counsel when dealing with difficult health care dilemmas.
2. Ethics committee should be structured to include a wide range of community leaders in positions of political stature, respect, and diversity.
3. The goals of the ethics committee are to:
   - Promote the rights of patients.
   - Promote shared decision making between patients and clinicians.
   - Assist the patient and family in coming to consensus when faced with ethical dilemmas.
4. The functions of ethics committees are multifaceted and include:
   - Policy and procedure development.
   - Staff and community education.
   - Consultation and conflict resolution.
     - A resource tool in resolving ethical dilemmas.
     - Patients and family should be encouraged to participate in addressing ethical dilemmas.
5. Decision making is difficult when there are:
   - A variety of value beliefs held by patients, family members, and caregivers.
   - Alternative choices that offer both good and bad outcomes.
   - Limited resources.
6. The resolution of ethical dilemmas is a perplexing task. Ethics committee member must be prepared to understand the challenge by actively participating in the decision-making process without bias.

TEST YOUR UNDERSTANDING

TERMINOLOGY

circular reasoning	health care ethics committee	reasoning and decision
conflict resolution	ethics consultation	making
ethical decision making	partial reasoning	

REVIEW QUESTIONS

1. What is the purpose of an ethics committee?

2. Discuss the functions of an ethics committee.

3. Explain the consultative role of the ethics committee.

4. Discuss the educational role of the ethics committee.

5. Discuss the ever-expanding role of ethics committees, including internal operational issues and external influences that affect internal operations.

6. Discuss what ethics members should take into consideration when addressing ethical dilemmas.

NOTES

1. *In re Quinlan*, 355 A.2d 647 (N.J. 1976).

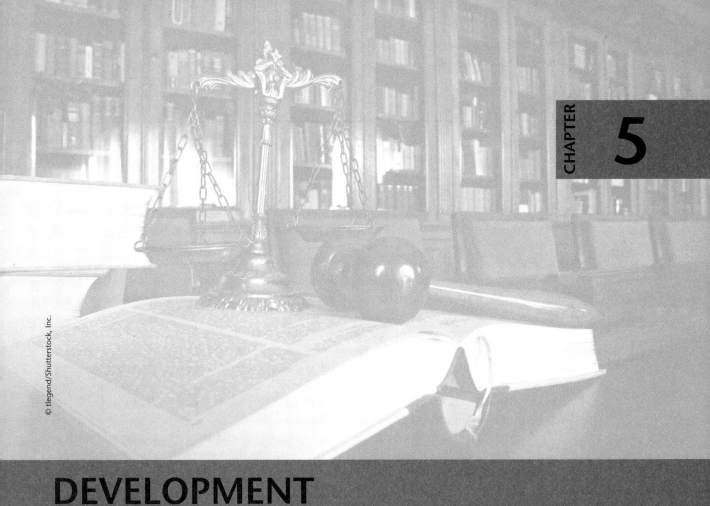

CHAPTER 5

DEVELOPMENT OF LAW

Laws are the very bulwarks of liberty; they define every man's rights, and defend the individual liberties of all men.

–J. G. HOLLAND (1819–1881)

LEARNING OBJECTIVES

Upon completion of this chapter, the reader will be able to:

- Understand the development and sources of law.
- Describe how the government is organized through the three branches of government.
- Explain the principle *separation of powers*.
- Describe what is meant by *conflict of laws*.
- Describe the functions of the Department of Health and Human Resources and its various operating divisions.

INTRODUCTION

In law a man is guilty when he violates the rights of others. In ethics he is guilty if he only thinks of doing so.

—IMMANUEL KANT

It is appropriate here to provide the reader with a background of the law, as it is the law that enables society to uphold what is right and punish those who transgress its intent—to protect the moral fiber upon which this nation was founded. This chapter introduces the reader to the development of American law, the functioning of the legal system, and the roles of the three branches of government in creating, administering, and enforcing the law in the United States. It is important to understand the foundation of the legal system before one can appreciate or comprehend the specific laws and principles relating to health care.

The law is rooted in tradition, culture, customs, and beliefs (e.g., religious influence—the Mosaic law). Laws constantly grow and change to meet the needs of the American culture, a mixture of many cultures. Familiarity with the vocabulary enables one to understand the ideas, concepts, and structure of the law. Laws continually evolve because of the ever-changing political, social, religious, and personal values of society, which is composed of many cultures that become more intertwined with each new generation.

Supreme Court Justice Oliver Wendell Holmes said that the law "is a magic mirror, wherein we see reflected not only our own lives but also the lives of those who went before us."[1] "The government of the United States has been emphatically termed a government of laws, and not of men. It will certainly cease to deserve this high appellation, if the laws furnish no remedy for the violation of a vested right."[2]

Most definitions of *law* define it as a system of principles and processes by which people in a society deal with their disputes and problems, seeking to solve or settle them without resorting to force. Laws are general rules of conduct that are enforced by government, which imposes penalties when prescribed laws are violated.

Laws govern the relationships between private individuals and organizations and between both of these parties and government. *Public law* deals with the relationships between individuals and government; *private law* deals with relationships among individuals. Laws regulate the activities and behaviors of individuals in international, federal, state, local, and municipal settings.

One important segment of public law is criminal law, which prohibits conduct deemed injurious to public order and provides for punishment of those proven to have engaged in such conduct. Public law also consists of countless regulations designed to advance societal objectives by requiring private individuals and organizations to adopt a specified courses of action in their activities and undertakings. The thrust of most public law is to attain what society deems to be valid public goals.

Private law is concerned with the recognition and enforcement of the rights and duties of private individuals and organizations. Tort and contract actions are two basic types of private law. In a tort action, one party asserts that the wrongful conduct of another has caused harm, and the injured party seeks compensation for the harm suffered. Generally, a contract action involves a claim by one party that another party has breached an agreement by failing to fulfill an obligation. Either remuneration or specific performance of the obligation may be sought as a remedy. It is clear that without an organized, clear system of laws that regulate society, anarchy would be the result.

The goal of this chapter is to help caregivers better understand the law and how it affects the difficulties they face while trying to do the right thing by making health care decisions that are both morally and legally acceptable.

SOURCES OF LAW

The basic sources of law are common law, which is derived from judicial decisions; statutory law, which emanates from the federal and state legislatures; and administrative law, prescribed by administrative agencies. In those instances in which written laws are either silent, vague, or contradictory to other laws, the judicial system often is called on to resolve those disputes until such time as appropriate legislative action can be taken to clear up a particular legal issue. In the following sections, the sources of law that formed the foundation of our legal system are discussed.

COMMON LAW

The term *common law* refers to the body of principles that have evolved and expanded from judicial decisions. Many of the legal principles and rules applied today by courts in the United States have their origins in English common law. Common law has its roots in "reason and justice" for all.

The judicial system is necessary because it is impossible to have a law that covers every potential human conflict that might occur in society. It not only serves as a mechanism for reviewing legal disputes that arise in the written law, but it also serves as an effective review mechanism for those issues on which the written law is silent or, in instances of a mixture of issues, involving both written law and common-law decisions.

During the colonial period, English common law began to be applied in the colonies. According to John Dickinson in his *Letters from a Farmer in Pennsylvania* in 1768:[3]

> The common law of England is generally received . . . but our courts *exercise a sovereign authority,* in determining what parts of the common and statute law ought to be extended: For it must be admitted, that the difference of circumstances necessarily requires us, in some cases to *reject* the determination of both. . . . Some of the English rules are adopted, others rejected.

Joseph Story, in an 1829 U.S. Supreme Court decision, wrote, "The common law of England is not to be taken in all respects to be that of America. Our ancestors brought with them its general principles, and claimed it as their birthright. But they brought with them, and adopted only that portion which was applicable to their situation."[4]

> The size of the country and the abundance of its natural resources made impossible the importation of the common law exactly as it had been developed in England. Measured by English standards, America had superabundant land, timber, and mineral wealth. American law had to serve the primary need of the new society to master the vast land areas of the American continent. The decisive facts upon which the law had to be based were the seemingly limitless expanses of land and the wealth and variety of natural resources.[5]

After the Revolution, each state, with the exception of Louisiana, adopted all or part of the existing English common law. Laws were added as needed. Louisiana civil law is based to a great extent on the French and Spanish laws and especially on the Napoleonic Code. As a result, there is no national system of common law in the United States, and common law on specific subjects may differ from state to state.

> Case law court decisions did not easily pass from colony to colony. There were no printed reports to make transfer easy, though in the 18th century some manuscript materials did circulate among lawyers. These could hardly have been very influential. No doubt custom and case law slowly seeped from colony to colony. Travelers and word of mouth spread knowledge of living law. It is hard to say how much; thus it is hard to tell to what degree there was a common legal structure.[6]
>
> Judicial review started to become part of the living law during the decade before the adoption of the federal Constitution. During that time American courts first began to assert the power to rule on the constitutionality of legislative acts and to hold unconstitutional statutes void.[7]

Cases are tried applying common-law principles unless a statute governs. Even though statutory law has affirmed many of the legal rules and principles initially established by the courts, new issues continue to arise, especially in private-law disputes that require decision making according to common-law principles. Common-law actions are initiated mainly to recover money damages and/or possession of real or personal property.

When a higher state court has enunciated a common-law principle, the lower courts within the state where the decision was rendered must follow that principle. A decision in a case that sets forth a new legal principle establishes a precedent. Trial courts or those on equal footing are not bound by the decisions of other trial courts. Also, a principle established in one state does not set precedent for another state. Rather, the rulings in one jurisdiction may be used by the courts of other jurisdictions as guides to the legal analysis of a particular legal problem. Decisions found to be reasonable will be followed.

The position of a court or agency, relative to other courts and agencies, determines the place assigned to its decision in the hierarchy of decisional law. The decisions of the Supreme Court of the United States are highest in the hierarchy of decisional law with respect to federal legal questions. Because of the parties or the legal question involved, most legal controversies do not fall within the scope of the Supreme Court's decision-making responsibilities. On questions of purely state concern—such as the interpretation of a state statute that raises no issues under the U.S. Constitution or federal law—the highest court in the state has the final word on proper interpretation. The following are explanations of some of the more important common-law principles:

- *Precedent*: A precedent is a judicial decision that can be used as a standard in subsequent similar cases. A precedent is set when a court decision is rendered that serves as a rule for future guidance when deciding similar cases.
- *Res judicata*: In common law, the term res judicata—which means "the thing is decided"— refers to that which has been previously acted on or decided by the courts. According to *Black's Law Dictionary,* it is a rule where "a final judgment rendered by a court of competent jurisdiction on the merits is conclusive as to the rights of the parties and their privies,

and, as to them, constitutes an absolute bar to subsequent action involving the same claim, demand, or cause of action."[8]

- *Stare decisis*: The common-law principle of stare decisis ("let the decision stand") provides that when a decision is rendered in a lawsuit involving a particular set of facts, another lawsuit involving an identical or substantially similar situation is to be resolved in the same manner as the first lawsuit. The resolution of future lawsuits is arrived at by applying the rules and principles of preceding cases. In this manner, courts arrive at comparable rulings. Sometimes, slight factual differences may provide a basis for recognizing distinctions between the precedent and the current case. In some cases, even when such differences are absent, a court may conclude that a particular common-law rule is no longer in accord with the needs of society and may depart from precedent. It should be understood that principles of law are subject to change, whether they originate in statutory or in common law. Common-law principles may be modified, overturned, abrogated, or created by new court decisions in a continuing process of growth and development to reflect changes in social attitudes, public needs, judicial prejudices, or contemporary political thinking.

STATUTORY LAW

Statutory law is written law emanating from federal and state legislative bodies. Although a statute can abolish any rule of common law, it can do so only by stating it in express words. States and local jurisdictions can enact and enforce only laws that do not conflict with federal law. Statutory laws may be declared void by a court; for example, a statute may be found unconstitutional because it does not comply with a state or federal constitution, because it is vague or ambiguous, or in the case of a state law, because it is in conflict with a federal law.

In many cases involving statutory law, the court is called on to interpret how a statute applies to a given set of facts. For example, a statute may state merely that no person may discriminate against another person because of race, creed, color, or gender. A court may then be called on to decide whether certain actions by a person are discriminatory and therefore violate the law.

Constitution of the United States

In civilized life, law floats on a sea of ethics.

–Earl Warren

The principles and rules of statutory law are set in hierarchical order. The *Constitution of the United States* adopted at the Constitutional Convention in Philadelphia in 1787 is highest in the hierarchy of enacted law. Article VI of the Constitution declares:

> This Constitution, and the Laws of the United States which shall be made in Pursuance thereof; and all Treaties made, or which shall be made, under the Authority of the United States, shall be the supreme Law of the Land; and the Judges in every State shall be bound thereby, any Thing in the Constitution or Laws of any State to the Contrary notwithstanding.[9]

The clear import of these words is that the U.S. Constitution, federal law, and federal treaties take precedence over the constitutions and laws of specific states and local jurisdictions. Statutory law may be amended, repealed, or expanded by action of the legislature.

Bill of Rights

The conventions of a number of the states, at the time of adopting the U.S. Constitution, expressed a desire to prevent the abuse of its powers. As a result of this concern, Congress ratified amendments to the Constitution of the United States. The *Bill of Rights,* the first 10 amendments to the constitution, was added to protect the rights of citizens. The amendments included the rights to privacy, equal protection, and freedom of speech and religion.

ADMINISTRATIVE LAW

Administrative law is the extensive body of public law issued by administrative agencies to direct the enacted laws of the federal and state governments. It is the branch of law that controls the administrative operations of government. Congress and state legislative bodies realistically cannot oversee their many laws; therefore, they delegate implementation and administration of the law to an appropriate administrative agency. Health care organizations in particular are inundated with a proliferation of administrative rules and regulations affecting every aspect of their operations.

The Administrative Procedures Act[10] describes the different procedures under which federal administrative agencies must operate.[11] The act prescribes the procedural responsibilities and authority of administrative agencies and provides for legal remedies for those wronged by agency actions. The regulatory power exercised by administrative agencies includes power to license, power of rate setting (e.g., Centers for Medicare and Medicaid Services), and power over business practices (e.g., National Labor Relations Board).

The rules and regulations established by an agency must be administered within the scope of the authority delegated to the agency by Congress. Agency regulations and decisions can be subject to judicial review.

U.S. GOVERNMENT ORGANIZATION

The government of the United States is a national constitutional republic covering 50 states, the nation's capital and its territories (e.g., Puerto Rico, Guam). The federal government is organized into three branches. The legislative, executive, and judicial branches of government are illustrated in **Figure 5-1**. The powers and duties of the three branches of government are described in the U.S. Constitution.

SEPARATION OF POWERS

A vital concept in the constitutional framework of government on both federal and state levels is the *separation of powers*. Essentially, this principle provides that no one branch of government is clearly dominant over the other two; however, in the exercise of its functions, each may affect and limit the activities, functions, and powers of the others. The concept of *separation of powers*—in effect, a system of checks and balances—is illustrated in the relationships

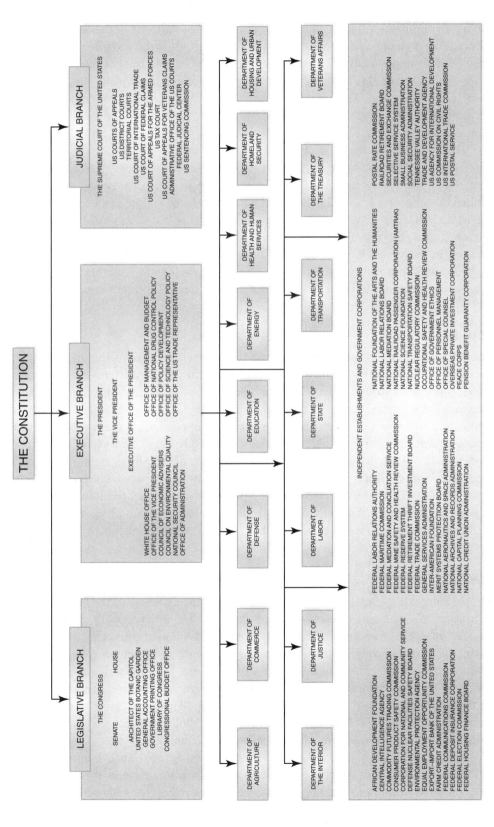

FIGURE 5-1   U.S. Government Organization.

among the branches of government with regard to legislation. On the federal level, when a bill creating a statute is enacted by Congress and signed by the president, it becomes law. If the president vetoes a bill, it takes a two-thirds vote of each house of Congress to override the veto. The president also can prevent a bill from becoming law by avoiding any action while Congress is in session. This procedure, known as a pocket veto, can temporarily stop a bill from becoming law and may permanently prevent it from becoming law if later sessions of Congress do not act on it favorably.

The Supreme Court may declare a bill that has become law invalid if the law violates the Constitution. "It is also not entirely unworthy of observation, that in declaring what shall be the Supreme law of the land, the Constitution itself is first mentioned; and not the laws of the United States generally, but those only which shall be made in pursuance of the Constitution, have that rank."[12]

Even though a Supreme Court decision is final regarding a specific controversy, Congress and the president may generate new, constitutionally sound legislation to replace a law that has been declared unconstitutional. The procedures for amending the Constitution are complex and often time consuming, but they can serve as a way to offset or override a Supreme Court decision.

CONFLICT OF LAWS

The various states and territories also have there own constitutions that must not be in conflict with the U.S. Constitution. When state and federal laws conflict, resolution can be sought in the appropriate federal court. The legal case, *Dorsten v. Lapeer County General Hospital*,[13] illustrates how federal and state laws can be in conflict. The plaintiff in this case brought an action against Lapeer General Hospital and certain physicians on the medical board alleging wrongful denial of her application for medical staff privileges. The plaintiff asserted claims under the U.S. Code for sex discrimination, violations of the Sherman Antitrust Act, and the like. The plaintiff filed a motion to compel discovery of peer-review reports to support her case. The U.S. District Court held that the plaintiff was entitled to discovery of peer-review reports despite a Michigan state law purporting to establish an absolute privilege barring access to peer-review reports conducted by hospital review boards.

LEGISLATIVE BRANCH

On the federal level, legislative powers are vested in the Congress of the United States, which consists of a Senate and a House of Representatives. The function of the legislative branch is to enact laws that may amend or repeal existing legislation and to create new legislation. It is the legislature's responsibility to determine the nature and extent of the need for new laws and for changes in existing laws. The work of preparing federal legislation is the responsibility of the various committees of both houses of Congress. There are 16 standing committees in the Senate and 19 in the House of Representatives. "The membership of the standing committees of each house is chosen by a vote of the entire body; members of other committees are appointed under the provisions of the measure establishing them."[14]

Legislative proposals are assigned or referred to an appropriate committee for study. The committees conduct investigations and hold hearings where interested persons may present their views regarding proposed legislation. These proceedings provide additional information to assist committee members in their consideration of proposed bills. A bill may be reported out of a committee in its original form or it may be reported out with recommended amendments, or the bill might be allowed to lie in the committee without action. Some bills eventually reach the full legislative body, where, after consideration and debate, they may be approved or rejected.

The U.S. Congress and all state legislatures are bicameral (consisting of two houses), except for the Nebraska legislature, which is unicameral. Both houses in a bicameral legislature must pass identical versions of a legislative proposal before the legislation can be brought to the chief executive.

JUDICIAL BRANCH

As I have said in the past, when government bureaus and agencies go awry, which are adjuncts of the legislative or executive branches, the people flee to the third branch, their courts, for solace and justice.

–JUSTICE J. HENDERSON, SUPREME COURT OF SOUTH DAKOTA[15]

The function of the judicial branch of government is adjudication— resolving disputes in accordance with law. As a practical matter, most disputes or controversies that are covered by legal principles or rules are resolved without resort to the courts.

Alexis de Tocqueville, a foreign observer commenting on the primordial place of the law and the legal profession, stated, "Scarcely any political question arises in the United States that is not resolved, sooner or later, into a judicial question."[16]

> It is emphatically the province and duty of the judicial branch to say what the law is. Those who apply the rule to particular cases must of necessity expound and interpret that rule. If two laws conflict with each other, the courts must decide on the operation of each.
>
> So if a law be in opposition to the constitution; if both the law and the constitution apply to a particular case, so that the court must either decide that case conformably to the law, disregarding the constitution; or conformably to the constitution, disregarding the law; the court must determine which of these conflicting rules govern the case. This is the very essence of judicial duty.
>
> . . . [I]t is apparent, that the framers of the constitution contemplated that instrument, as a rule for the government of courts, as well as of the legislature. Why otherwise does it direct the judges to take such an oath to support it?[17]

State Court System

Each state in the United States provides its own court system, which is created by the state's constitution and/or statutes. The oldest court in the United States, established in 1692, is the Supreme Judicial Court of Massachusetts.[18] Most of the nation's judicial business is reviewed and acted on in state courts. Each state maintains a level of trial courts that have original jurisdiction. This jurisdiction may exclude cases involving claims with damages less than a specified minimum, probate matters (e.g., wills and estates), and workers' compensation.

Different states have designated different names for trial courts (e.g., superior, district, circuit, or supreme courts). Also on the trial court level are minor courts such as city, small claims, and justice of the peace courts. States such as Massachusetts have consolidated their minor courts into a statewide court system.

There is at least one appellate court in each state. Many states have an intermediate appellate court between the trial courts and the court of last resort. Where this intermediate court is present, there is a provision for appeal to it, with further review in all but select cases. Because of this format, the highest appellate tribunal is seen as the final arbiter in cases that are important in themselves or for the particular state's system of jurisprudence.

Federal Court System

The trial court of the federal system is the U.S. District Court. There are 89 district courts in the 50 states (the larger states having more than one district court) and one in the District of Columbia. The Commonwealth of Puerto Rico also has a district court with jurisdiction corresponding to that of district courts in the different states. Generally, only one judge is required to sit and decide a case, although certain cases require up to three judges. The federal district courts hear civil, criminal, admiralty, and bankruptcy cases. The Bankruptcy Amendments and Federal Judgeship Act of 1984[19] provided that the bankruptcy judges for each judicial district shall constitute a unit of the district court to be known as the bankruptcy court.

The U.S. Courts of Appeals (formerly called Circuit Courts of Appeals) are appellate courts for the 11 judicial circuits. Their main purpose is to review cases tried in federal district courts within their respective circuits, but they also possess jurisdiction to review orders of designated administrative agencies and to issue original writs in appropriate cases. These intermediate appellate courts were created to relieve the U.S. Supreme Court of deciding all cases appealed from the federal trial courts.

The Supreme Court is the nation's highest court. It is the only federal court created directly by the Constitution.

> The judicial Power of the United States, shall be vested in one Supreme Court, and in such inferior Courts as the Congress may from time to time ordain and establish. The Judges, both of the supreme and inferior Courts, shall hold their Offices during good Behaviour, and shall, at stated Times, receive for their Services a Compensation, which shall not be diminished during their Continuance in Office.[20]

Eight associate justices and one chief justice sit on the Supreme Court. The court has limited original jurisdiction over the lower federal courts and the highest state courts. In a few situations, an appeal will go directly from a federal or state court to the Supreme Court, but in most cases today, review must be sought through the discretionary writ of certiorari, an appeal petition. In addition to the aforementioned courts, special federal courts have jurisdiction over particular subject matters. The U.S. Court of Claims has jurisdiction over certain claims against the government. The U.S. Court of Appeals for the Federal Circuit has appellate jurisdiction over certain customs and patent matters. The U.S. Customs Court reviews certain administrative decisions by customs officials. Also, there is a U.S. Tax Court and a U.S. Court of Military Appeals.

Executive Branch

The primary function of the executive branch of government on the federal and state level is to administer and enforce the law. The chief executive, either the President of the United States or the governor of a state, also has a role in the creation of law through the power to approve or veto legislative proposals.

The U.S. Constitution provides that "the executive Power shall be vested in a President of the United States of America. He shall hold his Office during the Term of four Years . . . together with the Vice President, chosen for the same Term."[21] The president serves as the administrative head of the executive branch of the federal government, which includes 15 executive departments, as well as a variety of agencies, both temporary and permanent.

The Cabinet, a creation of custom and tradition dating back to George Washington's administration, functions at the pleasure of the president. Its purpose is to advise the president on any subject on which he requests information (pursuant to Article II, section 2, of the Constitution).

The Cabinet is composed of the 15 executive departments.[22] Each department is responsible for a different area of public affairs, and each enforces the law within its area of responsibility. For example, the Department of Health and Human Services (DHHS) administers much of the federal health law enacted by Congress. Most state executive branches also are organized on a departmental basis. These departments administer and enforce state law concerning public affairs.

On a state level, the governor serves as the chief executive officer. The responsibilities of a state governor are provided for in the state's constitution. The Massachusetts State Constitution, for example, describes the responsibilities of the governor as follows:[23]

- To present an annual budget to the state legislature
- To recommend new legislation
- To veto legislation
- To appoint and remove department heads
- To appoint judicial officers
- To act as commander-in-chief of the state's military forces (the Massachusetts National Guard)

DEPARTMENT OF HEALTH AND HUMAN SERVICES

The Department of Health and Human Services (DHHS), a cabinet-level department of the executive branch of the federal government (**Figure 5-2**) responsible for developing and implementing appropriate administrative regulations for carrying out national health and human services policy objectives. It is also the main source of regulations affecting the health care industry. The secretary of the DHHS, serving as the department's administrative head, advises the president with regard to health, welfare, and income security plans, policies, and programs. The DHHS also is responsible for many health programs designed through its operating divisions and agencies to meet the health needs of the people.[24]

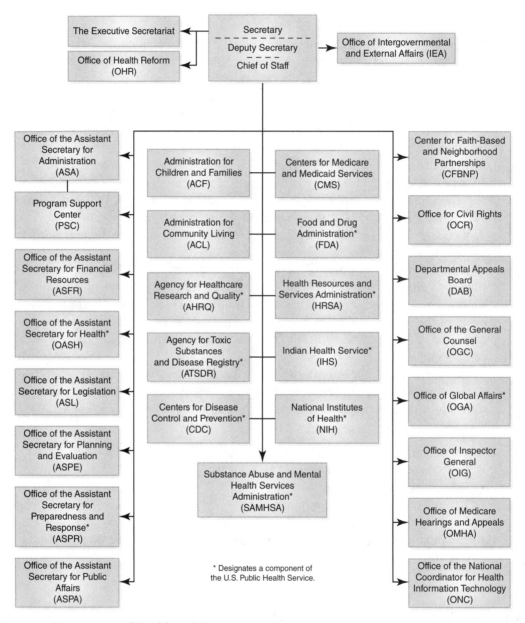

FIGURE 5-2　Department of Health and Human Services

CENTERS FOR MEDICARE AND MEDICAID SERVICES

The Centers for Medicare and Medicaid Services (CMS), formerly the Health Care Financing Administration, was created to combine under one administration the oversight of the Medicare program, the federal portion of the Medicaid program, the State Children's Health Insurance Program, and related quality-assurance activities.

Medicare is a federally sponsored health insurance program for persons older than 65 and certain disabled persons. It has two complementary parts: Medicare Part A helps cover the costs of inpatient hospital care and, with qualifying preadmission criteria, skilled nursing facility care, home health care, and hospice care. Medicare Part B helps pay for physicians' services and outpatient hospital services. It is funded through Social Security contributions (Federal Insurance Contributions Act payroll taxes), premiums, and general revenue. The program is administered through private contractors, referred to as intermediaries, under Part A and carriers under Part B. The financing of the Medicare program has received much attention by Congress because of its rapidly rising costs.

Medicaid, Title XIX of the Social Security Act Amendments of 1965, is a government program administered by the states that provides medical services (both institutional and outpatient) to the medically needy. Federal grants, in the form of matching funds, are issued to those states with qualifying Medicaid programs. In other words, Medicaid is jointly sponsored and financed by the federal government and several states. Medical care for needy persons of all ages is provided under the definition of need established by each state. Each state has set its own criteria for determining eligibility for services under its Medicaid program.

PUBLIC HEALTH SERVICE

The Public Health Service (PHS) is responsible for the protection of the nation's physical and mental health. The PHS accomplishes its mission by coordinating with the states in setting and implementing national health policy and pursuing effective intergovernmental relations; generating and upholding cooperative international health-related agreements, policies, and programs; conducting medical and biomedical research; sponsoring and administering programs for the development of health resources, the prevention and control of diseases, and alcohol and drug abuse; providing resources and expertise to the states and other public and private institutions in the planning, direction, and delivery of physical and mental health care services; and enforcing laws to ensure drug safety and protection from impure and unsafe foods, cosmetics, medical devices, and radiation-producing objects. Within the PHS are smaller agencies that are responsible for carrying out the purpose of the division and DHHS. The PHS is composed of the offices and agencies described next.

National Institutes of Health

The National Institutes of Health (NIH) is the principal federal biomedical research agency. It is responsible for conducting, supporting, and promoting biomedical research.

Centers for Disease Control and Prevention

The Centers for Disease Control and Prevention (CDC) is recognized as the lead federal agency for protecting the health and safety of people at home and abroad, providing credible information to enhance health decisions, and promoting health. The CDC serves as the national focus for developing and applying disease prevention and control, environmental health, and health promotion and education activities.

Food and Drug Administration

The Food and Drug Administration (FDA) supervises and controls the introduction of drugs, foods, cosmetics, and medical devices into the marketplace and protects society from impure and hazardous items. Although the intention of the FDA is to do good, as noted in the following news clipping, ethical conflicts can arise and be detrimental to the good intent of the agency.

Long Waits for Generics

Brand-name drug makers already pay hefty user fees to help speed their applications through the FDA. That money is expected to provide about a third of the agency's budget this year.

In general, we oppose user fees that allow a regulated industry to fund the regulators. A government agency can become dependent on the companies it's supposed to objectively regulate, which can influence decisions. In a 2006 survey . . . many FDA employees said they felt pressured to hastily and perhaps improperly approve user-fee drugs. And at least one felt the agency viewed industry, not the American public, as its client.

Jim Guest, Consumer Reports, *November 2010*

Discussion

1. Identify and describe the ethical issues of the FDA's funding practice.
2. Do you see any conflict in allowing private for-profit and not-for-profit hospital accreditation programs accredit hospitals on behalf of Medicare, noting that the hospitals pay the accrediting organization to conduct such surveys? Discuss your answer.

Substance Abuse and Mental Health Services Administration

The agency's mission is to reduce the impact of substance abuse and mental illness on America's communities.

Health Resources and Services Administration (HRSA)

The primary federal agency for improving access to health care services for people who are uninsured, isolated, or medically vulnerable. Its mission is to improve health and achieve health equity through access to quality services, a skilled health workforce, and innovative programs. HRSA takes a comprehensive approach to addressing HIV/AIDS with activities taking place across multiple bureaus and offices designed to deliver care to people living with HIV or AIDS, expand and strengthen the HIV care workforce, and improve access to and the quality of HIV care and treatment.

Agency for Healthcare Research and Quality

The Agency for Healthcare Research and Quality (AHRQ) provides evidence-based information on health care outcomes, quality, cost, use, and access. Information from AHRQ's research helps people make more informed decisions and improve the quality of health care services.

Agency for Toxic Substances and Disease Registry

The mission of the Agency for Toxic Substances and Disease Registry (ATSDR) is to prevent or mitigate harmful exposures and related disease by applying science, taking responsive action, and providing trustworthy health information.

Indian Health Service

Indian Health Service provides a comprehensive health service delivery system for approximately 2 million American Indians and Alaska Natives (AI/AN) who belong to 566 federally recognized tribes in 35 states.

CHAPTER REVIEW

1. A law is a general rule of conduct that is enforced by the government. When a law is violated, the government imposes a penalty.
   - *Public law* deals with the relationships between individuals and the government. Criminal law is a segment of public law.
   - *Private law* deals with relationships among individuals. Two types of private laws are tort and contract actions.
2. *Common law*
   - U.S. common law has as its roots in the English common-law system.
     - The first English royal court was established in the year 1178. There were few written laws at the time, and a collection of principles evolved from the decisions of the court. These principles, known as *common law*, were used to decide subsequent cases.
   - During the colonial period, the United States based its law on English common law, but states had the authority to modify their legal systems.
   - Lower courts must follow common-law principles established in a higher state court.
   - Trial courts or those otherwise on equal footing are not bound by the decisions of other trial courts.
   - A principle of law set in one state does not set precedent for another state.
   - Common-law principles can be modified, overturned, abrogated, or created by new court decisions.
3. *Statutory law* is written law that emanates from legislative bodies.
   - The Constitution is the highest level of enacted law.
   - Statutory law can be amended, repealed, or expanded by the legislature.
4. *Administrative law*
   - Public law issued by administrative agencies to administer the enacted laws of the federal and state governments.
   - Administrative agencies implement and administer the administrative law.
   - Rules and regulations established by an agency must be administered within the scope of the authority delegated by Congress.

5. Government organization
   - Three branches of government
     - *Legislative branch*, composed of the House of Representatives and the Senate, both enacts laws that can amend or repeal existing legislation and creates new legislation.
     - *Judicial branch* resolves disputes in accordance with the law.
     - Executive branch administers and enforces the law.
     - *Separation of powers* provides that no one branch of the government will be dominant over the other two.
     - States and local jurisdictions can enact and enforce only those laws that do not *conflict* with federal laws.
     - When state and federal laws conflict, resolution can be sought in an appropriate federal court.
6. The DHHS develops and implements administrative regulations for carrying out national health and human services policy objectives.
   - DHSS is the main source of regulations that affect the health care industry. Operating divisions of DHHS include the:
     - Centers for Medicare and Medicaid Services
     - Public Health Service
     - National Institutes of Health
     - Centers for Disease Control and Prevention
     - Food and Drug Administration
     - Substance Abuse and Mental Health Services Administration
     - Health Resources and Services Administration
     - Agency for Healthcare Research and Quality
     - Agency for Toxic Substances and Disease Registry
     - Indian Health Service

TEST YOUR UNDERSTANDING

TERMINOLOGY

administrative law	law	res judicata
Bill of Rights	Medicare	separation of powers
common law	precedent	stare decisis
Constitution of the United States	private law	statutory law
	public law	

REVIEW QUESTIONS

1. Define the term *law* and describe the sources from which law is derived.

2. Describe and contrast the legal terms *res judicata* and *stare decisis*.

3. Describe the function of each branch of government.

4. What is the meaning of separation of powers?

5. What is the function of an administrative agency?

6. Describe the various operating divisions and agencies within the DHHS.

NOTES

1. B. Schwartz, *The Law in America* 1 (1974).
2. *Marbury v. Madison,* 5 U.S. (Cranch) 137, 163 (1803).
3. Schwartz, supra note 1, at 29.
4. *Id.*
5. *Id.* at 30–31.
6. L. Friedman, *A History of American Law* 92 (1985).
7. Schwartz, supra note 1, at 51.
8. *Black's Law Dictionary* 1305 (6th. ed. 1990).
9. U.S. Const. art. VI, A4 1, cl. 2.
10. 5 U.S.C.S. A4A4 500–576 (Law. Co-op. 1989).
11. An "agency means each authority of the Government of the United States . . . but does not include (A) the Congress; the Courts of the United States . . ." 5 U.S.C.S. A4 551(1) (Law. Co-op. 1989).
12. *Marbury v. Madison,* 5 U.S. (Cranch) 137, 180 (1803).
13. 88 F.R.D. 583 (E.D. Mich. 1980).
14. Office of the Federal Register, National Archives and Records Administration, The United States Government Manual 2000/2001 29 (2000) [hereinafter Manual].
15. *Heritage of Yankton, Inc. v. South Dakota Dep't of Health*, 432 N.W.2d 68, 77 (S.D. 1988).
16. Schwartz, supra note 1, at 15.
17. *Marbury v. Madison*, 5 U.S. (Cranch) 137, 177–180 (1803).
18. Levitan, supra note 46, at 32.
19. 28 U.S.C. A4 151.
20. U.S. Const. art. III, A4 1.
21. U.S. Const. art. II, A41, cl. 1.
22. http://dir.yahoo.com/Government/U_S__Government/Executive_Branch/Departments_and_Agencies/.
23. D. Levitan, Your Massachusetts Government 14 (10th ed. 1984).
24. http://www.hhs.gov/about/foa/opdivs/.

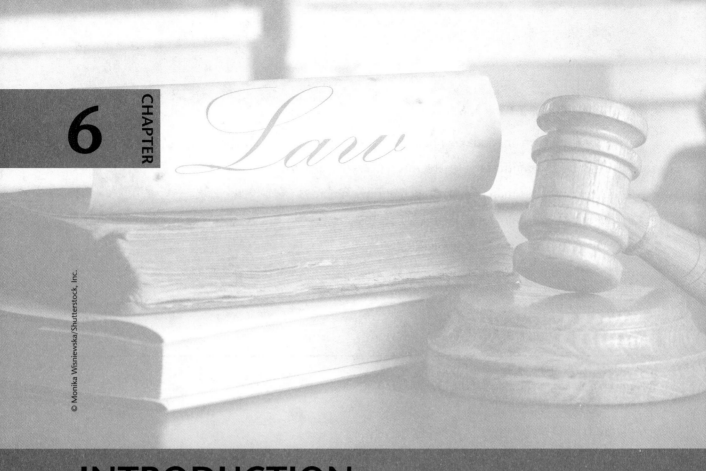

CHAPTER 6

INTRODUCTION TO LAW

Every instance of a man's suffering the penalty of the law, is an instance of the failure of that penalty in effecting its purpose, which is to deter from transgression.

—WHATELY

LEARNING OBJECTIVES

Upon completion of this chapter, the reader will be able to:

- Understand the meaning and objectives of tort law.
- Define negligence and understand the distinction and similarity between negligence and malpractice.
- Explain how the commission and omission of an act differ.
- Explain the elements necessary to prove a negligence case.
- Describe the importance of foreseeability in a negligence case.

- Describe what an intentional tort is and discuss several examples of intentional torts and how they might apply in various health care settings.
- Explain what a crime is and how various crimes are not so uncommon in the health care setting.
- Explain the various elements of a contract.
- Describe the pretrial procedures and the process of a trial.

INTRODUCTION

Laws are enacted to regulate human behavior for the benefit of society. They are designed to prevent harm to others while protecting the rights of individuals. In the law we are taught that we have a duty to care and that if we breach that duty and someone is injured as a result of that breach, there will be a penalty to pay, which could be financial loss, loss of license, and/or jail time to be served. This chapter introduces the reader to tort law, criminal law, contract law, and trial procedures. These are the areas of law that most often affect providers and patients.

TORT LAW

A *tort* is a civil wrong, other than a breach of contract, committed against a person or property (real or personal) for which a court provides a remedy in the form of an action for damages. Tort actions touch an individual on both a personal and a professional level, which is why those involved in the health care field should be armed with the knowledge necessary for them to be aware of their rights and responsibilities.

The objectives of tort law are as follows: preservation of peace (between individuals by providing a substitute for retaliation); culpability (to find fault for wrongdoing); deterrence (to discourage the wrongdoer [tort-feasor] from committing future torts); and compensation (to indemnify the injured person[s] of wrongdoing).

NEGLIGENCE

Negligence is a tort, a civil or personal wrong. It is the unintentional commission or omission of an act that a reasonably prudent person would or would not perform under given circumstances. Negligence is a form of conduct caused by heedlessness or carelessness that constitutes a departure from the standard of care generally imposed on reasonable members of society. It can occur where a person has considered the consequences of an act and has exercised his or her best possible judgment, fails to guard against a risk that should be appreciated, and engages in certain behavior expected to involve unreasonable danger to others.

Commission of an act includes, for example, the following acts:

- administering the wrong medication
- administering the wrong dosage of a medication
- administering a medication to the wrong patient
- performing a surgical procedure without patient consent

- performing a surgical procedure on the wrong patient
- surgically removing the wrong body part
- failing to assess and reassess a patient's nutritional needs

Omission of an act includes the following:

- failure to administer medication[s]
- failure to order required diagnostic tests per established hospital protocol for head trauma (e.g., CT scan)
- failure to follow up on abnormal test results
- failure to perform a "time-out" to ensure the correct surgical procedure is being conducted on the correct patient at the correct site

Malpractice is the negligence or carelessness of a professional person (e.g., a nurse, pharmacist, physician, or accountant). Criminal negligence is the reckless disregard for the safety of another (e.g., willful indifference to an injury that could follow an act). Negligence generally involves one of the following acts:

- *malfeasance* (execution of an unlawful or improper act [e.g., performing an abortion in the third trimester when such is prohibited by state law]);
- *misfeasance* (improper performance of an act, resulting in injury to another [e.g., wrong site surgery]), and
- *nonfeasance* (failure to act, when there is a duty to act as a reasonably prudent person would in similar circumstances [e.g., failing to order diagnostic tests or prescribe medications that should have been ordered or prescribed under the circumstances]).

ELEMENTS OF NEGLIGENCE

The four elements that must be present for a plaintiff to recover damages caused by negligence are (1) duty to care, (2) breach of duty, (3) injury, and (4) causation. All four elements must be present in order for a plaintiff to recover for damages suffered as a result of a negligent act.

Duty to Care

The first requirement in establishing negligence is that the plaintiff must prove the existence of a legal relationship between himself or herself and the defendant. *Duty* is defined as a legal obligation of care, performance, or observance imposed on one to safeguard the rights of others. This duty may arise from a special relationship such as that between a physician and a patient. The existence of this relationship implies that a physician–patient relationship was in effect at the time an alleged injury occurred. The duty to care can arise from a simple telephone conversation or out of a physician's voluntary act of assuming the care of a patient. Duty also can be established by statute or contract between the plaintiff and the defendant.

Duty to care is depicted in **Figure 6-1**, for example, where the pharmacy manager of General Hospital's pharmacy, prior to leaving work for the day, assigns responsibility to a recently hired pharmacist behind the counter, telling her, "You're in charge of the pharmacy, which includes the IV admixture room. Your duties and responsibilities are those as described in

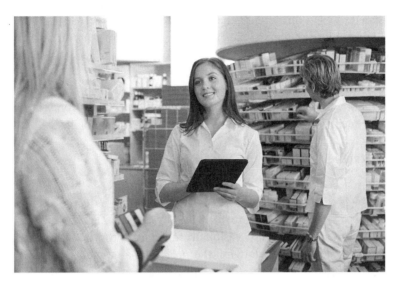

FIGURE 6-1 Duty to Care (© Tyler Olsen/Shutterstock, Inc.)

the pharmacy department policy and procedure manual. I will be leaving in an hour, so you should review them before I leave. If you have any questions after I leave, you can reach me on my cell phone."

This assignment established a duty on the part of the pharmacist to adhere to the policies and procedures in the department manual.

Standard of Care Expected

A duty of care carries with it a corresponding responsibility not only to provide care but also to provide it in an acceptable manner. Because of this obligation to conform to a recognized *standard of care*, the plaintiff must show that the defendant failed to meet the required standard of care. Just because an injury is suffered is not sufficient for imposing liability without proof that the defendant deviated from the practice of competent members of his or her profession.

The standard of care describes what conduct is expected of an individual in a given situation. The standard of care that must be exercised is that which a reasonably prudent person would adhere to when acting under the same or similar circumstances. A nurse, for example, who assumes the care of a patient has the duty to exercise that degree of skill, care, and knowledge ordinarily possessed and exercised by other nurses. If a patient's injury is the result of a negligent act of a physician, the standard of care required would be that degree of skill, care, and knowledge ordinarily possessed and exercised by other physicians. For an injury involving a specific specialty, the treating physician nurse, pharmacist, etc., would be expected to treat the patient in that same manner as the specialist in the field in which the caregiver is practicing.

The *reasonably prudent person* concept describes a nonexistent, hypothetical person who is put forward as the community ideal of what would be considered reasonable behavior. It is a measuring stick representing the conduct of the average person in the community under the circumstances facing the defendant at the time of the alleged negligence. The reasonableness of conduct is judged in light of the circumstances apparent at the time of injury and by reference to different characteristics of the actor (e.g., age, gender, physical condition, education, knowledge, training, and mental capacity).

The actual performance of an individual in a given situation will be measured against what a reasonably prudent person would or would not have done. Deviation from the standard of care will constitute negligence if there are resulting damages.

Ethicists and the Standard of Care

The standard of care required by a caregiver can in part be influenced by the principles of ethics that apply to the caregiver's profession. For example, a decision concerning termination of resuscitation efforts is an area in which the standard of care includes an ethical component. Under these circumstances, it occasionally may be appropriate for a medical expert to testify about the ethical aspects underlying the professional standard of care. In *Neade v. Portes,* 710 N.E.2d 418 (Ill. App. Ct. 1999), a physician expert was allowed to base an opinion on the breach of the standard of care based on violation of an ethical standard established by the American Medical Association.

Some duties are created by statute, which occurs when a statute specifies a particular standard that must be met. Many such standards are created by administrative agencies under the provisions of a statute. For liability to be established, based on a defendant's failure to follow the standard of care outlined by statute, the following elements must be present:

1. the defendant must have been within the specified class of persons outlined in the statute;
2. the plaintiff must have been injured in a way that the statute was designed to prevent; and
3. the plaintiff must show that the injury would not have occurred if the statute had not been violated.

Duty to Provide Timely Care

The surviving parents in *Hastings v. Baton Rouge Hospital*[1] brought a medical malpractice action for the wrongful death of their 19-year-old son. The action was brought against the hospital; the emergency department physician, Dr. Gerdes; and the thoracic surgeon on call, Dr. McCool. The patient had been brought to the emergency department at 11:56 p.m. because of two stab wounds and weak vital signs. Gerdes decided that a thoracotomy had to be performed. He was not qualified to perform the surgery and called McCool, who was on call that evening for thoracic surgery. Gerdes described the patient's condition, indicating that he had been stabbed in a major blood vessel. At trial, McCool claimed that he did not recall Gerdes saying that a major blood vessel could be involved. McCool asked Gerdes to transfer the patient to the Earl K. Long Hospital. Gerdes said, "I can't transfer this patient." McCool replied, "No. Transfer him." Kelly, an emergency department nurse on duty, was not comfortable with the decision to transfer the patient and offered to accompany him in the ambulance. Gerdes reexamined the patient, who exhibited marginal vital signs, was restless, and was draining blood from his chest.

The ambulance service was called at 1:03 a.m., and by 1:30 a.m. the patient had been placed in the ambulance for transfer. The patient began to fight wildly. The chest tube came out, and the bleeding increased. An attempt to revive him from a cardiac arrest was futile, and the patient died after having been moved back to the emergency department. The patient virtually bled to death.

The duty to care in this case cannot be reasonably disputed. Louisiana, by statute, imposes a duty on hospitals licensed in Louisiana to make emergency services available to all persons residing in the state regardless of insurance coverage or economic status. The hospital's own bylaws provided that no patient should be transferred without due consideration for his or her condition. Hospitals are required to stabilize the patient prior to transfer. In this case, there was a surgeon who was available to treat this patient. McCool decided to practice telephone medicine and made the unfortunate decision to transfer the patient, which resulted in risking the life of an unstable patient, resulting in his death.

Duty to Hire Competent Staff

Texas courts recognize that an employer has a duty to hire competent employees, especially if they are engaged in an occupation that could be hazardous to life and limb and requires skilled or experienced persons. For example, the appellant in *Deerings West Nursing Center v. Scott*[2] was found to have negligently hired an incompetent employee who it knew or should have known was incompetent, thereby causing unreasonable risk of harm to others.

Hopper testified that he was hired sight unseen over the telephone by the Deerings director of nursing. Even though the following day he went to the nursing facility to complete an application, he still maintained that he was hired over the phone. In his application, he falsely stated that he was a Texas-licensed vocational nurse (LVN). Additionally, he claimed that he had never been convicted of a crime. In reality, he had been previously employed by a bar, was not an LVN, had committed more than 56 criminal offenses of theft, and was on probation at the time of his testimony.

The duty of care in this case is clear. The appellant violated the very purpose of Texas licensing statutes by failing to validate whether or not Hopper had a current LVN license. The appellant then placed him in a position of authority and not only allowed him to dispense drugs but also made him a shift supervisor. This negligence eventually resulted in an inexcusable assault on an older woman.

Breach of Duty

After a duty to care has been established, the plaintiff must demonstrate that the defendant breached that duty by failing to comply with the accepted standard of care required. *Breach of duty*, the second element that must be present for a plaintiff to establish negligence, is the failure to conform to or the departure from a required obligation owed to a person. The obligation to perform according to a standard of care may encompass either performing or refraining from performing a particular act.

The court in *Hastings v. Baton Rouge Hospital*,[3] discussed earlier, found a severe breach of duty. Hospital regulations provide that when a physician cannot be reached or refuses a call, the chief of service is to be notified so that another physician can be obtained. This was not done. It is not necessary to prove that a patient would have survived if proper treatment

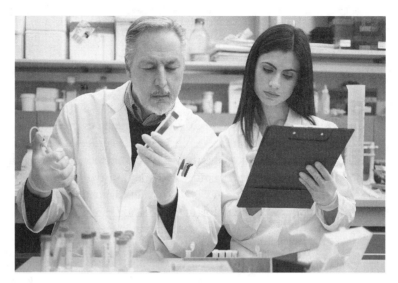

FIGURE 6-2 Breach of Duty (© Minerva Studio/Shutterstock, Inc.)

had been administered, only that the patient would have had a chance of survival. As a result of Dr. Gerdes' failure to make arrangements for another physician and Dr. McCool's failure to perform the necessary surgery, the patient had no chance of survival. The duty to provide for appropriate care under the circumstances was breached.

Breach of duty is illustrated in **Figure 6-2**, where the intravenous (IV) admixture room pharmacist checking the work of a pharmacy technician, fails to follow-up on his concern as to whether or not the medication in the IV bag had been diluted in the correct dosage. Failure to follow-up established a breach of duty.

Injury/Actual Damages

A defendant may be negligent and not incur liability if there is no injury or actual damages suffered by the plaintiff, the third element necessary to establish negligence. *Injury* includes more than physical harm. Without harm or injury, there is no liability. Injury is not limited to physical harm but includes loss of income or reputation and compensation for pain and suffering. The mere occurrence of an injury does not necessarily establish negligence for which the law imposes liability because the injury might be the result of an unavoidable accident or act of God, such as a lighting strike that is the direct cause of an injury.

The third element of negligence—injury—is portrayed in **Figure 6-3** where the death of an infant in General Hospital's nursery occurred 3 hours following administration of an improper dose of an IV medication.

In *Hastings*, the patient's death was a direct result of the breach of duty.

Causation/Proximate Cause

Causation, the fourth element necessary to establish negligence, requires that there be a reasonable, close, and causal connection between the defendant's negligent conduct and the resulting damages suffered by the plaintiff. In other words, the defendant's negligence must

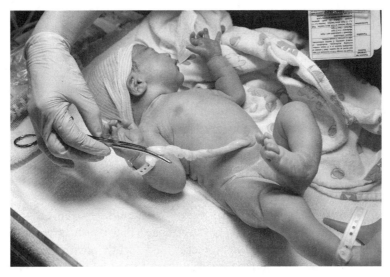

FIGURE 6-3   Injury Established (© Paul Hakimata Photography/Shutterstock, Inc.)

be a substantial factor causing the injury. *Proximate cause* is a term referring to the relationship between a breached duty and the injury. The breach of duty must be the proximate cause of the resulting injury.

Figure 6-4 portrays a defense attorney successfully arguing that the cause of death of an infant in General Hospital's nursery was due to the failure of the pharmacist to properly verify that the IV medication had been properly diluted and labeled by the pharmacy technician in the hospital's pharmacy. The IV solution, containing the medication, was delivered to the nursery, where the nurse checked the label, unaware that the medication left the pharmacy mislabeled and improperly diluted, administered it to the infant who subsequently died. Thus establishing the proximate cause of the injury, the fourth element of negligence—causation.

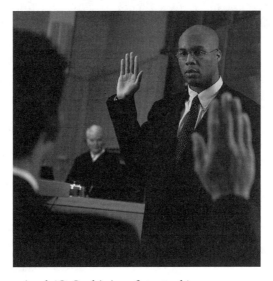

FIGURE 6-4   Causation Determined (© Corbis/age fotostock)

Causation in the *Hastings*[4] case was well established. In the ordinary course of events, a person does not bleed to death in a hospital emergency department over a 2-hour period without some surgical intervention to save the patient's life.

Foreseeability and Anticipation of Harm

Foreseeability is the reasonable anticipation that harm or injury is likely to result from an act or an omission of an act. As an aspect of causation in a negligence case, the test for foreseeability is whether a person of ordinary prudence and intelligence should have anticipated the danger to others caused by his or her negligent act. "The test is not what the wrongdoer believed would occur; it is whether he or she ought reasonably to have foreseen that the event in question, or some similar event, would occur."[5]

There is no expectation that a person can guard against events that cannot reasonably be foreseen. Foreseeability involves guarding against that which is probable and likely to happen, not against that which is only remotely and slightly possible. In *Hastings*, it was highly probable that the patient would die if the bleeding was not stopped. "The broad test of negligence is what a reasonably prudent person would foresee and would do in the light of this foresight under the circumstances."[6]

SUMMARY CASE

CASE: CURSORY EXAMS ARE RISKY

All of the elements necessary to establish negligence were well established in *Niles v. City of San Rafael*.[7] On June 26, 1973, at approximately 3:30 p.m., Kelly Niles, a young boy, got into an argument with another boy on the ball field. He was hit on the right side of his head. Kelly rode home on his bicycle and waited for his father, who was to pick him up for the weekend. At approximately 5:00 p.m., Kelly's father arrived. By the time they arrived in San Francisco, Kelly appeared to be in a great deal of pain. His father then decided to take him to Mount Zion Hospital, which was a short distance away. He arrived at the hospital emergency department at approximately 5:45 p.m.. On admission to the emergency department, Kelly was taken to a treatment room by a registered nurse. The nurse obtained a history of the injury and took Kelly's pulse and blood pressure. During his stay in the emergency department, he was irritable, vomited several times, and complained that his head hurt. An intern who had seen Kelly wrote "pale, diaphoretic, and groggy" on Kelly's chart. Skull X-rays were ordered and found to be negative except for soft tissue swelling that was not noted until later. The intern then decided to admit Kelly. A second-year resident was called, and he agreed with the intern's decision. An admitting clerk called the intern and indicated that Kelly had to be admitted by an attending physician. The resident went as far as to write "admit" on the chart and later crossed it out. A pediatrician who was in the emergency department at the time was asked to look at Kelly. The pediatrician was also the paid director of the Mount Zion Pediatric Out-Patient Clinic. The pediatrician asked Kelly a few questions and then decided to send him home. The physician could not recall what instructions he gave Kelly's father, but he did give the father his business card.

The pediatrician could not recall giving the father a copy of the emergency department's *Head Injury Instructions*, an information sheet that had been prepared for distribution to patients with head injuries. The sheet explained that patients should return to the emergency department should any of the following signs appear: a large, soft lump on the head, unusual drowsiness (cannot be awakened), forceful or repeated vomiting, a fit or convulsion (jerking or spells), clumsy walking, bad headache, and/or one pupil larger than the other.

Kelly was taken back to his father's apartment at about 7:00 p.m.. A psychiatrist friend stopped by and examined Kelly. He noted that one pupil was larger than the other. Kelly was taken back to the emergency department. A physician on duty noted an epidural hematoma during his examination and ordered that a neurosurgeon be called.

Today, Kelly can move only his eyes and neck. A lawsuit was brought against the hospital and pediatrician for $5 million. The city of San Rafael and public school district were included in the lawsuit as defendants. Expert testimony by two neurosurgeons during the trial indicated that Kelly's chances of recovery would have been very good if he had been admitted promptly. This testimony placed the proximate cause of the injury with the hospital. The final judgment was $4 million against the medical defendants, $2.5 million for compensatory damages, and another $1.5 million for pain and suffering.

Ethical and Legal Issues

The many lessons for discussion in *Niles v. City of San Rafael* include the following:

1. An organization can improve the quality of patient care rendered in the facility by establishing and adhering to policies, procedures, and protocols that facilitate the delivery of high-quality care across all disciplines.
2. The provision of high-quality health care requires collaboration across disciplines.
3. A physician must conduct a thorough and responsible examination and order the appropriate tests for each patient, evaluating the results of those tests before discharging the patient.
4. A patient's vital signs must be monitored closely and documented in the medical record. Corrective measures must be taken when a patient's medical condition signals a medical problem.
5. A complete review of a patient's medical record must be accomplished before discharging a patient.
6. Review of the record must include review of test results, nurses' notes, residents' and interns' notes, and the notes of any other physician or consultant who may have attended the patient.
7. Failure to fully review a patient's record can lead to an erroneous diagnosis, and the premature dismissal of a case can result in liability for both the organization and physician.

Duty to care involves a responsibility to do the "right thing." The right thing is based on an acceptable standard of care. If breaching the standard causes harm to the patient, not only is there a legal issue, there are ethical principles that have been violated. Nonmaleficence, for example, requires caregivers to avoid causing harm to patients.

INTENTIONAL TORTS

An *intentional tort* is one that is committed deliberately. Proof of intent is based on the premise that the defendant intended the harmful consequences of his or her behavior. An individual's reason to cause harm is irrelevant and does not protect him or her from responsibility for the damages suffered as the result of an intentional act.

Assault and Battery

It has long been recognized by law that a person possesses a right to be free from aggression and the threat of actual aggression against one's person. The right to expect others to respect the integrity of one's body has roots in both common and statutory law. The distinguishing feature between assault and battery is that *assault* effectuates an infringement on the mental security or tranquility of another, whereas *battery* constitutes a violation of another's physical integrity.

An assault is defined as the deliberate threat, coupled with the apparent present ability to do physical harm to another. No actual contact or damages are necessary. It is the deliberate threat or attempt to injure another or the attempt by one to make bodily contact with another without his or her consent. To commit the tort of assault, the following two conditions must be proven:

1. The person attempting to touch another unlawfully must possess the apparent present ability to commit the battery.
2. The person threatened must be aware of or have actual knowledge of an immediate threat of a battery and must fear it.

A *battery* is the intentional touching of another's person, in a socially impermissible manner, without that person's consent. It is intentional conduct that violates the physical security of another. The receiver of the battery does not have to be aware that a battery has been committed (e.g., a patient who is unconscious and has surgery performed on him or her without consent, either expressed or implied, is the object of a battery). The unwanted touching may give rise to a cause of action for any injuries brought about by the touching. No actual damages need be shown to impose liability.

False Imprisonment

False imprisonment is the unlawful restraint of an individual's personal liberty or the unlawful restraining or confining of an individual. The personal right to move freely and without hindrance is basic to our legal system. Any intentional infringement on this right may constitute false imprisonment. Actual physical force is not necessary to constitute false imprisonment. All that is necessary is that an individual who is physically confined to a given area experience a reasonable fear that force, which may be implied by words, threats, or gestures, will be used to detain the individual or to intimidate him or her without legal justification. Excessive force used to restrain a patient may produce liability for both false imprisonment and battery.

Defamation of Character

Defamation of character involves communications to someone other than the person defamed that tends to hold that person's reputation up to scorn and ridicule.

Slander is the oral form of defamation. For example, in *Eli v. Griggs County Hospital & Nursing Home*,[8] a nurse's aide was terminated as the result of an incident in the hospital dining room in which the aide, in the presence of patients and visitors, cursed at her supervisor and complained that personnel were working short staffed. Given the nature of her employment, such behavior justified her termination on a charge of reported breach of patient- and facility-specific information. No defamation resulted from the entry of such charges in the aide's personnel file because the record established that the charges were true.

Libel is the written form of defamation. Libel can be expressed in the form of signs, photographs, letters, cartoons, and various other forms of written communication. To be an actionable wrong, defamation must be communicated to a third person. Defamatory statements communicated only to the injured party are not grounds for an action. Truth of a statement is a complete defense.

Defamation on its face is actionable without proof of special damages. In certain cases, a court will presume that the words caused injury to the person's reputation. There are four generally recognized exceptions whereby no proof of actual harm to reputation is required to recover damages:

1. accusing someone of a crime
2. accusing someone of having a loathsome disease
3. using words that affect a person's profession or business
4. accusing someone of sexual misconduct

Invasion of Privacy

Invasion of privacy is a wrong that invades the right of a person to personal privacy. Absolute privacy has to be tempered with reality in the care of any patient, and the courts recognize this fact. Disregard for a patient's right to privacy is legally actionable, particularly when patients are unable to protect themselves adequately because of unconsciousness or immobility.

The *right to privacy* is implied in the Constitution. It is recognized as a right to be left alone—the right to be free from unwarranted publicity and exposure to public view, as well as the right to live one's life without having one's name, picture, or private affairs made public against one's will. Health care organizations and professionals may become liable for invasion of privacy if, for example, they divulge information from a patient's medical record to improper sources or if they commit unwarranted intrusions into a patient's personal affairs.

Patients have a right to personal privacy and a right to the confidentiality of their personal and clinical records. The information in a patient's medical record is confidential and should not be disclosed without the patient's permission. Those who come into possession of the most intimate personal information about patients have both a legal and an ethical duty not to reveal confidential communications. The legal duty arises because the law recognizes a right to privacy. An ethical duty is broader because it applies at all times. There are, however, occasions when there is a legal obligation or duty to disclose information. The law requires, for example, the reporting of communicable diseases, gunshot wounds, and the reasonable suspicion of patient abuse.

Infliction of Mental Distress

The intentional or reckless *infliction of mental distress* is characterized by conduct that is so outrageous that it goes beyond the bounds tolerated by a decent society. It is a civil wrong for which a tort-feasor can be held liable for damages. Mental distress includes mental suffering resulting from painful emotions such as grief, public humiliation, despair, shame, and wounded pride. Liability for the wrongful infliction of mental distress may be based on either intentional or negligent misconduct. A plaintiff may recover damages if he or she can show that the defendant intended to inflict mental distress and knew or should have known that his or her actions would give rise to it. Recovery generally is permitted even in the absence of physical harm.

CASE: THE COURT WAS APPALLED

In *Tomcik v. Ohio Dep't of Rehabilitation & Correction*,[9] the plaintiff, Tomcik, was in the custody of the defendant, a penal institution. Pursuant to the defendant's policy of medically evaluating all new inmates, on May 26, 1989, Dr. Evans gave Tomcik a medical examination. He testified that his physical evaluation included an examination of Tomcik's breasts; however, he stated that his examination was very cursory.

The day after her examination, Tomcik examined her own breasts. At that time, she discovered a lump in her right breast, which she characterized as being about the size of a pea. She then sought an additional medical evaluation at the defendant's medical clinic. Testimony indicated that fewer than half of the inmates who sign the clinic list are actually seen by medical personnel the next day. Also, inmates who are not examined on the day for which the list is signed are given no preference in being examined on the following day. In fact, their names are simply deleted from the daily list, and their only recourse is to continually sign the list until they are examined.

The evidence indicated that from May 27 on, Tomcik constantly signed the clinic list and provided the reason she was requesting medical care.

A nurse finally examined Tomcik on June 21. The nurse wrote in her nursing notes that Tomcik had a "moderate large mass in right breast." The nurse recognized that the proper procedure was to measure such a mass, but she testified that this was impossible because no measuring device was available. The missing "measuring device" to which she alluded was a simple ruler. The nurse concluded that Evans, the original doctor who had examined Tomcik, should examine her again.

On June 28, Evans examined Tomcik again. He recorded in the progress notes that she had "a mass on her right wrist. Will send her to hospital and give her Benadryl for allergy she has."[10] Evans meant to write "breast," not "wrist." He again failed to measure the size of the mass on Tomcik's breast.

Tomcik was transferred to the Franklin County Prerelease Center on September 28. On September 30, a nurse there examined Tomcik; the nurse recorded that she had a "golf ball–sized" lump in her right breast. Tomcik was transported to the hospital on October 27, where Dr. Walker treated her. A mammogram indicated that Tomcik's tumor was probably malignant. This diagnosis was confirmed by a biopsy performed on November 9. Tomcik was released from confinement on November 13.

On November 16, Dr. Lidsky, a surgeon employed outside of the penal institution, examined Tomcik. Lidsky noted the existence of the lump in her breast and determined that the size of the mass was approximately 4 to 5 centimeters and somewhat fixed. He performed a modified radical mastectomy on the plaintiff's right breast, removing nearly the entire breast.

Tomcik alleged that it was the delay in her examination that ultimately led to the removal of her right breast; had she been seen in a more timely manner, much of the breast could have been spared. The defendant, the corrections department, contended that even if its employees were negligent, Tomcik's cancer was so advanced when discovered that it would nevertheless have required removal of her breast.[11]

The Ohio Court of Appeals held that the delay in providing treatment to Tomcik fell below the medically acceptable standard of care. The court was *appalled* that the physician had characterized his evaluation as a medical examination and that what he described as a *cursory breast examination* should be considered medically sufficient. It seemed incredible to the court that a physician would deliberately choose not to take the additional few minutes or seconds to palpate thoroughly the sides of the breasts, which is a standard minimally intrusive cancer detection technique.

Ethical and Legal Issues

1. Do you agree with the court's decision? Discuss your answer.
2. Discuss why the court was appalled.
3. What ethical values were lacking by the caregivers?

CRIMINAL LAW

Laws were made to restrain and punish the wicked; the wise and good do not need them as a guide, but only as a shield against rapine and oppression; they can live civilly and orderly, though there were no law in the world.

—Owen Feltham (1602–1668)

What Went Wrong?

The son of a prominent Boston doctor . . . was on his way to becoming a leading surgeon in his own right when a bizarre blunder interrupted his climb: he left his patient on the operating table so he could cash his paycheck. A series of arrests followed, exposing a life of arrogance, betrayal, and wasted promise . . .

Reproduce from Neil Swidey, "What Went Wrong?" The Boston Globe, March 21, 2004.

Criminal law is society's expression of the limits of acceptable human behavior. A crime is any social harm defined and made punishable by law. The objectives of criminal law are to:

- maintain public order and safety
- protect the individual
- use punishment as a deterrent to crime
- rehabilitate the criminal for return to society

Crimes are generally classified as misdemeanors or felonies. The difference between a misdemeanor and a felony revolves around the severity of the crime committed and the punishment imposed. A *misdemeanor* is an offense punishable by less than 1 year in jail and/or a fine (e.g., petty larceny). A *felony* is a much more serious crime (e.g., rape, murder) and is generally punishable by imprisonment in a state or federal penitentiary for more than 1 year.

Peculiar to health care organizations is the fact that patients are often helpless and at the mercy of others. Health care facilities are far too often places where the morally weak and mentally deficient prey on the physically and sometimes mentally helpless. The very institutions designed to make the public well and feel safe can sometimes provide the setting for criminal conduct.

The topics in this section run counter to the ethics theory of *nonmaleficence*–to do no harm, as well as to the codes of professional ethics. For example, as noted in the grand jury indictment **Figure 6-5**, Dr. Gosnell snipped the spinal cords of infants delivered alive during abortion procedures. Crimes like his and others against society are not only legal wrongs, they are also ethically wrong.

The U.S. Department of Justice and state and local prosecutors are vigorously pursuing and prosecuting health care organizations and individuals for criminal conduct. Health care fraud, patient abuse, and other such crimes have caused law enforcement agencies to establish a zero-tolerance policy for such acts. This reality requires health care professionals to be observant in their environments and to report suspicious conduct, as appropriate.

CRIMINAL PROCEDURE

Criminal procedure deals with the set of rules governing the series of proceedings through which the government enforces criminal law as provided by municipalities, states, and the federal government, each of which have their own criminal codes that address and define conduct that constitute crimes. The following sections provide an overview of criminal procedure and the process for the prosecution of misdemeanors and felonies.

Arrest

Prosecutions for crimes generally begin with the arrest of a defendant by a police officer or with the filing of a formal action in a court of law and the issuance of an arrest warrant or summons. On arrest, the defendant is taken to the appropriate law enforcement agency for processing, which includes paperwork and fingerprinting. The police also prepare accusatory statements, such as misdemeanor information and felony complaints. Detectives are assigned to cases when necessary to gather evidence, interview persons suspected of committing a crime and witnesses to a crime, and assist in preparing a case for possible trial. After processing has been completed, a person is either detained or released on bond.

IN THE COURT OF COMMON PLEAS

FIRST JUDICIAL DISTRICT OF PENNSYLVANIA

CRIMINAL TRIAL DIVISION

IN RE: MISC. NO. 0009901-2008

COUNTY INVESTIGATING:

GRAND JURY XXIII: C-17

_____

REPORT OF THE GRAND JURY

_____

R. SETH WILLIAMS

District Attorney

This case is about a doctor who killed babies and endangered women. What we mean is that he regularly and illegally delivered live, viable, babies in the third trimester of pregnancy – and then murdered these newborns by severing their spinal cords with scissors. The medical practice by which he carried out this business was a filthy fraud in which he overdosed his patients with dangerous drugs, spread venereal disease among them with infected instruments, perforated their wombs and bowels – and, on at least two occasions, caused their deaths. Over the years, many people came to know that something was going on here. But no one put a stop to it.

There remained, however, a final difficulty. When you perform late-term "abortions" by inducing labor, you get babies. Live, breathing, squirming babies. By 24 weeks, most babies born prematurely will survive if they receive appropriate medical care. But that was not what the Women's Medical Society was about. Gosnell had a simple solution for the unwanted babies he delivered: he killed them. He didn't call it that. He called it "ensuring fetal demise." The way he ensured fetal demise was by sticking scissors into the back of the baby's neck and cutting the spinal cord. He called that "snipping."

❑ ❑ ❑

Gosnell's students parroted his grisly techniques. Massof himself admitted to us that, of the many spinal cords he cut, there were about 100 instances where he did so after seeing a breath or some sign of life. The shocking regularity of killing babies who were born alive, who moved and breathed, as testified to by Gosnell's employees, demonstrates that these murders were intentional and collaborative. In addition to the specific murder charges identified above, **we recommend that Kermit Gosnell, Lynda Williams, Sherry West, Adrienne Moton, and Steven Massof be charged with conspiracy to commit murder**.

❑ ❑ ❑

Section VII: Criminal Charges

Gosnell and his staff showed consistent disregard not only for the health and safety of their patients, but also for the laws of Pennsylvania. After reviewing extensive and compelling evidence of criminal wrongdoing at

FIGURE 6-5   Report of the Grand Jury

the clinic, the Grand Jury has issued a presentment recommending the prosecution of Gosnell and members of his staff for criminal offenses including:

- Murder of Karnamaya Mongar
- Murders of babies born alive
- Infanticide
- Violations of the Controlled Substances Act
- Hindering, Obstruction, and Tampering
- Perjury
- Illegal late-term abortions
- Violations of the Abortion Control Act
- Violations of the Controlled Substances Act
- Abuse of Corpse
- Theft by Deception
- Conspiracy
- Corrupt Organization
- Corruption of Minors

❏ ❏ ❏

15. The authorities responsible for overseeing, monitoring, or licensing Gosnell or his operation should conduct serious self-assessments to determine why their departments failed to protect the women and babies whose lives were imperiled at Gosnell's clinic. Employees who failed to perform their jobs of protecting the public should be held accountable.

The employees of the state and local health departments and the prosecutors for the Board of Medicine are charged with protecting the public health. Very few that we ran across in this investigation came even close to fulfilling that duty. These people seemed oblivious to the connection between their dereliction and the deaths and injuries that Gosnell inflicted under their watch.[i]

i   http://www.phila.gov/districtattorney/pdfs/grandjurywomensmedical.pdf.

FIGURE 6-5   Report of the Grand Jury (*Continued*)

Arraignment

The arraignment is a formal reading of the accusatory instrument and includes the setting of bail. The accused should appear with counsel or have counsel appointed by the court if he or she cannot afford his or her own. After the charges are read, the defendant pleads guilty or not guilty. A not guilty plea is normally offered on a felony. On a plea of not guilty, the defense attorney and prosecutor make arguments regarding bail. After arraignment of the defendant, the judge sets a date for the defendant to return to court. Between the time of arraignment and the next court date, the defense attorney and the prosecutor confer about the charges and the evidence in the possession of the prosecutor. At that time, the defense will offer any mitigating circumstances that it believes will convince the prosecutor to lessen or drop the charges.

Indictment

A felony complaint or an indictment commences a criminal proceeding. An individual may be tried for a felony after indictment by a grand jury unless the defendant waives presentment to the grand jury and pleads guilty by way of a superior court. Felony cases are presented to a grand jury by a district attorney or an assistant district attorney. The grand jury is presented with the prosecution's evidence, after which the grand jury may indict the target if they find reasonable cause to believe from the evidence presented all the elements of a particular crime are present. The grand jury may request that witnesses be subpoenaed to testify. A defendant may choose to testify and offer information if he or she wishes. Actions of a grand jury are handed up to a judge, after which the defendant is notified to appear to be arraigned for the crimes charged in the indictment.

Conference

If the defendant does not plead guilty, both felony and misdemeanor cases are taken to conference, and plea-bargaining commences with the goal of an agreed-on disposition. If no disposition can be reached, the case is adjourned, motions are made, and further plea-bargaining ensues. Generally after several adjournments, a case is assigned to a trial court.

Prosecution

The role of the prosecutor in the criminal justice system is well defined in *Berger v. United States*:[12]

> The United States Attorney is the representative not of an ordinary party to a controversy, but of a sovereignty whose obligation to govern impartially is as compelling as its obligation to govern at all; and whose interest, therefore, in a criminal prosecution is not that it shall win a case, but that justice will be done. As such, he is in a peculiar and very definite sense the servant of the law, the twofold aim of which is that guilt shall not escape or innocence suffer.

The potential of the prosecutor's office is not always fully realized in many jurisdictions. In many cities, the combination of the prosecutor's staggering caseload and small staff of assistants prevents sufficient attention being given to each case.[13]

Defense

The defense attorney generally sits in the proverbial hot seat, being perceived as the bad guy. Although everyone seems to understand the attorney's function in protecting the rights of those represented, the defense attorney often is not very popular.

> There is a substantial difference in the problem of representing the "run-of-the-mill" criminal defendant and one whose alleged crimes have aroused great public outcry. The difficulties in providing representation for the ordinary criminal defendant are simple compared with the difficulties of obtaining counsel for one who is charged with a crime which by its nature or circumstances incites strong public condemnation.[14]

Trial

Most of the processes of a criminal trial are similar to those of a civil trial. They include jury selection, opening statements, presentation of witnesses and other evidence, summations, instructions to the jury by the judge, jury deliberations, verdict, and opportunity for appeal to a higher court. In a criminal trial, the jury verdict must be unanimous, and the standard of proof is that guilt must be determined beyond a reasonable doubt whereas in a civil trial the plaintiff need only prove a claim by a preponderance of the evidence.

HEALTH CARE FRAUD

Executive's Medicare Scheme Had Lobbying Effort to Support It
He Franchised Fraud With Advocacy Group

Miami health-care executive Larry Duran orchestrated one of the largest Medicare frauds in U.S. history, submitting more than $205 million in phony claims and landing a record-breaking 50-year prison sentence for his crimes.

• • •

Patients often suffered from Alzheimer's disease, dementia or other conditions unsuited for therapy and were frequently left to urinate or defecate on themselves as they waited for treatment that never came, testimony showed.

"The people that were there were just kept there and run through like cattle," the judge in the case said.

Dan Eggen, The Washington Post, *October 5, 2011*

Health care fraud involves an unlawful act, generally deception for financial gain. It "encompasses an array of irregularities and illegal acts characterized by intentional deception."[15] The Federal Bureau of Investigation (FBI) reports that:

> Health care fraud costs the country an estimated $80 billion a year. And it's a rising threat, with national health care spending topping $2.7 trillion and expenses continuing to outpace inflation. *Recent cases also show that medical professionals are more willing to risk patient harm in their schemes.*[16]

The victims of health care frauds often include those who are physically and neurologically challenged. Senior citizens at the time in their life that they are most vulnerable are often the targets of perpetrators of fraud.

Investigation and Prosecution of Fraud

The primary agency for exposing and investigating health care fraud is the FBI. with jurisdiction over both federal and private insurance programs.[17] The Department of Justice-Health and Human Services Medicare Fraud Strike Force is a multiagency team of federal, state, and local investigators that is designed to combat Medicare fraud. Medicare fraud is estimated to cost the nation $80 billion dollars annually.[18] The success of cooperation of agencies on the federal and state levels was evident when the Medicare Fraud Strike Force charged 111 defendants in nine cities, including doctors, nurses, health care company owners and executives, and others, for their alleged participation in Medicare fraud schemes involving more than $225 million in false billing.[19]

> [T]he Department of Justice (DOJ) and HHS announced the expansion of Medicare Fraud Strike Force operations to two additional cities—Dallas and Chicago. Today's operation is the largest-ever federal health care fraud takedown. More than 700 law enforcement agents from the FBI, HHS-Office of Inspector General (HHS-OIG), multiple Medicaid Fraud Control Units, and other state and local law enforcement agencies participated in the operation. In addition to making arrests, agents also executed 16 search warrants across the country in connection with ongoing strike force investigations.[20]

The message is clear that those involved in health care fraud are being vigorously pursued. The federal government's initiative to investigate and prosecute health care organizations for criminal wrongdoing has resulted in the establishment of corporate compliance programs for preventing, detecting, and reporting criminal conduct. An effective corporate compliance program should include:

1. Developing appropriate policies and procedures
2. Appointing a compliance officer to oversee the compliance program
3. Communicating the organization's compliance program to employees
4. Providing for monitoring and auditing systems that are designed to detect criminal conduct by employees and other agents
5. Publicizing a reporting system whereby employees and other agents can report criminal conduct by others within the organization without fear of retribution
6. Taking appropriate steps to respond to criminal conduct and to prevent similar offenses
7. Periodically reviewing and updating the organization's corporate compliance program
8. Working with state and federal law enforcement and regulatory agencies and insurance companies to detect, prevent, and prosecute health care fraud
9. Developing appropriate policies and procedures
10. Appointing a compliance officer to oversee the compliance program
11. Communicating the organization's compliance program to employees
12. Providing for monitoring and auditing systems that are designed to detect criminal conduct by employees and other agents
13. Publicizing a reporting system whereby employees and other agents can report criminal conduct by others within the organization without fear of retribution
14. Taking appropriate steps to respond to criminal conduct and to prevent similar offenses
15. Periodically reviewing and updating the organization's corporate compliance program
16. Working with state and federal law enforcement and regulatory agencies and insurance companies to detect, prevent, and prosecute health care fraud

As noted in the following remarks by Attorney General Eric Holder, health care fraud continues to present significant risks to patient health and is a financial drain on the health care system leading to higher costs for legitimate care.

We are here to announce that Johnson & Johnson and three of its subsidiaries have agreed to pay more than $2.2 billion to resolve criminal and civil claims that they marketed prescription drugs for uses that were never approved as safe and effective—and that they paid kickbacks to both physicians and pharmacies for prescribing and promoting these drugs.

• • •

Put simply, this alleged conduct is shameful and it is unacceptable. It displayed a reckless indifference to the safety of the American people. And it constituted a clear abuse of the public trust, showing a blatant disregard for systems and laws designed to protect public health.

As our filings make clear, these are not victimless crimes. Americans trust that the medications prescribed for their parents and grandparents, for their children, and for themselves are selected because they are in the patient's best interest. Laws enacted by Congress—and the enforcement efforts of the Food and Drug Administration—provide important safeguards to ensure that drugs are approved for uses that have been demonstrated as safe and effective. Efforts by drug companies to introduce their drugs into interstate commerce for unapproved uses subvert those laws. Likewise, the payment of kickbacks undermines the independent medical judgment of health care providers. It creates financial incentives to increase the use of certain drugs, potentially putting the health of some patients at risk. Every time pharmaceutical companies engage in this type of conduct, they corrupt medical decisions by health care providers, jeopardize the public health, and take money out of taxpayers' pockets.

This settlement demonstrates that the Departments of Justice and Health and Human Services—working alongside a variety of federal, state, and local partners—will not tolerate such activities. No company is above the law. And my colleagues and I are determined to keep moving forward—guided by the facts and the law, and using every tool, resource, and authority at our disposal—to hold these corporations accountable, to safeguard the American people, and to prevent this conduct from happening in the future.[21]

Schemes to Defraud

A defendant is guilty of a scheme to defraud when he or she engages in an arrangement establishing a systematic ongoing course of conduct with intent to defraud more than one person or to obtain property from more than one person by false or fraudulent pretenses, representations, or promises, and so obtains property from one or more of such persons. To show intent in a scheme to defraud, one needs to establish the following elements:

• That on or about (date), in the county of (county), the defendant (defendant's name), engaged in a scheme constituting a systematic ongoing course of conduct;
• That the defendant did so with intent to defraud more than one person or to obtain property from more than one person by false or fraudulent pretenses, representations, or promises; and

- That the defendant so obtained property from one or more of such persons, at least one of whom has been identified.[22]

Health care fraud is committed when a dishonest provider or consumer intentionally submits or causes someone else to submit false or misleading information for use in determining the amount of health care benefits payable. Some examples of provider health care fraud include the following:

- *Billing for services not rendered*
- *Falsifying a patient's diagnosis* to justify tests, surgeries, or other procedures that are not medically necessary
- *Misrepresenting procedures performed* to obtain payment for noncovered services, such as cosmetic surgery
- *Upcoding services* (billing for a more costly service than the one actually performed)
- *Upcoding medical supplies and equipment* (billing for more expensive equipment than what was delivered to the patient)
- *Unbundling* (billing each stage of a procedure as if it were a separate procedure)
- *Billing for unnecessary* services (services that are not medically indicated)
- *Accepting kickbacks* for patient referrals
- *Waiving patient copays or deductibles*
- *Overbilling* the insurance carrier or benefit plan

Schemes to defraud are rampant on the Internet. Internet pharmacy is a risky business as noted in the next news clipping.

$12 Million in Medicaid Funds Went to Deceased in Illinois

The Illinois Medicaid program paid an estimated 12 million for medical services for people listed as the deceased in other state records, according to the internal state government memo.

• • •

Auditors identified overpayments for services to roughly 2,900 people after the date of their deaths.

Carla K. Johnson and Sara Burnett, The Washington Post, *April 20, 2014*

Renewed Criticism for Google Over Drug Sites

Several state attorneys general are pressing Google to make it harder for its users to find counterfeit prescription medicine and illegal drugs online, marking the second time in the past three years that the firm has drawn government scrutiny for its policies on rogue Internet pharmacies.

• • •

Google, which failed to persuade a California judge to dismiss the suits, entered settlement talks last month after attorneys for the shareholders obtained e-mails showing that top executives warned then-chief executive Eric Schmidt and co-founder Larry Page more than a decade ago about the risks of accepting such ads.

Matea Gold and Tom Hamburger, The Washington Post, *April 16, 2014*

Although Google reached a settlement to pay $500 million to avoid prosecution for aiding illegal online pharmaceutical ads, some state prosecutors want to see more from Google in preventing ads from unlicensed pharmacies. "Google acknowledged in the settlement that it had improperly and knowingly assisted online pharmacy advertisers allegedly based in Canada to run advertisements for illicit pharmacy sales targeting U.S. customers."[23]

A variety of schemes to defraud are noted in the following news clippings.

Medicare Fraud Crackdown Nabs 91 in 8 Cities Across U.S.

Among those charged in the coordinated series of arrests was a doctor in Detroit who allegedly billed Medicare for services provided to dead people and claimed that he performed psychotherapy treatments more than 24 hours a day. Other doctors, nurses and health-care company owners were charged in various schemes to get paid for services that were medically unnecessary or never provided, officials said.

"From Brooklyn to Miami to Los Angeles, the defendants allegedly treated the Medicare program like a personal piggy bank," Lanny A. Breuer, assistant attorney general for the Justice Department's criminal division, said at a news conference in Washington.

Jerry Markon, The Washington Post, *September 8, 2011*

Medicare Bilked of $77M "Like an ATM"

Over 7 years, the federal program for the elderly and disabled paid at least about $77 million—and possibly as much as $92 million—to purported medical equipment suppliers who used Medicare ID numbers of deceased physicians, says a report out today by congressional investigators. . . .

Despite learning of the problem in 2001, the government failed to fix it, the report says. Investigators reviewing billing data submitted by equipment suppliers from 2000 to 2007 using the ID numbers of 1,500 deceased doctors.

Julie Appleby, USA Today, *July 9, 2008*

Woman Guilty of Health Care Fraud

A Severna Park woman pleaded guilty yesterday to health care fraud, admitting she billed the government and insurance companies for more than $200,000 in services she never rendered. . . . A state-licensed clinical specialist in child and adolescent psychiatric and mental health, [she] now faces the possibility of 10 years in prison and $250,000 in fines.

To conceal the fraud, she used false information on medical forms and patient logs.

Scott Daugherty, The Capital, *July 3, 2008*

Healthy Dose of Fraud

In one example of fraud, patients were allegedly brought to California, where they were paid to undergo surgeries that they did not need. In the scam, agents say, recruiters bring "patients from across the nation to surgery centers in California where they give phony or exaggerated symptoms and doctors perform unnecessary operations on them. Then the surgery centers send inflated claims for the unnecessary procedures to the patients' insurance companies. When the insurers pay up, federal authorities say, the recruiters, the surgery centers and the patients split the proceeds."[24] Corporate fraud has become so rampant that the level of trust in and reputation of organizational leadership has reached an all-time low.

Home Care Fraud

Today, more Americans are living longer than ever before. As medicine has advanced, the average life expectancy has increased by 50%. An increasing number of older persons receive in-home care, dependent on family and health care providers to attend to their physical, financial, emotional, and health care needs. Medicare home health benefits allow individuals with restricted mobility to remain home, outside an institutional setting, by providing home care benefits. Home care services and supplies are generally provided by nurses, home nursing aides, speech therapists, and physical therapists under a physician-certified plan of care.

Home care is rapidly being recognized as a breeding ground for abuse. The numerous scams in home care fraud are caused by the difficulty in supervising services provided in the home, Medicare's failure to monitor the number of visits per patient, beneficiaries paying no copayments except for medical equipment, and the lack of accountability to the patient by failing to explain services provided.

Home care fraud is generally not easy to detect. It involves charging insurers for more services than patients received, billing for more hours of care than were provided, falsifying records, and charging higher nurses' rates for care given by aides. The trend toward shorter hospital stays has created a multibillion-dollar market in home care services. This new market brings many opportunities for fraud.

MANSLAUGHTER

Manslaughter is the commission of an unintentional act that results in the death of another person. It can be either voluntary or involuntary. Voluntary manslaughter is the intentional killing of another person in what is commonly referred to as the "heat of passion," which is caused by the provocation of the victim (e.g., found having an affair with the defendant's spouse). Involuntary manslaughter is the result of a negligent act (e.g., reckless driving).

MURDER

Murder is the unlawful killing of a person. It is a homicide, and it involves malice aforethought and the premeditated intent to kill another human being. First-degree murder involves the deliberate and premeditated killing of another with malice aforethought. Second-degree murder is not deliberate, nor is it premeditated; however, it is the killing of another with malice aforethought. The tragedy of murder in health care settings that are dedicated to the healing of the sick has all too frequently occurred, as noted in the following examples.

- In a highly publicized case, Dr. Kermit Gosnell was convicted of murdering newborn babies by snipping their spinal cords shortly after delivery. Following a 2-month trial and 10 days of deliberation the jury convicted Gosnell of murder. Although it was expected that prosecutors would seek the death penalty, Gosnell made a deal with prosecutors promising not to appeal the jury's decision in exchange for life in prison without parole.
- Cullen, a former nurse, pleaded guilty to 13 murders and attempting to kill two others in New Jersey and Pennsylvania.[25] Cullen had refused to cooperate with prosecutors unless they promised not to seek the death penalty. Cullen claimed responsibility for the deaths of 30 to 40 patients over a 16-year nursing career. "The case raises concerns about hospital oversight of medical errors, narcotics security, and background checks on prospective employees. Cullen was fired from five hospitals and resigned from two amid questions about his job performance."[26] Cullen had been found violating nursing standards from the beginning of his career. He had problems in every one of the 10 institutions that he worked for in New Jersey and Pennsylvania. Apparently not one of the institutions in which Cullen worked gave him a bad reference. "It amounted to a policy of 'see no evil, speak no evil'— one that gave Cullen, in effect, a license to kill."[27]
- Richard Angelo, an Eagle Scout and voluntary fireman, gained national attention as the "angel of death." He was a registered nurse on the cardiac/ intensive care unit at a Long Island hospital, where he murdered patients by injecting them with the drug Pavulon. Angelo was ultimately convicted of two counts of depraved indifference murder (second-degree murder), one count of second-degree manslaughter, one count of criminally negligent homicide, and six counts of assault with respect to five of the patients and was sentenced to 61 years to life.[28] Angelo had committed the murders in a bizarre scheme to revive the patients and be thought of as a hero. The attorney for the estate of one of the alleged victims had filed a wrongful death suit against Angelo and the hospital a day before the verdict was rendered by the jury.[29]

THEFT

Theft is the illegal taking of another person or organization's property. Health care organizations must be alert to the potential ongoing threat of theft by unscrupulous employees, physicians, patients, visitors, and trespassers. The theft of patient or resident valuables, supplies, drugs, and medical equipment is substantial and costs health care organizations millions of dollars each year.

Drug Theft by Employee

One day in October, the night shift charge nurse began to reconcile the narcotics inventory on the patient care unit with the evening charge nurse. All appeared to be okay and the reconciliation sheet was signed off by both charge nurses. An evening shift staff nurse walked over to the two charge nurses and reported suspicious activity as to the usage of Demerol and Percocet during the day shift. She reported that one of the day shift nurses had been signing out two narcotic medications for a 3-day postoperative C-section patient. The patient's medication record showed that the patient was administered Demerol at 8:30 a.m., 10:30 a.m., and 1:00 p.m.. The nurse also had written that Percocet and Tylenol 3 had been administered every 2 hours. The charge nurses recognized that it would be unusual for a patient to be administered both an injection and oral narcotic at the same time and unlikely every 2 hours. When three other evening shift nurses were queried about the suspicion of medication theft, they responded:

Nurse 1: "This has been going on for a long time."
Nurse 2: "I am not getting involved."
Nurse 3: "Do you think we should report this?"

The two charge nurses spoke to the hospital's night supervising nurse who reported the possibility of medication theft to the VP of nursing. The nurse in question had been suspected of medication theft in the past, but no one ever established sufficient evidence to confront her. The VP for nursing questioned the suspected RN the following day when she arrived for work. She denied involvement in the theft of drugs. The nurse was asked to undergo a drug test, which she refused. She was then suspended for a week. When she returned, she was not permitted to carry the narcotics lock keys for a week. Later, after she regained access to narcotic drugs, she was observed giving a patient two Motrin when Percocet had been prescribed. Although an incident report had been filed against her, she continued to work into January. As other nurses eventually became concerned that they might be implicated in drug theft, they went to the VP of nursing and reported their observations. Finally, the suspected nurse was terminated. Eventually she was listed in the state professional newsletter as having a suspended license.

Sadly, this young nurse (39 years of age) was in a vehicle accident 6 months later with two other passengers. They were speeding 75 mph around a 35-mph curve without seat belts. They hit the embankment and were thrown from the car. The nurse and one passenger died instantly. The nurse had drugs in her possession, and an autopsy confirmed the presence of alcohol and drugs in all three passengers.

If action had been taken sooner, this tragedy may never have occurred. Management had the opportunity to explain the responsibility of nurses to report suspicious activity but failed to do so.

This same scenario was reported to have occurred in another state when an LPN was caught stealing medications. Within 24 hours of being caught, she had a choice of admitting to the theft and her chemical dependency or walking out of the hospital in handcuffs with the police.

Distraught Nurse (edited)

The evidence presented in *People v. Lancaster*[30] was found to have provided a probable cause foundation for information charging felony theft of nursing home residents' money by the office manager. Evidence showed that on repeated occasions the residents' income checks were cashed or cash was otherwise received on behalf of residents; that the defendant, by virtue of her office, had sole responsibility for maintaining the residents' ledger accounts; and that cash receipts frequently were never posted to the residents' accounts.

In another case, *Miller v. Dunn*,[31] there was sufficient evidence to hold that a nurse assistant had misappropriated $15,000 from an 83-year-old nursing home resident. The record indicated that the funds were taken during those times when the resident made visits to the hospital for respiratory problems. The patient had been diagnosed with dementia, and the resident's confusion was increasing. The nursing assistant actively procured the check in question, filling in the date, amount, and her name as payee. As a result, the nursing assistant was placed on the Employee Disqualification List for misappropriating funds.

The following news clippings illustrate how rampant theft is in the health care industry.

Virginia Court Rules Identity Theft Victim to Get $532,000 from . . .

Sloane delivered her second child . . . unaware that her last name would prove too big a temptation for an employee of the hospital's accounting department, Shovana Sloan.

Sloan, who was hired for the department even though she was a felon, appropriated Sloane's identification and went on a $35,000 spending spree.

Alan Cooper, Daily Record and the Kansas City Daily News-Press, *September 23, 2006*[32]

Medical Theft Trend Sweeps Pennsylvania

A slew of hospital thefts nationwide—including close to $75,000 of equipment from Mount Nittany Medical Center in 2005—has opened investigators' eyes to a black market specializing in the swap of used medical instruments.

Krystle Kopacz, The Daily Collegian Online, *January 13, 2006*[33]

NHS Hospital Thefts Cost Millions

National Health Service (NHS) hospital wards in the UK are being targeted by thieves who steal tens of millions of pounds worth of medical equipment every year.

Hospital Healthcare.com, *June 26, 2008*[34]

Millions of Patient Billing Records Stolen from UT Hospital

Billing records for about 2.2 million patients and guarantors were stolen last week from the University of Utah Hospitals & Clinics, just one more in what appears to be a rapidly growing flood of identity theft incidents.

Anne Zieger, Fierce HealthIT, *June 14, 2008*[35]

Grady Hospital Battles Patient Thefts

"It's got to be clearly 180 degrees from what we expect in an institution of care and shelter," said Atlanta attorney Mark Spix, who says he represented a man whose wife lost an engagement ring after being flown to Grady in October 2004 with fatal injuries. "I just think that is unacceptable."

There were 260 thefts involving patients, employees and visitors in 2007, compared with 262 in 2006 and 279 in 2005, Grady spokeswoman Denise Simpson said.

Tim Eberly, The Atlanta Journal-Constitution, *July 24, 2008*[36]

CONTRACTS

A *contract* is a special kind of agreement, either written **(Figure 6-6)**, or oral, that involves legally binding obligations between two or more parties. A contract can also be implied such as when one or more persons provide emergency care and treatment to a comatose patient injured during an automobile accident. The major purpose of a contract is to specify, limit, and define the agreements that are legally enforceable.

ELEMENTS OF A CONTRACT

Whether contracts are executed in writing or agreed to orally, they must contain the following elements to be enforceable: (1) offer/communication, (2) consideration, and (3) acceptance.

Offer/Communication

An offer must be communicated to the other party so that it can be accepted or rejected. Unless the offeror specifically requires that the acceptance be received before a contract is formed, communication of the acceptance to the offeror is not necessary.

Consideration

An offer is a promise by one party to do (or not to do) something if the other party agrees to do (or not do) something. Not all statements or promises are offers. Generally, advertisements

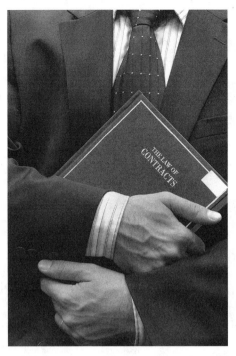

FIGURE 6-6   The Law of Contracts (© corgarashu/Shutterstock, Inc.)

of goods for sale are not offers but are invitations to the public to come to the place of business, view the merchandise, and be made an offer. An opinion is not an offer. Preliminary negotiations are not offers.

Acceptance

On proper acceptance of an offer, a contract is formed. It involves:

- *Meeting of the minds:* Acceptance requires a "meeting of the minds" (mutual assent). The parties must understand and then agree on the terms of the contract.
- *Definite and complete:* Acceptance requires mutual assent to be found between the parties. The terms must be so complete that both parties understand and agree to what has been proposed.
- *Duration:* Generally, the other party may revoke an offer at any time prior to a valid acceptance. When the offeror does revoke the proposal, the revocation is not effective until the offeree (the person to whom the offer is made) receives it. After the offeree has accepted the offer, any attempt to revoke the agreement is too late and is invalid.
- *Complete and conforming:* The traditional rule is that the acceptance must be the mirror image of the offer. In other words, the acceptance must comply with all the terms of the offer.

EMPLOYMENT CONTRACTS

An employer's right to terminate an employee can be limited by express agreement with the employee or through a collective bargaining agreement to which the employee is a beneficiary.

No such agreement was found to exist in *O'Connor v. Eastman Kodak Co.*,[37] in which the court held that an employer had a right to terminate an employee at will at any time, and for any reason or no reason. The plaintiff did not rely on any specific representation made to him during the course of his employment interviews, nor did he rely on any documentation in the employee handbook, which would have limited the defendant's common-law right to discharge at will. The employee had relied on a popular perception of Kodak as a "womb-to-tomb" employer.

EXCLUSIVE CONTRACTS

An *exclusive contract*, in the context of a hospital, is an agreement between two or more entities to deal only with each other regarding a specific area of business (e.g., hospital[s] and radiology physician[s] group). The essential feature of an exclusivity contract is the covenant not to engage in a particular business activity with other parties for a specified period of time.

An organization often enters into an exclusive contract with physicians and/or medical groups for the purpose of providing a specific service to the organization. Exclusive contracts generally occur within the organization's ancillary service departments (e.g., radiology, anesthesiology, and pathology). Physicians who seek to practice at organizations in these ancillary areas but who are not part of the exclusive group have attempted to invoke the federal antitrust laws to challenge these exclusive contracts. These challenges generally have been unsuccessful.

Exclusive Contract with Radiology Group

Tennessee code permitted the hospital authority to enter into an exclusive contract with a radiology group. The governing body's decision to close the staff of the imaging department did not violate medical staff bylaws, and the defendant radiologists were not legally or constitutionally entitled to a hearing if their privileges were terminated on entry of the hospital authority into an exclusive provider contract.[38]

Commercial Ethics and Noncompetition Agreements

The purpose in allowing noncompetition agreements is to foster "commercial ethics" and to protect the employer's legitimate interests by preventing unfair competition, not ordinary competition.

The respondent hospital in *Washington County Memorial Hospital v. Sidebottom*[39] employed the appellant/nurse practitioner from October 1993 through April 1998. Before beginning her employment, the nurse entered into an employment agreement with the hospital. The agreement included a noncompetition clause providing in part that the nurse "during the term of [the] Agreement and for a period of one (1) year after the termination of her employment . . . will not, anywhere within a fifty (50) mile radius . . . directly or indirectly engage in the practice of nursing . . . without the express direction or consent" of the hospital. In February 1994, the nurse requested the hospital's permission to work for the Washington County Health Department doing prenatal nursing care. Because the hospital was not then doing prenatal care, the hospital gave her permission to accept that employment but reserved the ability to withdraw the permission if the services the nurse was providing later came to be provided by the hospital. In January 1996, the nurse and the hospital entered into a second employment agreement that continued the parties' employment relationship through January

9, 1998. This agreement included a noncompetition clause identical to the 1993 employment agreement. It also provided for automatic renewal for an additional 2 years unless either party gave written termination notice no less than 90 days prior to the expiration of the agreement.

The hospital's interest lies in protecting its patient base as a primary source of revenue. The specific enforcement of the nurse's noncompetition clause is reasonably necessary to protect the hospital's interest. Actual damage need not be proven to enforce a covenant not to compete. Rather, the employee's opportunity to influence customers justifies enforcement of the covenant. Thus, the quality, frequency, and duration of an employee's exposure to an employer's customers are crucial in determining the covenant's reasonableness. The nurse had opportunity to influence the hospital's patients. Before her employment with the hospital, the nurse had never worked in Washington County, nor did she have a patient base there. The nurse helped to establish two rural health care clinics for the hospital, one of which she managed during her first year of employment. During almost 5 years of employment with the hospital, the nurse saw more than 3,000 patients. Pursuant to a collaborative practice agreement with a physician, the nurse treated patients, diagnosed illnesses and injuries, prescribed and dispensed medications, and ordered and interpreted laboratory tests. The nurse got to know the patients and families to whom she provided these services. At the clinic, she had her own telephone number, receptionist, appointment book, medical assistant, patient charts, laboratory, and examination rooms. Her offices were physically separated from those of the other medical practitioner at the clinic. Furthermore, during her employment, the hospital promoted the nurse as a nurse practitioner in the community by paying for advertisements with her picture and telephone number in the newspaper. In general, the nurse had a good rapport with her patients, and she had patients who requested her for medical services.

TRIAL PROCEDURE AND THE COURTROOM

This next section presents a brief review of the law as applied in the courtroom **(Figure 6-7)**. Although many of the procedures leading up to and followed during a trial are discussed in

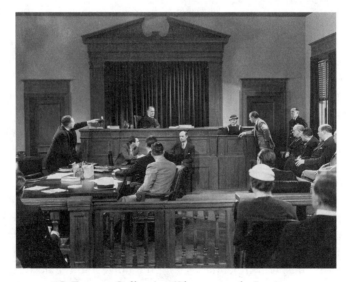

FIGURE 6-7   The Courtroom (© Everett Collection/Shutterstock, Inc.)

this chapter, civil procedure and trial practice are governed by each state's statutory requirements. Federal statutes govern cases on the federal level.

PLEADINGS

The pleadings of a case (e.g., summons and complaint), which include all the allegations of each party to a lawsuit, are filed with a court. The pleadings may raise questions of both law and fact. If only questions of law are at issue, the judge will decide the case based on the pleadings alone. If questions of fact are involved, the purpose of a trial is to determine those facts.

Summons and Complaint

The parties to a controversy are the plaintiff and the defendant. The plaintiff is the person who initiates an action by filing a complaint; the defendant is the person against whom a suit is brought. Many cases have multiple plaintiffs and defendants. Filing an order with a court clerk to issue a writ or summons commences an action.

Although the procedures for beginning an action vary according to jurisdiction, there are procedural common denominators. All jurisdictions require service of process on the defendant (usually through a summons) and a return to the court of that process by the person who served it. When a summons is not required to be issued directly by a court, an attorney, as an officer of the court, may prepare and cause a summons to be served without direct notice to or approval of a court. Notice to a court occurs when an attorney files a summons and complaint in a court, thereby indicating to the court that an action has been commenced.

The first pleading filed with the court in a negligence action is the complaint. The complaint identifies the parties to a suit, states a cause of action, and includes a demand for damages. It is filed by the plaintiff and is the first statement of a case by the plaintiff against the defendant. In some jurisdictions, a complaint must accompany a summons (an announcement to the defendant that a case has been commenced).

Answer

After service of a complaint, a response is required from the defendant in a document called the answer. In the answer, the defendant responds to each of the allegations contained in the complaint by stating his or her defense and by admitting to or denying each of the plaintiff's allegations. If the defendant fails to answer the complaint within the prescribed time, the plaintiff can seek judgment by default against the defendant.

Bill of Particulars

A bill of particulars in a civil case is a written demand for more detailed information concerning the alleged claim/s by the defendant/s. A bill of particulars is requested when there is generally insufficient information provided in the complaint to file an answer. If a counterclaim is filed, the plaintiff's attorney may request a bill of particulars from the defense attorney. In a criminal case the defendant/s attorney may request a bill of particulars in order to prepare their case.

Discovery

Discovery is the process of investigating the facts of a case before trial. The objectives of discovery are to:

- obtain evidence that might not be obtainable at the time of trial
- isolate and narrow the issues for trial
- gather knowledge of the existence of additional evidence that may be admissible at trial
- obtain leads to enable the discovering party to gather further evidence

The parties to a lawsuit have the right to discovery and to examine witnesses before trial.

Examination before trial (EBT) is one of several discovery techniques used to enable the parties of a lawsuit to learn more regarding the nature and substance of each other's case. An EBT consists of oral testimony under oath and includes cross-examination. A deposition, taken at an EBT, is the testimony of a witness that has been recorded in a written format. Testimony given at a deposition becomes part of the permanent record of the case. Each question and answer is transcribed by a court stenographer and may be used at the subsequent trial. Truthfulness and consistency are important because answers that differ from those given at trial will be used to attack the credibility of the witness.

PREPARATION OF WITNESSES

The manner in which a witness handles questioning at a deposition or trial is often as important as the facts of the case. Each witness should be well prepared before testifying. Preparation should include a review of all pertinent records. Helpful guidelines for witnesses undergoing examination in a trial or a court hearing include the following:

- Review the records (e.g., medical records and other business records) on which you might be questioned.
- Do not be antagonistic when answering the questions. The jury may already be somewhat sympathetic toward a particular party to the lawsuit; antagonism may serve only to reinforce such an impression.
- Be organized in your thinking and recollection of the facts regarding the incident.
- Answer only the questions asked.
- Explain your testimony in simple, succinct terminology.
- Do not overdramatize the facts you are relating.
- Do not allow yourself to become overpowered by the cross-examiner.
- Be polite, sincere, and courteous at all times.
- Dress appropriately and be neatly groomed.
- Pay close attention to any objections your attorney may have as to the line of questioning being conducted by the opposing counsel.
- Be sure to have reviewed any oral deposition in which you may have participated.
- Be straightforward with the examiner. Any answers designed to cover up or cloud an issue or fact will, if discovered, serve only to discredit any previous testimony that you may have given. Do not show any visible signs of displeasure regarding any testimony with which you are in disagreement.

- Be sure to have questions that you did not hear repeated and questions that you did not understand rephrased.
- If you are not sure of an answer, indicate that you are not sure or that you just do not know the answer.
- Remember that lawyers often get the answers they want by how they frame the questions they ask.

THE COURT

A case is heard in the court that has jurisdiction over the subject of controversy. The judge decides questions of law and is responsible for ensuring that a trial is conducted properly in an impartial atmosphere and that it is fair to both parties of a lawsuit. He or she determines what constitutes the general standard of conduct required for the exercise of due care. The judge informs the jury of what the defendant's conduct should have been, thereby making a determination of the existence of a legal duty.

The judge decides whether evidence is admissible, charges the jury (defines the jurors' responsibility in relation to existing law), and may take a case away from the jury (by directed verdict or judgment notwithstanding the verdict) if he or she believes that there are no issues for the jury to consider or that the jury has erred in its decision. This right on the part of the judge with respect to the role of the jury narrows the jury's responsibility with regard to the facts of the case. The judge maintains order throughout the suit, determines issues of procedure, and is generally responsible for the conduct of the trial.

Mother Loses Custody of Her Children—Because She Has Breast Cancer

A woman with terminal breast cancer says she has lost custody of her children because doctors do not know how long she will live.

A judge ruled that 37-year-old Alaina Giordano, from Durham, North Carolina, must give up both her children to her estranged husband after she was diagnosed with stage four breast cancer.

Durham County Family Court judge Nancy Gordon ruled that Mr. Snyder should get the children after a psychiatrist recommended that they should live with him because of the "deteriorating condition of the mother's health."

John Stevens, Daily Mail, *May 10, 2011*

A Facebook account was set up for Alaina, and within several weeks, 18,743 people linked to her page. The following is a sampling of the numerous posts on her Facebook page:

D.D. MAY GOD HAVE MERCY ON YOU AND I WILL PRAY FOR YOU AND YOUR CHILDREN. NO ONE HAS THE RIGHT TO TAKE WHAT GOD HAS GIVEN YOU . . . "YOUR CHILDREN"

M.A.B. she should not lose her family because she feel ill. Falling ill is not a lifestyle choice she made—it is a circumstance she is forced to endure she should not endure it without her children. mothers in prison may have their children with them for God's sake.

S.X. Came home to NC after a business trip to see this report. SHAMEFUL that a court and an "expert witness" could have so little compassion and rule like this. I'm shocked. I know the family. These kids belong with Mom!

"We have learned that the North Carolina Supreme Court has denied my motion for a stay—this means that now, my children will be moving to Chicago to start the school year with their father.

As I write today, I deal with the difficult recognition that my children will have to live 800 miles away from me, until my appeal can be heard. In the wake of this legal decision, my children and I now must grieve the pending loss of each other."

http://www.facebook.com/friendsofalaina

Comments by Danny

Alaina, I have been a hospital administrator and later inspected more that 500 hospitals and 100 ambulatory sites from Alaska to Puerto Rico. I have never experienced such a travesty by a Judge who apparently has little knowledge of the law or an understanding of the horrors you have been put through. Judges of this sort need some major training in ethics. I quote Earl Warren, Chief Justice of the United States (1891-1974), "In civilized life, law floats on a sea of ethics." The Judge in your case failed to understand and practice the teachings of this most Honorable judge—Earl Warren. I wish you love and happiness always . . . and know that you are loved.

Danny

Mother With Terminal Cancer Can Retain Child Custody, Judge Holds

In a case of first impression, a New Jersey judge has refused to strip a divorced mother of primary custody of her children even though she has terminal and inoperable breast cancer.

Ocean County Superior Court Judge Lawrence Jones said granting the father's motion for an emergency change in the children's primary residential status could cause them emotional harm.

"It would be fundamentally inequitable and inappropriate for this court to conclude that a person's illness, disability, or condition, even a condition as serious as Stage IV cancer, automatically renders a person unfit per se to continue serving as a custodial parent . . . ."

Michael Booth, New Jersey Law Journal, *November 22, 2013*[40]

Discussion

1. Make an argument supporting the judge's decision and one that opposes her decision.
2. Discuss both the moral and legal issues (e.g., the best interests of the child) you believe the judge may have failed to consider in this case.

THE JURY

The right to a trial by jury is a constitutional right in certain cases. Not all cases entitle the parties to a jury trial as a matter of right. For example, in many jurisdictions, a case in equity (a case seeking a specific course of conduct rather than monetary damages) may not entitle the parties to a trial by a jury. An example of an equity case is one that seeks a declaration as to the title to real property. Members of a jury are selected from a jury list. They are summoned to court by a paper known as the jury process. Impartiality is a prerequisite of all jurors. The number of jurors who sit at trial is 12 in common law. If there are fewer than 12, the number must be established by statute.

An individual may waive the right to a jury trial. If this right is waived, the judge acts as judge and jury, becomes the trier of facts, and decides issues of law.

Counsel for both parties of a lawsuit may question each prospective jury member for impartiality, bias, and prejudicial thinking. This process is referred to as the *voir dire*, the examination of jurors. After members of the jury are selected, they are sworn in to try the case.

The jury makes a determination of the facts that have occurred, evaluating whether the plaintiff's damages were caused by the defendant's negligence and whether the defendant exercised due care. The jury makes a determination of the particular standard of conduct required in all cases in which the judgment of reasonable people might differ. The jury must pay close attention to the evidence presented by both sides of a suit in order to render a fair and impartial verdict.

The jury also determines the extent of damages, if any, and the degree to which the plaintiff's conduct may have contributed to any injuries suffered.

SUBPOENAS

A *subpoena* is a legal order requiring the appearance of a person and/or the presentation of documents to a court or administrative body. Attorneys, judges, and certain law enforcement and administrative officials, depending on the jurisdiction, may issue subpoenas.

- A *subpoena ad testificandum* orders the appearance of a person at a trial or other investigative proceeding to give testimony. Witnesses have a duty to appear and may suffer a penalty for contempt of court should they fail to appear.
- A *subpoena duces tecum* is a written command to bring records, documents, or other evidence described in the subpoena to a trial or other investigative proceeding. The subpoena is served on a person able to produce such records.

OPENING STATEMENTS

During the opening statement, the plaintiff's attorney outlines what he or she intends to prove. The opening statement by the plaintiff's attorney provides in capsule form the facts of the case, what he or she intends to prove by means of a summary of the evidence to be presented, and a description of the damages to his or her client.

The defense attorney makes his or her opening statement indicating the position of the defendant and the points of the plaintiff's case he or she intends to refute. The defense attorney summarizes the facts as they apply to the case for the defendant.

BURDEN OF PROOF

The *burden of proof* requires that the plaintiff's attorney show that the defendant violated a legal duty by not following an acceptable standard of care and that the plaintiff suffered injury because of the defendant's breach. If the evidence presented does not support the allegations made, the case is dismissed.

EVIDENCE

Evidence consists of the facts proved or disproved during a lawsuit. The law of evidence is a body of rules under which facts are proved. To be admitted at trial, evidence must be competent, relevant, and material.

Direct Evidence

Direct evidence is proof offered through direct testimony. It is the jury's function to receive testimony presented by witnesses and to draw conclusions in the determination of facts.

Demonstrative Evidence

Demonstrative (real) evidence is evidence furnished by things themselves. It is considered the most trustworthy and preferred type of evidence. It consists of tangible objects to which testimony refers (e.g., medical instruments and broken infusion needles) that can be requested by a jury. Demonstrative evidence is admissible in court if it is relevant, has probative value, and serves the interest of justice. It is not admissible if it will prejudice, mislead, confuse, offend, inflame, or arouse the sympathy or passion of the jury. Other forms of demonstrative evidence include photographs, motion pictures, computer generated information, drawings, human bodies as exhibits, pathology slides, fetal monitoring strips, safety committee minutes, infection committee reports, medical staff bylaws, rules and regulations, nursing policy and procedure manuals, census data, and staffing patterns.

A plaintiff's injuries are admissible as an exhibit if the physical condition of the body is material to the complaint. The human body is considered the best evidence as to the nature and extent of the alleged injury/injuries. If there is no controversy about either the nature or the extent of an injury, presenting such evidence could be considered prejudicial and an objection can be made as to its presentation to a jury.

Documentary Evidence

Documentary evidence is written evidence capable of making a truthful statement (e.g., drug manufacturer inserts, autopsy reports, birth certificates, and medical records). Documentary evidence must satisfy the jury as to authenticity. Proof of authenticity is not necessary if the opposing party accepts its genuineness. In some instances, concerning wills, for example, witnesses are necessary. In the case of documentation, the original of a document must be produced unless it can be demonstrated that the original has been lost or destroyed, in which case a properly authenticated copy may be substituted.

EXAMINATION OF WITNESSES

After conclusion of the opening statements, the judge calls for the plaintiff's witnesses. An officer of the court administers an oath to each witness, and direct examination begins. On cross-examination by the defense, an attempt is made to challenge or discredit the plaintiff's witness. The plaintiff's attorney may ask the same witness more questions in an effort to overcome the effect of the cross-examination. Re-cross-examination may also take place if necessary for the defense of the defendant.

Expert Witness

Laypersons are quite able to render opinions about a great variety of general subjects, but for technical questions, the opinion of an expert is necessary. At the time of testifying, each expert's training, experience, and special qualifications are explained to the jury. The experts are asked to give an opinion concerning hypothetical questions based on the facts of the case. Should the testimony of two experts conflict, the jury will determine which expert opinion to accept. Expert witnesses may be used to assist a plaintiff in proving the wrongful act of a defendant or to assist a defendant in refuting such evidence. In addition, expert testimony may be used to show the extent of the plaintiff's damages or to show the lack of such damages.

DEFENSE OF ONE'S ACTIONS

The defendant's case is presented to discredit the plaintiff's cause of action and prevent recovery of damages. Principles of law that may relieve a defendant from liability include assumption of a risk, comparative negligence, contributory negligence, Good Samaritan laws, ignorance of fact, unintentional wrongs, the statute of limitations, and sovereign immunity.

Assumption of a Risk

Assumption of a risk is knowing that a danger exists and voluntarily accepting the risk by exposing oneself to it, knowing that harm might occur. Assumption of a risk may be implicitly assumed, as in alcohol consumption, or expressly assumed, as in relation to warnings found on cigarette packaging.

This defense provides that the plaintiff expressly has given consent in advance, relieving the defendant of an obligation of conduct toward the plaintiff and taking the chances of injury from a known risk arising from the defendant's conduct. For example, one who agrees to care for a patient with a communicable disease and then contracts the disease would not be entitled to recover from the patient for damages suffered. In taking the job, the individual agreed to assume the risk of infection, thereby releasing the patient from all legal obligations.

The following two requirements must be established in order for a defendant to be successful in an assumption of risk defense:

1. the plaintiff must know and understand the risk that is being incurred; and,
2. the choice to incur the risk must be free and voluntary.

Comparative Negligence

A defense of *comparative negligence* provides that the degree of negligence or carelessness of each party to a lawsuit must be established by the finder of fact and that each party then is responsible for his or her proportional share of any damages awarded. For example, if a plaintiff suffers injuries of $10,000 from an accident and is found to be 20% negligent and the defendant is found to be 80% negligent, the defendant would be required to pay $8,000 to the plaintiff. Thus, with comparative negligence, the plaintiff can collect for 80% of the injuries, whereas an application of contributory negligence would deprive the plaintiff of any monetary judgment. This doctrine relieves the plaintiff from the hardship of losing an entire claim when a defendant has been successful in establishing that the plaintiff has contributed to his or her own injuries.

Contributory Negligence

Contributory negligence can be defined as any lack of ordinary care on the part of the person injured that, combined with the negligent act of another, caused the injury. A person is contributorily negligent when that person does not exercise reasonable care for his or her own safety. As a general proposition, if a person has knowledge of a dangerous situation and disregards the danger, then that person is contributorily negligent.

Good Samaritan Laws

The various states have enacted *Good Samaritan laws* that relieve health care professionals, and in some instances laypersons, from liability in certain emergency situations. Good Samaritan legislation encourages health care professionals to render assistance at the scene of emergencies. Good Samaritan statutes provide a standard of care that delineates the scope of immunity for those persons eligible under the law.

Ignorance of the Law and Unintentional Wrongs

Ignorance of the law excuses no man; not that all men know the law, but because 'tis an excuse every man will plead, and no man can tell how to confute him.

–JOHN SELDEN (1584–1654)

The defendant cannot use ignorance of the law to excuse his or her negligent actions; otherwise, pleading ignorance would reward an individual. Arguing that a negligent act is unintentional is no defense. If such a defense were acceptable, all defendants would use it.

Because a defense of ignorance or "I didn't know what I was doing" is not an acceptable answer in a courtroom, you need to learn and understand the potential consequences of your actions in the health care setting. This text lays the foundation for understanding your legal and ethical rights and responsibilities.

Statute of Limitations

The *statute of limitations* refers to legislatively imposed time constraints that restrict the period of time after an injury occurs during which a legal action must be commenced. Should a cause of action be initiated later than the period of time prescribed, the case cannot proceed. The statutory period begins when an injury occurs, although in some cases (usually involving foreign objects left in the body during surgery) the statutory period commences when the injured person discovers or should have discovered the injury.

Many technical rules are associated with statutes of limitations. Computation of the period when the statute begins to run in a particular state may be based on any of the following factors:

- The date that the physician terminated treatment
- The time of the wrongful act
- The time when the patient should have reasonably discovered the injury
- The date that the injury is discovered
- The date when the contract between the patient and the physician ended

Sovereign Immunity

Sovereign immunity refers to the common-law doctrine by which federal and state governments historically have been immune from liability for harm suffered from the tortious conduct of employees. For the most part, both federal and state governments have abolished sovereign immunity.

CLOSING STATEMENTS

Closing statements give attorneys an opportunity to summarize for the jury and the court what they have proven. They may point out faults in their opponent's case and emphasize points they want the jury to remember.

JUDGE'S CHARGE TO THE JURY

After the attorneys' summations, the court charges the jury before the jurors recess to deliberate. Because the jury determines issues of fact, it is necessary for the court to instruct the jury with regard to applicable law. This is done by means of a charge. The charge defines the responsibility of the jury, describes the applicable law, and advises the jury of the alternatives available to it.

JURY DELIBERATION

After the judge's charge, the jury retires to the jury room and deliberates as to whether or not the defendant is liable. The jury returns to the courtroom upon reaching a verdict, and its determinations are presented to the court.

If a verdict is against the weight of the evidence, a judge may dismiss the case, order a new trial, or set his or her own verdict. At the time judgment is rendered, the losing party has an opportunity to motion for a new trial. If a new trial is granted, the entire process is repeated; if not, the judgment becomes final, subject to review of the trial record by an appellate court.

DAMAGES

Damages suffered by plaintiffs can be awarded as compensation for loss or injury as a result of the negligence of the defendants.. Damages can be sought for emotional distress, physical pain and suffering, and economic loss. *Punitive damages* are sometimes awarded over and above that which is intended to compensate the plaintiff for economic losses resulting from the injury. Punitive damages cover such items as physical disability, mental anguish, loss of a spouse's services, physical suffering, injury to one's reputation, and loss of companionship. Punitive damages are referred to as "that mighty engine of deterrence" in *Johnson v. Terry*.[41] In *Estes Health Care Centers v. Bonnerman,* it was found that:[42]

> While human life is incapable of translation into a compensatory measurement, the amount of an award of punitive damages may be measured by the gravity of the wrong done, the punishment called for by the act of the wrongdoer, and the need to discourage similar wrongs.

APPEALS

An appellate court reviews a case on the basis of the trial record as well as written briefs and, if requested, concise oral arguments by the attorneys. A brief summarizes the facts of a case, testimony of the witnesses, laws affecting the case, and arguments of counsel. The party making the appeal is the appellant. The party answering the appeal is the appellee. After hearing the oral arguments, the court takes the case under advisement until such time as the judges consider it and agree on a decision. An opinion is then prepared, explaining the reasons for a decision. The appellate court may modify, affirm, or reverse the judgment or may order a new trial on appeal.

CHAPTER REVIEW

1. *Tort* is a civil wrong committed against a person or property for which a court provides a correction in the form of an action for damages.
   - Objectives of tort law
     - Preservation of peace (between individuals by providing a substitute for retaliation)
     - Culpability—find fault for wrongdoing.
     - Deterrence—to discourage the wrongdoer (tort-feasor) from committing future torts.
     - Compensation—to indemnify the injured person[s] of wrongdoing.
2. *Negligence* is the unintentional *commission* or *omission* of an act that a reasonably prudent person would *or would not perform under given circumstances.*
   - *Malpractice*
     - Negligence or carelessness of a professional person
   - Forms of negligence
     - *Malfeasance,* execution of an unlawful or improper act
     - *Misfeasance,* improper performance of an act that results in injury to another
     - *Nonfeasance,* failure to act when there is a duty to do so

- Elements of negligence
  - *Duty to care*—obligation to conform to a recognized standard of care
  - *Breach of duty*—failure to meet a prevailing standard of care
  - *Injury*—actual damages must be established
  - *Causation*—defendant's departure from the standard of care must be the cause of the plaintiff's injury.
    - *Foreseeability*—reasonable anticipation that harm or injury will result from an act or a failure to act.
    - The test for foreseeability is whether or not one should have reasonably anticipated that the event in question or a similar event would occur.

3. *Intentional tort* is a wrong involves an act that violates another person's interests.
   - Assault and battery
     - *Assault* is the infringement on the mental security or tranquility of another person.
     - *Battery* is the violation of another person's physical integrity.
   - False imprisonment
     - The unlawful restraint of an individual's personal liberty or the unlawful restraint or confinement of an individual
   - Defamation of character
     - A false oral or written communication to someone other than the individual defamed, subjecting that individual's reputation to scorn and ridicule
       - *Libel*—written defamation
       - *Slander*—spoken defamation
   - Invasion of privacy
   - Infliction of mental distress
     - Characterized by conduct that is so outrageous that it goes beyond the bounds tolerated by a decent society

4. *Criminal law* is society's expression of the limits of acceptable human behavior.
   - *Crime*, a social harm defined and made punishable by law
     - *Misdemeanor* is an offense punishable by less than 1 year in jail and/or a fine.
     - *Felony* is generally punishable by imprisonment in a state or federal prison for a period of more than 1 year.
     - *Criminal negligence*, the reckless disregard for the safety of others and willful indifference to an injury that could result from an act. It differs from tort liability in that it provides for a more specific lack of care commonly characterized as "gross negligence" and "recklessness."
   - Objectives of criminal law
     - Maintain public order and safety
     - Protect individuals and society from harm
     - Provide punishment as a deterrent to crime
     - Rehabilitate criminals for return to society
   - Criminal procedure
     - Arrest
     - Arraignment
     - Indictment
     - Conference

- - ○ Prosecution
    - ○ Defense
    - ○ Trial
  - Health care fraud
  - Manslaughter
  - Murder
  - Theft
5. *Contract*, a written or oral agreement that involves legally binding obligations between two or more parties.
   - Elements of a contract
     - ○ Offer/communication
     - ○ Consideration
     - ○ Acceptance
   - *Exclusive contracts* allow organizations to contract with physicians and/or medical groups to provide specific services to the organization.
     - ○ Employment contracts
     - ○ Exclusive contracts
     - ○ Commercial ethics and noncompetitive agreements
6. Trial procedures
   - Pleadings
     - ○ *Summons and complaint*
     - ○ *Answer*
     - ○ *Bill of particulars*
     - ○ Discovery
       - ○ Investigation of facts.
       - ○ Examination Before Trial (EBT).
     - ○ Process that allows for witnesses to be examined prior to trial
   - Preparation of witnesses
   - Court
   - Jury
     - ○ Determines the facts in a case.
     - ○ Makes a determination of the particular standards of conduct required in which the judgment of reasonable people might differ.
   - Subpoenas
   - Opening statements
   - Burden of proof
   - Evidence
     - ○ *Direct evidence*, proof offered via direct testimony
     - ○ *Demonstrative evidence*, proof offered by objects themselves
     - ○ *Documentary evidence*, written evidence capable of making a truthful statement
   - Examination of witnesses
     - ○ *Expert witness* used to resolve issues in a case outside the understanding or experience of the average juror
   - Defending one's actions in a negligence case
     - ○ *Assumption of a risk*

- ○ *Comparative negligence*
- ○ *Contributory negligence*
- ○ *Good Samaritan laws*
- ○ *Ignorance of the law and unintentional wrongs*
- ○ *Statute of limitations*
- ○ *Sovereign Immunity*
- Closing statements
- Judge's charge to the jury
- Jury deliberation
- Damages
  - ○ Nominal damages,
  - ○ Compensatory damages,
  - ○ Punitive damages.
- Appeals process

TEST YOUR UNDERSTANDING

TERMINOLOGY

assault	evidence	murder
assumption of a risk	exclusive contract	negligence
battery	false imprisonment	nonfeasance
breach of duty	felony	nonmaleficence
burden of proof	foreseeability	omission
causation	Good Samaritan laws	proximate cause
commission	infliction of mental distress	punitive damages
comparative negligence	injury	reasonably prudent person
contract	intentional tort	right to privacy
contributory negligence	invasion of privacy	slander
damages	libel	sovereign immunity
defamation of character	malfeasance	standard of care
demonstrative evidence	malpractice	statute of limitations
direct evidence	manslaughter	subpoena
documentary evidence	misdemeanor	theft
duty to care	misfeasance	tort

REVIEW QUESTIONS

1. Describe the objectives of tort law.

2. Discuss the distinctions among negligent torts, intentional torts, and strict liability.

3. Explain the difference between a *commission* and *omission* of a negligent act.

4. Explain the difference between negligence and malpractice.

5. What are the elements that must be proven in order to be successful in a negligence suit? Illustrate your answer with a case. (The facts of the case can be hypothetical.)

6. Describe the categories of intentional torts.

7. How does slander differ from libel? Give an example of each.

8. Describe the objectives of criminal law.

9. Describe the difference between a misdemeanor and a felony. Give an example of each.

10. Discuss why physicians have been so reluctant to remove a patient's life-support systems.

11. Describe a scheme to defraud.

12. Explain the elements of a contract.

13. Describe why exclusive contracts are so controversial.

14. Describe the trial process, including pretrial motions and the functions of the judge, jury, and attorneys.

15. Describe the kinds of evidence that a plaintiff can present in order to establish a negligent act.

16. What defenses can a defendant present in order to refute a plaintiff's evidence?

17. Describe how statutes of limitations favor defendants in a lawsuit.

18. Describe the various types of damages that can be awarded a plaintiff.

19. Explain why either the plaintiff or defendant may wish to appeal a jury's verdict.

NOTES

1. 498 So. 2d 713 (La. Ct. App. 1986).
2. 787 S.W.2d 494 (Tex. Ct. App. 1990).
3. 498 So. 2d 713 (La. Ct. App. 1986).
4. 498 So. 2d 713 (La. Ct. App. 1986).
5. *Clark v. Wagoner*, 452 S.W.2d 437, 440 (Tex. 1970).
6. 57A Am. Jur.2d Torts § 134 (1989).
7. 116 Cal. Rptr. 733 (Cal. Ct. App. 1974).
8. 385 N.W.2d 99 (N.D. 1986).
9. *Tomcik v. Ohio Dep't of Rehabilitation & Correction*, 598 N.E.2d 900 (Ohio Ct. App. 1991).
10. *Id.* at 904.
11. *Id.*

12. 295 U.S. 78, 88 (1935).

13. J. Kaplan, *Criminal Justice Introductory Cases and Materials* 228 (1973).

14. *Id.* at 259.

15. http://www.osc.state.ny.us/localgov/pubs/red_flags_fraud.pdf.

16. http://www.fbi.gov/about-us/investigate/white_collar/health-care-fraud/.

17. *Id.*

18. *Id.*

19. *U.S. Department of Health and Human Services*, News Release, *February 17, 2011.*

20. *Id.*

21. *Attorney General Eric Holder*, Attorney General Eric Holder Delivers Remarks at the Johnson and Johnson Press Conference, The United States Department of Justice, *November 4, 2013.* http://www.justice.gov/iso/opa/ag/speeches/2013/ag-speech-131104.html.

22. New York State Unified Court System, "Scheme to Defraud in the Second Degree," http:// www.nycourts.gov/cji/2-PenalLaw/190/190.60.pdf.

23. Thomas Catan, *Con Artist Starred in Sting That Cost Google Millions, The Wall Street Journal,* January 25, 2012. http://online.wsj.com/news/articles/SB10001424052970204624204577176964003660658.

24. Huge Medical Insurance Scam Alleged, ABC News, *March 18*; http://abcnews.go.com/Primetime/story?id=131894&page=1#.TswWoWB-Tbp.

25. *USA Today*, November 30, 2004, at 3A.

26. *USA Today*, November 29, 2004, at 3A.

27. http://www.cbsnews.com/stories/2004/08/13/60minutes/main635860.shtml.

28. Charles Montaldo, "Profile of serial killer Richard Angelo," About.com; http://crime.about.com/od/serial/a/richardangelo.htm.

29. Collwell, *The Verdict of Angelo*, 50(103) *Newsday* 1989, at 3.

30. 683 P.2d 1202 (Colo. 1984).

31. 184 S.W.3d 122 (Mo. App. 2006).

32. Alan Cooper, "Virginia court rules identity theft victim to get $532,000 from credit agency," CBS Interactive Business Network Resource Library.

33. http://www.collegian.psu.edu/archives/article_a90522a0-e00a-57bc-9c67-2eb64b1018ba.html.

34. HospitalHealthcare.com, "NHS hospital theft costs millions," June 6, 2008; http:// www.hospitalhealthcare.com/default.asp?page=article.display&title=NHShospital theftscostmillions&article.id=11504.

35. Anne Zieger, "Millions of patient billing records stolen from UT hospital," FierceHealthIT, June 14, 2008; http://www.fiercehealthit.com/story/millions-patient-billing-records-stolen-uthospital/2008-06-14-0.

36. Tim Eberly, "Grady Hospital battles patient thefts," *Atlanta Journal-Constitution,* July 24, 2008.

37. 492 N.Y.S.2d 9 (N.Y. 1985).

38. *City of Cookeville*, No. M2001-00695-SC-R11-CV (Tenn. 2004).

39. 7 S.W.3d 542 (Mo. App. 1999).

40. http://www.njlawjournal.com/id=1202629427960&Mother_With_Terminal_Cancer_Can_Retain_Child_Custody_Judge_Holds.

41. No. 537-907 (Wis. Cir. Ct. Mar. 18, 1983).

42. 411 So. 2d 109, 113 (Ala. 1982).

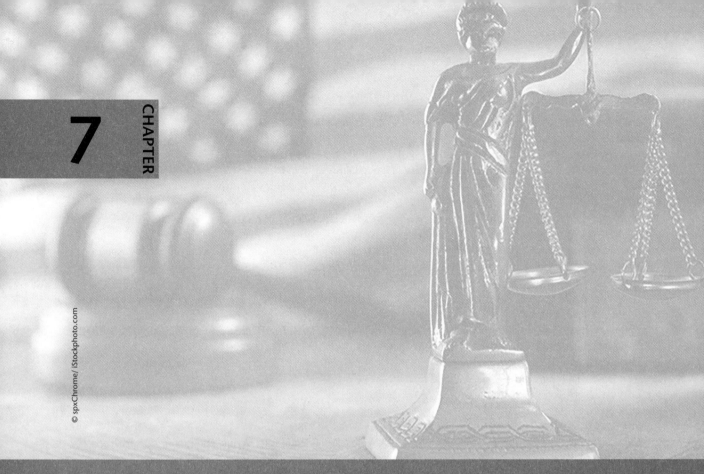

GOVERNMENT ETHICS AND THE LAW

Nothing is politically right which is morally wrong.

–DANIEL O'CONNELL (1775–1847)[1]

LEARNING OBJECTIVES

Upon completion of this chapter, the reader will be able to:

- Describe some of the reasons why there has been a loss of trust in government.
- Explain the purpose of various government committees on ethics.
- Discuss how public policy protects the rights of citizens.
- Describe federal laws designed to protect each individual's rights.
- Explain the concept of political malpractice.
- Understand the importance of ethics in public service.

INTRODUCTION

Let every American, every lover of liberty, every well wisher to his posterity, swear by the blood of the Revolution, never to violate in the least particular, the laws of the country; and never to tolerate their violation by others. As the patriots of seventy-six did to the support of the Declaration of Independence, so to the support of the Constitution and Laws, let every American pledge his life, his property, and his sacred honor—let every man remember that to violate the law, is to trample on the blood of his father, and to tear the character of his own, and his children's liberty. Let reverence for the laws, be breathed by every American mother, to the lisping babe, that prattles on her lap—let it be taught in schools, in seminaries, and in colleges; let it be written in Primers, spelling books, and in Almanacs—let it be preached from the pulpit, proclaimed in legislative halls, and enforced in courts of justice. And, in short, let it become the political religion of the nation; and let the old and the young, the rich and the poor, the grave and the gay, of all sexes and tongues, and colors and conditions, sacrifice unceasingly upon its altars.[2]

−ABRAHAM LINCOLN

The words of Abraham Lincoln, so passionately spoken, resonate true today. Political corruption, antisocial behavior, declining civility, Veterans Administration hospitals misrepresenting wait times for veterans to get doctors' appointments, and rampant unethical conduct have heightened discussions over the nation's moral decline and decaying value systems. The numerous instances of questionable political decisions, executives with shocking salaries, dishonesty at work and school, sexually explicit websites, and the entertainment media have contributed to this decline. Legislators, investigators, prosecutors, and the courts have been quick to speak moral truths but continue to be slow in action. Can this boat be turned around, or are we just plugging the holes with new laws and creating more leaks in a misguided sinking ship?

The question remains: Can the decline in ethical behavior be reversed as citizens struggle with a broken legal system inundated with new laws? The answer is more likely to be a return to practicing the virtues and values upon which this nation was founded. Ethics and the law are not mutually exclusive—they are intertwined throughout the text, providing an overview of government agencies designed to protect each individual's rights (e.g., the right to privacy and self-determination).

U.S. OFFICE OF GOVERNMENT ETHICS

The *Office of Government Ethics* (OGE) is an agency within the executive branch of government whose mission and goals is to foster high ethical standards for employees in the executive branch of government. Common ethical issues that come under the committee's purview include gifts from outside sources, gifts between employees, conflicting financial interests, remedies for financial conflicts of interest, impartiality in performing official duties, seeking other employment, misuse of position, outside activities, postemployment, representation to government agencies and courts, supplementation of salary, financial disclosure, informal advisory letters and memoranda and formal opinions, DAEOgrams (memoranda to Designated Agency Ethics Officials providing guidance on how to interpret and comply with modifications or new issuances of ethics laws, policies, and procedures; copies of the memoranda released since 1992 are available in the DAEOgrams section of the OGE website), and contractors in the workplace.[3]

HOUSE OF REPRESENTATIVES COMMITTEE ON ETHICS

I weep for the liberty of my country when I see at this early day of its successful experiment that corruption has been imputed to many members of the House of Representatives, and the rights of the people have been bartered for promises of office.

—ANDREW JACKSON

The Committee on Ethics is designated the "supervising ethics office" for the House of Representatives. The jurisdiction of the Committee on Ethics is derived from authority granted under House Rules and federal statutes.

> The Committee on Ethics is unique in the House of Representatives. Consistent with the duty to carry out its advisory and enforcement responsibilities in an impartial manner, the Committee is the only standing committee of the House of Representatives with its membership divided evenly by party. These rules are intended to provide a fair procedural framework for the conduct of the Committee's activities and to help ensure that the Committee serves the people of the United States, the House of Representatives, and the Members, officers, and employees of the House of Representatives.[4]

The scope of the committee's jurisdiction under the various authorizing rules and statutes involves duties and responsibilities related to:

- Jurisdiction over all bills, resolutions, and other matters relating to the Code of Official Conduct.
- Recommendations of administrative actions to establish or enforce standards of official conduct.
- Investigation of alleged violations of the Code of Official Conduct or of any applicable rules, laws, or regulations governing the performance of official duties or the discharge of official responsibilities.
- Reports to appropriate federal or state authorities substantial evidence of a violation of any law applicable to the performance of official duties that may have been disclosed in a committee investigation.
- Consideration of requests for written waivers of the gift rule.
- Oversight over foreign gifts and gifts to superiors and other federal employees.
- Prohibition of members, officers, and employees of the House of Representatives from soliciting or receiving gifts.[5]

SENATE SELECT COMMITTEE ON ETHICS

(a) The ideal concept of public office, expressed by the words, "a public office is a public trust," signifies that the officer has been entrusted with public power by the people; that the officer holds this power in trust to be used only for their benefit and never for the benefit of himself or of a few; and that the officer must never conduct his own affairs so as to infringe on the public interest. All official conduct of Members of the Senate should be guided by this paramount concept of public office.[6]

The U.S. Senate Select Committee on Ethics consists of six members of the Senate, of whom three shall be selected from members of the majority party and three shall be selected from members of the minority party.[7] The committee is responsible for investigating complaints involving a violation of the Franking statute, Financial Disclosure Statements and for Outside Employment with respect to members, officers, and employees of the Senate, foreign gifts and decorations, gifts to an official superior or receiving gifts from employees with a lower salary level, prohibitions against members, officers, and employees of the Senate soliciting or receiving gifts.[8]

The Senate Select Committee on Ethics is authorized to receive and investigate allegations of improper conduct which may reflect upon the Senate, violations of law, violations of the Senate Code of Official Conduct, and violations of rules and regulations of the Senate; recommend disciplinary action; recommend additional Senate rules or regulations to insure proper standards of conduct; and report violations of law to the proper federal and state authorities.[9]

OFFICE OF CONGRESSIONAL ETHICS

The Office of Congressional Ethics (OCE) was created in March 2008 as an independent, nonpartisan office governed by a board composed of private citizens that provides more public review and insight into the ethical conduct of members of the House of Representatives. The OCE reviews allegations of misconduct against members, officers, and staff of the House and, when appropriate, refers matters to the House Committee on Ethics. The OCE is not authorized to determine if a violation occurred nor it is it authorized to sanction members, officers, or employees of the House or to recommend sanctions. The OCE is not able to provide advice or education on the rules and standards of conduct applicable to members, officers, and employees of the House.[10] The mission of the OCE and its board is to assist the House in upholding high standards of ethical conduct for its members, officers, and staff and, in so doing, to serve the American people. The board of directors consists of eight members, which are private citizens and cannot serve as members of Congress or work for the federal government.[11] As the reader will note, there are a variety of laws and agencies that provide oversight and regulations that are designed to protect the right and safety of all citizens. Government is a reflection of the people it serves. Failure of the many to participate in the political process leads to government for the few who do.

U.S. JUDICIAL CODE OF CONDUCT

As with other branches of government federal judges are expected to abide by a code of conduct that includes ethical principles and guidelines. "The Code of Conduct provides guidance for judges on issues of judicial integrity and independence, judicial diligence and impartiality, permissible extra-judicial activities, and the avoidance of impropriety or even its appearance."[12]

PUBLIC POLICY

Public policy is the principle of law that holds that no one can lawfully do that which tends to be injurious to the public or against the public good. The sources of public policy "include legislation; administrative rules, regulations, or decisions; and judicial decisions. In certain instances, a professional code of ethics may contain an expression of public policy."[13]

Ethics and the law are not mutually exclusive—they are intertwined. Without the two, we would become a lawless land. The following pages present an overview of laws, influenced by ethical principles, designed to protect each individual's rights (e.g., the right to privacy and self-determination).

VETERANS ADMINISTRATION

The House Committee on Veterans' Affairs reviews veteran programs, examines current laws, and reports bills and amendments to strengthen existing laws concerning veterans and the Department of Veterans Affairs (VA), such as health care and disability compensation. Jeff Miller (R-FL) chairs the committee.[14] The news clippings below describe a variety of concerns with care veterans are receiving in Veterans Hospitals. Although there is undoubtedly excellent care in the VA system, there is a need to improve the care for every veteran, as noted by committee chairman Jeff Miller:

> A pattern of heartbreaking veteran deaths, suicides and a host of other patient safety issues have cast a dark shadow over VA medical centers around the country. For months we have tried in vain to compel VA leaders to take meaningful steps to prevent future adverse incidents by holding accountable VA employees and managers responsible for letting patients fall through the cracks. Unfortunately, department officials seem more intent on issuing bureaucratic slaps on the wrist than the sort of serious punishments required to send a message that substandard care for veterans will not be tolerated. What's more, patient deaths apparently aren't even enough to prevent failing VA executives from receiving huge performance bonuses and glowing performance reviews. Because these issues are long-standing, systemic, and evidently immune to the current structure of accountability within VA, I believe President Obama's direct involvement and leadership is required to help us end the culture of complacency that is engulfing the Veterans Health Administration and compromising patient safety." [15]

With growing concerns that certain VA hospitals have been misrepresenting wait times for veterans to schedule medical appointments, Veterans Affairs Secretary Eric Shinseki, under increasing pressure by Congress, resigned his position. President Obama nominated Robert A. McDonald for the position, which was confirmed by Congress on July 29, 2014.[16]

VA, Heal Thyself, Agency is Told at Hearing Filled with Pained Testimony

The House Committee on Veteran's Affairs met in Pittsburgh on Monday to hear testimony about problems with health care at agency facilities in that city and others.

• • •

Miller said the "the vast majority of the departments more than 300,000 employees are dedicated and hard-working, and many veterans are satisfied with the medical care they received from the VA."

But he and others sharply doubted the ability of the department's leadership to avoid "heartbreaking situations" like those reported to the committee.

"By now," he said, "It's abundantly clear to most people that a culture change at VA is in order."

Joe Davidson, The Washington Post, *September 13, 2013*

Atlanta VA Exec Scored Bonuses While Audits Found Lapses

The former top administrator at the Atlanta VA Medical Center received $65,000 in performance bonuses over a four-year span as internal audits revealed lengthy wait times for mental health care and mismanagement that led to three deaths.

Daniel Malloy, The Atlanta Journal – Constitution, *April 26, 2013*

"Too trapped in a war to be at peace"

Shortly before his death on June 10, Army veteran Daniel Somers wrote a note for his family, asking his wife, Angel, to share it as she saw fit.

"I am left with basically nothing," he typed on his laptop at their Phoenix townhouse. "Too trapped in a war to be at peace, too damaged to be at war."

His service in Iraq, including multiple combat missions as a turret gunner, left him with severe post–traumatic stress disorder and traumatic brain injury. But the government, he wrote, had "turned around and abandoned me."

Steve Vogel, The Washington Post, *August 24, 2013*

Daniel Somers eventually saw a caregiver. Unfortunately for Daniel, the caregiver retired. He attempted to make a new appointment. That is when he ran into the all too common roadblock, being told that there was a shortage of caregivers and that he would be notified when he could be scheduled for his next appointment.

The following *reality check* is believed by some to be an all too common experience by inspectors of not only VA hospitals but many hospitals across the country.

VA Hospital

And so there we were in a VA hospital, sent to survey the quality of patient care services provided to veterans. During the survey, there seemed to be a lack of interest in constructive suggestions as to how the hospital could improve services. Survey team members who wrote negative findings had been watched closely as though they were the ones being surveyed throughout the process. The real concern of management seemed to be more how the surveyors would score the hospital's delivery of care to veterans, then how they could improve services. They seemed pleasant when things were going well, argumentative when they were not. The surveyors were between a rock and a hard place. Not only do the surveyors score the hospital, the hospital scores the surveyors as required by the surveyors' employer. Down score the hospital and the inspectors could often expect to be down scored. The problem comes down to the integrity of the surveyor and the hospital. If a hospital views a survey as an opportunity to learn and improve patient care services, it is likely that it can be a win-win situation for both the surveyors and the hospital, ultimately benefiting the patient.

Anonymous

The next *reality check* illustrates how the majority of veterans standing outside a major VA hospital waiting for the clinics to open viewed their care. As I approached them and inquired about their care, it was reassuring that these veterans were extremely positive as to the care they were receiving.

Veterans Lack Insurance Benefits

Marc had a chat with some veterans about their health care benefits. Most seemed satisfied. Joe, one of the veterans, opening his mouth wide to show me, said, "Look at my teeth. [He had but a few teeth in his mouth.] They won't fix them because they are not considered a war-related injury." He turned his head sideways, and Marc noticed that an ear was missing. Joe continued, "Now this ear is gone. I lost it during the Viet Nam war. I was, however, able to get a prosthesis. It needs some work, so I didn't wear it. I guess they will provide me with a new one. I am able to get care for it because it is a war-related injury, but I really could use some teeth."

Marc queried the hospital about Joe's teeth. They said that because of policy and the fact that Joe's teeth were not related to a war injury, there was nothing that they could do for him. They did however suggest Joe could go to the University Hospital and get a set of false teeth that should be relatively inexpensive. Marc asked to see the hospital's dental area. Following a tour of the dental suite, Marc commented, "This is the most modern dental facility I have ever seen." The staff was happy that Marc was pleased with the facility. After observing ample staff, workspace, modern equipment, top of the line dental chairs, and unoccupied rooms, he asked, "Are you open? Where are the patients?" The staff in unison responded, "Oh yes, we are open but we don't have any patients at the moment. We should have a few later." The staff proceeded to discuss with enthusiasm the wide variety of dental procedures they could provide, including complicated extractions, implants, preparation of dentures, and so on.

Discussion

1. Would you consider this to be a form of political malpractice? Discuss your answer.
2. Because hospital staff was able to make suggestions to a veteran for care outside the Veterans Administration health care system, how would you respond if you were the veteran?

FOURTEENTH AMENDMENT TO THE CONSTITUTION

According to the Fourteenth Amendment to the Constitution, a state cannot act to deny any person equal protection of the laws. If a state or a political subdivision of a state, whether through its executive, judicial, or legislative branch, acts in such a way as to deny unfairly to any person the rights accorded to another, the amendment has been violated.

Section 1. All persons born or naturalized in the United States, and subject to the jurisdiction thereof, are citizens of the United States and of the state wherein they reside. No State shall make or enforce any law, which shall abridge the privileges or immunities of citizens of the United States; nor shall any State deprive any person of life, liberty, or property, without due process of law; nor deny to any person within its jurisdiction the equal protection of the laws

Section 5. The Congress shall have power to enforce, by appropriate legislation, the provisions of this article.

TITLE VI: CIVIL RIGHTS ACT

Civil rights are those rights ensured by the U.S. Constitution and by the acts of Congress and the state legislatures. Generally, the term includes all the rights of each individual in a free society.

Congress and the federal courts have dealt with discriminatory practices in health care organizations. Discrimination in the admission of patients and segregation of patients on racial grounds are prohibited in any organization receiving federal financial assistance. Pursuant to Title VI of the *Civil Rights Act* of 1964, the guidelines of the Department of Health and

Human Services (HHS) prohibit the practice of racial discrimination by any organization or agency receiving money under any program supported by HHS. This includes all "providers of service" receiving federal funds under Medicare legislation.

SHERMAN ANTITRUST ACT

The *Sherman Antitrust Act*, named for its author, Senator John Sherman of Ohio, prescribes that every contract, combination in the form of trust or otherwise, or conspiracy in restraint of trade or commerce among the several states is declared to be illegal. Those who attempt to monopolize, combine, or conspire with any other person or persons to monopolize any part of the trade or commerce can be deemed guilty of a felony.[17] Areas of concern for health care organizations include reduced market competition, price fixing, actions that bar or limit new entrants to the field, preferred provider arrangements, and exclusive contracts.

A health care organization must be cognizant of the potential problems that may exist when limiting the number of physicians that it will admit to its medical staff. Because closed staff determinations can effectively limit competition from other physicians, the governing body must ensure that the decision-making process in granting privileges is based on legislative, objective criteria and is not dominated by those who have the most to gain competitively by denying privileges. Physicians have attempted to use state and federal antitrust laws to challenge determinations denying or limiting medical staff privileges. Generally, these actions claim that the organization conspired with its medical staff to ensure that the complaining physician would not obtain privileges in order to reduce competition.

PRIVACY ACT

The *Privacy Act of 1974*, Title 5 United States Code (U.S.C.) 552, was enacted to safeguard individual privacy from the misuse of federal records, to give individuals access to records concerning themselves that are maintained by federal agencies, and to establish a Privacy Protection Safety Commission. Section 2 of the Privacy Act reads as follows:

> [a] The Congress finds that (1) the privacy of an individual is directly affected by the collection, maintenance, use, and dissemination of personal information by Federal agencies; (2) the increasing use of computers and sophisticated information technology, while essential to the efficient operations of the Government, has greatly magnified the harm to individual privacy that can occur from any collection, maintenance, use, or dissemination of personal information; (3) the opportunities for an individual to secure employment, insurance, and credit, and his right to due process, and other legal protections are endangered by the misuse of certain information systems; (4) the right to privacy is a personal and fundamental right protected by the Constitution of the United States; and (5) in order to protect the privacy of individuals identified in information systems maintained by Federal agencies, it is necessary and proper for the Congress to regulate the collection, maintenance, use, and dissemination of information by such agencies. [b] The purpose of this Act is to provide certain safeguards for an individual against an invasion of personal privacy by requiring Federal agencies, except as otherwise provided by law, to (1) permit an individual to determine what records pertaining to him are collected, maintained, used, or disseminated by such agencies; (2) permit an individual to prevent records pertaining to him

obtained by such agencies for a particular purpose from being used or made available for another purpose without his consent; (3) permit an individual to gain access to information pertaining to him in Federal agency records, to have a copy made of all or any portion thereof, and to correct or amend such records; (4) collect, maintain, use, or disseminate any record of identifiable personal information in a manner that assures that such action is for a necessary and lawful purpose, that the information is current and accurate for its intended use, and that adequate safeguards are provided to prevent misuse of such information . . .

HEALTH INSURANCE PORTABILITY AND ACCOUNTABILITY ACT (HIPAA)

The *Health Insurance Portability and Accountability Act* (HIPAA) of 1996 (Public Law 104–191) was designed to protect the privacy, confidentiality, and security of patient information. HIPAA standards are applicable to all health information in all of its formats (e.g., electronic, paper, verbal). It applies to both electronically maintained and transmitted information. HIPAA privacy standards include restrictions on access to individually identifiable health information and the use and disclosure of that information, as well as requirements for administrative activities such as training, compliance, and enforcement of HIPAA mandates.

EMERGENCY MEDICAL TREATMENT AND ACTIVE LABOR ACT (EMTALA)

In 1986, Congress passed the *Emergency Medical Treatment and Active Labor Act* (EMTALA), which forbids Medicare-participating hospitals from "dumping" patients out of emergency departments. The act provides that:

In the case of a hospital that has a hospital emergency department, if any individual (whether or not eligible for benefits under this subchapter) comes to the emergency department and a request is made on the individual's behalf for examination or treatment for a medical condition, the hospital must provide for an appropriate medical screening examination within the capability of the hospital emergency department, including ancillary services routinely available to the emergency department, to determine whether or not an emergency medical condition . . . exists.[18]

EMTALA was clearly violated in the *Burditt* case reviewed next.

CASE: EMTALA VIOLATED

In *Burditt v. U.S. Department of Health and Human Services*,[19] EMTALA was violated by a physician when he ordered a woman with dangerously high blood pressure (210/130) and in active labor with ruptured membranes transferred from the emergency department of one hospital to another hospital 170 miles away. The physician was assessed a penalty of $20,000. Dr. Louis Sullivan, secretary of HHS at that time, issued a statement: "This decision sends a message to physicians everywhere that they need to provide quality care to everyone in need of emergency treatment who comes to a hospital. This is a significant opinion and we are pleased with the result."[20] The American Public Health Association, in filing an amicus curiae brief, advised the appeals court that "if Burditt wants to ensure that he will never be asked to treat a patient not of his choosing, then he ought to vote with his feet by affiliating only with hospitals that do not accept Medicare funds or do not have an emergency department."[21]

Ethical and Legal Issues

1. What are the main issues in this case?
2. What ethical theories, principles, and values are of concern? Describe them.
3. What action can be taken to prevent similar occurrences in the future?
4. What could have been done to prevent the ethical and legal issues from occurring in the first place?
5. If you were the judge in this case, what would you do in light of the American Public Health Association's comments?
6. Describe both the hospital and physician's ethical and legal responsibilities.

HEALTH CARE QUALITY IMPROVEMENT ACT

The *Health Care Quality Improvement Act* of 1986 (HCQIA) was enacted in part to provide those persons giving information to professional review bodies and those assisting in review activities limited immunity from damages that may arise as a result of adverse decisions that affect a physician's medical staff privileges. Before enacting the HCQIA, Congress found that "[t]he increasing occurrence of medical malpractice and the need to improve the quality of medical care . . . [had] become nationwide problems," especially in light of "the ability of incompetent physicians to move from State to State without disclosure or discovery of the physician's previous damaging or incompetent performance" (42 U.S.C. § 11101). The problem, however, could be remedied through effective professional peer review combined with a national reporting system that made information about adverse professional actions against physicians more widely available. HCQIA was enacted by Congress to "facilitate the frank exchange of information among professionals conducting peer review inquiries without the fear of reprisals in civil lawsuits. The statute attempts to balance the chilling effect of litigation on peer review with concerns for protecting physicians improperly subjected to disciplinary action."

CASE: FAILURE TO MEET ETHICAL STANDARDS

Meyers applied for medical staff privileges at a hospital. Shortly thereafter, the Credentials Committee and the Medical Executive Committee (MEC) and the board of the hospital approved Meyers for appointment to the medical staff. All initial appointments to the medical staff were provisional for 1 year. At the end of that year, the physician was required to be reevaluated for advancement from associate to active staff.

The Credentials Committee began to evaluate Meyers for advancement to active staff privileges. The committee was concerned about Meyers's history: moving from hospital to hospital after disputes with hospital staff, his failure to disclose timely and fully disciplinary and corrective action taken against him in another state, and the quality of his patient care. The MEC voted to accept a Credentials Committee recommendation to revoke Meyers's staff privileges. The MEC was to consider the recommendation from the Credentials Committee and make a recommendation to the board, which had the ultimate authority to grant or deny advancement, or terminate Meyers's privileges.

The board informed Meyers that it was assuming responsibility for determining his reappointment and advancement to active staff because of concerns with the manner in which the peer review process was being handled. Three members of the board, acting as a Credentials Committee, conducted an independent review. This committee discussed concerns about Meyers's behavior and his inability to get along with others, in addition to questions about his surgical technique. The committee questioned Meyers about several incident reports concerning disruptive behavior, his history of problems at other hospitals, his failure to complete medical records timely, his hostility toward the operation room staff, reports of breaking the sterile field, and his failure to provide appropriate coverage for patients while he was away. Meyers acknowledged that he had a personality problem.

The three-member committee of the board voted to deny Meyers's appointment to active staff. The reasons cited for the committee's decision were Meyers's failure to satisfy requirements that he "abide by the ethics of the profession," work cooperatively with others, timely complete medical records, and abide by hospital standards. The committee outlined Meyers's pattern of rude, abusive, and disruptive behavior that included, but was not limited to, temper tantrums, attempted interference with the right of an attending physician to refer a patient to the surgeon of his choice or to transfer the patient, condescending remarks toward women, refusal to speak to a member of his surgical team during surgical procedures, and several instances of throwing a scalpel during surgery. The committee informed Meyers that this behavior could have an adverse effect on the quality of patient care. As for his failure to complete medical records timely, the committee stated "delinquent medical records can put patients at risk by being inaccurate or incomplete if needed to assist in later diagnosis and treatment of a patient."

A Fair Hearing Committee issued its recommendation that Meyers not be reappointed to the hospital's staff because of his failure to meet "ethical standards" and his inability to work cooperatively with others. In May, the board adopted and affirmed the Fair Hearing Committee's recommendation. Ultimately, after further appeals the board revoked Meyers's privileges.

Meyers brought suit in seeking a permanent injunction to require the hospital to reinstate him to staff. The court denied the motion for an injunction that would require the hospital to reinstate Meyers's privileges.

The court agreed with hospital defendants that the behavior of Meyers had the potential of affecting the health and welfare of patients, despite the fact that no patients were actually injured. High-quality patient care demands that doctors possess at least a reasonable ability to work with others. Clearly, the hospital defendants were acting with a reasonable belief that the professional review action was in the furtherance of quality health care. They were concerned that Meyers's behavior would continue until a patient was injured as a result of his actions.[22]

Ethical and Legal Issues

1. Describe the ethical theories, principles, and values of concern in this case.
2. Describe what steps the organization could take to prevent similar occurrences in the future.

Agency for Healthcare Research and Quality

The *Agency for Healthcare Research and Quality* (AHRQ), established in 1989, is charged with researching ways to improve the quality of health care, reduce its costs, and broaden access to essential services. The AHRQ was created as a result of the mistakes that have occurred and continue to occur in the delivery of care. The pain, misery, and financial drain on the injured, their families, and society have taken its toll. The numerous ethical and legal issues that have evolved spawned the need for the AHRQ.

Ethics in Patient Referral Act

In 1989, the *Ethics in Patient Referral Act* was enacted, prohibiting physicians who have ownership interest or compensation arrangements with a clinical laboratory from referring Medicare patients to that laboratory. The law also requires all Medicare providers to report the names and provider numbers of all physicians or their immediate relatives with ownership interests in the provider entity prior to October 1, 1991.

Patient Self-Determination Act

The *Patient Self-Determination Act* of 1990 (PSDA)[23] was enacted to ensure that patients are informed of their rights to execute advance directives and accept or refuse medical care. On December 1, 1991, the PSDA[24] took effect in hospitals, skilled nursing facilities, home health agencies, hospice organizations, and health maintenance organizations serving Medicare and Medicaid patients. As a result of implementation of the PSDA,[25] health care organizations participating in the Medicare and Medicaid reimbursement programs must address patient rights regarding life-sustaining decisions and other advance directives. Health care organizations have a responsibility to explain to patients, staff, and families that patients have a legal right to direct their own medical and nursing care as it corresponds to existing state law, including right-to-die directives. A person's right to refuse medical treatment is not lost when his or her mental or physical status changes. When a person is no longer competent to exercise his or her right of self-determination, the right still exists, but the decision must be delegated to a surrogate decision maker. Those organizations that do not comply with a patient's medical directives or those of a legally authorized decision maker are exposing themselves to the risk of a lawsuit.

Each state is required under the PSDA to provide a description of the law in the state regarding advance directives to providers, whether such directives are based on state statutes or judicial decisions. Providers must ensure that written policies and procedures with respect to all adult individuals regarding advance directives are established as follows:[26]

(A) to provide written information to each such individual concerning

(i) an individual's rights under State law (whether statutory or as recognized by the courts of the State) to make decisions concerning such medical care, including the right to accept or refuse medical or surgical treatment and the right to formulate advance directives . . . and

(ii) written policies of the provider organization respecting the implementation of such rights;

(B) to document in the individual's medical record whether or not the individual has executed an advance directive;

(C) not to condition the provision of care or otherwise discriminate against an individual based on whether or not the individual has executed an advance directive;

(D) to ensure compliance with requirements of State law (whether statutory or recognized by the courts of the State) respecting advance directives at the facilities of the provider or organization; and

(E) to provide (individually or with others) for education for staff and the community on issues concerning advance directives.

Although the PSDA is being cheered as a major advancement in clarifying and nationally regulating this often obscure area of law and medicine, there are continuing problems and new issues that must be addressed.

SARBANES-OXLEY ACT

The sense of somehow me beating up on Wall Street, I think most folks on Main Street feel like they got beat up on. . . . There's a big chunk of the country that thinks that I have been too soft on Wall Street. That's probably the majority, not the minority.

If you're making a billion dollars a year after a very bad financial crisis where eight million people lost their jobs and small businesses can't get loans, then I think that you shouldn't be feeling put upon.

The notion that somehow me saying maybe you should be taxed more like your secretary when you're pulling home a billion dollars or a hundred million dollars a year, I don't think is me being extremist or being anti-business.

—PRESIDENT BARACK OBAMA

The *Sarbanes-Oxley Act* was signed by President George W. Bush on July 30, 2002, in response to the Enron debacle and high-profile cases of corporate financial mismanagement. The act requires top executives of public corporations to vouch for the financial reports of their companies. The act encourages self regulation and the need to promote due diligence, select a leader with morals and core values, examine incentives, constantly monitor the organization's culture, build a strong, knowledgeable governing body, be on the alert for conflicts of interest, focus attention on the right things, and have the courage to speak out.

PATIENT PROTECTION AND AFFORDABLE CARE ACT (2010)

The *Patient Protection and Affordable Care Act* (PPACA) is a federal statute that contains a set of health care reforms passed by Congress and signed into law by President Barack Obama on March 23, 2010. After several challenges as to the constitutionally of the PPACA, the United States Supreme Court determined in 2012 that the PPACA was constitutional.

The PPACA was designed to expand medical insurance coverage to Americans that did not already have it by offering affordable and competitive rates through a newly created Health Insurance Marketplace, providing subsidies to individuals based on ability to pay.

The law was set to bring insurance coverage to over 30 million Americans who never had coverage. The PPACA includes provisions for reform of the private health insurance market, providing better coverage for people with preexisting conditions, improving prescription drug coverage in Medicare, and extending the life of the Medicare trust fund by at least 12 years.

The website www.healthcare.gov has been set up to assist those who wish to purchase health insurance. The website has been fraught with problems in connecting and signing up for insurance. Glitches in the system should come as no surprise with such a far-reaching program considering a population of over 317 million. As with a wedding of 300 people, there are glitches and often times a lot of angry people who were invited to the church but not the reception, food was cold, the wedding was on an island in the South Pacific, you preferred to sit at a different table then the one you were assigned, you were placed to far away from the bride and groom's table, you were forgotten when the family picture was taken, and yet you were the grandparents, etc. In the end there is a happily married couple. The plan for the PPACA is to provide a more affordable and accessible health care system. Unfortunately, the political battles over the PPACA continue to disrupt the democratic process.

Congress continues to make decisions on a bipartisan basis, often, seemingly, without regard to the needs of the people. There are those who consider health care a right and others who consider it a privilege. Many believe, for Congress, it seems, health care is a right, as noted by their superior health insurance plans at reduced costs due to lucrative subsidized health insurance premiums paid by the people. The costs associated with PPACA are without question fraught with numerous ethical dilemmas. Responsibility for reducing the costs associated with PPACA lies in part with each individual and their chosen style of life, which includes the abuse of addictive substances.

POLITICAL MALPRACTICE

I hate all the bungling as I do sin, but particularly bungling in politics, which leads to the misery and ruin of many thousands and millions of people.

—JOHANN WOLFGANG VON GOETHE

Political malpractice is negligent conduct by an elected or appointed political official. Ronald Brownstein wrote in a news column in the *St. Petersburg Times*, "Practical steps are possible to help millions of low income families live healthier lives and receive more effective care when they need it. Ignoring that opportunity, while waiting for consensus on coverage, would be a form of political malpractice."[27]

The likelihood of a successful negligence case against a member of Congress is doubtful. If such a case ever got through a courtroom door the following four elements of negligence would have to be proven:

1. The first element necessary to prove political malpractice requires that the plaintiff/s be able to establish there is *a duty to care*. Establishing this first element of negligence for a senator, for example, would be a difficult hurdle to jump. The oath of office for a senator is so amorphous that it would be difficult to establish a duty to care, as illustrated in the following quotes.

Oath of Office

I do solemnly swear (or affirm) that I will support and defend the Constitution of the United States against all enemies, foreign and domestic; that I will bear true faith and allegiance to the same; that I take this obligation freely, without any mental reservation or purpose of evasion; and that I will well and faithfully discharge the duties of the office on which I am about to enter: So help me God.[28]

Looking beyond the oath of office:

For nearly three-quarters of a century, that oath served nicely, although to the modern ear it sounds woefully incomplete. Missing are the soaring references to bearing "true faith and allegiance"; to taking "this obligation freely, without any mental reservation or purpose of evasion"; and to "well and faithfully" discharging the duties of the office.[29]

Should a plaintiff be able to overcome this first element of negligence, thus proving a duty to care, the remaining elements could be just as difficult to establish.

2. The second element of political malpractice requires the plaintiff to prove that the *duty to care was breached*. Arguably, politicians, for example, who agree to veto any program the President supports while he is in office is contrary to the spirit of the law. The dilemma here requires the plaintiff/s to prove what specific duty to care was breached.
3. The third element of political malpractice requires proof of harm.
4. The fourth element requires proof of a *causal connection* between the politician's breach of duty and harm suffered. In other words, the plaintiff/s must prove that the breach of duty was the proximate cause of the plaintiff's injury.

Like medical malpractice, political malpractice involves a failure to offer professional services to help prevent the travesties that take place daily, as illustrated by the following anonymous true story.

The Coal Miner

Jimmy was a coal miner who had black lung disease. I had introduced myself to him as the administrator. Jimmy introduced himself to me and then turned to a man who was on the opposite side of his bed and said, "This is my brother Bill." I asked, as he turned looking back at me, "Are we taking good care of you?" He said, "Yes." Bill, looking at me, choked up and asked, "Can you help my brother? He has given up the will to live. Please help my brother want to live." I looked at Jimmy lying there in his bed, fragile and struggling to breathe between each word, as he said, "I can no longer carry on this way. I am ready to move on. I'm a tired old man. I have fought so long. I've needed benefits for so many years for my family and myself. No one was able to help me. You see, I have black lung disease. I can barely breathe." He then turned, looking over to Bill, and said, "My brother also has black lung disease. We worked together in the coalmines for many years. This is our reward." I looked at Jimmy and slowly back to Bill and said, "I will help you." As we said our goodbyes, I thought to myself, as I left the room, this man has fought so long. He has asked for so little, a man forgotten by a cruel system of corrupt government and greedy corporations. I remember this day all too well. It brings tears to my eyes as I recall the sadness of that day.

Administrator

Discussion

1. Explain what action you would take to help Jimmy.
2. Describe the ethical principles that apply to this case.

CHAPTER REVIEW

1. Government Ethics Committees
   - U.S. Office of Government Ethics
     ○ Agency within the executive branch of government.
   - House of Representatives Committee on Ethics
   - Senate Select Committee on Ethics
   - Office of Congressional Ethics
   - U.S. Judicial Code of Conduct
2. Public Policy Protecting the Rights of Citizens—Principle of law that holds that no one can lawfully do that which tends to be injurious to the public or against the public good.
   - Veterans Administration
   - Fourteenth Amendment to the Constitution
     ○ A state cannot act to deny any person equal protection of the laws.
   - Title VI of the Civil Rights Act of 1964
     ○ HHS prohibits the practice of racial discrimination by any organization or agency receiving money under any program supported by HHS.
   - Sherman Antitrust Act
   - The Privacy Act of 1974, Title 5 United States Code (U.S.C.) 552
     ○ Enacted to safeguard individual privacy from the misuse of federal records.
     ○ Provide individuals access to records concerning themselves that are maintained by federal agencies.
     ○ Establish a Privacy Protection Safety Commission.
   - HIPAA (Public Law 104-191)
     ○ Designed to protect the privacy, confidentiality, and security of patient information.
     ○ HIPAA standards are applicable to all health information in all of its formats (e.g., electronic, paper, verbal). It applies to both electronically maintained and transmitted information.
   - EMTALA
     ○ Forbids Medicare-participating hospitals from "dumping" patients out of emergency departments.

- HCQIA
  - Enacted in part to provide those persons giving information to professional review bodies and those assisting in review activities limited immunity from damages that may arise as a result of adverse decisions that affect a physician's medical staff privileges.
- AHRQ
  - Charged with researching ways to improve the quality of health care, reduce its costs, and broaden access to essential services.
- Ethics in Patient Referral Act of 1989
  - Prohibits physicians who have ownership interest or compensation arrangements with a clinical laboratory from referring Medicare patients to that laboratory.
- PSDA
  - Enacted to ensure that patients are informed of their rights to execute advance directives and accept or refuse medical care. Each state is required under the PSDA to provide a description of the law in the state regarding advance directives to providers, whether such directives are based on state statutes or judicial decisions.
- Sarbanes-Oxley Act
  - Executives of public corporations to vouch for the financial reports and encourages self-regulation.
3. Political malpractice
   - Negligent or unethical conduct on the part of an elected official.

TEST YOUR UNDERSTANDING

TERMINOLOGY

Agency for Healthcare Research and Quality

Civil Rights Act

Emergency Medical Treatment and Active Labor Act

Ethics in Patient Referral Act

Health Care Quality Improvement Act

Health Insurance Portability and Accountability Act

Office of Government Ethics

Patient Protection and Affordable Care Act

Patient Self-Determination Act

political malpractice

Privacy Act of 1974

public policy

Sarbanes-Oxley Act

Sherman Antitrust Act

REVIEW QUESTIONS

1. Discuss how the various branches of government address ethical issues.

2. Discuss how public policy protects individual rights (e.g., privacy and self-determination).

3. Discuss the legal and ethical implications of the public policy acts presented here.

4. Describe how the concept of "political malpractice" is similar to "medical malpractice" as discussed in this chapter.

NOTES

1. Irish politician.
2. http://www.abrahamlincolnonline.org/lincoln/speeches/lyceum.htm.
3. http://oge.gov/About/Mission-and-Responsibilities/Mission—Responsibilities/.
4. Committee on Ethics, Committee Rules, http://ethics. house.gov/about/committee-rules.
5. Committee on Ethics, Jurisdiction, http://ethics.house.gov/jurisdiction.
6. U.S. Senate Select Committee on Ethics, Jurisdiction, http://www.ethics.senate.gov/public/index.cfm/jurisdiction.
7. U.S. Senate Select Committee on Ethics, Rules of Procedure, http://www.ethics.senate.gov/public/index.cfm/files/serve?File_id=551b39fc-30ed-4b14-b0d3-1706608a6fcb.
8. U.S. Senate Select Committee on Ethics, Jurisdiction, http://www.ethics.senate.gov/public/index.cfm/jurisdiction.
9. *Id.*
10. Office of Congressional Ethics, Frequently Asked Questions, http://oce.house.gov/faq.html.
11. *Id.*
12. http://www.uscourts.gov/RulesAndPolicies/CodesOfConduct.aspx.
13. *Pierce v. Ortho Pharmaceutical Corp.*, 417 A.2d 505, 512 (N.J. 1980).
14. http://veterans.house.gov/about.
15. Rep. Jeff Miller, Chairman, House Committee on Veterans Affairs, *July 11, 2013* http://veterans.house.gov/press-release/miller-president-obama-must-help-stop-patient-deaths-bring-accountability-to-va.
16. http://www.va.gov/opa/bios/secretary.asp.
17. 15 U.S.C. § 1 (1982).
18. 42 U.S.C.A. § 1395dd(a) (1992).
19. 934 F.2d 1362 (5th Cir. Tex. 1991).
20. Courts Uphold Law, *Regulations against Patient Dumping*, Nation's Health, August 1991, at 1.
21. *Id.* at 17.
22. *Meyers v. Logan Mem. Hosp.*, 82 F. Supp. 2d 707 (2000).
23. 42 U.S.C. 1395cc(a)(1).
24. Public Law 101–508, November 5, 1990, sections 4206 and 4751 of the Omnibus Budget Reconciliation Act.
25. 42 U.S.C. § 1395 (1992).
26. 42 U.S.C. § 1395cc (1992).
27. *Health Care Safety Net Stretched Thin*, Ronald Brownstein, *St. Petersburg Times*, June 4, 2004, Section A, at 13a.
28. http://www.senate.gov/artandhistory/history/common/briefing/Oath_Office.htm.
29. *Id.*

ORGANIZATIONAL ETHICS AND THE LAW

It is of utmost importance that each organization recognizes that its success lies with its ability to assure the staff, community and patients that it holds itself accountable to ensuring the highest standards of quality professional care and the well-being of all that enter its hallowed halls.

—Gᴘ

LEARNING OBJECTIVES

Upon completion of this chapter, the reader will be able to:

- Describe corporate structure.
- Describe a code of ethics for organizations.
- Discuss organizational misconduct.
- Explain *respondeat superior* and *corporate negligence*.
- Describe corporate duties and responsibilities.
- Describe strategies to restore organizational trust.

INTRODUCTION

Legal and ethical issues in the health care setting are being carefully scrutinized across the nation by state and federal regulatory agencies. Organizations, like individuals, must comply with rules of law and ethical conduct. This chapter introduces the reader to corporate authority, contents for codes of ethics for organizations, and the ethical and legal risks to which health care organizations and their governing bodies can be exposed. There is an overview of corporate negligence, respondeat superior, and independent contractor. The emphasis of this chapter is on the duties and responsibilities of health care organizations.

CORPORATE AUTHORITY

The typical health care organization is incorporated under state law as a freestanding for-profit or not-for-profit corporation. The corporation has a governing body that has ultimate responsibility for the decisions made in the organization. The existence of this authority creates certain duties and liabilities. The governing body, having ultimate responsibility for the operation and management of the organization, generally delegates responsibility for the day-to-day operations of the organization to the organization's chief executive officer.

Although health care organizations may operate as sole proprietorships or partnerships, most function as corporations. Thus, an important source of law applicable to governing boards and to the duties and responsibilities of their members is state corporation laws. An incorporated health care organization is a legal person with recognized rights, duties, powers, and responsibilities. Because the legal "person" is in reality a "fictitious person," there is a requirement that certain people are designated to exercise the corporate powers and that they are held accountable for corporate decision making.

Health care corporations—governmental, charitable, or proprietary— have certain powers expressly or implicitly granted to them by state statutes. Generally, the authority of a corporation is expressed in the law under which the corporation is chartered and in the corporation's articles of incorporation. The existence of this authority creates certain duties and liabilities for governing bodies and their individual members. Members of the governing body have both express and implied *corporate authority*.

EXPRESS CORPORATE AUTHORITY

Express corporate authority is authority specifically delegated by statute. Health care corporations derive authority to act from the laws of the state in which they are incorporated. The articles of incorporation set forth the purposes of each corporation's existence and the powers that the corporation is authorized to exercise to carry out its purposes.

IMPLIED CORPORATE AUTHORITY

Implied corporate authority is the authority to perform any and all acts necessary to exercise a corporation's expressly conferred authority and to accomplish the purposes for which it was created. Generally, implied corporate authority arises where there is a need for corporate powers not specifically granted in the articles of incorporation. A governing body, at its own discretion, may enact new bylaws, rules, and regulations; purchase or mortgage property; borrow money; purchase equipment; select personnel; adopt corporate resolutions that delineate decision-making responsibilities; and so forth. These powers can be enumerated in the articles of incorporation and, in such cases, would be categorized as express rather than implied corporate authority.

ULTRA VIRES ACTS

Ultra vires is a Latin term meaning "beyond the powers." *Ultra vires acts* are those acts conducted by a corporation that lies beyond its scope of authority to perform. A governing body can be held liable for acting beyond its scope of authority, which is either expressed (e.g., in its articles of incorporation) or implied in law. The governing body acts on behalf of the corporation. If any action is in violation of a statute or regulation, it is illegal. An example of an illegal act would be the "known" employment of an unlicensed person in a position that by law requires a license. The state, through its attorney general, has the power to prevent the performance of an *ultra vires act* by means of an injunction.

CODE OF ETHICS FOR ORGANIZATIONS

Codes of ethics for organizations provide guidelines for behavior that help carry out an organization's mission, vision, and values. Organizational codes of ethics build trust, increase awareness of ethical issues, guide decision-making, and encourage staff to seek advice and report misconduct when appropriate. The following list provides some value statements that should be considered when preparing an organization's code of ethics.

1. Employees and staff members will comply with the organization's code of ethics, which includes compassionate care; an understanding and acceptance of the organization's mission, vision, and values; and adherence to one's professional code of conduct.
2. Ethics training will be provided as required training for all employees.
3. Ethics competencies will be reviewed at the time of each employee's initial ethics training and scheduled evaluation.
4. The organization will be honest and fair in dealings with employees.
5. The organization will develop and maintain an environment that fosters the highest ethical and legal standards.
6. Corporate officers, managers, and employees will be impartial when personal interests conflict with those of the organization and fellow employees.
7. Employees will be free to speak up without fear of retribution or retaliation.
8. A compliance officer will be available to protect employees who wish to speak-up as to unprofessional practices he or she observes in the organization. The compliance officer will be held accountable for maintaining the confidentiality of the employee's identity. Failure to do so will result in the immediate termination of the compliance officer.

9. The pitfalls of groupthink will not be acceptable conduct in the organization. The preservation of harmony will not become more important than the critical evaluation of ideas by *all* employees.

10. Employees and patients will be provided with a safe environment (e.g., freedom from sexual harassment) within which to work.

11. The drive to increase revenues will not be tied to unethical activities, such as workforce cutbacks as a means to discharge employees when they are encouraged to speak up and then blacklisted because of their honesty.

12. Employees will avoid conflict-of-interest situations by not favoring one's own interests over those of others, including the organization.

13. Patients will be provided with care that is of the highest quality regardless of the setting.

14. All patients will be treated with honesty, dignity, respect, and courtesy.

15. Patients will be informed as to the risks, benefits, and alternatives to care.

16. Patients will be treated in a manner that preserves their rights, dignity, autonomy, self-esteem, privacy, and involvement in their care.

17. Each patient's culture, religion, and heritage will be respected and addressed as appropriate.

18. The organization will provide for a patient advocacy program.

19. The organization will provide appropriate support services for those with physical disabilities (e.g., those with language barriers and those who are hearing- or seeing-impaired).

20. Patients will be provided with a "Patient's Bill of Rights and Responsibilities" on admission to the hospital.

21. Each patient's right to execute advance directives will be honored.

UNPROFESSIONAL CONDUCT

Unprofessional conduct continues to plague the health care system. Complex health care fraud schemes, for example, resulting in losses of billions of dollars annually impede advances in medicine and deny high-quality health care to the people. Enforcing and bringing to justice the number of individuals and organizations who defraud the government simply add to the losses. This section introduces the reader to a variety of ethical and legal risks associated with such conduct. Unprincipled behavior and conduct includes: lack of trust and integrity; false advertising; failure to disclose financial incentives, and concealing mistakes.

TRUST AND INTEGRITY

Trust and integrity cannot always be presumed. Organizations must encourage patients to ask questions and seek second opinions both for peace of mind and to aid in determining the best course of treatment. As noted in the next news clipping, some health care providers consider their financial interests more important then the welfare of their patients.

Settlement Reached in St. Joe's Medical Malpractice Case

A federal investigation and hospital review that began in 2010 found hundreds of cases between 2007 and 2009 in which Midei allegedly profited by placing stents in patients' arteries that weren't medically necessary.

● ● ●

During opening statements in the case, lawyers for the plaintiffs said the coronary unit at St. Joe's was completely out of control and that patients were given stents they did not need. They said Midei and the hospital consciously decided to break the rules and look the other way, profiting from an abnormally high number of procedures.

WBAL TV 11, *May 3, 2013*[1]

FALSE ADVERTISING

False or misleading advertising by health care entities continues to confuse and mislead the public in the search for high-quality care. Hospitals, for example, at a time when the Joint Commission provided hospitals with numerical scores advertised their perfect or nearly perfect accreditation scores. Scores as high as 100 were often posted on billboards and/or in local newspapers. The intent of such advertisements was to associate high scores with a higher quality of care then hospitals receiving lower scores. Following numerous complaints by health care organizations and surveyors, numerical scoring was discontinued, arguably due in part to the misuse of scores for advertising purposes. Some hospitals seemed to be more concerned with scores than complying with the standards required for accreditation purposes. From both an ethical and legal point of view, health care organizations should not advertise misleading information to encourage public confidence in the quality of care provided by the organization over that of another.

Advertising Unintentionally Misleading

Imagine you are an off-duty EMT on vacation driving down a four-lane highway and suddenly you observe a car swerving off the road and flipping onto its side. You stop and see a young man lying on the grass and a young lady hysterical and afraid. Her friend appears to have hit his head on the windshield. There are no streetlights or cell phone connections, and there are no car lights in the distance. Not knowing the extent of the injuries, you gently place the victims in the car and start driving to the nearest exit. You observe a sign advertising "Anytown Hospital—Accreditation Survey Score 100, Exit 11-A" and another billboard advertising "General Medical Center—Accreditation Survey Score 89, Exit 11-B." You just passed exit 10. Luck was on your side. Knowing that a score of 100 sounded better than a score of 88, you decided to take Exit 11-A. You followed the emergency sign.

You stopped the car in front of the emergency department entrance, jumped out and ran to the door. There was a sign that said ring bell if you need help. You quickly learned that you just arrived at a behavioral health hospital. General Medical Center Exit-B turned out to be a major teaching hospital. Anytown Hospital's advertisement was not intended to mislead the public but to advertise how well they did during their survey. After all, the community was well aware of the services each hospital offered.

Discussion

1. Discuss what action the hospitals should take to prevent confusion in advertising.
2. Describe a principle of ethics that has been violated if no action is taken to prevent similar incidents.

CASE: BAIT AND SWITCH ADVERTISING

An action was filed against the defendant, Managed Care, alleging claims of false advertising in connection with Managed Care's sale, marketing, and rendering of medical services. The plaintiff alleged that he was an enrollee in Managed Care's health plan. He also alleged that through misleading and deceptive material representations and omissions, Managed Care had employed a fraudulent, unfair scheme to induce people to enroll in its plan by misrepresenting that its primary commitment was to maintain and improve the quality of health care. The plaintiff alleged that Managed Care had been aggressively engaged in implementing undisclosed systemic internal policies that were designed to discourage its primary care physicians from delivering medical services and to interfere with the medical judgment of its health care providers. The result of these policies, he alleged, was a reduction in the quality of health care that is directly contrary to Managed Care's representations.

The plaintiff claimed that Managed Care's false advertising reduced the quality of medical services available to the enrollees and decreased the monetary value of their health coverage. The plaintiff requested restitution, refund, or reimbursement of monies paid by or on behalf of enrollees that resulted from excessive and ill-gotten monies obtained by Managed Care as a result of its unlawful, fraudulent, and unfair business practices and misleading advertisements.

Ethical and Legal Issues

1. Describe the ethical issues in this case.
2. Describe the value of a corporate compliance program and how it could help prevent false advertising.

CONCEALING MISTAKES

Mistakes in medicine are common occurrences that often result in extended hospital stays, higher costs, injury, disability, or death. The Joint Commission in its accreditation process requires that patients be informed when a mistake has been made.

22. The licensed independent practitioner responsible for managing the patient's care, treatment, and services, or his or her designee, informs the patient about unanticipated outcomes of care, treatment, and services related to sentinel events when the patient is not already aware of the occurrence or when further discussion is needed. [2014] Hospital Accreditation Standards, Standard RI.01.02.01.]

Unfortunately for patients, organizations sometimes cover up their mistakes as noted in the following case.

CASE: WRONG SURGICAL PROCEDURE COVER-UP

The physician–petitioner in *In re Muncan*[2] did not review either the patient's CT or MRI images prior to surgery. In addition, he did not have the images with him in the operating room on the day of surgery. Had he done so, he would have discovered that the CT scan report erroneously stated there was a mass in the patient's left kidney when in fact the mass was located in the patient's right kidney. During surgery, the physician did not observe any gross abnormalities or deformities in the left kidney and was unable to palpate any masses. Nonetheless, he removed the left kidney.

The Supreme Court of New York, Appellate Division, Third Department held that the evidence was sufficient to support an inference of fraud. The physician knew he removed the wrong kidney and instead of taking steps to rectify the situation, intentionally concealed his mistake.

Statistical reports can knowingly be inaccurate and give patients a false sense of comfort when selecting a hospital for care, as noted in the following *reality check.*

Appearance May Not Be Reality

General Hospital's staff aggregated its infection rate data for comparison purposes with four other hospitals in the community. The staff members were aware that the data were flawed. They presented a false perception that General Hospital's postoperative infection rates were lower than those of peer hospitals. The comparison data were published in the local newspaper.

The Jones family, believing the data to be correct and concerned about the number of deaths related to hospital-acquired infections, relied on the data in selecting General Hospital as their preferred hospital.

Anonymous

Ethical and Legal Issues

1. Describe how organizational and professional codes of ethics were violated in this case.
2. Describe what role an organization's ethics committee could play in addressing this or similar issues.

CORPORATE NEGLIGENCE

Corporate negligence occurs when a corporation fails to perform those duties it owes directly to a patient or to anyone else to whom a duty may extend. If such a duty is breached and a patient is injured as a result of that breach, the organization can be held culpable under the theory of corporate negligence.

> Corporate negligence is a doctrine under which the hospital is liable if it fails to uphold the proper standard of care owed the patient, which is to ensure the patient's safety and well-being while at the hospital. This theory of liability creates a nondelegable duty which the hospital owes directly to a patient. Therefore, an injured party does not have to rely on and establish the negligence of a third party.[3]

Liability extends to nonemployees who act as a hospital's ostensible agents. For example, in *Thompson v. Nason Hospital*,[4] a Pennsylvania court recognized that hospitals are more than mere conduits through which health care professionals are brought into contact with patients. Hospitals owe some nondelegable duties directly to their patients independent of the negligence of their employees, such as duties to use reasonable care in the maintenance of safe and adequate facilities and equipment; select and retain only competent physicians; oversee all persons who practice medicine within their walls as to patient care; and formulate, adopt, and enforce adequate rules and policies to ensure the best quality care for their patients. *Darling v. Charleston Community Memorial Hospital*, discussed next, has had a major impact on the liability of health care organizations for patient injuries suffered within their walls. The immunity status of nonprofit hospitals was no longer an acceptable defense against a plaintiff's negligence claims.

CASE: DARLING—HEALTH CARE'S BENCHMARK CASE

In 1965, the landmark case *Darling v. Charleston Community Memorial Hospital*[5] had a major impact on the liability of health care organizations. The court enunciated a "corporate negligence doctrine" under which hospitals have a duty to provide adequately trained medical and nursing staff. A hospital is responsible, in conjunction with its medical staff, for establishing policies and procedures for monitoring the quality of medicine practiced within the hospital.

Darling involved an 18-year-old college football player who was preparing for a career as a teacher and coach. The patient, a defensive halfback for his college football team, was injured during a play. He was rushed to the emergency department of a small, accredited community hospital where the only physician on emergency duty that day was Dr. Alexander, a general practitioner. Alexander had not treated a major leg fracture for 3 years.

The physician examined the patient and ordered an X-ray that revealed that the tibia and the fibula of the right leg had been fractured. The physician reduced the fracture and applied a plaster cast from a point 3 or 4 inches below the groin to the toes. Shortly after the cast had been applied, the patient began to complain continually of pain. The physician split the cast and continued to visit the patient frequently while the patient remained in the hospital. Not thinking that it was necessary, the emergency department physician did not call in a specialist for consultation.

After 2 weeks, the student was transferred to a larger hospital and placed under the care of an orthopedic surgeon. The specialist found a considerable amount of dead tissue in the fractured leg. During the next 2 months, the specialist removed increasing amounts of tissue in a futile attempt to save the leg until it became necessary to amputate the leg 8 inches below the knee. The student's father did not agree to a settlement and filed suit against the emergency department physician and the hospital. Although the physician later settled out of court for $40,000, the case continued against the hospital.

The documentary evidence relied on to establish the standard of care included the rules and regulations of the Illinois Department of Public Health under the Hospital Licensing Act; the standards for hospital accreditation, today known as the Joint Commission; and the bylaws, rules, and regulations of Charleston Hospital. These documents were admitted into evidence without objection. No specific evidence was offered that the hospital had failed to conform to the usual and customary practices of hospitals in the community.

The trial court instructed the jury to consider those documents, along with all other evidence, in determining the hospital's liability. Under the circumstances in which the case reached the Illinois Supreme Court, it was held that the verdict against the hospital should be sustained if the evidence supported the verdict on any one or more of the 20 allegations of negligence. Allegations asserted that the hospital was negligent in its failure to (1) provide a sufficient number of trained nurses for bedside care of all patients at all times, in this case, nurses who were capable of recognizing the progressive gangrenous condition of the plaintiff's right leg, and (2) failure of its nurses to bring the patient's condition to the attention of the hospital administration and staff so that adequate consultation could be secured and the condition rectified.

Although these generalities provided the jury with no practical guidance for determining what constitutes reasonable care, they were considered relevant to helping the jury decide what was feasible and what the hospital knew or should have known concerning hospital responsibilities for the proper care of a patient. There was no expert testimony characterizing when the professional care rendered by the attending physician should have been reviewed, who should have reviewed it, or whether the case required consultation.

Evidence relating to the hospital's failure to review Alexander's work, to require consultation or examination by specialists, and to require proper nursing care was found to be sufficient to support a verdict for the patient. Judgment was eventually returned against the hospital in the amount of $100,000.

The Illinois Supreme Court held that the hospital could not limit its liability as a charitable corporation to the amount of its liability insurance.

[T]he doctrine of charitable immunity can no longer stand . . . a doctrine which limits the liability of charitable corporations to the amount of liability insurance that they see fit to carry permits them to determine whether or not they will be liable for their torts and the amount of that liability, if any.[6]

In effect, the hospital was liable as a corporate entity for the negligent acts of its employees and physicians. Among other things, the Darling case indicates the importance of instituting effective credentialing and continuing medical evaluation and review programs for all members of a professional staff.

Ethical and Legal Issues

1. Describe the legal issues in this case.
2. Describe how the hospital failed in its ethical duty to the patient.

DOCTRINE OF *RESPONDEAT SUPERIOR*

Respondeat superior (let the master respond) is a legal doctrine holding employers liable, in certain cases, for the wrongful acts of their agents (employees). This doctrine has also been referred to as vicarious liability, whereby an employer is answerable for the torts committed by employees. In the health care setting, an organization, for example, is liable for the negligent acts of its employees, even though there has been no wrongful conduct on the part of the organization. For liability to be imputed to the employer:

1.   A master–servant relationship must exist between the employer and the employee; and
2.   The wrongful act of the employee must have occurred within the scope of his or her employment.

The question of liability frequently rests on whether persons treating a patient are independent agents (responsible for their own acts) or employees of the organization. The answer to this depends on whether the organization can exercise control over the particular act that was the proximate cause of the injury. The basic rationale for imposing liability on an employer developed because of the employer's right to control the physical acts of its employees. It is not necessary that the employer actually exercise control, only that it possesses the right, power, and authority to do so.

When filing a lawsuit, the plaintiff's attorney generally names both the employer and employee. This occurs because the employer is generally in a better financial condition to cover the judgment. The employer is not without remedy if liability has been imposed against the organization due to an employee's negligent act. The employer can seek indemnification from the employee. Although it would be highly unlikely for a hospital to seek recovery from an employee, the ever-increasing number of employed physicians could give rise to a hospital to seek indemnification from a physician who is the cause of a negligent injury and carries his own malpractice insurance policy.

INDEPENDENT CONTRACTOR

Independent contractors are responsible for their own negligent acts. The independent contractor relationship is established when the principal has no right of control over the manner in which the agent's work is to be performed. However, some cases indicate that an organization can be held liable for an independent contractor's negligence. For example, in *Mehlman v. Powell,*[7] the court held that a hospital could be found vicariously liable for the negligence of an emergency department physician who was not a hospital employee but who worked in the emergency department in the capacity of an independent contractor. The court reasoned that the hospital maintained control over billing procedures, maintained an emergency department, and represented to the patient that the members of the emergency department staff were its employees, which might have caused the patient to rely on the skill and competence of the staff.

CORPORATE DUTIES AND RESPONSIBILITIES

Along with the corporate authority that is granted to the governing body, duties are attached to its individual members. These responsibilities are considered duties because they are imposed by law and can be enforced in legal proceedings. Governing body members are considered by law to have the highest measure of accountability. They have a fiduciary duty that requires acting primarily for the benefit of the corporation. The general duties of a governing body are both implied and express. Failure of a governing body to perform its duties may constitute mismanagement to such a degree that the appointment of a receiver to manage the affairs of the corporation could be warranted.

The duty to supervise and manage is applicable to the trustees as it is to the managers of any other business corporation. In both instances, there is a duty to act as a reasonably prudent person would act under similar circumstances. The governing body must act prudently in administering the affairs of the organization and exercise its powers in good faith. Various duties and responsibilities of hospital organizations are reviewed here.

APPOINTMENT OF A CEO

The governing body is responsible for appointing a chief executive officer (CEO) to act as its agent in the management of the organization. The CEO is responsible for the day-to-day operations. The individual selected as CEO must possess the competence and the character necessary to maintain satisfactory standards of patient care.

The responsibilities and authority of the CEO should be expressed in an appropriate job description, as well as in any formal agreement or contract that the organization has with the CEO. Some state health codes describe the responsibilities of administrators in broad terms. They generally provide that the CEO/administrator shall be responsible for the overall management of the organization.

The general duty of a governing body is to exercise due care and diligence in supervising and managing the organization. This duty does not cease with the selection of a CEO. A governing body can be liable if the level of patient care becomes inadequate because of the governing body's failure to supervise properly the management of the organization. CEOs, like board members, can be personally liable for their own acts of negligence that injure others.

CEO CHALLENGES AND RESPONSIBILITIES

Among the many responsibilities that apply to CEOs are the following:

- Uphold the organization's and one's professional code of ethics.
- Show support and respect to all physicians and staff, knowing that as a team they are the ones who provide bedside care.
- Make daily rounds in the organization. Fix the things they can and find a way to fix the things they think they cannot.
- Develop friendships and supporters who can help the organization to meet those extraordinary goals.
- Implement community outreach programs. Reach out, teach, and educate members of the community on preventative care.
- Not be influenced by power brokers simply because of their position. CEOs and managers must do the right thing, all the time—not in a vacuum, but as a team.
- Show respect to all persons. Treat consultants, accreditation representatives, and inspectors on all levels (e.g., federal, state, local, and private) with respect, knowing that they are all there to help the organization become better in its delivery of patient care.

CEO CODE OF ETHICS

The following is the preamble to the Code of Ethics of the American College of Healthcare Executives (ACHE):[8]

> The purpose of the Code of Ethics of the American College of Healthcare Executives is to serve as a standard of conduct for members. It contains standards of ethical behavior for health care executives in their professional relationships. These relationships include colleagues, patients, or others served; members of the health care executive's organization and other organizations, the community, and society as a whole.
>
> The Code of Ethics also incorporates standards of ethical behavior governing individual behavior, particularly when that conduct directly relates to the role and identity of the health care executive.
>
> The fundamental objectives of the health care management profession are to maintain or enhance the overall quality of life, dignity, and well-being of every individual needing health care service and to create a more equitable, accessible, effective, and efficient health care system.
>
> Health care executives have an obligation to act in ways that will merit the trust, confidence, and respect of health care professionals and the general public. Therefore, health care executives should lead lives that embody an exemplary system of values and ethics.

Maintain Moral Integrity

The CEO must reflect moral integrity in fulfilling the duties and responsibilities of his or her position. There will often be decisions that may be costly to one's career path, as noted in the following *reality checks*.

Ensuring Integrity

Jim, the administrator of General Hospital, was reviewing his mail and reports placed in his inbox by Carol, his secretary. He noticed a copy of correspondence that had been forwarded to him from the corporate office. The letter, describing a donation that had been made, read:

Dear John,

The care received at your East campus was outstanding. As a result, I am forwarding to your offices a check in the amount of $500,000.

Sincerely,

After reading his morning mail and reports, Jim placed the letter in his outbox for filing. Carol later picked up Jim's mail and other reports from his outbox. Later that afternoon, Carol walked back into Jim's office and inquired, "Did you read this letter forwarded to you from the corporate office?" Handing it to Jim, he replied, "Yes, I read it." Carol then asked, "Do you see anything that piqued your curiosity in this letter?" Jim replied that he had not. Carol, pointing at a strip of whiteout tape, urged Jim to look more closely. She then asked Jim to turn the letter over and read the words the tape was covering. He turned the letter over, noting what the letter had said. It appeared that only a copy had been meant for Jim, not the original correspondence. With the missing words inserted, the correspondence read:

> *Dear John,*
>
> *The care received at your East campus was outstanding. As a result, I am forwarding to your offices a check in the amount of $500,000, earmarked for capital projects at your East campus.*
>
> *Sincerely,*
>
> *Anonymous*

Discussion

1. Discuss why the whiteout tape might have been placed over the words, "earmarked for capital projects at your East campus." Take into account the comma placed prior to the word "earmarked."
2. What action should Jim take? Remember that Jim could not absolutely determine who placed the whiteout tape on the correspondence, the letter's author or some other unknown person.
3. Assuming Jim sent a memo to the corporate chief financial officer (CFO) to inquire what happened to the donated funds, should the CFO respond to Jim? In what way?
4. Assuming that the CFO failed to respond to Jim, should Jim take any further action, and, if so, what action should he consider?

Discrimination: Behind Closed Doors

It was a Monday morning. Jack remembers it well. As an administrator of a hospital in a multihospital system, Jack was settling into his office when his secretary put through a call from Gerard, the system CEO who was in the corporate office. Gerald asked Jack about interviews of candidates for the emergency department director. Jack replied that the emergency department director search committee has three interviews scheduled for that afternoon. Gerard replied, "The director has to be Christian." Jack interrupted saying, "Are you serious?" Gerard responded, "This is what the board wants. There are too many Jewish medical directors." Jack replied, "This is what the board wants?" Gerard, again quickly interrupting, "Well no, it's what I want." Jack, not believing that Gerard made this decision on his own, replied, "First of all, the selection of director is being conducted by a search committee that includes myself and the other medical directors as well as representatives from the general medical staff. The final decision is the consensus of that committee." Gerard replied, "You are the administrator, and you can pick who you want." Jack responded, "Who I want is the most qualified person for the position." Gerard replied, "You got my message," and abruptly hung up the phone.

That afternoon after interviewing the final candidates, the entire search committee unanimously agreed to select the physician they considered most qualified, a person who happened to be Jewish.

Later that week, Jack decided to take a vacation day to celebrate the Feast of San Gennaro in New York City. He received a call on his cell phone. Jack answered, and his secretary said, "Gerard wants to see you in his office on Monday morning." Jack said, "I can tell from your voice: it sounds ominous?" She said, "I think it is."

On Monday morning, Gerard said, "I am planning to move you to the corporate office. I need your skills here." The corporate office often was jokingly referred to as the deep dark hole. This was a place where people seemed to disappear from the face of the earth, never to be heard from again.

Jack said, "I really prefer to stay at the hospital as the administrator." Gerard replied, "That's not an option." Jack said, "Is this about the selection of the emergency department director? Because the doctor is Jewish?" Gerard said, "Now why would you think that?" Gerard, pausing for a moment, continued, "I really need your skills here." Jack replied, "Do you remember the previous administrator recorded all his telephone calls?" Gerard replied, "What are you getting at?" Jack continued, "I never disconnected the recorder. Your conversation about the selection of an emergency room director was very clear." Gerard replied angrily, "Are you threatening me." Jack said, "No, I just wanted you to understand that the recorder was never disconnected."

Anonymous

Discussion

1. Discuss what you believe are the ethical issues of this case.
2. What should Jack do, assuming he really did tape the conversation?
3. If Jack had not taped the conversation, would that change your mind as to what he should do?

Truthfulness Can Shed Light on Character

A CEO rudely left a briefing being conducted by a group of consultants. The consultants had been contracted by the governing body to review the quality of care being delivered at the hospital where he was employed. The CEO was unhappy with the report because it contained a list of things that needed to be addressed to improve the quality of patient care. As the CEO started to leave the room, he abruptly turned and said, "This is not just about the hospital! This is about my job!" His managers then rose and followed him out of the room, without looking back—no goodbyes with stone-cold faces.

Anonymous

Discussion

1. Discuss what codes of ethics were violated in this case.
2. Explain how you would handle this incident if you were a member of the board.

Screen Job Applicants

All job applicants must be closely screened prior to employment, regardless of the responsibilities for which they are seeking employment. The screening process is generally the responsibility of the human resources department and hospital managers. As noted in the news clippings that follow, failure to adequately screen applicants can lead to damaging consequences for both patients and the hospital.

Job Applicants Not Always Screened

Despite the danger of hiring an employee who might jeopardize assisted living residents, some facilities neglect background screening of new workers.

More than 1 in 10 facilities inspected by state regulators in seven states during a two-year period within 2000–2002 picked up at least one citation for neglecting background checks on prospective caregivers. . . .

Kevin McCoy, USA Today, *May 26, 2004*

Did Hospitals "See No Evil"?

When police in New Jersey arrested a male nurse named Charles Cullen last year, he made a terrible claim. He said he'd killed as many as 40 patients during the course of his nursing career.

The question remains: How could Cullen have worked at 10 different hospitals in New Jersey and Pennsylvania, over a period of 16 years—despite the fact that at seven of those hospitals, he was under investigation, fired or forced to resign?

Apparently, not one of those institutions gave Cullen a bad reference, or told other hospitals he was trouble. It amounted to a policy of "See no evil-speak no evil"—one that gave Cullen, in effect, a license to kill.

Rebecca Leung, CBSNews.com, *April 4, 2004*[9]

CREDENTIALING, APPOINTMENT, AND PRIVILEGING

The governing body is ultimately responsible for the credentialing, appointment, and privileging process of the organization's professional staff. The duty to select members of the professional staff is legally vested in the governing body charged with managing the organization. Although cognizant of the importance of professional staff membership, the governing body must meet its obligation to maintain high standards of practice and fairness. The governing board of a hospital must therefore be given great latitude in prescribing the necessary qualifications for potential applicants. Because no court should substitute its evaluation of professional competency for that of a hospital board, a court's review should be limited to ensuring that the qualifications imposed by a board are reasonably related to the operation of the hospital and fairly administered. Moreover, courts are generally reluctant to get involved with the internal affairs of a hospital or professional society unless any sanctions they impose violate public policy.

Credentialing is a process for validating the background of health care professionals and assessing their qualifications to provide health care services. The process is an objective evaluation of a professional's current licensure, training, or experience; competence; and ability to perform the services or procedures requested. Credentialing occurs during both the initial appointment and reappointment process. The *delineation of clinical privileges* is the process by which the medical staff determines precisely what procedures a physician is authorized to perform. This determination is based on the credentials necessary to competently perform the privileges requested.

The medical staff is responsible to the governing body for the quality of care rendered by members of the medical staff. The hospital's governing body has a duty to ensure that a mechanism is in place for the medical staff to evaluate, counsel, and when necessary take disciplinary action against physicians who pose an unreasonable risk of harm to patients.

Ensure Competency

Hospitals have a responsibility to take reasonable steps to ensure that physicians are qualified for the privileges granted. Failure to screen a medical staff applicant's credentials properly can lead to liability for injuries suffered by patients as a result of that omission. Hospitals must adhere to procedures established under both their own bylaws and state statutes. The measure of quality and the degree of quality control exercised in a hospital are the direct responsibilities of the medical staff. Hospital supervision of the manner of appointment of physicians to its staff is mandatory, not optional.

False Statements

In *Hoxie v. Ohio State Med. Bd.,* it was determined that a physician had made false statements concerning his criminal history when he stated in a deposition that he had never been arrested. There was sufficient evidence presented to support permanent revocation of his license to practice medicine. Certified records held by the state of California indicated that the physician had been arrested or detained by the Los Angeles Police Department multiple times in the 1970s and 1980s for possessing marijuana and PCP, for driving under the influence of alcohol and/or drugs, and for driving with a suspended license. Although the physician asserted that documentation of his criminal past had been fabricated by police and was not credible, law enforcement investigation reports are generally admissible. The physician himself added to the reliability of the records by verifying all significant identifying information contained within the documents and records.[10]

Masquerading as a Physician

An action was brought against Canton (who was masquerading as a physician, Dr. LaBella), the hospital, and others in *Insinga v. LaBella*[11] for the wrongful death of a 68-year-old woman whom Canton had admitted. The patient died while she was in the hospital. Canton was found to be a fugitive from justice in Canada, where he was under indictment for the manufacture and sale of illegal drugs. He fraudulently obtained a medical license from the state of Florida and staff privileges at the hospital by using the name of LaBella, a deceased physician. Canton was extradited to Canada without being served process. The U.S. District Court for the Southern District of Florida directed a verdict in favor of the hospital. On appeal, the Florida Supreme Court held that the corporate negligence doctrine imposes on hospitals an implied duty to patients to select competent physicians who, although they are independent practitioners, would be providing in-hospital care to their patients through staff privileges. Hospitals are in the best position to protect their patients and consequently have an independent duty to select competent independent physicians.

DISCIPLINE OF PHYSICIANS

Although the governing body has ultimate responsibility for disciplining members of the professional staff (e.g., disruptive behavior, incompetence, psychological problems, substance abuse), responsibility for disciplinary actions are generally delegated to the administrator and various department directors and managers. Depending on the seriousness of alleged misconduct, disciplinary action may require board involvement for resolution, such as those occurrences noted in the following news clipping.

The Joint Commission as far back as 2008 responded to complaints of disruptive physician behavior that can place patient care at risk and increase medical errors. The standards made it mandatory for hospitals to establish written policies designed to address behavior that is demeaning, aggressive, uncivil, or hostile in the patient care setting.[12] The American Medical Association (AMA) has defined disruptive behavior as a style of interaction with physicians, hospital personnel, patients, family members, or others that interferes with patient care.[13]

The discipline of a physician is sometimes difficult without adequate support of the medical staff, as noted in the following *reality check*.

Physicians Reluctant to Discipline Physicians

Anytown Hospital has an outstanding reputation for surgical services. The operating room supervisor and a surgical nurse told Bob Wright that Dr. Flipton, an anesthesiologist, is abusing the use of anesthesia gases in the hospital's dental suite. He was reportedly seen by operating staff administering nitrous oxide (laughing gas) by holding a mask against his face for short periods of time. This scene would be followed by a string of silly, seemingly meaningless jokes. Bob has repeatedly discussed this matter with the medical executive committee. The medical executive committee refused to take any action without definitive action by the department chair. Bob suspects that if he pursues the matter further with the governing board, he could end up without a job. The governing body is generally unable to resolve disciplinary actions against a physician without support of the medical executive committee.

Ethical and Legal Issues

1. What do you believe the ethical issues are for Bob? For Bob, doing the right thing and survival are competing concerns.
2. Which of the following would you do if you were in Bob's position, with two children in college and hefty mortgage payments?
   - Voluntarily leave my job
   - Aggressively pursue the problem
   - Secretly enlist the aid of the medical staff
   - Confront Dr. Flipton
   - Other option (explain)

A hospital and its governing body were determined to be immune from liability under the federal Health Care Quality Improvement Act of 1986 in *Taylor v. Kennestone Hosp.*,[14] for claims arising out of their decision to deny a physician's application to renew his medical staff privileges. A peer review board found that reasonable investigation had adduced evidence demonstrating that the physician had a history of sexual misconduct toward both nurses and patients. He admitted that he had sexual harassment problems, that he stopped seeing patients at the hospital, and that he sought psychiatric treatment. He admitted that he failed to comply fully with his own psychiatrist's plan of care before he resumed seeing patients in the hospital. The evidence established that the peer reviewers could reasonably believe that their actions were warranted and that those actions furthered the quality of health care.

CASE: PHYSICIAN PRIVILEGES SUSPENDED

A physician received a letter from a hospital informing him that his clinical privileges at the hospital had been summarily suspended. The medical executive committee reviewed the suspension and recommended that it be upheld. The hospital board ultimately revoked the physician's staff privileges. The physician received a hearing before a fair hearing panel, which recommended that he be reinstated. The board, however, upheld the revocation.

The physician alleged, among other things, wrongful termination and intentional infliction of emotional distress. The defendants argued that the courts do not have jurisdiction to review staffing decisions made by private, nonprofit hospitals.

The Court of Civil Appeals of Oklahoma, Division II, found that judicial tribunals are not equipped to review the action of hospital boards in selecting or refusing to appoint physicians to their medical staffs. The authorities of hospitals endeavor to serve in the best possible manner the sick and the afflicted. Not all professionals have identical ability, competence, experience, character, and standards of ethics. The mere fact that a physician is licensed to practice a profession does not justify any inference beyond the conclusion that a physician has met the minimum requirements for that purpose.

Without regard to the absence of any legal liability, the hospital in granting a physician privileges to practice in its facilities extends a moral or official approval to him in the eyes of the public. Not all professionals have personalities that enable them to work in harmony with others, and to inspire confidence in their peers and in patients. Courts should not substitute their evaluation in such matters. It is the board, not the court, that is charged with the responsibility of providing a competent staff of physicians. The board has chosen to rely on the advice of its medical staff, and the court cannot surrogate for the medical staff in executing this responsibility. Human lives are at stake, and the board must be given discretion in its selection so that it can have confidence in the competence and moral commitment of its staff.[15]

Ethical and Legal Issues

1. Do you agree with the court's decision? Explain.
2. Discuss under what circumstances you believe a court should become involved in an organization's disciplinary processes (e.g., age discrimination).

PROVIDE ADEQUATE STAFF

Staffing shortages for both hospitals and nursing homes continue to plague the health care industry. Because the quality of care provided by nursing homes is subject to substantial scrutiny, American families face difficult decisions about whether to move a loved one into such a setting.

Under federal law, nursing facilities must have sufficient nursing staff to provide nursing and related services adequate to attain and maintain the highest practicable physical, mental, and psychosocial well-being of each resident, as determined by resident assessments and individual plans of care. As nursing facilities are increasingly filled with older, disabled residents with complex care needs, the demands for highly educated and trained nursing personnel continue to grow.

PROVIDE ADEQUATE SUPPLIES AND EQUIPMENT

The governing body must ensure that there are adequate supplies and equipment on hand in each of its facilities. If the board is unable to provide the necessary supplies and equipment, it must consider finding the funds necessary to fulfill its mission or scaling back operations and, if necessary, consider other options, such as filing for bankruptcy or selling the organization's assets to a competing organization.

Hospital's Challenge to Survive

Brad was concerned with what he considered little opportunity for advancement at Blooming Hospital. He had been there for 8 years and there were two administrators in line for Woody's position as chief executive officer. As far as Brad knew, Woody had no plans to leave Blooming Hospital. He was well liked, competent, and to this day the best boss anyone could hope to have.

Because of financial needs, Brad discussed his concerns with Margaret, the chief operating officer at Hope Hospital, one of several hospitals in a multihospital system. A few months later Margaret called Brad and said, "I am leaving Hope Hospital and moving to another hospital in the system as CEO. Are you interested in applying for my job?" Brad replied that he was interested. He applied and was offered the job.

Brad found it difficult to approach Woody. As he walked towards Woody's office, he felt a veil of despair and second thoughts but knew it would be financially difficult not to accept the position at Hope Hospital. Woody had an open door policy and Brad entered his office unannounced. Woody said, "Hi Brad." Brad replied, "Hi Woody. I find it hard to tell you but I was offered a job at Hope Hospital in the number two position." Woody asked, "Are you sure this is what you want to do?" Brad replied that it was. Woody appeared disappointed as Brad left his office. Later that afternoon Woody went to Brad's office and described how the system Brad was about to enter could be problematic for him. As Woody stood in the doorway, he continued, "Hope Hospital has a reputation of being intensely political." Woody was not one to use many words but again he looked disappointed. After a few moment of silence, Woody turned and left the room. Brad could have asked for a raise but was uncomfortable to ask and felt Woody might have misgivings towards him.

Brad, after giving a months notice, had left Blooming Hospital. The CEO at Hope Hospital was a kind gentleman. He, however, resigned his position just 9 months after Brad's arrival. Brad was appointed the interim CEO as the board conducted a search for a new CEO. Brad threw his resume into the mix. Following a lengthy search and interviews, Brad was appointed CEO of Hope Hospital.

Brad was happy to be managing a profitable hospital, however he quickly faced challenges on many fronts, including a continuing battle to obtain supplies from vendors due to the transfer of funds from his hospital by corporate leadership to prop up other failing entities in the system outside the state where his hospital was located. The following timeline documents his struggle to keep the hospital afloat:

July 2010—Phone Message from the Director of Procurement

Proctor and Gamble has cut us off from all delivery of supplies. Johnson & Johnson has cut off all deliveries of supplies. Scott Labs and Anthony Medical have cut us off from all deliveries. If we don't soon get supplies, the lab will be forced to close.

August 2010—Lack of OR Sutures

Dr. Plastics entered Brad's office and said, "I can't perform surgery without the proper suture materials. I have a patient on the table and they don't have the sutures I prefer to close the surgical incision." He then turned to return to the OR, looking back and apologizing, "I know you don't control where the money goes."

Brad discussed the lack of sutures material with Marcy, the OR supervisor. Marcy, in tears, said, "Brad, supply shortages are making my job difficult enough and now the physicians are taking out their frustrations on me. Dr. Plastics, who complained to you, had other suture options, but like all surgeons, he had his own preferences, probably, I suspect, based on a salesman's pressure." Brad replied, "I can't second-guess the surgeon's selection of sutures; however, I understand your frustrations and I will continue to bring them up with the corporate CEO. I can assure you that the board members are well aware of the continuing supply shortages."

August 2010—Lack of X-ray Film

One Friday at 5:00 p.m. a radiologist went to Brad's office to report, "I know you are under a lot of pressure, but we do not have sufficient X-ray film to get through the weekend!" After Brad arranged to borrow X-ray film from a local state hospital, he called the corporate accounts payable department to inquire about payment of the vendor—a task that was beginning to be a daily occurrence for Brad.

September 2010—Message Relayed from Administrative Secretary

"Dr. Wild stormed in. He is furious! The fetal monitor machine is out of commission. He was lied to and told it was working but it wasn't. This is a life-saving instrument and failure to have it fixed is intolerable (and a few more adjectives I couldn't get down in shorthand) and inexcusable *and a legal matter*—this is just the tip of the iceberg. If things don't start to improve he will pull his entire practice out of the hospital."

April 2011—Memo from the President of the Medical/Dental Staff

We have been reduced to using menstrual pads for abdominal dressings. On two occasions last week a major disaster was narrowly averted in the Operating Room only because of the proximity of . . . City Hospital and their willingness to supply us with emergency equipment.

March 2012—Input from Department of Supply Procurement

The director of supply procurement wrote a memo stating that the acute shortages of OR material and X-ray film were putting patients at risk at this facility. The memo recommended considering an orderly closing of the facility. Those present at a meeting to discuss the issue unanimously agreed that without immediate intervention regarding the specific needs, closing of the hospital should begin on a specified date. Ms. Nurse added that ensuring an adequate supply of sutures was critical.

June 2012—Phone Message from Dr. Orthopedics

Dr. Orthopedics called at noon today (6/12). He said about a week ago he was here at night and there were no finger splints. Dr. Orthopedics said he had to resort to the use of popsicle sticks that he obtained in the hospital coffee shop for splints.

September 2012—Memo from Dr. ER

Over the past 3 to 4 weeks the supply of orthopedic-related supplies in the emergency room has dwindled to a dangerous level. Something must be done soon.

October 2012—Letter from Dr. Peds

I was on call for the emergency room . . . on Friday, October 23, 2012. I was disappointed to note that important casting materials were not available. . . . I can repeat what others have said: if the hospital is to continue to provide high-quality care, a certain minimum level of supplies must be available.

January 2013—Memo from Dr. Orthopedics

Once again, I am forced to bring to your attention the abysmal state of affairs with reference to your credit ratings with various surgical vendors. It is a continual source of embarrassment to me to have to call in personal favors with salesmen and vendors so as to provide my patients with prostheses and equipment they need for their optimal health care.

April 2013—Board Minutes

Father Smith (board member who chaired the physicians relations committee) requested that Brad and the president of the medical staff work together in locating the areas of greatest concern with regard to supply shortages. Father Smith asked that this information be available at the next board meeting.

May 2013—Brad speaks with the Corporate CEO

Brad called the corporate office to discuss the ongoing seriousness of the supply issues. The purchase, storage, and distribution of supplies had been centralized in a corporate location off site. At the same time, Accounts Payable was also centralized and was accused of paying vendors on the basis of who screamed the loudest rather than on patient need.

June 2013—Administrator and Medical Staff President Joint Memo to the Board

We sincerely believe that as a result of the supply shortages, the negative impact on morale of patients and employees during the past 5 years is substantial. The serious nature of these concerns are noted in the following paragraphs.

Major Vendors requiring advance payment

2010	18
2011	53
2012	129
2013	350

The system CEO was distressed that Brad had provided this information to the board, complaining to him, "You're out to get me." Brad responded, "I am complying with the board's request, and it's in the board minutes. Besides, I gave you an advance copy of the memorandum."

Discussion

1. Discuss the ethical issues that this case raises.
2. Are there any circumstances in which CEOs should attempt to keep information from their boards?
3. Brad is in a multihospital system making major profits but cannot control the flow of funds out of the community hospital. The governing body is aware of the serious nature of the supply crisis. What should the board do?
4. If you were Brad or on the board, what action would you take?

ALLOCATE SCARCE RESOURCES

It is the responsibility of the governing body, and not the legal system, to provide appropriate staffing and provide adequate supplies and equipment for patients. Although the courts do not overlook the importance of maintaining adequate levels of patient care, it is not the job of the courts to referee disagreements. For example, a disagreement between the governing body and the local community as to how to allocate limited resources is not a question for the courts to settle. Questions of this sort often involve ethical principles and values. How to spend limited resources that provide good for the many is a value judgment, not a legal decision. Hospitals are in the business of serving patients with many kinds of illnesses and disabilities. Recognizing that the medical community is best equipped to conduct the balancing that medical resource allocations inevitably require, Congress has declined to give courts a mandate to arbitrate allocation disputes.[16]

The following news clippings describe how some hospitals have been negatively affected when resources are not wisely distributed.

MDs Weigh Action Over Hospital $$

A suit may be in the offing blocking the . . . [multi-system corporation] from pumping profits made by its [community hospital] into the . . . [system's] two financially-ailing sister hospitals....

"It's a matter of going to the operating room and finding that a particular piece of equipment isn't working, or finding that certain items are not up to date."

Although . . . [system] officials would not comment, sources close to the scene say the . . . [system] will maintain that it has the right to spend as it sees fit.

Vicky Penner Katz, Smithtown News, *July 24, 1980*

... Says Hospitals Won't Fail

The . . . [system] has been siphoning funds from the financially stable . . . hospital to make up deficits at the two other hospitals, which have a large volume of charity cases. The drain has angered . . . [community] physicians, who complain that it has caused staff and supply shortages.

Nearly 100 vendors have stopped dealing with the hospital. . . .

Neil S. Rosenfeld, Newsday, *January 22, 1981*

Multihospital System's Allocation of Scarce Resources

At a time when many hospitals were on the brink of bankruptcy and struggling to survive, Brad, the administrator of a hospital in a multihospital system had a positive bottom line in the millions. The hospital was located in an upscale, affluent community. Unfortunately, the money was siphoned off to support the operations and capital projects of other hospitals in the system. Meanwhile, Brad's hospital was suffering from lack of supplies and funds for local capital projects.

Physicians and many community members, aware of the positive bottom line, were disturbed that the hospital's funds from operations and donations were being earmarked to fund the day-to-day operations of the system's failing hospitals. In addition, at a time when these hospitals were losing money, funds from Brad's hospital were being earmarked for major building projects in these hospitals, as well as corporate office projects.

It was like trying to squeeze blood out of a stone to get people to donate to their own community hospital. The community had no trust their donations would stay in the community.

Corporate leadership was expanding its capital projects, expanding nonrevenue-producing projects, relocating corporate offices to a more expensive site, building lavish suites, adding staff with vague job descriptions that served only to burden and penalize the revenue-producing entities, and jeopardizing patient care with their pet projects by deluging hospital staff with paperwork so they could produce even more paperwork to justify their own existence. Hospital staff felt that corporate staff had become an obstacle to the provision of high-quality patient care. No relief from battlefield fatigue seemed to be on the horizon.

Brad was able to work with some local community leaders (e.g., banker, lawyer, physician, newspaper editor, real estate agent) to establish a fundraising board whose mission was to oversee the local fundraising process and ensure the proper allocation of community funds to the local hospital. Although many corporate leaders privately objected to the concept, the corporate board reluctantly recognized the community board's existence, hoping to make inroads into the pockets of the wealthy. With half-hearted support by the corporation's leadership, the death of many of the founding fathers of the community board, and the resignation of Brad, who had developed the trust and provided the leadership, the community board slowly faded out of existence under the leadership of the administrators that followed him.

Anonymous

Discussion

1. Discuss the ethical issues related to Brad's dilemma regarding cash flow to other entities in the corporation. Do you consider this an isolated incident or an all too frequent occurrence with the rise of multihospital systems? Explain your answer.
2. Discuss what steps you would take to resolve the resource allocation issues if you were in Brad's position.
3. Discuss the community's reluctance to donate to the local hospital. What would you do?

COMPLY WITH RULES AND REGULATIONS

The governing body in general and its agents are responsible for compliance with federal, state, and local rules and regulations regarding the operation of the organization. Depending on the scope of the wrong committed and the intent of the governing body, failure to comply could subject board members and/or their agents to civil liability and, in some instances, to criminal prosecution. The following *reality check* describes what can happen when an organization fails to comply with the provisions of the Family Medical Leave Act (FMLA).

Noncompliance with the FMLA

The FMLA of 1993 was enacted to grant temporary medical leave to employees up to a total of 12 workweeks of unpaid leave during any 12-month period for such things as the birth and care of an employee's child, the care of an immediate family member with a serious health condition, or inability to work because of a serious health condition. After an FMLA leave, the employee's job—or an equivalent job with equivalent pay, benefits, and other terms and conditions of employment—must be restored.

Ten CEOs and human resource directors were randomly queried to determine their compliance with the FMLA. Specifically, in 9 of the 10 organizations queried, a nurse, for example, would be returned to the same or similar position without financial penalty (e.g., prorated salary increase) after her return from family leave.

One organization chose to penalize an employee's employment status by removing the employee's part-time status for the remainder of the year in which family leave had been granted and taken. In addition, this same organization's leaders prorated the employee's salary increase. In effect, this was a penalty that would be compounded each year the employee worked in the organization.

On appeal by the employee to the United States Department of Labor, this organization was required to reimburse the employee for lost wages unlawfully withheld from the employee during the year in which family leave had been taken.

Discussion

1. Discuss what recourse the employee has when faced with discriminatory practices, both within the corporation (e.g., register a complaint with the human resources department and/or corporate compliance officer) and outside the organization (e.g., file a complaint with the Department of Labor).
2. Such activities raise both legal (e.g., interpretation of the law) and ethical issues (e.g., nonmaleficence).

COMPLY WITH ACCREDITATION STANDARDS

Accredited hospitals are responsible for compliance with their accrediting body's standards (e.g., the Joint Commission). Failure to follow safe practices identified in accreditation standards can result in patient injuries such as noted in the following news clipping where patient equipment was disconnected because alarms were annoying to staff who became desensitized to the alarms—often as a result of frequent false alarms.

"Alarm Fatigue" Poses Risk for Hospital Patients

The sheer number—several hundred alarms per patient per day—can cause alarm fatigue. Nurses and other workers, overwhelmed or desensitized by the constant barrage, sometimes respond by turning down the volume on the devices, shutting them off or simply ignoring them—actions that can have serious, potentially fatal, consequences.

Clinicians and patient-safety advocates have warned of alarm fatigue for years, but the issue is taking on greater urgency as hospitals invest in more-complex, often-noisy devices meant to save lives. Last month, the Joint Commission, which accredits hospitals, directed facilities to make alarm safety a top priority or risk losing their accreditation.

Lena H. Sun, The Washington Post, *July 8, 2013*

Noncompliance with accreditation standards can lead to an organization's loss of accreditation, which in turn would provide grounds for third-party reimbursement agencies (e.g., Medicare) to deny payment for treatment. The following case describes how a patient alarm was disabled, resulting in the death of a patient.

CASE: MONITOR ALARM DISCONNECTED

In *Odom v. State Department of Health and Hospitals*,[17] the appeals court held that the decedent's cause of death was directly related to the absence of a heart monitor. Jojo was born 12 weeks prematurely at the HPL Medical Center. Jojo remained in a premature infant's nursery and was eventually placed into two different foster homes prior to his admission to Pinecrest foster home. While Jojo was a Pinecrest resident, Mr. and Mrs. Odom adopted Jojo. He was unable to feed himself and was nourished via a gastrostomy tube. Because he suffered from obstructive apnea, he became dependent on a tracheostomy (trach) tube.

At Pinecrest, Jojo was assigned to Home 501. While making patient rounds, Ms. Means found Jojo with his trach tube out of the stoma. She called for help, and Ms. Wiley, among others, responded. Wiley immediately took the CPR efforts under her control. She noticed that Jojo was breathless and immediately reinserted the trach tube. She then noticed that Jojo was still hooked to a monitor.

No one had heard the heart monitor's alarm sound. Means asserts that the monitor was on, because she saw that the monitor's red lights were blinking, indicating the heart rate and breathing rate. She stated that she took the monitor's leads off of Jojo to put the monitor out of the way, but the alarm did not sound. CPR efforts continued while Jojo was placed on a stretcher and sent by ambulance to HPL. Jojo was pronounced dead at HPL's emergency department at 7:02 p.m.

The Odoms filed a petition against Pinecrest, alleging that Jojo's death was caused by the negligence and fault of Pinecrest, its servants, and employees. Judgment was for the plaintiffs. The trial court's reasons for judgment were enlightening because it stated that the monitor should have been on but was, however, disconnected by the staff and that this was the cause, in fact, of Jojo's injury. The appeals court found that the record supported the trial court's findings. There was overwhelming evidence upon which the trial court relied to find that the monitor was turned off, in breach of the various physicians' orders with which the nurses should have complied. The monitor was supposed to be on Jojo to warn the nurses of any respiratory distress episodes that he might experience. A forensic pathologist's report showed the cause of Jojo's death to be hypoxia, secondary to respiratory insufficiency, secondary to apnea episodes. Thus, Jojo's cause of death was directly related to the absence of a heart monitor.

The accreditation process of a health care organization is a major event in its day-to-day operations. Organizations are expected to maintain a culture that supports patient safety and an environment that fosters respect, honesty, and compassionate care. The accreditation process is one of many tools that help ensure that high-quality care is being provided. As the following *reality check* illustrates, there are times when a wake-up call is necessary to alert leadership that the provision of high-quality care is no trivial event when your goal is to heal another human being.

Accreditation is Serious Business

Three field consultants were assigned by their employer, the National Accreditation Association (NAA), to review the quality of care being delivered at Newtown Medical Center and its three outpatient centers. Newtown was larger and even more complex than the consultants had anticipated, offering multiple services. On the first day of the consulting assignment, only three of the six assigned consultants reported to the medical center for duty. Patrick, the team leader, called the corporate office to discuss the need for additional help. Mike, the manager responsible for addressing field requests, did not return Patrick's call. Despite the lack of a follow-up call from Mike, the team covered the assigned task.

On the fourth day of the 5-day survey Cheri, Newtown's survey coordinator, asked Patrick if there was anything that needed to be covered prior to the exit conference to be held the following afternoon. Patrick replied, "Yes there is. At the leadership conference this morning there was no representation from the governing body. I find it difficult to score the various aspects of leadership since no one attended the scheduled interview."Somewhat concerned about the outcome of the quality review the following day when the consultants presented their report, Cheri said, "The medical center's leadership has not taken these surveys very seriously in the past. It has been an uphill battle to get them involved. Let me see what I can do to arrange for a leadership conference in the morning. We have 36 members on our board, hopefully I can find a few to attend." The following morning Cheri approached Michael and said, "I was able to convince two board members to meet with you at 11:00 a.m."

Michael met with the two board members along with the CEO. After the meeting had ended, a board member approached Michael and said, "You sure are persistent. But I must say it was truly a worthwhile meeting."

Discussion

1. Do you agree with Michael's persistence in conducting the leadership interview? Discuss your answer.
2. Because the survey team was short three consultants, would you consider this a meaningful survey as to the quality of care being rendered at Newtown Medical Center? Discuss your answer.
3. Do you think the CEO would complain about being billed for six consultants when only three were present to conduct the survey? Discuss your answer knowing that the results of the survey were positive and that three additional consultants could have added to the number of findings resulting in a more negative report and an unhappy board.

ACCREDITATION AND CONFLICT OF INTEREST

The mission of accrediting bodies is to improve the quality of care rendered in the nation's hospitals through its survey process. Accrediting bodies depend upon the hospitals they survey to reimburse them for the costs of those surveys. This obligates the accrediting body to maintain satisfied clients, and in so doing, a *conflict of interest* arises. How credible can a survey be when the accrediting body is dependent upon satisfied customers for financial survival? Further, hospitals evaluate the performance of the surveyors. Surveyors are expected to score an organization's performance knowing that organizations often challenge a surveyor's findings, which can lead to character assassination in the worst case scenario and/or a poor performance review of the surveyor by the organization. Conflicting interests here encourage surveyors/inspectors to be cautious about what they score because of fear of retaliation by both the organizations surveyed and the accrediting body that may side with the organization. Because of the financial implications for both the accrediting body and the surveyed organization, surveys are far from effective in protecting the consumer from human errors that result in more than 100,000 deaths and injuries annually in the nation's hospitals.

The food inspection process is remarkably similar to the hospital accreditation surveys:

- Food makers often know when inspectors will audit their facilities, and they vigorously prepare for those inspections. This was also true with hospitals until the Joint Commission, for example, decided to conduct unannounced surveys. This change occurred mostly because of criticism from surveyors, the Centers for Medicare and Medicaid, the public, and some of the surveyed organizations. But the wheels of change move slowly; more than a decade passed before the Joint Commission submitted to the long overdue change.
- Most food makers score high in their inspections and still have recalls and outbreaks.
- As with hospitals, the food companies typically pay food industry inspectors, creating a conflict of interest for inspectors who might fear they will lose business if they do not hand out high ratings.

Hospital scores were eventually discontinued in the accreditation process because of criticism on numerous occasions from both its own surveyors and accredited hospitals. Because of the competition among hospitals, the surveyors were pressured to provide high scores by the organizations it surveyed. As noted in the following *reality check* patients who passed away in high-scoring hospitals were not all pleased with the scores some hospitals were receiving.

One Family's Experience

It was early winter and Mary Ann had continuous headaches for more than a year. Dr. Fastrack, her family physician, examined her and diagnosed her with migraines. Handing her a prescription for ibuprofen, Dr. Fastrack said, "Mary Ann, it is stress related. Maybe some meditation would be helpful." That following summer Mary Ann went to the Jersey shore, where she had been going on vacation for several years. While she was there she experienced excruciating headaches. She went to a local emergency room where they also diagnosed her with a severe migraine. Mary Ann returned home and was eventually examined by a neurologist who ordered a brain scan. She was diagnosed with a brain tumor in her right frontal lobe, the same area of the head she hit when she went through a car window 17 years earlier. About a year following radiation treatment she was told she was in remission. It was Christmas and she immediately called her brother who was at his in-laws, to tell him the good news. Mary Ann never saw another Christmas. Several years following her death, her daughter, my niece said, "Can you believe the hospital where my mom died had advertised in our local newspaper that it scored 100 on a hospital accreditation survey. There wasn't even a physician on duty in the emergency room. I wouldn't take my dog to that hospital. They killed my mom."

Anonymous

Clearly, the banking industry, food industry, and health care industry all share one major disturbing characteristic: there is a blatant conflict of interest between the inspecting agencies and the entities they are inspecting. As noted in the following *reality check*, someone needs to regulate the regulators.

Integrity Can Be Lost Through Greed

Forever Anonymous, Inc. (FA) employees are prohibited from consulting with accredited health care organizations during their employment with FA. In addition, employees are prohibited, for 3 years following termination, from consulting with any organizations they may have surveyed during their tenure with FA.

It is believed that not all members of FA's leadership have been following this policy after termination of their employment. Employees were questioning among themselves, does this policy apply only to rank-and-file employees, or does it include FA's leadership? Should the FA board investigate what organizations former FA leaders have been consulting with and in what capacity? Should FA's board investigate what members of leadership have consulted and/or continue to consult? And what is the propriety of such consultations?

The importance of this policy is apparent. During a survey, some hospitals through their leadership, often let it be known to the inspectors, accidentally of course, what former members of FA's leadership they have been consulting with to prepare for their survey, expecting some leniency will be shown by the surveyors during the survey process. Yes, unfortunately, there are often some members of an organization's leadership who are more concerned about the results of a survey and how it might affect their jobs than about how it affects the quality of patient care in their organization.

Anonymous

Discussion

1. Describe how the FA board could address this issue.
2. Identify the ethical issues in this *reality check*.

PROVIDE TIMELY TREATMENT

VA, Heal Thyself, Agency Is Told at Hearing Filled with Pained Testimony

VA officials in Pittsburgh knew of an outbreak of Legionnaires' disease, "but they kept it a secret for more than a year."

VA staff in Buffalo potentially exposed patients to hepatitis and HIV by reusing disposable insulin injection pens. "At least 18 veteran patients have tested positive for hepatitis so far."

VA workers, patients and family members had "a series of allegations" regarding "poor care" at the Dallas VA medical center.

Employee whistleblowers at the VA medical center in Jackson, Miss., reported "poor sterilization procedures, understaffing and misdiagnoses" to the Office of Special Counsel, an independent federal watchdog.

Joe Davidson, The Washington Post, *September 13, 2013*

Health care organizations are expected to provide timely treatment to patients. Hospitals can be liable for delays in treatment that result in injuries to their patients. For example, the patient in *Heddinger v. Ashford Memorial Community Hospital*[18] filed a malpractice action against a hospital and its insurer, alleging that a delay in treating her left hand resulted in the loss of her little finger. Medical testimony presented at trial indicated that if proper and timely treatment had been rendered, the finger would have been saved. The U.S. District Court entered judgment on a jury verdict for the plaintiff in the amount of $175,000. The hospital appealed, and the U.S. Court of Appeals held that even if the physicians who attended the patient were not employees of the hospital but were independent contractors, the risk of negligent treatment was clearly foreseeable by the hospital.

The following *reality check* describes one consultant's experience in the VA hospital system.

Veterans' Care Unconscionably Delayed

I surveyed more than 500 hospitals. At one point I asked not to be placed on Veterans hospital accreditation surveys. Not all but some of the Veterans Administration (VA) hospitals were very argumentative fearing the possibility of written citations. So much so that on a ride from one VA hospital in Pennsylvania to a Pittsburgh VA the referring VA hospital sent three staff members to chauffeur me to the Pittsburgh VA. They all argued my concerns that a veteran on a 6-month waiting list for a neurological consult was too long. They kept arguing, not discussing, that if he needed immediate attention he would have been referred to a local civilian hospital for care. I said, "In my opinion, if he needs a neurological consult, he needs it now. Not 6 months from now."

Anonymous

Discussion

1. Based on this *reality check*, what action should the VA leadership take in order to prevent such occurrences in the future?
2. Discuss how this situation might have been different if the veteran was a relative of one of the employees accompanying the surveyor in the car.

AVOID CONFLICTS OF INTEREST

Suspicious Consulting Fees

About 800,000 Americans will get a new hip or knee this year, up 63% from 491,000 in 2001. Now a U.S. Department of Justice investigation reveals that many orthopedic surgeons have been pocketing hundreds of thousands of dollars in "consulting fees" with the understanding that they would implant a particular company's device—even if it wasn't the best choice for a patient.

The country's top five medical device makers, which account for nearly 95% of the knee and hip implants on the market, have been implicated.

Catherine Guthrie, Oprah Magazine, *May 2008*

A conflict of interest involves situations where a person has the opportunity to promote self-interests that could have a detrimental effect on an organization with which he or she has a special relationship (e.g., employee, board member). The potential for conflict of interest exists for individuals at all levels within an organization. Disclosure of potential conflicts of interest should be made so that appropriate action may be taken to ensure that such conflict does not inappropriately influence important organization and health care decisions. Board members, physicians, and employees are required by most organizations to submit a form disclosing potential conflicts of interest that might negatively affect the organization's reputation or financial resources.

CASE: CORPORATE COVER-UP

The case of *Advocat, Inc. v. Sauer*[19] involved the care of Mrs. Sauer, a 93-year-old nursing facility patient. On July 19, 1998, her vital signs began to decline, and the nursing staff reported this to her treating physician, who ordered that she be taken to the emergency department at a nearby medical center. She arrived at the hospital in a semicomatose condition and died about 16 hours later.

Nursing notes indicated that Sauer had lost 15 pounds in the previous month and was in need of a feeding tube. There were signs of bedsores on her body caused by lying in urine and excrement. Sauer's estate sued for damages.

The trial began and lasted 8 days, with 28 witnesses testifying and 24 binders of exhibits. At the trial's conclusion, the jury retired to consider four counts: ordinary negligence, medical malpractice, breach of contract, and wrongful death. The jury returned a verdict for the Sauer Estate on all counts. Total damages amounted to more than $78 million. On appeal, the appellants argued that the damage awards for negligence and medical malpractice were grossly excessive.

The appellants argued that long-term care surveys conducted at the facility had been admitted into evidence over their objection. They claimed that the survey results inflamed the jury because the surveys were replete with statements that there was not enough help in the nursing home to feed, bathe, or clean residents.

They further argued that testimony submitted by witnesses that the nursing home had engaged in "false charting" to show more staff than were actually present was prejudicial, because it suggested that the appellants had staffing inadequacies that they tried to conceal from the state.

Sauer died of severe malnutrition and dehydration. There was evidence presented that she was found at times with dried feces under her fingernails from scratching herself while lying in her own excrement. At other times, staff did not get her out of her bed as they should have. Often, Sauer's food tray was found in her room, untouched, because there was no staff member at the nursing home available to feed her. She was not provided with range-of-motion assistance when the facility was short of staff.

Sauer had pressure sores on her back, lower buttock, and arms. A former staff member remembered seeing Sauer at one time with an open pressure sore the size of a softball. At times, she had no water pitcher in her room, nor did she receive a bath for a week or more because of shortage of staff. Sauer was found to suffer from poor oral hygiene, having caked food and debris in her mouth.

The appellate court found that the jury verdicts were not based on passion or prejudice. There was ample testimony and evidence to demonstrate that plaintiff's decedent suffered considerably and was not properly cared for in the nursing home, that the home was short-staffed, and that the home tried to cover this up by "false charting" and by bringing in additional employees on state inspection days. All of that served to support the estate's case that the nursing home knew it had staffing problems and committed negligence as to the decedent because it was short-staffed due to cutbacks.

The appellate court found that the circuit court abused its discretion by not granting a new trial due to excessive damages.

Ethical and Legal Issues

1. Describe the legal and ethical issues presented this case.
2. According to a federal study, nearly 90% of the nation's nursing homes are poorly staffed and find it difficult to provide basic services, such as cleaning, dressing, grooming, and feeding their residents.[20] Assuming the accuracy of this number, discuss how you would distribute limited dollars to address this issue. Consider how your decision may affect the allocation of funds to other health-related programs (e.g., immunizations, prenatal care, and preventative medicine). Assume that no new dollars can be allocated for the new health care budget year.

PROVIDE A SAFE ENVIRONMENT

Hospitals are required to provide a safe environment for patients, visitors, and staff. Safety concerns in hospitals flow from general mechanical safety to direct patient care in the operating room.

Efforts to End Surgeries on Wrong Patient or Body Part Falters

"Health care has far too little accountability for results. . . . All the pressures are on the side of production; that's how you get paid," said Hopkins's [Peter] Pronovost [safety expert and medical director of the John Hopkins Center for Innovation in Quality Patient Care], who adds that increased pressure to turn over operating rooms quickly has trumped patient safety, increasing the chance of error.

Sandra G. Boodman, Kaiser Health News, *June 20, 2011*[21]

Employers are required by law and accreditation standards to provide a safe environment for patients, visitors, and employees. Although one cannot guard against the unforeseeable, a health care organization is liable, as noted in the next case, for injuries resulting from dangers that it knowingly failed to guard against or those that it should have known about and failed to guard against. An organization has a duty to safeguard the welfare of its patients, even from harm by third persons, and that duty is measured by the ability of the patient to provide for his or her own safety.

CASE: CHALLENGING THE OBVIOUS—RUNAWAY ELEVATOR

Approximately 100 years ago, the Maryland Court of Appeals held that one who "is engaged in the undertaking of running an elevator as a means of personal transportation" is required to use the "highest degree of care and diligence practicable under the circumstances," which is the same standard that common carriers are required to meet.

On August 30, 2000, Jane Correia was a passenger in an elevator owned and operated by Johns Hopkins Health Services Company and Johns Hopkins Hospital. The elevator came to a sudden stop because of a mechanical defect. Due to injuries allegedly caused by this malfunction, Mrs. Correia and her husband sued Johns Hopkins, and others, in the Circuit Court for Baltimore City for negligence. A jury considered the matter in October 2005.

The Correias introduced evidence that showed that, in the 6 months prior to the accident, Johns Hopkins had received 32 complaints about the elevator Mrs. Correia was in when the accident occurred. The 32 complaints, if accurate, indicated that at various times prior to the accident the elevator was dropping, jumping, jerking, skipping, and sometimes trapping passengers.

At the end of a 9-day trial, the court gave the jury the following instruction:

The owner of a passenger elevator, in this case . . . Johns Hopkins is the owner of the passenger elevator, is bound to exercise to the highest degree of care and skill and diligence . . . practicable under the circumstances to guard against injury to individuals riding on those elevators. This rule of law applies to the owner of the elevator only. It does not apply to the service company [codefendant] Schindler [Elevator Company].

The jury returned a verdict in favor of Mrs. Correia in the amount of $264,500 and a separate $35,500 verdict in favor of Mr. and Mrs. Correia, jointly, for loss of consortium. Both verdicts were against Johns Hopkins; the jury found that codefendant Schindler Elevator Company was not negligent.

Johns Hopkins appealed, contending, among other things, that the trial judge committed reversible error in giving the instruction quoted previously.

On appeal, the Maryland Court of Appeals held that, from the record, it did not appear that this was a "close case" as to whether Johns Hopkins exercised the highest degree of care for Mrs. Correia's safety. There was strong evidence that it had not met its duty, especially in light of the numerous complaints about the elevator in the 6 months prior to the accident. The case, it appears, was "close" as to the issue of causation in that there was room for doubt as to whether an abrupt stop of a low-speed elevator could have caused the extensive injuries claimed.

The Court of Special Appeals of Maryland determined that the trial judge did not abuse his discretion in denying the motion for mistrial. The judgment was affirmed, with costs to be paid by Johns Hopkins Hospital and John Hopkins Health Service Company.[22]

Ethical and Legal Issues

1. Do you believe that this case should have been settled out of court? Discuss your answer.
2. Explain how would you have handled this case. Discuss your answer.

PREVENTION OF FALLS

The patient in *Thomas v. Sisters of Charity of the Incarnate Word*[23] fell three stories to his death after he became locked out on the hospital roof and sat on a ledge in an apparent attempt to attract someone to get assistance. The trial court found that the fire exit configuration that allowed the patient access to the roof created an unreasonable risk of harm that was in fact the cause of his death.

There was testimony that the lack of signage violated both the Life Safety and 1988 Standard Building Codes. Standard building code required that signs direct an individual to the exit discharge or ultimate exit to the outside of the building. A lack of signage also violated hospital policy requiring that the roof should have been marked as a restricted area. The exit configuration was unsafe for either ordinary or emergency use because of the confusion encountered by an individual locked out of the building without any direction or instruction on where to go. Given the hospital's duty regarding this exit, its breach of that duty was clear. The door to the roof contained no warning that it would lock the patient out of the building if he exited. Whether the patient exited the building voluntarily or out of momentary confusion, the hospital breached its duty to warn him that he would be locked out and to direct him across the catwalk to the fire exit stairwell.

PROTECT PATIENTS AND STAFF FROM SEXUAL ASSAULT

Hospitals are expected to protect patients and staff from sexual assault. A claim that a hospital was negligent in preventing such an assault will succeed only if such an assault is foreseeable. Such was not the case in following example.

CASE: SEXUAL ASSAULT IN THE RECOVERY ROOM

The plaintiff was recovering from vaginal surgery. A surgical resident, employed by the hospital sexually assaulted her during her recovery. There is no dispute about the assault or the resident's liability. The question here is whether the hospital may be liable under a theory of vicarious liability or for negligence in its duty to protect the plaintiff.

The plaintiff, under the effects of anesthesia following surgery, was placed in a small four-bed recovery room. Nurse R, accompanied by another nurse, admitted the plaintiff to the unit and monitored her vital signs. Minutes later, the nurses turned their attention to a second patient who had been placed on an adjacent bed two feet away and were soon joined by Nurse G, their supervisor. Privacy curtains between the plaintiff and the second patient had not been drawn.

A surgical resident wearing hospital scrubs and an identification badge entered the recovery room and went to the plaintiff's bed. He was not one of the physicians listed on the plaintiff's chart, and none of the nurses knew him. According to the plaintiff, she awoke to find the resident pulling up her hospital gown and performing an "internal pelvic exam," which was contraindicated in light of the nature of the plaintiff's surgery. The plaintiff tried to sit up and cover herself with the gown and repeatedly asked him to stop. On her third plea, the physician hastily began to leave the recovery room. After the plaintiff complained to the nurses about what had taken place, the supervising nurse confronted the resident, who admitted that he had examined the plaintiff without the presence of a female witness, as required by hospital policy. The hospital terminated the resident following an investigation.

The Appellate Division Majority reasoned that a direct negligence claim must fail because the resident's misconduct was not foreseeable. The court also dismissed the vicarious liability claim against the hospital because the physician was acting outside the scope of his authority.

Two dissenting judges disagreed with the majority. They noted that the majority's holding on the direct negligence cause of action failed to consider the actual foreseeability of harm, indicated by observations the hospital staff could or should have made at the time immediately preceding the actual wrongdoing.

Nurse R had acknowledged that residents were not directly assigned to the recovery room. Her deposition testimony further indicated that she was aware of the identity of all of the plaintiff's physicians and that the resident was not one of those assigned to the plaintiff's care. In fact, all of the nurses in the recovery room were unacquainted with the resident. All of the nurses knew of the hospital's policy requiring the presence of a female staff member during a male physician's pelvic examination of a female patient.

Despite the nurses' assertions that they saw or heard nothing, an additional key question of credibility arises from the inference created by the undisputed close proximity of all of the nurses to the plaintiff's bed.

In contrast to the Appellate Division majority opinion, the dissenting judges considered that this confluence of factors provided a sufficient basis from which a jury could determine that the nurses unreasonably disregarded that which was readily there to be seen and heard, alerting them to the risk of misconduct against the plaintiff by the resident, which could have been prevented. Accordingly, the Appellate Division order was modified by remitting the case to the Supreme Court (trial court in New York) for further proceedings.[24]

Ethical and Legal Issues

1. Describe the ethical and legal issues presented in this case.
2. Describe how the physician's professional code of ethics was breached.

DECISIONS THAT COLLIDE WITH PROFESSIONAL ETHICS

Management's financial decisions can at times be on a collision course with practice and professional codes of ethics. The principles of autonomy, beneficence, and justice and the ability to practice what is right according to such principles often collide when organizations have to, for example, ration scarce resources. Such rationing may require managers to cut costs at the expense of quality.

A LIFE NEEDLESSLY SHORTENED

An action filed against a health insurance company alleged that the way the insurer handled the insured's chemotherapy needlessly shortened her life, causing her last days to be more painful than they should have been. The jury awarded the plaintiff $49 million. The punitive damages award was considered excessive under Ohio law, and the trial court's failure to find as such was so unreasonable as to constitute abuse of discretion. A $30 million award was appropriate given the profits of the corporations involved and appropriate in the scheme of past punitive damages awards in Ohio.[25]

FINANCIAL INCENTIVE SCHEMES

The managed care industry has historically failed to acknowledge the practice of denying medical claims at the expense of the patient's health, while at the same time benefiting managed care organizations. Dr. Linda Peeno, a Medical Reviewer for Humana, exposed this practice during her testimony before Congress, which stated in part:[26]

> I wish to begin by making a public confession: In the spring of 1987, as a physician, I caused the death of a man.
>
> Although this was known to many people, I have not been taken before any court of law or called to account for this in any professional or public forum. In fact, just the opposite occurred: I was "rewarded" for this. It bought me an improved reputation in my job, and contributed to my advancement afterwards. Not only did I demonstrate I could indeed do what was expected of me, I exemplified the "good" company doctor: I saved a half million dollars!
>
> Since that day, I have lived with this act, and many others, eating into my heart and soul. For me, a physician is a professional charged with the care, or healing, of his or her fellow human beings. The primary ethical norm is: do no harm. I did worse: I caused a death. Instead of using a clumsy, bloody weapon, I used the simplest, cleanest of tools: my words. The man died because I denied him a necessary operation to save his heart. I felt little pain or remorse at the time. The man's faceless distance soothed my conscience. Like a skilled soldier, I was trained for this moment. When any moral qualms arose, I was to remember: I am not denying care; I am only denying payment.
>
> • • •
>
> For me, "ethics" must be done close range. Distance blurs the complexities of human experiences. Those who argue that "the further removed, the clearer the thinking" are those who too often use "ethics" as legalism, public relations, or high-sounding rationalization. I would argue that, at least in medicine, one's ethical "authority" diminishes the further one is from the frontlines of patient experiences.[27]

Dr. Peeno came forward with her story and dedicated her career to helping others in a compassionate manner working in the field of health care ethics.

> As part of this effort, I chair a hospital ethics committee (University of Louisville Hospital), for which I do consultation, education and policy development. I am the executive director of an international academic society (International Society for the Systems Sciences), and as chair of its Medicine and Healthcare group, I work on ethical issues in international health care systems. I serve on the national board of Citizen Action, a nonpartisan consumer organization, through which I work toward equitable health reform. I am the founder of the CARE Foundation, a nonprofit group organized to promote consumer education, public accountability, and ethical responsibility in managed care. I am here to represent the largest interest group in our health care system: those affected by its design and operations, those who validate its consequences within their lives.[28]

Greg Ganske addressed the House of Representative on March 28, 2000:

Let me give my colleagues one example out of many of a health plan's definition of medically necessary services. "Medical necessity means the shortest, least expensive or least intense level of treatment, care or service rendered or supply provided as determined by us." Well, Mr. Speaker, contracts like this demonstrate that some health plans are manipulating the definition of medical necessity to deny appropriate patient care by arbitrarily linking it to saving money, not the patient's medical needs.[29]

Recently, the medical community has turned its attention to the authority of state medical boards to police improper physician expert testimony in medical malpractice actions. The discussion has been broadened to consider whether the presentation of testimony constitutes the carrying out of the practice of medicine. Depending on the state, some cases have held that the "carrying out" requirement means that the medical judgment must affect or have the possibility of affecting the patient. For example, in *Murphy v. Board of Medical Examiners*,[30] an Arizona court held that a physician performing prospective utilization review was practicing medicine because his decisions "could affect" a patient's health. Dr. Peeno was engaging in prospective utilization review; however, several federal courts have held that neither prospective nor retrospective review constituted the practice of medicine.[31] The public does, however, have the right to expect expert physicians to be accurate and truthful when giving testimony. If the profession cannot police itself, then the states will be forced to intervene in order to protect the public.

The patient in *Shea v. Esensten*[32] died after suffering a heart attack. Although the patient had recently visited his primary care physician and presented with symptoms of cardiac problems and the patient also had a family history of cardiac trouble, the physician did not refer the patient to a cardiologist. The patient's widow sued the health management organization for failing to disclose the financial incentive system it provided to its physicians to minimize referrals to specialists. The United States Court of Appeals for the Eighth Circuit agreed that knowledge of financial incentives that affect a physician's decisions to refer patients to specialists is material information requiring disclosure. The appeals court reversed a lower court's dismissal of the claim.

RESTORING TRUST

The lack of trust is slowly deteriorating the people's faith in the nation's health care system. A lack of trust in the physician, hospital, and insurer is pervasive throughout the health care system. The horror stories in newspapers, malpractice suits, and the Institute of Medicine's report on health care mistakes identify problems and provide a catalyst for encouraging lawsuits.

Organizations need to make a concerted effort to develop strategies to build and restore trust in the health care industry. The following strategies assist in building consumer trust:

- Conduct business in compliance with applicable laws, rules, and regulations.
- Adhere to ethical standards.

- Provide cost-effective care.
- Fairly and accurately represent the organization's capabilities when treating a patient's ailments.
- Maintain a uniform standard of care throughout the organization, regardless of a person's ability to pay, race, creed, color, and/or national origin.
- Consider patient values and preferences as part of recognizing the organization's legal responsibilities.
- Inform patients of their rights and responsibilities.
- Develop and recommend guidelines that assist and support patients and their families in exercising their rights.
- Describe the process to patients by which hospital staff interact and care for them.

Trust must begin within the organization between management and employees. As the following *reality check* describes, organizations can often become dysfunctional and cause employee turnover and resentment among employees.

Equal Pay for Equal Work?

The annual Health Systems Consulting conference was held at the New York City Hilton. During the closing session on Friday, the company's leadership sat onstage summarizing the week's training and conducting a question-and-answer period. Prior to the session, Frank, an administrator consultant, had asked his manager, "The grapevine is telling me that nurses have been placed at a higher pay rate than administrators. Is that true?" His manager replied, "You asked a direct question, so I will answer it, even though per company policy we don't generally share such information.

The answer is yes. It was implemented several weeks ago. The consulting process is more and more clinical and therefore nurses are getting a higher starting salary." Frank answered, "That is true, but we still all do the same work." His manager replied, "That's the way it is," and walked away.

Anonymous

Discussion

1. Because employment law requires equal pay for equal work, what ethical concerns do you see in this case?
2. If you were Frank, what action would you pursue, if any?

Questions Solicited Not Always Welcomed

When you question a company policy, even after company insistence that all questions are welcomed, there can be a price to be paid. Gerard asked anyway, "Since the health survey process is leaning more toward the clinical side of care and we are attempting to get more physician involvement in the patient care review process, why aren't physicians the team leaders? After all, they have the best clinical judgment."

The leadership were basically at a loss about what to say but in the end gave the usual response by stating they would look into it. One physician stood and said, "Nurses are better at this process than physicians." The room became silent and the physician received some glares from his colleagues. The leadership quickly moved on to the next question.

Gerard later received several conflicting comments from his colleagues in the lobby:

Nurse Consultant 1: "I knew you were an ****. Now, I know you are an ****. I will give you the dirtiest work on the survey when you are on a consulting job with me!"

Nurse 2: "You're senile!"

Nurse 3: "You had the courage to say what you think."

AF Nurse practitioner/Consultant 4: "You stood up for something you believed in. I admire you for that."

Nurse Consultant 5: "Nurses are more clinically adept than physicians."

Nurse 6: "Gerard, some of those nurses were pretty awful to you. Why don't you join us for something to eat?"

Nurse 7: "We don't agree with all you said, but we respect your opinion."

Nurse 8: "You had the courage to say what you think."

Physician Consultant 1: "You will most likely find a horse's head in your bed in the morning."

Physician Consultant 3: "Gerard, I agreed with you, but was it really worth it?"

Physician Consultant 4: "I see you're still alive."

Gerard, somewhat despondent, walked away and into the lobby gift shop. He spotted an article in the *Washington Post*.

The Role of Nurses Extends Beyond the Hospital Ward

A nurse is a doctor's best friend, according to Marvin M. Lipman, Consumers Union's chief medical adviser. This advice was given to him by a hospital ward's head nurse when he was a third-year medical student making contact with patients for the first time, along with the suggestion that he'd do well not to forget it.

Over the years, those words continued to echo in Lipman's mind. In part because hospital nurses work for the institution and many doctors work for themselves, occasional conflicts between the two are inevitable. When encountering such situations, he has generally tended to take the side of the nurses, sometimes to the chagrin of his fellow physicians. But he explains that his loyalty comes from the many times he has seen nurses go that extra step to make a patient more comfortable or more at ease.

Consumers Union of United States Inc., The Washington Post, May 30, 2011

Discussion

1. Gerard is a congenial, humorous, and respected person. His colleagues know that he does give his opinion if he sees a wrong that should be righted, whether it is for him or others. Should he have spoken up or remained silent? Discuss your answer.
2. Based on the *Washington Post* article, do you think Gerard might have had second thoughts about his concerns?
3. Describe the actions of Gerard's colleagues and what ethical theories might apply.

EFFECTIVE COMMUNICATION BUILDS TRUST

Effective communication spawns trust and is commonly acknowledged as a deciding factor in building a harmonious organization. All the players must work together and understand the role each plays. As in an orchestra **(Figure 8-1)**, the instruments must work together to produce harmony. The better the musicians play, the more satisfied the audience. Even if you were able to play all the instruments in the orchestra, you can play only one at a time. During an interview with PBS Dr. William Edwards Deming, an American author, professor, and consultant, stated that in a "140 piece orchestra, everybody supports the other 139. He's not there to play a solo. He's not to play as loud as he can play to attract attention. He's there to support the other 139. The job of the conductor is to optimize their talents, their abilities."[33] And so it is with health care workers; they are there to support one another and *each caregiver trusts the other to play his or her part well.* The better the teamwork in the health care setting the better the care, which in turn breeds satisfied patients, families, and staff.

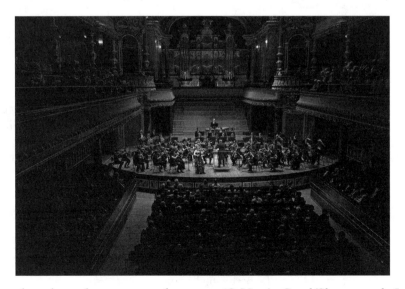

FIGURE 8-1   Together, the orchestra creates harmony. (© Martin Good/Shutterstock, Inc.)

CHAPTER REVIEW

1. This chapter introduces the reader to the ethical responsibilities and legal risks of health care organizations.
2. Authority of a corporation is expressed in the law under which the corporation is chartered.
   - Governing body
     - *Express* corporate authority
       - *Verbal*
       - *Written*
     - *Implied* corporate authority
     - *Ultra vires acts*
       - Acts violate a corporation's scope of authority.
3. Organization code of ethics
   - Provides guidelines for behavior that help carry out an organization's mission, vision, and values.
   - Builds trust.
   - Increases awareness of ethical issues.
   - Guides decision making.
   - Encourages staff to seek advice and report organizational misconduct.
4. Unethical organizational conduct
   - Trust and Integrity
   - False Advertising
   - Concealing Mistakes
   - Financial Incentive Schemes
5. Corporate negligence
   - Failure to perform duties owed directly to a patient or anyone else to whom a duty may extend.
   - *Theory of corporate negligence*—if a corporate duty is breached and a patient is injured as a result of that breach, the organization can be held liable for the injuries suffered.
6. Doctrine of *Respondeat superior*
   - A legal doctrine holding an employer liable for the wrongful acts of its agents (employees).
   - *Respondeat superior* has also been referred to as *vicarious liability*, whereby an employer is answerable for the torts committed by its employees.
   - *Darling v. Charleston Community Memorial Hospital*[34] is the benchmark case, which has had a major impact on the liability of health care organizations.
   - The court here enunciated a "corporate negligence doctrine," under which hospitals have a duty to provide adequately trained medical and nursing staff.
7. Independent contractors
   - Responsible for their own negligent acts.
   - Occurs when the principal has no right of control over the manner in which the agent's work is to be performed.

8. Corporate duties and responsibilities
   * Appointment of a CEO
   * Credentialing, appointments, and privileging of professional staff
   * Provide adequate staff
   * Provide adequate supplies and equipment
   * Allocation of scarce resources
   * Comply with rules and regulations
   * Comply with accreditation standards
   * Provide timely treatment
   * Avoid conflicts of interest
   * Provide a safe environment
   * Protect patients and staff from sexual assault
9. Build and restore trust through effective communications.

TEST YOUR UNDERSTANDING

TERMINOLOGY

codes of ethics for organizations

conflict of interest

corporate authority

corporate negligence

credentialing

Darling v. Charleston Community Memorial Hosp.

delineation of clinical privileges

express corporate authority

implied corporate authority

independent contractor

respondeat superior

ultra vires acts

REVIEW QUESTIONS

1. Discuss the governing body's decision-making authority.

2. Explain what an *ultra varies act* is.

3. Describe the important aspects of a code of ethics for organizations.

4. Discuss the various forms of professional misconduct discussed here.

5. Describe the relationship between *corporate negligence, respondeat superior,* and *independent contractor.*

6. Describe the duties and responsibilities of health care organizations and how the failure to adhere those duties and responsibilities can result in both legal and ethical issues.

7. Discuss how an organization's decisions can collide with professional ethics.

8. Discuss the importance of effective communications in building trust in the health care setting.

NOTES

1. http://www.wbaltv.com/news/maryland/baltimore-county/settlement-reached-in-st-joes-medical-malpractice-case/-/10136486/19985154/-/91thi9z/-/index.html
2. 745 N.Y.S.2d 304 (N.Y. App. Div. 2002).
3. *Thompson v. Nason Hosp.,* 591 A.2d 703, 707 (Pa. 1991).
4. *Id.*
5. 211 N.E.2d 253 (Ill. 1965).
6. Id. at 260.
7. 46 U.S.I.W. 2227 (Md. 1977).
8. http://www.ache.org/abt_ache/code.cfm.
9. CBSNews.com, "Did hospitals 'see no evil'?" April 4, 2004; http://www.cbsnews.com/stories/2004/04/02/60minutes/main610047.shtml
10. No. 05AP-681 (Ohio App. 2006).
11. 543 So. 2d 209 (Fla. 1989).
12. http://www.jointcommission.org/jc_physician_blog/revisiting_disruptive_and_inappropriate_behavior/.
13. http://www.ama-assn.org/ama/pub/physician-resources/medical-ethics/code-medical-ethics/opinion9045.page.
14. No. A03A2308 (Ga. App. 2004).
15. *Medcalf v. Coleman,* No. 98906 (2003).
16. *Freilich v. Upper Chesapeake Health, Inc.,* 313 F.3d 205 (2002).
17. 733 So. 2d 91 (La. App. 3 Cir. 1999).
18. 734 F.2d 81 (1st Cir. 1984).
19. 111 S.W.3d 346 (2003).
20. Christopher Newton, "90% of nursing homes providing substandard care–federal report," *Seattle Times,* February 20, 2002, at A1.
21. Sandra G. Boodman, "Effort to end surgeries on wrong patient or body part falters," June 20, 2011; http://www.kaiserhealthnews.org/Stories/2011/June/21/wrong-site-surgery-errors.aspx.
22. *The Johns Hopkins Hospital, et al. v. Jane E.S. Correia, et ux.,* 174 Md. App. 359, 921 A.2d 837 (2007).
23. No. 38,170 (La. App. 2004).
24. *N.X. v. Cabrini Med. Ctr.,* 765 N.E.2d 844 (2002).
25. 107 F.3d 625 & 8th Circuit (1997).
26. Available at http://wn.com/Linda_Peeno.
27. http://www.thenationalcoalition.org/DrPeenotestimony.html#c6.
28. http://www.thenationalcoalition.org/DrPeenotestimony.html#c6.
29. House of Representatives, "Important issue facing House-Senate Conference on Health Care Reform," March 28, 2000; http://www.fenichel.com/Ganske.shtml.
30. 949 P2d 530,535 (Ariz. Ct. App. 1997).
31. *Adnan Varol, M.D., P.C. v. Blue Cross Blue Shield of Mich.,* 708 F. Supp. 826 (E.D. Mich. 1989); *Corcoran v. United Health Care,* 956 F.2d 1321 (5th Cir. 1992).
32. http://biotech.law.lsu.edu/cases/hmo/shea_v_esensten.htm
33. http://www.getbig.com/boards/index.php?topic=179701.0.
34. *Dardinger, Exr. v. Anthem Blue Cross and Blue Shield,* 2002 Ohio 7113 (Ohio 2002).

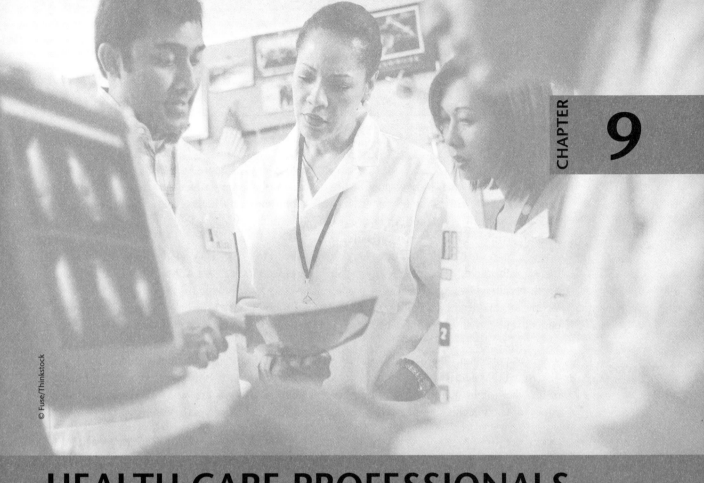

© Fuse/Thinkstock

CHAPTER 9

HEALTH CARE PROFESSIONALS LEGAL–ETHICAL ISSUES

Ethics is nothing else than reverence for life.

—ALBERT SCHWEITZER

LEARNING OBJECTIVES

Upon completion of this chapter, the reader will be able to:

- Identify a variety of ethical and legal issues that arise in selected health care professions (e.g., nursing, emergency services, laboratory, pharmacy, radiology).
- Explain how practicing one's professional code of ethics can assist in resolving day-to-day issues that arise during patient care.
- Explain the difference between the certification and licensure of a health care professional.
- Identify helpful suggestions that help caregivers provide high-quality care.

INTRODUCTION

My life is my message.

—MAHATMA GANDHI

This chapter presents an overview of how ethics and the law affect a variety of health care professions. The ethical codes for each profession demand a high level of integrity, honesty, and responsibility. Codes of ethics are designed to facilitate the resolution of common ethical dilemmas that arise in one's profession.

The contents of codes of ethics vary depending on the risks associated with a particular profession. Ethical codes for psychologists, for example, define relationships with clients in greater depth because of the personal one-to-one relationship they have with their clients. Laboratory technicians and technologists, on the other hand, generally have little or no personal contact with patients but can have a significant impact on their care. Laboratory technologists in their ethical code pledge accuracy and reliability in the performance of tests. The importance of this pledge was borne out in a March 11, 2004, report by the *Baltimore Sun* wherein state health officials discovered that a hospital's laboratory personnel overrode controls in testing equipment showing results that might be in error and then mailed them to patients anyway.[1] The various codes of ethics for each health care profession are accessible by profession on the Internet.

NURSES—ETHICS AND LEGAL ISSUES

To Be a Nurse: Swedish Hospital, Seattle, Washington

- *In memory of all those patients that have enriched my life and blessed me with their spirit of living—while they are dying.*
- *Nursing is the honor and privilege of caring for the needs of individuals in their time of need. The responsibility is one of growth to develop the mind, soul, and physical well-being of oneself as well as the one cared for.*
- *Excellence is about who we are, what we believe in, what we do with everyday of our lives. And in some ways we are a sum total of those who have loved us and those who we have given ourselves to.*
- *I have been with a number of people/patients when they die and have stood in awe. Nursing encompasses the sublime and the dreaded. We are regularly expected to do the impossible. I feel honored to be in this profession.*
- *To get well I knew I had to accept the care and love that were given to me—when I did healing washed over me like water.*
- *Through all of this I was never alone.*
- *In the caring for one another both are forever changed.*
- *A friend takes your hand and touches your heart.*
- *To all of you whose names were blurred by the pain and the drugs.*
- *Don't ever underestimate your role in getting patients back on their feet.*
- *Will I lose my dignity? Will someone care? Will I wake tomorrow from this nightmare?*
- *You exist as women living between heaven and hell. Inside a machine that demands absolute vigilance. I hated every minute of my stay with you; however, I totally realize the value of your efforts. Please accept my heartiest thank you.*

—UNKNOWN AUTHORS

The nurse is generally the one medical professional the patient sees more than any other. Consequently, the nurse is in a position to monitor the patient's illness, response to medication, display of pain and discomfort, and general condition. This section provides an overview of the ethical responsibilities and legal issues of nursing practice. Although nurses traditionally have followed the instructions of attending physicians, physicians realistically have long relied on nurses to exercise independent judgment in many situations.[2] Patients in hospitals, nursing homes, or at home learning to manage a chronic condition are often at their most vulnerable moments. Nurses are the health care providers they are most likely to encounter; spend the greatest amount of time with; and often depend on for care. Research is now beginning to document what physicians, patients, other health care providers, and nurses themselves have long known: how well we are cared for by nurses affects our health and sometimes can be a matter of life or death.[3]

The more than a decade old nursing shortage continues to require hospitals to search for foreign-trained registered nurses. New immigration laws have complicated the hiring and immigration process. Many countries are facing similar shortages, thus raising ethical dilemmas when recruiting foreign nurses from countries with shortages of their own.

Higher salaries and incentives have done little to resolve the nursing shortage. The unemployment rate would be expected to provide some incentive for students to enter the nursing profession, but the shortage persists. The Secretary of Health and Human Services (HHS), Kathleen Sebelius, announced that $55.5 million in funding was awarded in FY 2013 to strengthen training for health professionals and increase the size of the nation's health care workforce.

> These grants and the many training programs they support have a real impact by helping to create innovative care delivery models and improving access to high-quality care," Secretary Sebelius said.
>
> More than 270 grants will address health workforce needs in nursing, public health, behavioral health, health workforce development, and dentistry. The grants are managed by HHS' Health Resources and Services Administration (HRSA).
>
> A majority of the funding, $45.4 million, will support nursing workforce development in the following areas:
>
> * Increasing the number of nurse faculty ($22.1 million)—provides low-interest loans to nurses to train to become faculty and loan cancellation for service as faculty.
> * Improving nursing diversity ($5.2 million)—expands educational opportunities for students from disadvantaged backgrounds, including racial and ethnic minorities who are underrepresented among registered nurses.
> * Increasing nurse anesthetist traineeships ($2.2 million) —supports nurse anesthetist programs to provide traineeships to licensed registered nurses enrolled as full-time students in a master's or doctoral nurse anesthesia program.
> * Promoting interprofessional collaborative practice ($6.7 million)—brings together interprofessional teams of nurses and other health professionals to develop and implement innovative practice models for providing care.
> * Supporting advanced nursing education ($9.2 million)—funds advanced nursing programs that support registered nurses in becoming nurse practitioners, nurse midwives and other practice nurses.[4]

50 and You Lived Your Life?

I recall teaching an ethics course to nurses in a master's degree program in New York. As we were discussing care for the elderly, a young nurse, about 23 years of age, said, "I think we should not be providing expensive tests and treatments for patients over 50 years of age. People at that age have basically lived their lives." Although most of the nurses in the class were in their late 40s and early 50s, there was silence across the room. My assumption is the nurse was unaware of the age group in the class, as she was the youngest nurse. As to the older nurses, I am not sure as to why they remained so silent. To my surprise, no one uttered a word and the class moved on as though nothing was said. I must say that I, being 33, was speechless.

Anonymous

Discussion

1. Discuss the ethical issues here that concern you.
2. Describe how you might have responded if you were instructing the class.

REGISTERED NURSE

A *registered nurse* is one who has passed a state registration examination and has been licensed to practice nursing. The scope of practice of a registered professional nurse includes patient assessment, analyzing laboratory reports, patient teaching, health counseling, executing medical regimens, and operating medical equipment as prescribed by a physician, dentist, or other licensed health care provider. The nursing profession "is in a period of rapid and progressive change in response to the advances in technology, changes in patterns of demand for health services, and the evolution of professional relationships among nurses, physicians and other health professions."[5] Although most states have similar definitions of nursing, differences generally revolve around the scope of practice permitted.

ADVANCED PRACTICE NURSES

An *advanced practice nurse* (APRN) is a registered nurse having education beyond that of a registered nurse. APRNs include nurse practitioners, clinical nurse specialists, nurse anesthetists, and nurse midwives. They often play a critical role as primary care providers for patients who live in remote areas or have difficulty obtaining a primary care physician. APRNs are certified by a nationally recognized professional organizations in their nursing specialty or meet other criteria established by a board of nursing that sets education, training, and experience requirements.

Nurse Practitioner

The Role of Nurses Extends Beyond the Hospital Ward

Nurse practitioners . . . Studies have found that their ability to diagnose illnesses, order and interpret tests, and treat patients is equivalent to that of primary-care physicians. They also tend to spend more time with patients during routine office visits than physicians, and they are more likely to discuss preventative health measures. As of 2010, 140,000 NPs were working in the United States.

Nurse practitioners are poised to become even more visible with the passage last year of the Patient Protection and Affordable Care Act, which could add nearly 35 million people to the ranks of the insured.

Consumers Union of United States Inc., The Washington Post, *May 30, 2011*

A *nurse practitioner* (NP) is a registered nurse who has completed the necessary education to engage in primary health care decision making. The NP is trained in the delivery of primary health care and the assessment of psychosocial and physical health problems, such as performing routine examinations and ordering routine diagnostic tests. The NP provides primary health care services in accordance with state nurse practice laws.

Clinical Nurse Specialist

The *clinical nurse specialist* (CNS) is a professional registered nurse with an advanced academic degree, experience, and expertise in a clinical specialty (e.g., obstetrics, pediatrics). The clinical nurse specialist functions in a leadership capacity as a clinical role model, assisting the nursing staff to continuously evaluate patient care. The CNS acts as a resource for the management of patients with complex needs and conditions, participates in staff development activities related to his or her clinical specialty, and makes recommendations for establishing standards of care for patients. The CNS functions as a change agent by influencing attitudes, modifying behavior, and introducing new approaches to nursing practice, and collaborates with other members of the health care team to develop and implement the therapeutic plan of care for patients.

Nurse Anesthetist

Administration of anesthesia by a *nurse anesthetist* requires special training and certification. Nurse-administered anesthesia was the first expanded role for nurses requiring certification. Oversight and availability of an anesthesiologist are required by most organizations. The major risks for nurse anesthetists include improper placement of an airway, failure to recognize significant changes in a patient's condition, and the improper use of anesthetics (e.g., wrong anesthetic, wrong dose, wrong route).

Nurse Midwife

Nurse midwives provide comprehensive prenatal care, including delivery for patients who are at low risk for complications. For the most part, they manage normal prenatal, intrapartum, and postpartum care. Provided that there are no complications, normal newborns are also cared for by a nurse midwife. Nurse midwives often provide primary care for women's health issues from puberty to postmenopause.

SPECIAL DUTY NURSE

A *special duty nurse* is a nurse employed by a patient or patient's family to perform nursing care for the patient. An organization is generally not liable for the negligence of a special duty nurse unless a master–servant relationship can be determined to exist between the organization and the special duty nurse. If a master–servant relationship exists between the organization and the special duty nurse, the doctrine of respondeat superior may be applied to impose liability on the organization for the nurse's negligent acts. Although the patient employs the special duty nurse and the organization has no authority to hire or fire the nurse, the organization does have the responsibility to protect the patient from incompetent or unqualified special duty nurses.

FLOAT NURSE

Float nurses are designated as such because they are rotated from unit to unit based on staffing needs. They often cover nursing units with unusually burdensome workloads that often involve complex patients. Float nurses can present a liability to the organization if they are assigned to work in an area where they are not qualified and competent to perform the assigned duties. Failure to match skills with work assignments can be risky business for both the patient and the health care professional. Behavioral health nurses, for example, usually does not have the skills or competencies to cover for surgical nurses in the operating room. Failure to make assignments based on a nurse's skills presents a legal risk if a patient is injured as the result of a nurse's negligent act. The standard of care required in order to establish negligence would be based on the skills and competencies required of the assigned task. In addition to legal implications, it is clear that assignment of a professional to a task he or she is not competent to perform is ethically and morally wrong. The New York State Nurses Association in a position statement on float nurses states in part:

> Adequate staffing (appropriate number, mix and competency of nursing staff) is critical to ensure quality patient care.
>
> The nursing profession has an obligation to evaluate and monitor patient assignments to ensure the delivery of safe, quality care.
>
> The state has a responsibility to hold healthcare employers accountable for the provision of appropriate and timely orientation and training for staff expected to float to unfamiliar units.
>
> The optimum solution to emergency staffing, such as in a sudden fluctuation in census or unexpected increase in absenteeism, is the establishment of an internal pool

of competent personnel whose credentials have been reviewed and who have been oriented to the facility's units and current policies.

All professional nurses must continually assess their own knowledge, ability, and experience and access appropriate resources when needed.

RNs have the right and responsibility to express their concerns and protest an assignment if placed in a potentially unsafe practice situation.[6]

Joint Commission standards require that, "Those who work in the hospital are competent to complete their assigned tasks."[7] It is the responsibility of the hospital's leadership to ensure that nurses are competent to perform the duties and responsibilities to which they are assigned. Not only is the employee responsible for a negligent act, the hospital can be found liable for assigning an employee to a duty that he or she is not competent to perform. This applies not strictly to float nurses but to all staff members.

AGENCY PERSONNEL

Health care organizations are at risk for the negligent conduct of agency personnel. Because of this risk, it is important to ensure that agency workers have the necessary skills and competencies to carry out the duties and responsibilities assigned by the organization.

NURSING ASSISTANTS

A *nursing assistant* is an aide who has been certified and trained to assist patients with activities of daily living. The nursing assistant provides basic nursing care to nonacutely ill patients and assists in the maintenance of a safe and clean environment under the direction and supervision of a registered nurse or licensed practical nurse. The nursing assistant helps with positioning, turning, and lifting patients and performs a variety of tests and treatments. The nursing assistant establishes and maintains interpersonal relationships with patients and other hospital personnel while ensuring confidentiality of patient information. Common areas of negligence for nursing assistants include failure to follow or improperly perform procedures; failure to assist patients and prevent falls, unsafe placement, or positioning of equipment; failure to maintain equipment properly; failure to observe a patient and take vital signs at appropriate intervals; failure to chart pertinent information regarding a patient's changing condition (e.g., vital signs); and failure to respond to a patient's call for help (e.g., call bells).

STUDENT NURSES

Student nurses are entrusted with the responsibility of providing nursing care to patients. When liability is being assessed, a student nurse serving at a health care facility is considered an agent of the facility. Student nurses are personally liable for their own negligent acts, and the facility is liable for their acts on the basis of *respondeat superior.*

A student nurse is held to the standard of a competent professional nurse when performing nursing duties. The courts have taken the position that anyone who performs duties customarily performed by a professional nurse is held to the standard of care required of a professional nurse. Every patient has the right to expect competent nursing services even if students provide the care as part of their clinical training.

NEGLIGENT ACTS IN NURSING

The following cases illustrate some of the acts or omissions constituting negligence that all nurses should be aware of. They are by no means exhaustive and merely represent the wide range of potential legal pitfalls in which nurses might find themselves.

Nurse Assessments and Diagnosis Valid

The defendant physicians in *Cignetti v. Camel*[8] ignored a nurse's assessment of a patient's diagnosis, which contributed to a delay in treatment and injury to the patient. The nurse had testified that she told the physician that the patient's signs and symptoms were not those associated with indigestion. The defendant physician objected to this testimony, indicating that such a statement constituted a medical diagnosis by a nurse. The trial court permitted the testimony to be entered into evidence. Section 335.01(8) of the Missouri Revised Statutes (1975) authorizes a registered nurse to make an assessment of persons who are ill and to render a nursing diagnosis. On appeal, the Missouri Court of Appeals affirmed the lower court's ruling, holding that evidence of negligence presented by a hospital employee, for which an obstetrician was not responsible, was admissible to show the events that occurred during the patient's hospital stay.

Ambiguous Medication Order

A nurse is responsible for making an appropriate inquiry if there is uncertainty about the accuracy of a physician's medication order in a patient's record. The medication order in *Norton v. Argonaut Insurance Co.*,[9] as entered in the medical record, was incomplete and subject to misinterpretation. Believing the order to be incorrect because of the dosage, the nurse asked two physicians present on the patient care unit whether the medication should be given as ordered. The two physicians did not interpret the order as the nurse did and therefore did not share the same concern. They advised the nurse that the attending physician's instructions did not appear out of line. The nurse did not contact the attending physician but instead administered the misinterpreted dosage of medication. As a result, the patient died due to a fatal overdose of the medication.

The nurse was negligent by failing to consult with the attending physician before administering the medication. The nurse was held liable, as was the physician who wrote the ambiguous order that led to the fatal dose. In discussing the standard of care expected of a nurse who encounters an apparently erroneous order, the court stated that not only was the nurse unfamiliar with the medication in question, but she also violated the rule generally followed by members of the nursing profession in the community, which requires that the prescribing physician be called when there is doubt about an order. The court noted that it is the duty of a nurse to make absolutely certain what the physician intended regarding both dosage and route.

Wrong Dosage of a Medication

State Cites Safety Drug Lapses at Cedars-Sinai

Cedars-Sinai Medical Center's handling of high-risk drugs placed its pediatric patients in immediate jeopardy of harm, the state said Wednesday in its response to an overdose involving the newborn twins of actor Dennis Quaid.

In a 20-page report, the California Department of Public Health said the prestigious Los Angeles hospital gave the twins and another child 1,000 times the intended dosage of the blood thinner heparin Nov. 18.

"This violation involved multiple failures by the facility to adhere to established policies and procedures for safe medication use," state inspectors wrote.

Charles Ornstein, Los Angeles Times, *January 10, 2008*

More Heparin Overdoses, This Time in Texas

Add at least 17 Texas infants to the number of children mistakenly given overdoses of heparin in the hospital. At least one of those infants died, and an autopsy is planned to determine whether the blood thinner played a role. Another is still in critical condition.[10]

Tami Dennis, Los Angeles Times, *July 9, 2008*

The nurse in *Harrison v. Axelrod*[11] administered the wrong dosage of Haldol to the patient on seven occasions while employed at a nursing facility. The patient's physician had prescribed a 0.5-mg dosage of Haldol. The patient's medication record indicated that the nurse had been administering doses of 5 mg, which were being sent to the patient care unit by the pharmacy. The nurse had admitted that she administered the wrong dosage and that she was aware of the facility's medication administration policy, which she breached by failing to check the dosage supplied by the pharmacy against the dosage ordered by the patient's physician. The commissioner of the Department of Health made a determination that the administration of the wrong dosage of Haldol on seven occasions constituted patient neglect.

Medicating the Wrong Patient

A patient's identification bracelet must be checked before administering any medication. To ensure that the patient's identity corresponds to the name on the patient's bracelet, the nurse should address the patient by name when approaching the patient's bedside to administer any medication. Should a patient unwittingly be administered another patient's medication, the attending physician should be notified and appropriate documentation placed in the patient's chart.

Failure to Note an Order Change

Failure to review a patient's record before administering a medication to ascertain whether an order has been modified may render a nurse liable for negligence. The physician in *Larrimore v. Homeopathic Hospital Association*[12] wrote an instruction on the patient's order sheet changing the method of administration from injection to oral medication. The nurse mistakenly gave the medication by injection. Perhaps the nurse had not reviewed the order sheet after being told by the patient that the medication was to be given orally; perhaps the nurse did not notice the physician's entry. Either way, the nurse's conduct was held to be negligent. The court went on to say that the jury could find the nurse negligent by applying ordinary common sense to establish the applicable standard of care.

Failure to Follow Instructions

Failure of a nurse to follow the instructions of a supervising nurse to wait for her assistance prior to performing a procedure can result in the revocation of the nurse's license. The nurse in *Cafiero v. North Carolina Board of Nursing*[13] failed to heed instructions to wait for assistance before connecting a heart monitor to an infant. The incorrect connection of the heart monitor resulted in an electrical shock to the infant.

> [6] Ms. Cafiero put the leads on Jami's [sic] chest, and inserted the end of the leads into a cord attached to the back of the monitor. Ms. Cafiero then plugged the machine into the wall. A click was heard, and Jami [sic] was noted to be balled up in a fetal position, trembling, with a red color, and "looked hard." Mrs. Moss screamed and told Ms. Cafiero to turn the monitor off, that she was shocking her baby. Ms. Cafiero told her everything would be o.k. in a minute. Mrs. Moss then saw a black cord on the bed next to Jami [sic] and she unplugged the leads from this black cord. Jami [sic] then fell back on the bed. Ms. Moss went into the hall calling for assistance from a physician.
>
> Gretchen Baughman, RN, Charge Nurse on this shift, came to the room and initiated cardio-pulmonary resuscitation. Jami [sic] was successfully resuscitated, and transferred to the Pediatric Intensive Care Unit (PICU). She did sustain two burns on her chest and one burn on her stomach from this incident. Jamie's parents were later told by the Risk Manager that Jami [sic] was electrocuted by the Neonatal Monitor . . . .[14]

The board of nursing, under the Nursing Practice Act, revoked the nurse's license. The board had the authority to revoke the nurse's license even though her work before and after the incident had been exemplary. The dangers of electric cords are within the realm of common knowledge. The record showed that the nurse failed to exercise ordinary care in connecting the infant to the monitor.

Failure to Report Physician Negligence

An organization can be liable for the failure of nursing personnel to take appropriate action when a patient's personal physician is clearly unwilling or unable to cope with a situation that threatens the life or health of the patient. In a California case, *Goff v. Doctors General Hospital,*[15] a patient was bleeding seriously after childbirth because the physician failed to suture her properly. The nurses testified that they were aware of the patient's dangerous condition and that the physician was not present in the hospital. Both nurses knew the patient would die if nothing was done, but neither contacted anyone except the physician. The hospital was liable for the nurses' negligence in failing to notify their supervisors of the serious condition that caused the patient's death. Evidence was sufficient to sustain the finding that the nurses who attended the patient and who were aware of the excessive bleeding were negligent and that their negligence was a contributing cause of the patient's death. The measure of duty of the hospital toward its patients is the exercise of that degree of care used by hospitals generally. The court held that nurses who knew that a woman they were attending was bleeding excessively were negligent in failing to report the circumstances so that prompt and adequate measures could be taken to safeguard her life.

Failure to Question Patient Discharge

A nurse has a duty to question the discharge of a patient if he or she has reason to believe that such discharge could be injurious to the health of the patient. Jury issues were raised in *Koeniguer v. Eckrich*[16] by expert testimony that the nurses had a duty to attempt to delay the patient's discharge if her condition warranted continued hospitalization. By permissible inferences from the evidence, the delay in treatment that resulted from the premature discharge contributed to the patient's death. Summary dismissal of this case against the hospital by a trial court was found to have been improper.

Failure to Observe Patient's Changing Condition

Failure to observe changes in a patient's condition can lead to liability on the part of the nurse and the organization. The recovery room nurse in *Eyoma v. Falco*[17] (who had been assigned to monitor a postsurgical patient) left the patient and failed to recognize that the patient had stopped breathing. Nurse Falco had been assigned to monitor the patient in the recovery room. She delegated that duty to another nurse and failed to verify that the other nurse accepted that responsibility.

Nurse Falco admitted she never got a verbal response from the other nurse, and, when she returned, there was no one near the decedent. She acknowledged that Dr. Brotherton told her to watch the decedent's breathing but claimed that she was not told that the decedent had been given narcotics. She maintained that on her return she checked the decedent and observed his respirations to be eight per minute.

Thereafter, Brotherton returned and inquired about the decedent's condition. Falco informed the doctor that the patient was fine; however, on his personal observation, Brotherton realized that the decedent had stopped breathing. Decedent, because of oxygen deprivation, entered a comatose state and remained unconscious for over a year until his death.[18]

The jury held the nurse to be 100% liable for the patient's injuries. The court held that there was sufficient evidence to support the verdict.

Charting Observations

The patient's care, as well as the nurse's observations, should be recorded on a regular basis. The nurse should comply promptly and accurately with the physician orders written in the record. Should the nurse have any doubt as to the appropriateness of a particular order, he or she is expected to verify with the physician the intent of the prescribed order.

Failure to Remove Endotracheal Tube

The court in *Poor Sisters of St. Francis v. Catron*[19] held that the failure of nurses and an inhalation therapist to report to the supervisor that an endotracheal tube had been left in the plaintiff longer than the customary period of 3 or 4 days was sufficient to allow the jury to reach a finding of negligence. The patient experienced difficulty speaking and underwent several operations to remove scar tissue and open her voice box. At the time of trial, she could not speak above a whisper and breathed partially through a hole in her throat created by a tracheotomy. The hospital was found liable for the negligent acts of its employees and the resulting injuries to the plaintiff.

CHIROPRACTOR

Chiropractors are required to exercise the same degree of care, judgment, and skill exercised by other reasonable chiropractors under like or similar circumstances. They are expected to maintain the integrity, competency, and standards of their profession, as well as avoid even the appearance of professional impropriety.

Chiropractors have a duty to determine whether a patient is treatable through chiropractic means and to refrain from chiropractic treatment when a reasonable chiropractor would or should be aware that a patient's condition will not respond to chiropractic treatment. Failure to conform to the standard of care can result in liability for any injuries suffered.

CASE: POOR JUDGMENT

The chief medical officer of the Nebraska Department of Health and Human Services Regulation and Licensure in *Poor v. State*[20] entered an order revoking Poor's license to practice as a chiropractor in the state of Nebraska.

Poor engaged in a conspiracy to manufacture and distribute a misbranded substance and introduced into interstate commerce misbranded and adulterated drugs with the intent to defraud and mislead. He was arrested for driving under the influence and was convicted of that offense. In addition, Poor knowingly possessed cocaine. He conceded that these factual determinations were understood as beyond dispute.

The district court's determination that Poor had engaged in "grossly immoral or dishonorable conduct" was not based on "trivial reasons." The appeals court found that Poor's conduct clearly fell within the plain and ordinary meaning of grossly immoral or dishonorable conduct. In its order finding Poor to be unfit, the district court relied in part on Poor's denial of conduct underlying a previous felony conviction. The court stated, "Poor's denial now, after taking advantage of a plea bargain, that he committed any of the acts he admitted to in the United State[s] District Court is disturbing and is not consistent with the integrity and acceptance of responsibility expected by persons engaged in a professional occupation."

Chiropractic medicine is a regulated health care profession. Patients necessarily rely on a chiropractor's honesty, integrity, sound professional judgment, and compliance with applicable governmental regulations. Poor argued that there was absolutely no testimony or evidence to the effect that anything he did constituted a threat of harm to his patients.

The Supreme Court of Nebraska determined that due to the seriousness of Poor's felony conviction and its underlying conduct, his subsequent lack of candor with respect to that conduct, as well as his lack of sound judgment demonstrated by his driving-under-the-influence conviction, revocation of Poor's license was an appropriate sanction.

Ethical and Legal Issues

1. Did the chiropractor in this case violate his professional code of ethics? Explain your answer.
2. Describe how an individual's personal life can affect one's professional career.

DENTISTRY

Hawaii Family Sues Dentist for Root Canal that Left 3-Year-Old Girl BRAIN DEAD

A Hawaii family has sued a dentist for root canal gone horribly wrong that left a 3-year-old girl brain dead.

The lawsuit brought by the Boyle family against Island Dentistry in Honolulu alleges staff bungled the Dec. 3 procedure on little Finley Boyle and were unprepared for the emergency 26 minutes into her multiple root canal, local news station KITV reported.

The child "went into respiratory and cardiac arrest due to an overdose given to her during her treatment," Finley's family wrote on an online fundraiser.

Stephen Rex Brown, New York Daily News, *January 3, 2014*

Dentists are expected to respect patient rights and to avoid harm to their patients. They are expected to treat patients within their scope of practice. Such did not occur in the following cases.

CASE: PRACTICING OUTSIDE THE SCOPE OF PRACTICE

Practicing outside one's scope of practice involves both ethical and legal issues. For example, plaintiff Brown, in *Brown v. Belinfante,*[21] sued a dentist for performing several elective cosmetic procedures, including a facelift, eyelid revision, and facial laser resurfacing. He was licensed to practice dentistry in Georgia. Brown claims that after the cosmetic procedures, she could not close her eyes completely, developed chronic bilateral eye infections, and required remedial corrective surgery. Brown alleged that the dentist's performance of the cosmetic procedures constituted negligence because he exceeded the scope of the practice of dentistry.

The primary purposes of the Georgia Dental Act are to define and regulate the practice of dentistry. The statute limits the scope of the practice of dentistry. Such limitation protects the health and welfare of patients who submit themselves to the care of dentists by guarding against injuries caused by inadequate care or by unauthorized individuals. Brown falls within that class of persons the statute was intended to protect, and the harm complained of was of the type the statute was intended to guard against. In performing the elective cosmetic procedures, the dentist violated the Dental Practice Act by exceeding the statutory limits of the scope of dentistry.

Ethical and Legal Issues

1. Describe the ethical issues presented here.
2. Describe the legal issues in this case.

CASE: INAPPROPRIATE SEXUAL CONDUCT

Revocation of a dentist's license on charges of professional misconduct was properly ordered in *Melone v. State Education Department*[22] on the basis of substantial evidence that while acting in a professional capacity the dentist had engaged in physical and sexual contact with five different male patients within a 3-year period. Considering the dentist's responsible position, the extended time period during which the sexual contacts occurred, the age and impressionable nature of the victims (7 to 15 years of age), and the possibility of lasting effects on the victims, the penalty was not shocking to the court's sense of fairness.

Ethical and Legal Issues

1. Describe the ethical and legal issues of this case.
2. Describe what procedures could be implemented in a dentist's office to help reduce the likelihood of sexual abuses.

DENTAL HYGIENIST

Dental hygienists are expected to treat patients with respect and to disclose all relevant information so that they can make informed choices about their care. Patient information must be kept confidential. Dental hygienists have an obligation to provide services in a manner that protects all patients and minimizes harm to them.

CASE: UNLAWFUL ADMINISTRATION OF NITROUS OXIDE

This case[23] arises from a complaint by a dental hygienist against a former employer, Lowenberg and Lowenberg Corporation. The dental hygienist alleged that the defendant allowed dental hygienists to administer nitrous oxide to patients. Under state law, dental hygienists may not administer nitrous oxide. The Department of Education's Office of Professional Discipline investigated the complaint by using an undercover investigator. The investigator made an appointment for teeth cleaning. At the time of her appointment, she requested that nitrous oxide be administered. Agreeing to the investigator's request, the dental hygienist administered the nitrous oxide. There were no notations in the patient's chart indicating that she had been administered nitrous oxide.

A hearing panel found the dental hygienist guilty of administering nitrous oxide without being properly licensed. In addition, the hearing panel found that the dental hygienist had failed to record accurately in the patient's chart that she had administered nitrous oxide.

The New York Supreme Court, Appellate Division, held that the investigator's report provided sufficient evidence to support the hearing panel's determination. There is adequate evidence in the record to support a finding that the dentist's conduct was such that it could reasonably be said that he permitted the dental hygienist to perform acts that she was not licensed to perform.

Ethical and Legal Issues

1. Discuss how the ethical values listed in the Pillars of Moral Strength were violated in this case.
2. Explain how both legal and ethical issues are intertwined in this case.

CASE: PATIENT INJURED DURING PROCEDURE

The plaintiff in *Hickman v. Sexton Dental Clinic*[24] brought a malpractice action against a dental clinic for a serious cut under her tongue. The dental assistant, without being supervised by a dentist, placed a sharp object into the patient's mouth, cutting her tongue while taking impressions for dentures. The court of common pleas entered a judgment on a jury verdict in favor of the plaintiff, and the clinic appealed. The court of appeals held that the evidence presented was sufficient to infer without the aid of expert testimony that there was a breach of duty to the patient. The testimony of Dr. Tepper, the clinic dentist, was found pertinent to the issue of the common knowledge exception in which the evidence permits the jury to recognize breach of duty without the aid of expert testimony. Tepper presented the following testimony regarding denture impressions:[25]

Q. You also stated that you have taken, I believe, thousands?

A. Probably more than that.

Q. Of impressions?

A. Yes, sir.

Q. This never happened before?

A. No, sir, not a laceration.

Q. Would it be safe and accurate to say that if someone's mouth were to be cut during the impression process, someone did something wrong?

A. Yes, sir.

Ethical and Legal Issues

1. Do you see any ethical issues in this case? Explain your answer.
2. Describe the legal issues of this case.

DIETARY

Good nutrition is crucial to the recovery of the patient. A nurse performs nutritional screenings at the time of a patient's hospital admission. A screening tool is used to help determine when a full assessment is necessary. The screenings are based on specific questions asked of the patient. The results of a screening can trigger a more thorough nutritional assessment, which is conducted by a registered dietitian. A patient's nutritional needs are often neglected because of poorly designed screening tools that often fail to trigger a full assessment. A patient's short hospital stay also contributes to poor screenings and assessments.

Patient's Diet Order Inappropriate

Mom had colon cancer and was told she would be placed on a soft diet following surgery. One evening following surgery I was visiting mom. The diet aide entered the room, laid down mom's food tray on her bedside table, and left the room. Mom lifted the cover off her plate. There on her plate laid a dried-out pork chop with mashed potatoes and broccoli. She looked up at me and said, "Do you want my meal? I can't eat that." I walked to the nurses' station and asked, "Why does my mom have pork chops on her plate. She was told she would be on a soft diet following surgery." The nurse said, "Let me look at her record. After a few moments searching the record, the nurse looked up at me and said, "Yes, it's right here written by the doctor. 'Regular diet for Mrs. Dively.' I can't change her diet. I will have to get an order change from her physician." The nurse continued, "Your mom will have to remain on a regular diet until the doctor writes a new order." I asked, "And how long will that take?" The nurse replied, "When he comes in to visit her on rounds. Probably tomorrow because he just saw her earlier." I then asked to speak to the dietitian. She came to the floor and said, "I understand your dilemma, but I can't change your mom's diet without an order from the physician." I asked for the evening nursing manager, who eventually talked to me on the nursing station phone. She was eventually able to get an order change from the physician who had not returned her call until later that evening.

Anonymous

Dietitians are expected to exercise professional judgment and practice dietetics based on scientific principles and current practice. Yet few health care organizations have fully integrated them into their *patient care teams*. Although the participation of pharmacists in the patient care setting is becoming the norm on patient care units, participation of dietitians is yet to be at an optimal level.

CASE: PATIENT SUFFERS MALNUTRITION

Health care organizations must provide each patient with a nourishing, palatable, well-balanced diet that meets the daily nutritional and special dietary needs of each patient. Failure to do so can lead to negligence suits. The deceased patient's daughter in *Lambert v. Beverly Enterprises, Inc.*,[26] filed an action claiming that her father had been mistreated. The notice of intent to sue indicated that the deceased suffered various injuries and malnutrition as a direct result of the acts or omissions of dietary personnel and that the plaintiff's father suffered actual damages that included substantial medical expenses and mental anguish because of the injuries he sustained. A motion to dismiss the case was denied.

Ethical and Legal Issues

1. Identify the ethical issues in this case.
2. How might the dietitians' professional ethical code have been violated in this case?

The inability of hospitals and ambulatory care centers to provide adequate staff to address the nutritional needs of patients is due in part to financial constraints. Rural outpatient centers are generally understaffed and barely have time to address the patient's presenting complaints. Staffing to address the unique nutritional needs of many patients often goes unchecked. Frequently patients with poor nutritional habits often return over the years with more severe, costly, and debilitating medical conditions (e.g., diabetes and heart disease), as discussed in the following *reality check*.

Patient's Nutritional Status Not Addressed

Jeb, a 12-year-old 175-pound boy came with his mother to General Hospital's ambulatory care clinic to be treated for poison ivy. When Brad, a physician's assistant, was completed with his assessment, he provided Jack's mother with a prescription and gave instructions for caring for her son. He then asked, "Do you have any questions?" She replied that she had none. After she and her son left the treatment room I asked, as a resident assigned to the clinic for training, "Brad, do you know if anyone ever discussed Jack's nutritional status with his mother and the future risks associated with his weight."

Brad looked in Jack's medical record and noted that he had been a patient in the clinic since birth. He could not find any notations indicating there was any discussion over the years regarding his weight. He did note that there was a height and weight chart in the record by age and that Jack's height was in the norm for his age, however, his weight was as he put it, "Off the scale." He looked at me and said, "The problem here is, the mother, as you may have observed, has a weight problem as well. We have been asking for a registered dietitian to schedule a morning once a week for referral purposes. It like singing in the wind and nobody is listening."

Anonymous

Discussion

1. Balancing the financial constraints of the clinic and the long-term health risks that Jeb faces, discuss what creative action you would take in order to provide nutritional consultations for clinic patients, assuming the hospital has no available resources to provide for nutritional counseling.
2. What are the ethical issues of treating poison ivy and seemingly ignoring Jeb's risks of developing diabetes and/or heart disease?

INCIDENCE AND RECOGNITION OF MALNUTRITION

The importance of diet is often not given sufficient consideration in health care settings, which was noted by J. P. McWhirter and C. R. Pennington in a study conducted to determine the incidence and recognition of malnutrition in a hospital. The results of the study were printed in the British Medical Journal.[27] Although not totally conclusive of what the findings would be in a larger sampling, the results of this study are somewhat perplexing. The abstract of the McWhirter and Pennington study is presented here.

Abstract

Objectives: To determine incidence of malnutrition among patients on admission to hospital, to monitor their changes in nutritional status during stay, and to determine awareness of nutrition in different clinical units.

Design: Prospective study of consecutive admissions.

Setting: Acute teaching hospital.

Subjects: 500 patients admitted to hospital: 100 each from general surgery, general medicine, respiratory medicine, orthopaedic surgery, and medicine for the elderly.

Main Outcome Measures: Nutritional status of patients on admission and reassessment on discharge, review of case notes for information about nutritional status.

Results: On admission, 200 of the 500 patients were undernourished (body mass index less than 20) and 34% were overweight (body mass index >25). The 112 patients reassessed on discharge had mean weight loss of 5.4% with greatest weight loss in those initially most undernourished. But the 10 patients referred for nutritional support showed mean weight gain of 7.9%. Review of case notes revealed that, of the 200 undernourished patients, only 96 had any nutritional information documented.

Conclusion: Malnutrition remains a largely unrecognized problem in hospital and highlights the need for education on clinical nutrition.

J. P. McWhirter and C. R. Pennington, "Incidence and Recognition of Malnutrition in Hospital," BMJ *308:945, April 9, 1994*

EMERGENCY SERVICES

Wait Times Lengthen at Emergency Rooms

Emergency-room patients are waiting ever longer to see a doctor, a potentially dangerous development as rising numbers of uninsured and underinsured Americans turn to ERs for medical care.

Theo Francis, The Wall Street Journal, *January 15, 2008*

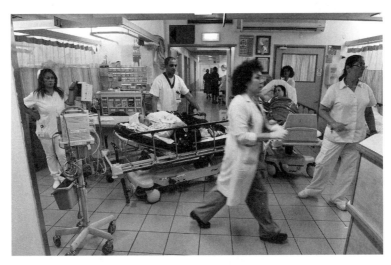

FIGURE 9-1   Teamwork in Action (© ChameleonsEye/Shutterstock, Inc.)

Federal and state statutes impose a duty on hospitals to provide emergency care. The statutes require hospitals to provide some degree of emergency service. If the public is aware that a hospital furnishes emergency services and relies on that knowledge, the hospital has a duty to provide those services to the public.

Treatment rendered by hospitals is expected to be commensurate with that available in the same or similar communities or in hospitals generally. In *Fjerstad v. Knutson,*[28] the South Dakota Supreme Court found that a hospital could be held liable for the failure of an on-call physician to respond to a call from the emergency department. An intern, who attempted to contact the on-call physician and was unable to do so for 3 1/2 hours, treated and discharged the patient. The hospital was responsible for assigning on-call physicians and ensuring that they would be available when called. The patient died during the night in a motel room as a result of asphyxia resulting from a swelling of the larynx, tonsils, and epiglottis that blocked the trachea. Testimony from the laboratory director indicated that the emergency department's on-call physician was to be available for consultation and was assigned that duty by the hospital. Expert testimony also was offered that someone with the decedent's symptoms should have been hospitalized and that such care could have saved the decedent's life. The jury could have believed that an experienced physician would have taken the necessary steps to save the decedent's life.

CASE: ON-CALL PHYSICIAN FAILS TO RESPOND

Hospitals are expected to notify specialty on-call physicians when their particular skills are required in the emergency department. An on-call physician who fails to respond to a request to attend a patient can be liable for injuries suffered by the patient because of his or her failure to respond. In *Thomas v. Corso,*[29] a Maryland court sustained a verdict against the hospital and physician. The patient had been brought to the hospital emergency department after being struck by a car. A physician did not attend to him even though he had dangerously low blood pressure and was in shock. There was some telephone contact between the nurse in the emergency department and the physician who was providing on-call coverage. The physician did not act on the hospital's call for assistance until the patient was close to death, and the patient did die. The court reasoned that expert testimony was not even necessary to establish what common sense made evident: that a patient who had been struck by a car may have suffered internal injuries and should have been evaluated and treated by a physician. Lack of attention in such cases is not reasonable care by any standard. The concurrent negligence of the nurse, who failed to contact the on-call physician after the patient's condition had worsened, did not relieve the physician of liability for his failure to come to the emergency department at once. Rather, under the doctrine of *respondeat superior*, the nurse's negligence was a basis for holding the hospital liable as well.

Ethical and Legal Issues

1. Describe how both the physician and nurse failed in their ethical responsibilities to the patient.
2. Describe what actions the hospital can take to prevent future occurrences of this nature.
3. What are the legal and ethical concerns for the physician, nurse, and hospital?

Timely Response May Require a Phone Call

Hospitals are not only required to care for emergency patients but also required to do so in a timely fashion. In *Marks v. Mandel*,[30] a Florida trial court was found to have erred in directing a verdict against the plaintiff. It was decided that the relevant inquiry in this case was whether the hospital and the supervisor should bear ultimate responsibility for failure of the specialty on-call system to function properly. Jury issues had been raised by evidence that the standard for on-call systems was to have a specialist attending the patient within a reasonable time of being called.

Emergency rooms are aptly named and vital to public safety. There exists no other place to find immediate medical care. The dynamics that drive paying patients to a hospital's emergency rooms are well known. A sudden injury occurs, a child breaks his arm, an individual suffers a heart attack, an existing medical condition worsens, a diabetic lapses into a coma, demanding immediate medical attention at the nearest emergency room. The catchphrase in legal nomenclature "time is of the essence" takes on real meaning. Generally, one cannot choose to pass by the nearest emergency room, and after arrival, it would be improvident to depart in hope of finding one that provides services through employees rather than independent contractors. The patient is there and must rely on the services available and agree to pay the premium charged for those services.[31]

The public not only relies on the medical care rendered by emergency departments but also considers the hospital as a single entity providing all of its medical services. A set of commentators observed:[32]

> [T]he hospital itself has come to be perceived as the provider of medical services. According to this view, patients come to the hospital to be cured, and the doctors who practice there are the hospital's instrumentalities, regardless of the nature of the

private arrangements between the hospital and the physician. Whether or not this perception is accurate seemingly matters little when weighed against the momentum of changing public perception and attendant public policy.

The change in public reliance and public perceptions, as well as the regulations imposed on hospitals, has created an absolute duty for hospitals to provide competent medical care in their emergency departments.

Given the cumulative public policies surrounding the operation of emergency departments and the legal requirement that hospitals provide emergency services, hospitals must be accountable in tort for the actions of caregivers working in their emergency departments.

Emergency Department Lifeline

Emergency departments are the lifelines for millions of people around the nation each day. For those with and those without insurance, each day we know someone out there cares. Often forgotten is the compassion that caregivers show each day. One such occurrence was observed when a young man walked into the emergency room at General Hospital. He described symptoms of severe chest pain. He was afraid but was soon rushed to a room where he was attended to by a physician, a nurse, an EKG technician, and a laboratory technician. He had blood drawn, an EKG, and a history and physical. As I watched, his fear turned to gratitude as treatment was administered and his pain alleviated. Fear faded away and the young man left with instructions for follow-up care. Fear turned to happiness for this young man. His smile spoke a million words.

Anonymous

PARAMEDICS

Many states have enacted legislation that provides civil immunity to *paramedics* who render emergency lifesaving services. In *Morena v. South Hills Health Systems,*[33] the Pennsylvania Supreme Court held that paramedics were not negligent in transporting a victim of a shooting to the nearest available hospital, rather than to another hospital located 5 or 6 miles farther away where a thoracic surgeon was present. The paramedics were not capable, in a medical sense, of accurately diagnosing the extent of the decedent's injury. Except for the children's center and the burn center, no emergency trauma centers are specifically designated for the treatment of particular injuries.

The plaintiff, in *Riffe v. Vereb Ambulance Service, Inc.,*[34] alleged that, while responding to an emergency call an emergency medical technician began administering lidocaine to the patient, as ordered over the telephone by the medical command physician at the defendant hospital. While en route to the hospital, the patient was administered 44 times the normal dosage of lidocaine. Consequently, normal heart function was not restored, and the patient was pronounced dead at the hospital shortly thereafter. At trial, the superior court held that the liability of medical technicians could not be imputed to the hospital. The court noted the practical impossibility of the hospital carrying ultimate responsibility for the quality of care and treatment given patients by emergency medical services.

LABORATORY

Laboratory medical technologists are expected to protect the welfare of patients and the tests conducted above all else. They are expected to avoid dishonest and unethical conduct. An organization's laboratory provides data that are vital to a patient's treatment. Among its many functions, the laboratory monitors therapeutic ranges, measures blood levels for toxicity, places and monitors instrumentation on patient units, provides education for the nursing staff (e.g., glucose monitoring), provides valuable data used in research studies, supplies data on the most effective and economical antibiotic for treating patients, serves in a consultative role, and provides important data as to the nutritional needs of patients.

ETHICS AND INACCURATE LAB RESULTS

Ethics codes for both health care organizations and their professionals are written to protect patients, as well as, employees and their employers. The American Society for Clinical Laboratory Science in its code of ethics states as to the duty owed to patients:

> Clinical laboratory professionals are accountable for the quality and integrity of the laboratory services they provide. This obligation includes maintaining individual competence in judgment and performance and striving to safeguard the patient from incompetent or illegal practice by others.
> Clinical laboratory professionals maintain high standards of practice. They exercise sound judgment in establishing, performing and evaluating laboratory testing.
> Clinical laboratory professionals maintain strict confidentiality of patient information and test results. They safeguard the dignity and privacy of patients and provide accurate information to other health care professionals about the services they provide.[35]

Lab tests are not always accurate, sometimes due to human error or faulty test results. According to an article in the *Baltimore Sun* on March 11, 2004, approximately 640 patients at Maryland General Hospital may have received incorrect HIV and hepatitis test results. Some patients might have been told they were HIV-negative when in fact they were positive and vice versa, and the hospital failed to notify the patients of the problem. A former hospital employee had apparently filed a complaint. State health officials discovered in January that the hospital's laboratory personnel overrode controls in the testing equipment that showed the results might be in error and then mailed them to patients anyway.[36] Licensure and certification of laboratory staff is necessary in order to help prevent incidents of this nature. The American Society for Clinical Pathology in a policy statement on State Licensure of Laboratory Personnel, Policy (Number 05-02) states that:

> Due to the complexity of laboratory medicine and its importance in quality patient care, it is imperative that medical laboratory personnel possess the qualifications necessary to ensure their professional competence. Licensure and certification programs

not only set minimum standards for medical laboratory personnel working in clinical laboratories; they also help ensure quality laboratory testing and proper patient care.[37]

Inaccurate lab tests are not uncommon occurrences and the headlines of inaccurate reporting continue to come to public attention, as noted in the next news clipping.

Spokane Woman Suing over False HIV Diagnosis

A Spokane woman is suing a Pennsylvania-based plasma donation company saying she was falsely told she had hepatitis and HIV after donating plasma at a clinic in Hayden, Idaho.

Melissa Bloom filed the lawsuit against BioLife Plasma Services alleging the clinic acted negligently when employees informed her she had the viruses after a combination of blood samples from several donors tested positive.

Bloom is seeking damages for emotional stress and punitive damages, saying she was informed of the positive test in April and went immediately to her doctor's office for tests that determined she did not have the viruses.

KOMONEWS.com, Associated Press, *December 26, 2013*[38]

REFUSAL TO PERFORM HIV TESTING

Stepp, a laboratory staff technician, refused to perform tests on AIDS-contaminated fluids for which she was eventually terminated by the hospital. The Review Board of the Indiana Employment Security Division upheld the hospital's decision to terminate the technician. The technician appealed the board's decision. The Court of Appeals of Indiana, in *Stepp v. Review Board of the Indiana Employment Security Division*,[39] held that the technician was dismissed for just cause and that the laboratory did not waive its right to compel employees to perform assigned tasks. The technician had been warned, suspended, and discharged for her refusal to perform the tests. She told her supervisors that she refused to perform the tests because "AIDS is God's plague on man and performing the tests would go against God's will."[40] The technician argued that that the employer hospital failed to provide a safe place to work. Under Section 11(c)(1) of the Occupational Safety and Health Act of 1970 (OSHA) an employer is prohibited from discharging any employee who exercises any right afforded by OSHA, which provides "the right of an employee to choose not to perform his assigned task because of a reasonable apprehension of death or serious injury coupled with a reasonable belief that no less drastic alternative is available." The Supreme Court in *Whirlpool Corp. v. Marshall*, 445 U.S. 1 (1980) laid out a two-part test. "First, an employee must reasonably believe the working conditions pose an imminent risk of serious bodily injury, and second, the employee must have a reasonable belief there is not sufficient time or opportunity either to seek effective redress from his employer or to apprise OSHA of the danger."[41] Stepp failed to successfully argue both parts of this test.

Although Stepp's case involved legal issues for the courts to decide, there are a variety of moral issues for health care professionals to consider when refusing to perform tests that are required to determine a patient's diagnosis. Of major applicability in this case is the principle of *nonmaleficence*—first, do no harm. Suppose for a moment that a technician was working alone at night on a weekend and was the only hospital employee that could perform cardiac enzyme blood tests to determine if the patient had a cardiac event. The blood sample arrives in the laboratory with an AIDS warning label attached. Should the laboratory technician refuse to perform the test, the legal and moral principles of ethics and applicable codes would not support the technician's refusal to perform the tests so urgently needed to determine the patient's treatment regimen.

MEDICAL ASSISTANT

A *medical assistant* is an unlicensed person who provides administrative, clerical, and/or technical support to a licensed practitioner. A licensed practitioner is generally required to be physically present in the treatment facility, medical office, or ambulatory facility when a medical assistant is performing procedures.[42] Employment of medical assistants is expected to continue to grow over time. This growth is due in part to technological advances in medicine and a growing and aging population. Increasing use of medical assistants in the rapidly growing health care industry will most likely result in continuing employment growth for the occupation.[43]

Medical assistants work in physicians' offices, clinics, nursing homes, and ambulatory care settings. The duties of medical assistants vary from office to office, depending on the location and size of the practice and the practitioner's specialty. In small practices, medical assistants usually are generalists, handling both administrative and clinical duties. Those in large practices tend to specialize in a particular area, under supervision. Administrative duties often include answering telephones, greeting patients, updating and filing patients' medical records, filling out insurance forms, handling correspondence, scheduling appointments, arranging for hospital admission and laboratory services, and handling billing and bookkeeping. Clinical duties vary according to state law and include assisting in taking medical histories, recording vital signs, explaining treatment procedures to patients, preparing patients for examination, and assisting the practitioner during examinations. Medical assistants collect and prepare laboratory specimens or perform basic laboratory tests on the premises, dispose of contaminated supplies, and sterilize medical instruments. They instruct patients about medications and special diets, prepare and administer medications as directed by a physician, authorize drug refills as directed, provide telephone prescriptions to a pharmacy, prepare patients for X-rays, perform electrocardiograms, remove sutures, and change dressings.

Medical assistants who work in the various medical specialties often have additional duties. Podiatric medical assistants, for example, make foot molds and assist podiatrists in surgery. Ophthalmic medical assistants help ophthalmologists provide eye care. They conduct diagnostic tests, measure and record vision, and test eye muscle function. They also teach patients how to insert, remove, and care for contact lenses. Under the direction of the physician, ophthalmic medical assistants may administer eye medications. They also maintain optical and surgical instruments and may assist the ophthalmologist in surgery.[44]

CASE: LOOKING FOR HELP

On July 12, Jill had severe pain in the left side of her head while at work. She was not speaking coherently and eventually lost consciousness for a few moments. She was taken to her physician's office by a coworker. Jill's physician ordered some tests at the hospital's outpatient imaging center to rule out a transient ischemic attack (TIA). A medical assistant at the imaging center explained to Jill that her tests could not be scheduled until July 14.

Dan drove his wife Jill to her appointment. They arrived early on July 14 for her imaging test. On their arrival at the imaging center, Dan dropped Jill off at the front entrance while he searched for a parking space. Meanwhile Jill went into the center and handed her prescription to Carol, a medical assistant at the front desk. Carol said to Jill, "I am sorry, but we cannot perform your test. Your doctor faxed us an unsigned and undated order sheet. It is confusing as to what imaging studies he wants. He checked a box on the physician's order sheet indicating that he wanted a CT scan of the head. In addition, there was a handwritten note on the form indicating that your physician wants an MRI to rule out a TIA. We are not sure if he wants one or both tests. You will have to get clarification from the physician as to exactly what procedure he wants." Dan, after having parked his wife's car, arrived at the front desk and saw his wife somewhat distressed. Carol explained the problem to Dan. He asked Carol, "Could you please contact the physician and ask him to clarify and fax back to the center what tests he wants?" Carol replied, "We are very busy; however, you can use our phone and ask the physician to clarify his order and have him fax us a new order." Jill interrupted, appearing somewhat agitated, and asked, "What is your fax number?" Carol (pointing to a wall) replied, "It is posted there on the wall by the phone. You can use that phone." Carol suggested to Jill that she complete the patient intake paperwork while Dan contacted Jill's physician. Dan was able to get a new faxed order. As they waited for Jill to be called for her tests, with her eyes tearing up, she turned to Dan and said, "This is how my last 6 years of life have been, fighting this horrendous disease. What would I do without you?"

Ethical and Legal Issues

1.　Should the medical assistant have clarified the physician's order prior to the patient's arrival? Consider in your answer how Carol might have reacted if she was the patient, or her spouse, parent, or child was the patient?

2.　Discuss what ethical issues you would be concerned with and what action would you take if you were a member of the governing body sitting in the waiting room observing this incident.

CASE: UNTIMELY DIAGNOSIS

The patient–plaintiff in *Follett v. Davis*[45] discovered a lump in her right breast in the spring of 1988. She made an appointment to see Dr. Davis, her obstetrician/gynecologist, to see if she should be concerned about the breast lump she had discovered. The clinic had no record of her appointment. The clinic's employees directed her to radiology for a mammogram. A technician examined the plaintiff's breast and confirmed the presence of a lump in her right breast. Neither Dr. Davis nor any other physician at the clinic offered the plaintiff an examination. In addition, she was not scheduled for a physician's examination as a follow-up to the mammogram. The plaintiff was instructed that she would hear from Dr. Davis if there were any concerns with her mammogram.

The radiologist explained in his deposition that the mammogram was not normal. Dr. Davis received and reviewed the mammogram report and considered it to be negative for malignancy. He did not know this was a new breast lump because none of the clinic employees had informed him about it. Neither clinic staff nor Dr. Davis contacted the plaintiff about her lump or the mammogram. The plaintiff called the clinic on April 6, 1990. She was told that there was nothing to worry about unless she heard from Dr. Davis. On September 24, 1990, the plaintiff returned to the clinic after she had developed pain associated with the same lump. A mammogram performed on that day gave results consistent with cancer. Three days later, Dr. Davis made an appointment for the plaintiff with a clinic surgeon for a biopsy and treatment. She kept her appointment with the surgeon. Nevertheless, this was her last visit with the clinic, as she subsequently transferred her care to other physicians. In October 1990, the biopsy confirmed the diagnosis of cancer.

In August 1992, the plaintiff filed a lawsuit. The evidence showed that after the patient found a lump in her breast, she went to Dr. Davis, and clinic for help. Dr. Davis and the clinic, through the clinic's employees and agents, undertook to treat her ailment. That undertaking ended when the clinic's surgeon performed the biopsy and therefore was continuous in nature. The evidence demonstrated that had clinic procedures been followed, Dr. Davis or another physician at the clinic would have made a more timely diagnosis.

Ethical and Legal Issues

1. Describe the legal and ethical issues presented in this case.
2. Discuss what action the clinic's leadership should take in order to prevent similar incidents in the future.

MEDICAL RECORDS

Health care organizations are required to maintain a medical record for each patient in accordance with accepted professional standards and practices. The main purposes of the medical record are to provide a planning tool for patient care; to record the course of a patient's treatment and the changes in a patient's condition; to document the communications between the practitioner responsible for the patient and any other health care professional who contributes to the patient's care; to assist in protecting the legal interests of the patient, the organization, and the practitioner; to provide a database for use in statistical reporting, continuing education, and research; and to provide information necessary for third-party billing and regulatory agencies. Medical records must be complete, accurate, current, readily accessible, and systematically organized.

PHARMACY

The practice of pharmacy essentially includes preparing, compounding, dispensing, and retailing medications. These activities may be carried out only by a pharmacist with a state license or by a person exempted from the provisions of a state's pharmacy statutes. The entire stock of drugs in a pharmacy is subject to strict government regulation and control. The pharmacist is responsible for developing, coordinating, and supervising all pharmacy activities and reviewing the drug regimens of each patient.

Because of the immense variety and complexity of medications now available, it is impossible for nurses or physicians to keep up with all of the information required for safe medication use. The *pharmacist* has become an essential resource in modern hospital practice.[46]

Medication errors are considered a leading cause of patient injury. Antibiotics, chemotherapeutic drugs, and anticoagulants are the three categories of drugs responsible for most drug-related adverse events. The prevention of medication errors requires recognition of common causes and the development of practices to help reduce the incidence of errors. With thousands of drugs, many of which look alike and sound alike, it is understandable that medication errors are so common. The more common types of medication errors include prescription errors, transcription errors (often caused by illegible handwriting and improper use of abbreviations), dispensing errors, and administration errors. As noted in the following news clippings, medication errors are all to common occurrences.

Hospital Errors Common and Underreported

Sorrel King's 18-month-old daughter Josie was recovering from second degree burns at Johns Hopkins Hospital in Baltimore when a communication breakdown caused a deadly misstep.

As King watched, a nurse gave Josie a methadone injection despite verbal orders to the contrary, assuring King that the order had been changed. Josie, who was about to be released from the hospital, went into cardiac arrest. "I took one look at her, ran into the hallway, and screamed for help," King said. Josie died 2 days later . . . .

As many as one-third of hospital visits leads to hospital-related injuries, according to a report published today in *Health Affairs*.

Katie Moisse, ABC News Medical Unit, *April 7, 2011*[47]

Drug Overuse Threatens Nursing Home Residents

More than five years after the federal government warned that drugs routinely prescribed to nursing-home residents posed serious threats, including an increased risk of death, inappropriate use remains high, according to a recent analysis by the American Society of Health-System Pharmacists (ASHP).

Consumer Reports, *December 2010*

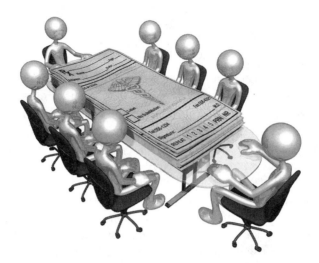

FIGURE 9-2   Prescription Errors Reviewed (© Scott Maxwell/LuMaxArt/Shutterstock, Inc.)

DISPENSING AND ADMINISTRATION OF DRUGS

The dispensing of medications is the processing of a drug for delivery or for administration to a patient pursuant to the order of a health care practitioner. It consists of checking the directions on the label with the directions on the prescription or order to determine accuracy; selecting the drug from stock to fill the order; counting, measuring, compounding, or preparing the drug; placing the drug in the proper container; and adding to a written prescription any required notations.

The administration of medications is the act of giving a single dose of a prescribed drug to a patient by an authorized person in accordance with federal and state laws and regulations. The complete act of administration includes removing an individual dose from a previously dispensed, properly labeled container (including a unit dose container); verifying it with the physician's order; giving the individual dose to the proper patient; and recording the time and dose given.

Licensed persons, in accordance with state regulations, may administer medications. Each dose of a drug administered must be recorded on the patient's clinical records. A separate record of narcotic drugs must be maintained. The record must contain a separate sheet for each narcotic of different strength or type administered to the patient. The narcotic record must contain the following information: date and time administered, physician's name, signature of person administering the dose, the balance of the narcotic drug on hand, and the proper recording of any drugs wasted/destroyed.

In the event that an emergency arises requiring the immediate administration of a particular drug, the patient's record should be documented properly, showing the necessity for administration of the drug on an emergency basis. Procedures should be in place for handling emergency situations.

DRUG SUBSTITUTION

Drug substitution may be defined as the dispensing of a different drug or brand in place of the drug or brand ordered. "All states permit generic interchange to one extent or another."[48] Health care organizations use a "formulary system" whereby physicians and pharmacists create a formulary listing drugs used in the institution. The formulary contains the brand names and generic names of drugs. Under the formulary system, a physician agrees that his or her prescription calling for a brand name drug may be filled with the generic equivalent of that drug (e.g., a drug that contains the same active ingredients in the same proportions). When a formulary system is in use, the prescribing physician can request the use of a particular brand name drug, when he or she deems it necessary or desirable for patient safety, by expressly prohibiting the use of the formulary system.

Hospitals are watchful for any abuses by physicians who circumvent the formulary for no valid patient safety reason. The ever-escalating costs of pharmaceutical products necessitates that hospitals become more vigilant in order to rein in costs.

EXPANDING ROLE OF THE PHARMACIST

Historically, the role of the pharmacist was centered on management of the pharmacy and accurate preparation and dispensing of drugs. The duties and responsibilities of pharmacists have, however, moved well beyond the scope of filling prescriptions and dispensing medications. Pharmacists do much more than this. They are increasingly playing an ever-expanding clinical role on various hospital specialty units (e.g., cardiology and oncology). They provide patient and staff education, consultation, and evaluation and selection of medications for placement in the hospital formulary; review medication errors; and report adverse drug reactions. Schools of pharmacy, recognizing the ever-expanding role of pharmacists in the clinical aspects of patient care have raised the educational requirements for new graduates by requiring a Doctor of Pharmacy (Pharm.D.) degree.

Duty to Monitor Patient's Medications

In *Baker v. Arbor Drugs, Inc.*,[49] a Michigan court imposed a duty on a pharmacist to monitor a patient's medications. Three different prescriptions were prescribed by the same physician and filled at the same pharmacy. The pharmacy maintained a computer system that detected drug interactions. The pharmacy advertised to consumers that it could, through the use of a computer monitoring system, provide a medication profile of a customer for adverse drug reactions. Because the pharmacy advertised and used the computer system to monitor the medications of a customer, the pharmacist voluntarily assumed a duty of care to detect the harmful drug interaction that occurred.

Warning Patients About Potential for Overdose

A Pennsylvania court held that a pharmacy failed to exercise due care and diligence because the patient was not warned about the maximum dosage of a medication.[50] This failure resulted in an overdose, causing the patient permanent injuries. Expert testimony focused on the fact that a pharmacist who receives inadequate instructions as to the maximum recommended dosage of a medication has a duty to ascertain whether the patient is aware of the limitations concerning the use of the drug or, alternatively, to contact the prescribing physician regarding the inadequacy of the prescription.

Refusal to Honor a Questionable Prescription

In *Hooks v. McLaughlin*,[51] the Indiana Supreme Court held that a pharmacist had a duty to refuse to refill prescriptions at an unreasonably faster rate than prescribed pending directions from the prescribing physician. The Indiana Code provides that a pharmacist is immune from civil prosecution or civil liability if he or she, in good faith, refuses to honor a prescription because, in his or her professional judgment, honoring of the prescription would aid or abet an addiction of habit.[52]

BILLING FRAUD

Pharmacists have a duty to act with honesty and integrity in their professional relationships as noted in the following excerpt from their Code of Ethics for ethical behavior.

> *IV. A pharmacist acts with honesty and integrity in professional relationships.*
>
> A pharmacist has a duty to tell the truth and to act with conviction of conscience. A pharmacist avoids discriminatory practices, behavior or work conditions that impair professional judgment, and actions that compromise dedication to the best interests of patients.[53]

The following legal cases illustrate how not only did the pharmacists break the law; they also failed to adhere to their own code or professional ethics.

The court of appeals in *State v. Beatty*[54] upheld a lower court's finding that the evidence submitted against the defendant pharmacist was sufficient to sustain a conviction for Medicaid fraud. The state was billed for medications that were never dispensed, for more medications than some patients received, and in some instances, for the more expensive trade name drugs when cheaper generic drugs were dispensed.

The pharmacists in *People v. Kendzia*[55] were convicted of selling generic drugs in vials with brand name labels. Investigators, working undercover, were provided with Medicaid cards and fictitious prescriptions requiring brand name drugs to be dispensed as written. Between April and October 1979, the investigators had taken the prescriptions to the pharmacy, where they were filled with generic substitutions in vials with the brand name labels.

PHYSICAL THERAPY

Physical therapy is the art and science of preventing and treating neuromuscular or musculoskeletal disabilities through the evaluation of an individual's disability and rehabilitation potential and the use of physical agents—heat, cold, electricity, water, and light—and neuromuscular procedures that, through their physiologic effect, improve or maintain the patient's optimum functional level. Because of different physical disabilities brought on by various injuries and medical problems, physical therapy is an extremely important component of a patient's total health care. As the following cases illustrate, there can be both ethical and legal issues when a therapist incorrectly interprets a physician's orders for physical therapy.

INCORRECTLY INTERPRETING PHYSICIAN'S ORDERS

Pontiff, in *Pontiff v. Pecot & Assoc.*,[56] filed a petition for damages against Pecot and Associates and Morris. Pontiff alleged that Pecot and Associates had been negligent in failing to train, supervise, and monitor its employees properly, including Morris, and that Pecot and Associates was otherwise negligent. Pontiff alleged that employee Morris failed to exercise the degree of care and skill ordinarily exercised by physical therapists, failed to heed his protests that he could not perform the physical therapy treatments she was supervising, and failed to stop performing physical therapy treatments after he began to complain he was in pain. Pontiff claimed he felt a muscle tear while he was exercising on the butterfly machine, a resistive exercise machine.

Pontiff's expert, Boulet, a licensed practicing physical therapist, testified that Pecot deviated from the standard of care of physical therapists by introducing a type of exercise that, according to her, was not prescribed by Dr. deAraujo, the treating physician. She stated that Pecot had added resistive or strengthening exercises to Pontiff's therapy and that these were not a part of the physician's prescription. Pecot argued that resistive exercises were implicitly part of the prescription, even if her interpretation of the prescription was not reasonable.

Legally, under Louisiana law, a physical therapist may not treat a patient without a written physical therapy prescription. *Ethically*, the Physical Therapists' Code of Ethics, Principle 3.4, states "any alteration of a program or extension of services beyond the program should be undertaken in consultation with the referring practitioner." Because resistive exercises were not set forth in the original prescription, Boulet stated that consultation with the physician was necessary before Pontiff could be advanced to that level. Only in the case where a physician has indicated on the prescription that the therapist is to "evaluate and treat" would the therapist have such discretion. There was no such indication on the prescription written by Dr. deAraujo.

Davis, a physical therapist in private practice and Pecot's expert witness, testified that the program that Pecot designed for Pontiff was "consistent with how she interpreted the prescription for therapy that the physician wrote." Davis, however, did not at any time state that Pecot's interpretation was a reasonable one. In fact, Davis herself would not have interpreted the prescription in the manner that Pecot did. Davis testified only that Pecot's introduction of resistive exercises was reasonable based on her interpretation of the prescription.

It is clear that Pecot, as a licensed physical therapist, owed a duty to Pontiff, her client. Pecot's duty is defined by the standard of care of similar physical therapists and the American Physical Therapy Association. If Pecot found the prescription to be ambiguous, she had a duty to contact the prescribing physician for clarification. The appeals court found that the trial court was correct in its determination that Pontiff presented sufficient evidence to show that this duty was breached and that Pecot's care fell below the standard of other physical therapists.

RESIDENT NEGLECT

The physical therapist in the following case not only fail the legal system but also failed to adhere to the professional code of ethics for physical therapists, which provides:

> 2B. Physical therapists shall provide physical therapy services with compassionate and caring behaviors that incorporate the individual and cultural differences of patients/clients.

In *Zucker v. Axelrod*,[57] a physical therapist had been charged with resident neglect for refusing to allow an 82-year-old nursing facility resident to go to the bathroom before starting his therapy treatment session. Undisputed evidence at a hearing showed that the petitioner refused to allow the resident to be excused to go to the bathroom. The petitioner claimed that her refusal was because she assumed that the resident had gone to the bathroom before going to therapy and that the resident was undergoing a bladder-training program. The petitioner had not mentioned when she was interviewed after the incident or during her hearing testimony that she considered bladder training a basis for refusing to allow the resident to go to the bathroom. It is uncontroverted that the nursing facility had a policy of allowing residents to go to the bathroom whenever they wished to do so. The court held that the evidence supported resident neglect.

Multidisciplinary Approach to Patient Care

Do patients believe that care is always well coordinated? Are patients at times treated based on short "handwritten notes" by the prescribing physician? Are mistakes sometimes made because of illegible handwriting? Is it helpful to the radiologist if the ordering physician notes on the order sheet why a particular imaging study is required? Do nurses sometimes find it necessary to clarify medication orders? Do pharmacists find it necessary to contact the physician when there are dosing questions? Would it be helpful for the prescribing physician to discuss a patient's needs with the treating therapist? Would it be helpful if the physician reviewed the imaging studies of his or her patient with serious neck injuries, prior to treatment by a therapist? Does understaffing affect the quality of care?

Jill recently visited a pain center where the medical director had integrated a pain therapist into the hospital's pain management program. After several visits to the hospital's pain management program, Jill complimented the staff as to their multidisciplinary approach to her care.

The medical director stated that the success of the hospital's pain management program was due to the multidisciplinary approach practiced in the hospital. He stated that pain management is often poorly practiced because of the failure of the treating physician to become more involved in the patient's therapy. A patient's pain is often exacerbated because of a superficial treatment plan that fails to include the physician, and the failure to provide the images to the treating therapist. Both the physician and treating therapist, and most important the patient's care, are optimized when there is ongoing communication among caregivers. The medical director further stated that professionalism and satisfaction among caregivers improve when communications flow freely.

Jill again complimented the staff and stated that she would not hesitate to recommend the hospital's pain management program to her family and friends.

The next time a caregiver treats a patient, the patient should ask: What records have you seen? Have you discussed my treatment plan with my physician? What were my physician's specific orders? May I see them? What precautions have you been asked to follow with me? Have you seen my imaging studies? Has anyone discussed them with you?

My pledge as a patient: I will ask myself, am I being treated in an assembly-line fashion, assembled in a room like cattle, without privacy in cramped corridors by a caregiver who, because of understaffing, is frantically moving from patient to patient, or am I truly getting individualized care and treatment in a style worthy of the words "I am receiving good quality care"?

Discussion

1. Regardless of your profession or health care setting, discuss how the multidisciplinary approach to patient care might be improved in your organization.
2. Consider and discuss what questions you might ask if you were the patient undergoing treatment.

PHYSICIAN ASSISTANT

Physician assistants (PAs) are health care professionals who "practice medicine on a team under the supervision of physicians and surgeons. "There are more than 90,000 nationally certified PAs, according to the National Commission on Certification of Physician Assistants."[58] They are formally educated to examine patients, diagnose injuries and illnesses, and provide treatment. PAs work in physicians' offices, hospitals, and other health care settings."[59] They are subject to the licensing laws within the state they are qualified to practice. As the role of PAs continues to expand, it is mandatory that they review and understand applicable state licensing laws. In addition, PAs must work within the scope of practice as defined by their employers.

PAs are responsible for their own negligent acts. Further, an employer of a PA can be held liable for a PA's negligent acts on the basis of *respondeat superior*. Physicians who delegate tasks to PAs that licensing laws stipulate a physician must perform can be held liable for assignment of an unauthorized task that results in an injury to a patient. If there is no proof that a PA breached the applicable standard of care for a PA, liability will not accrue to the PA. However, if the physician was negligent in making the assignment to the PA that led to the injury, liability could accrue to the physician.

The plaintiff in *Cox v. MA Primary and Urgent Care Clinic*[60] sued for injuries she allegedly suffered as a result of a PA's failure to diagnose her condition accurately. The patient was eventually diagnosed with cardiomyopathy. A mitral valve repair and mitral valve replacement were ultimately performed. The patient sued the PA for failure to readily diagnose her condition. The Tennessee Supreme Court after reviewing the case held:

> The professional standard of care applicable to physician assistants is distinct from that applicable to physicians. Because Plaintiff introduced no expert proof as to any violation of the applicable standard of care, the trial court was correct in its ruling that Defendants are entitled to summary judgment.[61]

To limit the potential risk of liability for a PA's negligent acts, PAs should be monitored and supervised by a physician. Moreover, guidelines and procedures should also be established to provide a standard mechanism for reviewing a PA's performance.

PSYCHOLOGY

Psychologists are expected to safeguard the welfare and rights of those with whom they interact professionally. They must establish relationships of trust with those with whom they work. They must uphold professional standards of conduct, clarify their professional roles and obligations, and accept responsibility for their behavior.

UNETHICAL CONDUCT

Sturm, a licensed psychologist who has taught professional ethics since 1985 and who served on the ethics committee of the Oregon Psychological Association for 6 years, testified that testimony about the best interests of children in a custody dispute by a therapist who had not observed both parents' interactions with the children was unethical. Sturm further stated that a psychologist has an obligation to adopt an impartial stance and to avoid actions that would escalate an adversarial nature of the relationship between the parents. Sturm explained that psychologists have "an ethical responsibility to anticipate the possible purposes" behind a request to prepare an affidavit to be used in a custody dispute in order to prevent misuse of the evaluation and agreed that practices such as making evaluative statements about persons or relationships not observed directly are blatantly unethical. The petitioner's affidavit made such statements, and it was not until the show cause hearing that petitioner admitted to her bias toward her patient.[62]

SEXUAL HARASSMENT

The *Ethical Principals of Psychologists and Code of Conduct*, in standard 3.02 on sexual harassment states that:

> Psychologists do not engage in sexual harassment. Sexual harassment is sexual solicitation, physical advances or verbal or nonverbal conduct that is sexual in nature, that occurs in connection with the psychologist's activities or roles as a psychologist and that either (1) is unwelcome, is offensive or creates a hostile workplace or educational environment, and the psychologist knows or is told this or (2) is sufficiently severe or intense to be abusive to a reasonable person in the context. Sexual harassment can consist of a single intense or severe act or of multiple persistent or pervasive acts.[63]

The Board of Psychologist Examiners in *Gilmore v. Board of Psychologist Examiners*[64] revoked a psychologist's license because of sexual improprieties. The psychologist petitioned for judicial review. She argued that therapy had terminated before the sexual relationships began. The court of appeals held that evidence supported the board conclusion that the psychologist had violated an ethical standard in caring for her patients. When a psychologist's personal interests intrude into the practitioner–client relationship, the practitioner is obliged to seek objectivity through a third party. The board's findings and conclusions indicated that the petitioner failed to maintain that objectivity.

REPORTING CHILD ABUSE

Two children were placed in the temporary custody of a foster family. One child was referred to a licensed psychologist for evaluation. After two interviews, the psychologist formed the professional opinion that the child had been sexually molested. Based in part on statements made by the child, the psychologist further believed that the perpetrator of the suspected molestation was the father. At a hearing before the juvenile court, the court determined that the evidence did not support a finding the child had been abused by his father. Custody was returned to the parents. The child's parents subsequently initiated an action for medical malpractice against the psychologist. The psychologist claimed immunity from liability, as provided by a state child abuse reporting statute. The trial court and the parents appealed, arguing that the immunity provisions of the statute do not apply to the psychologist because she was not a "mandatory reporter" under that statute.[65]

The Georgia Court of Appeals held that the statute's grant of immunity from liability extended to the psychologist. The evidence did not establish bad faith on the part of the psychologist so as to deprive her of such immunity. The statute provides that any person participating in the making of a report or participating in any judicial proceeding or any other proceeding resulting in a report of suspected child abuse is immune from any civil or criminal liability that might otherwise be incurred or imposed, provided such participation pursuant to the statute is made in good faith. The grant of qualified immunity covers every person who, in good faith, participates over time in the making of a report to a child welfare agency. Proof of negligent reporting or bad judgment is not proof that the psychologist refused to fulfill her professional duties out of some harmful motive or that she consciously acted for some dishonest purpose. There was no competent evidence that the psychologist acted in bad faith.

RADIOLOGY

Radiology technologists are expected to conduct themselves in a professional manner, respond to patient needs, and support colleagues and associates in providing quality patient care. The American Society of Radiologic Technologists Code of Ethics provides in part that "The radiologic technologist assesses situations; exercises care, discretion and judgment; assumes responsibility for professional decisions; and acts in the best interest of the patient."[66] The technologist failed to exercise discretion in the following case by not making sure the patient was secured to the table prior to the examination to prevent the patient from falling.

FAILURE TO RESTRAIN CAUSES PATIENT FALL

The plaintiff in *Cockerton v. Mercy Hospital Medical Center*[67] was admitted to the hospital for the purpose of surgery. Her physician ordered postsurgical X-rays for her head and face to be taken the next day. A hospital employee took the plaintiff from her room to the X-ray department by wheelchair. A nurse had assessed her condition as slightly "woozy" and drowsy. An X-ray technician took charge of the plaintiff in the X-ray room. After the plaintiff was taken inside the X-ray room, she was transferred from a wheelchair to a portable chair for the procedure. After being moved, the plaintiff complained of nausea. The technician did not use the restraint straps to secure the plaintiff to the chair. At some point during the procedure, the plaintiff had a fainting seizure. The technician called for help. When another hospital employee entered the room, the technician was holding the plaintiff in an upright position. She appeared nonresponsive. The plaintiff only remembered being stood up and having a lead jacket placed across her back and shoulders. The technician maintains that the plaintiff did not fall. At the time the plaintiff left the X-ray room, her level of consciousness was poor. The plaintiff's physician noticed a deflection of the plaintiff's nose but had difficulty assessing it because of the surgical procedure from the day before.

The following day, the deflection of the plaintiff's nose was much more evident. A specialist was contacted, and an attempt was made to correct the deformity. The specialist made an observation that it would require a substantial injury to the nose to deflect it to that severity.

The plaintiff instituted proceedings against the hospital, alleging that the negligence of the nurses or technicians allowed her to fall during the procedure and subsequently caused injury. The jury concluded that the hospital was negligent in leaving the plaintiff unattended or failing to restrain her, which proximately caused her fall and injury.

The X-ray technician testified that during the X-ray the plaintiff appeared to have a "seizure episode." She also testified that she left the plaintiff unattended for a brief period of time and that she did not use the restraint straps that were attached to the portable X-ray chair. Using the restraint straps would have secured the plaintiff to the portable chair during the X-ray examination.

RESPIRATORY CARE

Respiratory care involves the treatment, management, diagnostic testing, and control of patients with cardiopulmonary deficits. A *respiratory therapist* (RT) is a person employed in the practice of respiratory care who has the knowledge and skill necessary to administer respiratory care. As with other health care professions, respiratory RTs are expected to comply with their professional code of ethics. The American Association for Respiratory Care in its Statement of Ethics and Professional Conduct requires that RTs "Demonstrate behavior that reflects integrity, supports objectivity, and fosters trust in the profession and its professionals."[68] That code was violated in *State University v. Young.*[69] In this case the RT was suspended for using the same syringe for drawing blood from a number of critically ill patients. The therapist had been warned several times of the dangers of that practice and that it violated the state's policy of providing quality patient care.

Although an RT is responsible for the negligent acts, the employer is can be held responsible for the negligent acts of the therapist under the legal doctrine of *respondeat superior.*

CASE: RESTOCKING THE CODE CART

In *Dixon v. Taylor,* 111 N.C. App. 97, 431 S.E.2d 778 (1993), Dixon had been admitted to the hospital and was diagnosed with pneumonia in her right lung. Dixon's condition began to deteriorate, and she was moved to the intensive care unit (ICU). A code blue was eventually called, signifying that her cardiac and respiratory functions were believed to have ceased. During the code, a decision was made to intubate by inserting an endotracheal tube into Dixon so that she could be given respiratory support by a mechanical ventilator.

As Dixon's condition stabilized, Dr. Taylor, Dixon's physician at that time, ordered that she be gradually weaned from the respirator. Blackham, a respiratory therapist employed by the hospital, extubated Dixon at 10:15 p.m. Taylor left Dixon's room to advise her family that she had been extubated.

Blackham decided an oxygen mask would provide better oxygen to Dixon but could not locate a mask in the ICU; thus, he left ICU and went across the hall to the critical care unit. When Blackham returned to Dixon's room with the oxygen mask and placed it on Dixon, he realized that she was not breathing properly. Blackham realized that she would have to be reintubated as quickly as possible.

A second code was called and Shackleford, a nurse in the cardiac critical care unit, responded to the code. Shackleford recorded on the code sheet that she arrived in Dixon's room at 10:30 p.m. She testified that Blackham said he had too short of a blade and he needed a medium, a Number 4 MacIntosh laryngoscope blade which was not on the code cart. The code cart is a cart equipped with all the medicines, supplies, and instruments needed for a code emergency. The code cart in the ICU had not been restocked after the first code that morning; thus, Shackleford was sent to obtain the needed blade from the critical care unit across the hall.

When Shackleford returned to the ICU, the blade was passed to Taylor, who had responded to the code and was attempting to reintubate Dixon. After receiving the blade, Taylor was able to quickly intubate Dixon. Dixon was placed on a ventilator, but she never regained consciousness. After the family was informed there was no hope that Dixon would recover the use of her brain, the family requested that no extraordinary measures be taken to prolong her life.

A medical negligence claim was filed against Taylor and the hospital. The jury found that Taylor was not negligent. Evidence presented at trial established that the hospital's breach of duty in not having the code cart properly restocked resulted in a 3-minute delay in the intubation of Dixon. Reasonable minds could accept from the testimony at trial that the hospital's breach of duty was a cause of Dixon's brain death, without which the injury would not have occurred. Foreseeability on the part of the hospital can be established from the evidence introduced by the plaintiff that the written standards for the hospital require every code cart be stocked with a Number 4 MacIntosh blade. This evidence permits a reasonable inference that the hospital should have foreseen that the failure to have the code cart stocked with the blade could lead to critical delays in intubating a patient. Accordingly, there was substantial evidence that the failure to have the code cart stocked with the proper blade was a proximate cause of Dixon's fatal injuries.

Ethical and Legal Issues

1. Describe the ethical issues involved in this case.
2. Explain how the elements of negligence are meet in this case.
3. What steps could be implemented to prevent similar occurrences in the future?

SOCIAL WORK

Social workers in the hospital setting assist patients and families with: psychosocial issues; obtaining insurance coverage; making difficult care decisions; and, assisting the patient and family in planning for postdischarge care. As with many professions, social workers are often overlooked and underused when it comes to the team approach to health care. It has, over the years, been a low priority with hospitals to hire an effective team, adequately staffed to address the myriad of issues that need to be addressed in the delivery of patient care.

The National Association of Social Workers Code of Ethics specifies the following six purposes:[70]

1. The Code identifies core values on which social work's mission is based.
2. The Code summarizes broad ethical principles that reflect the profession's core values and establishes a set of specific ethical standards that should be used to guide social work practice.
3. The Code is designed to help social workers identify relevant considerations when professional obligations conflict or ethical uncertainties arise.
4. The Code provides ethical standards to which the general public can hold the social work profession accountable.
5. The Code socializes practitioners new to the field to social work's mission, values, ethical principles, and ethical standards.
6. The Code articulates standards that the social work professional itself can use to assess whether social workers have engaged in unethical conduct. NASW has formal procedures to adjudicate ethics complaints filed against its members. [For information on NASW adjudication procedures, see NASW Procedures for the Adjudication of Grievances.] In subscribing to this Code, social workers are required to cooperate in its implementation, participate in NASW adjudication proceedings, and abide by any NASW disciplinary rulings for sanctions based on it.

As with any profession, legal and moral concern social workers as well, as noted in the following news clipping.

Caseworker Fired after Baby Dies

A District of Columbia social worker was fired Tuesday following the death of a baby who was reported as neglected, city officials said.

The city's Child and Family Service Agency received a call about the 6-month-old boy in March, but the social worker assigned to the case never visited the child, interim Attorney General Peter Nickles said.

Nikita Stewart, The Washington Post, July 8, 2008

CERTIFICATION OF HEALTH CARE PROFESSIONALS

The *certification* of health care professionals is the recognition by a governmental or professional association that an individual's expertise meets the standards of that group. Some professional groups establish their own minimum standards for certification in those professions that are not licensed by a particular state. Certification by an association or group is a self-regulation credentialing process.

LICENSING OF HEALTH CARE PROFESSIONAL

Licensure can be defined as the process by which some competent authority grants permission to a qualified individual or entity to perform certain specified activities that would be illegal without a license. As it applies to health care personnel, licensure refers to the process by which licensing boards, agencies, or departments of the several states grant to individuals who meet certain predetermined standards the legal right to practice in a health care profession and to use a specified health care practitioner's title. The commonly stated objectives of licensing laws are to limit and control admission to the different health care occupations and to protect the public from unqualified practitioners by promulgating and enforcing standards of practice within the professions. Health professions commonly requiring licensure include dentists, nurses, pharmacists, PAs, osteopaths, physicians, and podiatrists.

The authority of states to license health care practitioners is explicit in their regulatory powers. Implicit in the power to license is the right to collect licensing fees, establish standards of practice, require certain minimum qualifications and competency levels of applicants, and impose on applicants other requirements necessary to protect the general public welfare. This authority, which is vested in the legislature, may be delegated to political subdivisions or to state boards, agencies, and departments. In some instances, the scope of the delegated power is made specific in the legislation; in others, the licensing authority may have wide discretion in performing its functions. In either case, however, the authority granted by the legislature may not be exceeded.

SUSPENSION AND REVOCATION OF LICENSE

Licensing boards have the authority to suspend or revoke the license of a health care professional found to have violated specified norms of conduct. Such violations may include procurement of a license by fraud; unprofessional, dishonorable, immoral, or illegal conduct; performance of specific actions prohibited by statute; and malpractice. Suspension and revocation procedures are most commonly contained in a state's licensing act; in some jurisdictions, however, the procedure for suspension and revocation of a license is left to the discretion of the licensing board.

HELPFUL ADVICE FOR CAREGIVERS

- Break down the barriers between departments and work as a team.
- Abide by the ethical code of one's profession.
- Do not criticize the professional skills of others.
- Maintain complete medical records.
- Provide each patient with medical care comparable with national standards.
- Seek the aid of professional medical consultants when indicated.
- Obtain informed consent for diagnostic and therapeutic procedures.
- Inform the patient of the risks, benefits, and alternatives to proposed procedures.
- Practice the specialty in which you have been trained.
- Participate in continuing education programs.
- Keep patient information confidential.

- Check patient equipment regularly, and monitor it for safe use.
- When terminating a professional relationship, give adequate written notice to the patient.
- Authenticate all telephone orders.
- Obtain a qualified substitute when you will be absent from your practice.
- Be a good listener, and allow each patient sufficient time to express fears and anxieties.
- Develop and implement an interdisciplinary plan of care for each patient.
- Safely administer patient medications.
- Closely monitor each patient's response to treatment.
- Provide education and teaching to patients.
- Foster a sense of trust and feeling of significance.
- Communicate with the patient and other caregivers.
- Provide cost-effective care without sacrificing quality.

CHAPTER REVIEW

1. The contents of codes of ethics vary depending on the risks associated with a particular profession.
   - Ethical codes for psychologists, for example, define relationships with clients in greater depth because of the personal one-to-one relationship they have with their clients.
   - Practicing outside one's scope of practice has both ethical and legal concerns.
2. Legislation in many states imposes a duty on hospitals to provide emergency care. If the public is aware that a hospital furnishes emergency services and relies on that knowledge, the hospital has a duty to provide those services to the public.
3. Hospitals are expected to notify specialty on-call physicians when their particular skills are required in the emergency department. A physician who is on call and fails to respond to a request to attend a patient can be liable for injuries suffered by the patient because of his or her failure to respond.
4. There can be both ethical and legal repercussions if a professional incorrectly interprets a physician's orders.
5. A defense that sexual improprieties with clients did not take place during treatment sessions is unacceptable conduct.
6. Scope of practice refers to the permissible boundaries of practice for health care professionals, as is often defined in state statutes, which define the actions, duties, and limits of professionals in their particular roles.
7. A professional who exceeds his or her scope of practice as defined by state practice acts can be found to have violated licensure provisions or to have performed tasks that are reserved by statute for another health care professional.
8. The power and authority to regulate drugs and their products, packaging, and distribution rest primarily with federal and state governments.
9. Certification of health care professionals is the recognition by a governmental or professional association that an individual's expertise meets the standards of that group.
10. Licensure can be defined as the process by which some competent authority grants permission to a qualified individual or entity to perform certain specified activities that would be illegal without a license.

TEST YOUR UNDERSTANDING

TERMINOLOGY

advanced practice nurse	licensure	pharmacist
certification	medical assistant	physical therapy
chiropractor	nonmaleficence	physician assistant
clinical nurse specialist	nurse anesthetist	psychologist
dentist	nurse midwife	radiology technologists
dietitian	nurse practitioner	registered nurse
float nurse	nursing assistant	respiratory therapist
laboratory medical technologists	paramedic	social workers
	patient care teams	special duty nurse

REVIEW QUESTIONS

1. Describe how ethics and the law have an impact on the various health care professions discussed in this chapter.

2. Discuss the ethical and legal implications of practicing outside one's scope of practice.

3. Discuss the circumstances under which a hospital has a duty to provide emergency services to the public?

4. Are sexual improprieties acceptable with clients as long as they do not take place during treatment? Explain your answer.

5. Consider under what circumstances a professional's legal responsibilities may overlap with his or her ethical duties.

6. Describe how and why the scope of practice for various professionals (e.g., nurses and pharmacists) is changing.

7. Discuss what action a caregiver should take, if any, if a physician's written orders appear questionable.

8. Describe a professional's responsibilities when a patient's condition takes a turn for the worse.

9. Describe the difference between the certification and licensing of a health care professional.

NOTES

1. Walter F. Roche, Jr., "City hospital's HIV testing manipulated," *Baltimore Sun,* March 11, 2004; http://www.baltimoresun.com/news/local/bal-lab0311,0,6183061.story?coll5bal-localheadlines.

2. *Fraijo v. Hartland Hosp.,* 160 Cal. Rptr. 252 (Ct. App. 1979).

3. Institute of Medicine, "Keeping patients safe: Transforming the work environment of nurses." Washington, DC: The National Academies Press, at 2. Available at http://www.nap.edu/openbook.php?isbn=0309090679.

4. http://www.hhs.gov/news/press/2013pres/12/20131205a.html.

5. Department of Health, Education & Welfare, "Extending the scope of nursing practice: A report of the Secretary's Committee to Study Roles for Nurses," Pub. No. (HSM) 73-2037, 8 (1971).

6. http://www.nysna.org/practice/positions/floating.htm.

7. 2014 Hospital Accreditation Standards, LD.03.06.04 at LD – 20.

8. 692 S.W.2d 329 (Mo. Ct. App. 1985).

9. 144 So. 2d 249 (La. Ct. App. 1962).

10. Tami Dennis, "More heparin overdoses, this time in Texas," *Los Angeles Times,* July 9, 2008; http://latimesblogs. latimes.com/booster_shots/2008/07/more-heparin-ov.html.

11. *Harrison v. Axelrod,* 599 N.Y.S.2d 96 (N.Y. App. Div. 1993).

12. 181 A.2d 573 (Del. 1962).

13. 403 S.E.2d 582 (N.C. Ct. App. 1991).

14. *Id* at 584-585.

15. 333 P.2d 29 (Cal. Ct. App. 1958).

16. 422 N.W.2d 600 (S.D. 1988).

17. 589 A.2d 653 (N.J. Super. App. Div. 1991).

18. Id. at 655.

19. 435 N.E.2d 305 (Ind. Ct. App. 1982).

20. *Poor v. State*, No.S-02-472, 266 Neb. 183 (Neb. 2003).

21. 557 S.E.2d 339 (2001).

22. 495 N.Y.S.2d 808 (N.Y. App. Div. 1985).

23. *Lowenberg v. Sobol*, 594 N.Y.S.2d 874 (N.Y. App. Div. 1993).

24. 367 S.E.2d 453 (S.C. 1988).

25. Id. at 455–456.

26. 753 F. Supp. 267 (W.D. Ark. 1990).

27. http://www.ncbi.nlm.nih.gov/pmc/articles/PMC2539799/.

28. 271 N.W.2d 8 (S.D. 1978).

29. 288 A.2d 379 (Md. 1972).

30. 477 So. 2d 1036 (Fla. Dist. Ct. App. 1985).

31. *Baptist Mem'l Hosp. Sys. v. Sampson*, 969 S.W.2d 945, 947 (Tex. 1998).

32. Martin C. McWilliams, Jr. & Hamilton E. Russell, III, Hospital Liability for Torts of Independent Contractor Physicians, 47 S.C. L. reV. 431, 473 (1996).

33. 462 A.2d 680 (Pa. 1983).

34. 650 A.2d 1076 (Pa. Super. 1994).

35. http://www.ascls.org/about-us/code-of-ethics.

36. Walter F. Roche, Jr., "City hospital's HIV testing manipulated," *The Baltimore Sun*, March 11, 2004, http://www. baltimoresun.com/news/maryland/bal-lab0311,0,3643424.story.

37. https://www.ascp.org/pdf/StateLicensureofLaboratoryPersonnel.aspx.

38. http://www.komonews.com/news/local/Spokane-woman-suing-over-false-HIV-diagnosis-237318161.html.

39. 521 N.E.2d 350 (Ind. Ct. App. 1988).

40. *Id.* at 352.

41. *Id.* at 353.

42. See Certmedassistant.com, "Certified medical assistant," http://www.certmedassistant.com/what-medical-assistant.html.

43. U.S. Department of Labor, Bureau of Labor Statistics, "Occupational outlook handbook, 2010-11 edition"; http://www.bls.gov/ooh/<URL not found 8/1/2014.

44. Ibid.

45. 636 N.E.2d 1282 (Ind. Ct. App. 1994).

46. Institute of Medicine, "To err is human: Building a safer health system," supra note 1, at 194.

47. Katie Moisse, "Hospital errors common and underreported," ABC News, April 7, 2011; http://abcnews.go.com/Health/hospital-errors-common-underreported-study/story?id=13310733.

48. http://legacy.uspharmacist.com/index.asp?show=article&page=8_1129.htm.

49. 544 N.W.2d 727 (Mich. Ct. App. 1996).

50. *Riff v. Morgan Pharmacy*, 508 A.2d 1247 (Pa. Super. Ct. 1986).

51. 642 N.E.2d 514 (Ind. 1994).

52. Ind. Code A4 25-26-13-16(b)(3) (1993).

53. http://www.pharmacist.com/code-ethics.

54. 308 S.E.2d 65 (N.C. Ct. App. 1983).

55. 478 N.Y.S.2d 209 (N.Y. App. Div. 1984).

56. 780 So. 2d 478 (2001).

57. 527 N.Y.S.2d 937 (N.Y. App. Div. 1988).

58. http://www.aapa.org/the_pa_profession/quick_facts/resources/item.aspx?id=3848.

59. http://www.bls.gov/ooh/Healthcare/Physician-assistants.htm.

60. 313 SW 3d 240 - Tenn: Supreme Court 2010.

61. *Id.* 262.

62. *Loomis v. Board of Psychologist Exam'rs,* 954 P.2d 839 (1998).

63. http://www.apa.org/ethics/code/index.aspx#.

64. 725 P.2d 400 (Or. Ct. App. 1986).

65. *Michaels v. Gordon,* 439 S.E.2d 722 (Ga. Ct. App. 1993).

66. http://www.asrt.org/docs/practice-standards/codeofethics.pdf.

67. 490 N.W.2d 856 (Iowa Ct. App. 1992).

68. http://www.aarc.org/resources/position_statements/ethics.html.

69. 566 N.Y.S.2d 79 (N.Y. App. Div. 1991).

70. http://socialworkers.org/pubs/code/code.asp.

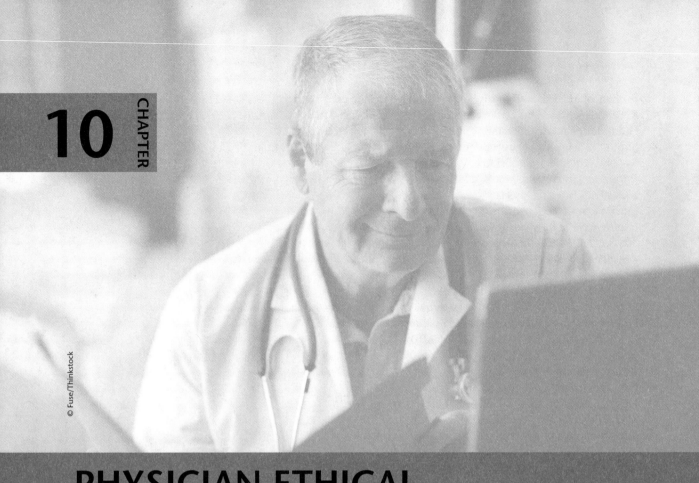

10

PHYSICIAN ETHICAL AND LEGAL ISSUES

LEARNING OBJECTIVES

Upon completion of this chapter, the reader will be able to:

- Apply the *Hippocratic Oath* to modern codes of medical ethics.
- Understand how the law and ethics intertwine in patient care.
- Describe common medical errors and ethical issues relative to physician practice.
- Describe important guidelines for developing positive physician–patient relations.

INTRODUCTION

The Hippocratic Oath

I SWEAR by Apollo the physician, and Aesculapius, and Health, and All-heal, and all the gods and goddesses, that, according to my ability and judgment, I will keep this Oath and this stipulation—to reckon him who taught me this Art equally dear to me as my parents, to share my substance with him, and relieve his necessities if required;

to look upon his offspring in the same footing as my own brothers, and to teach them this art, if they shall wish to learn it, without fee or stipulation; and that by precept, lecture, and every other mode of instruction, I will impart a knowledge of the Art to my own sons, and those of my teachers, and to disciples bound by a stipulation and oath according to the law of medicine, but to none others. I will follow that system of regimen which, according to my ability and judgment, I consider for the benefit of my patients, and abstain from whatever is deleterious and mischievous. I will give no deadly medicine to any one if asked, nor suggest any such counsel; and in like manner I will not give to a woman a pessary to produce abortion. With purity and with holiness I will pass my life and practice my Art. I will not cut persons laboring under the stone, but will leave this to be done by men who are practitioners of this work. Into whatever houses I enter, I will go into them for the benefit of the sick, and will abstain from every voluntary act of mischief and corruption; and, further from the seduction of females or males, of freemen and slaves. Whatever, in connection with my professional practice or not, in connection with it, I see or hear, in the life of men, which ought not to be spoken of abroad, I will not divulge, as reckoning that all such should be kept secret. While I continue to keep this Oath unviolated, may it be granted to me to enjoy life and the practice of the art, respected by all men, in all times! But should I trespass and violate this Oath, may the reverse be my lot![1]

This chapter provides the reader with an overview of common medical errors and ethical issues relative to the practice of medicine. The medical profession has long subscribed to a body of ethical principals. One of Hippocrates' gifts to medicine, among many, was the *Hippocratic Oath* for physicians, which has been modified and adopted by various medical schools such as John Baylor College of Medicine, Johns Hopkins Medical School, and Tufts University School of Medicine[2] as noted in the following extract:

I swear to fulfill, to the best of my ability and judgment, this covenant:

I will respect the hard-won scientific gains of those physicians in whose steps I walk, and gladly share such knowledge as is mine with those who are to follow.

I will apply, for the benefit of the sick, all measures which are required, avoiding those twin traps of overtreatment and therapeutic nihilism.

I will remember that there is art to medicine as well as science, and that warmth, sympathy, and understanding may outweigh the surgeon's knife or the chemist's drug.

I will not be ashamed to say "I know not," nor will I fail to call in my colleagues when the skills of another are needed for a patient's recovery.

I will respect the privacy of my patients, for their problems are not disclosed to me that the world may know. Most especially must I tread with care in matters of life and death. If it is given me to save a life, all thanks. But it may also be within my power to take a life; this awesome responsibility must be faced with great humbleness and awareness of my own frailty. Above all, I must not play at God.

I will remember that I do not treat a fever chart, a cancerous growth, but a sick human being, whose illness may affect the person's family and economic stability. My responsibility includes these related problems, if I am to care adequately for the sick.

I will prevent disease whenever I can, for prevention is preferable to cure.

I will remember that I remain a member of society, with special obligations to all my fellow human beings, those sound of mind and body as well as the infirm. If I do not violate this oath, may I enjoy life and art, respected while I live and remembered with affection thereafter. May I always act so as to preserve the finest traditions of my calling and may I long experience the joy of healing those who seek my help.

Source: *Louis Lasagna, 1964, Academic Dean of the School of Medicine at Tufts University, and used in many medical schools today.*

Although there is no direct punishment for violating the Hippocratic oath, medical malpractice suits often involve a physician's failure to adhere to the oath and/or other applicable medical codes of ethics. Malpractice suits can lead to financial awards to the injured party.

CODE OF MEDICAL ETHICS

The American Medical Association in the footsteps of Hippocrates describes the code of ethical conduct for physicians:

I. A physician shall be dedicated to providing competent medical care, with compassion and respect for human dignity and rights.

II. A physician shall uphold the standards of professionalism, be honest in all professional interactions, and strive to report physicians deficient in character or competence, or engaging in fraud or deception, to appropriate entities.

III. A physician shall respect the law and also recognize a responsibility to seek changes in those requirements that are contrary to the best interests of the patient.

IV. A physician shall respect the rights of patients, colleagues, and other health professionals, and shall safeguard patient confidences and privacy within the constraints of the law.

V. A physician shall continue to study, apply, and advance scientific knowledge; maintain a commitment to medical education; make relevant information available to patients, colleagues, and the public; obtain consultation; and use the talents of other health professionals when indicated.

VI. A physician shall, in the provision of appropriate patient care, except in emergencies, be free to choose whom to serve, with whom to associate, and the environment in which to provide medical care.

VII. A physician shall recognize a responsibility to participate in activities contributing to the improvement of the community and the betterment of public health.

VIII. A physician shall, while caring for a patient, regard responsibility to the patient as paramount.

IX. A physician shall support access to medical care for all people.

Source: Code of Medical Ethics, A9 2001, American Medical Association.[3]

LAW AND ETHICS INTERTWINE

This section introduces the reader to how the law and ethics intertwine in patient care. The law provides that injury to a patient due to a negligent act can result in financial penalties imposed by the courts to compensate the injured party and hopefully deter similar acts. *Nonmaleficence* in medical ethics is a central guiding principle of the ethical practice of medicine; first expressed by Hippocrates, and translated into Latin as *primum non nocere*, first do no harm. It is medicine's most fundamental axiom that aptly describes where the law and ethics unite—*first do no harm*. The injury of a patient due to an avoidable negligent act often involves both principles of law and ethics.

HIPPOCRATIC OATH AND AMA CODE OF ETHICS VIOLATED

The Thompsons in *Scripps Clinic v. Superior Ct.*[4] alleged negligent treatment of Patricia Thompson's broken clavicle. A medical malpractice claim was filed against Dr. Thorne and Dr. Carpenter, both of whom were affiliated with Scripps, a group medical practice. At the time the malpractice action was filed, Patricia was no longer being treated by Thorne and Carpenter, but was being treated by other Scripps physicians: Drs. Botte and Froenke for the broken clavicle and Dr. Harkey for endometriosis.

Binford, a Scripps employee, sent a letter to the Thompsons informing them that Scripps had been notified about the legal action the Thompsons had taken against the group. Because of the legal action, the Scripps Clinic requested that Health Net immediately terminate the Thompsons with the Scripps Clinic and transfer their membership to another medical group.

When Patricia received Binford's letter, she immediately requested Health Net to reassign the couple to a new medical group. Health Net transferred the Thompsons to the San Diego Medical Group. As the result of Scripps's actions, Patricia had to cancel a follow-up visit with Dr. Harkey that had been scheduled near the end of June even though Patricia was still suffering severe pain and bleeding. Before Patricia could be referred to a new gynecologist at University of California, San Diego Medical Group, she had to schedule a visit with her new primary care physician and receive authorization. Patricia's care was also delayed until the San Diego Medical Group received her medical records from Scripps.

Scripps contends that it gave adequate notice to the Thompsons. The court disagreed. There was a 2-week hiatus between the time Scripps denied the Thompsons access to its physicians for nonemergency services and the time the Thompsons were assigned to the San Diego Medical Group.

The court rejected Scripps's contention the court should have granted summary adjudication of the negligent infliction of emotional distress and breach of fiduciary duty causes of action. The court denied the motion because the Thompsons raised a triable issue of fact as to breach, based upon the declaration of Dr. David Goldstein, the Thompsons' expert. Goldstein declared Scripps breached the standard of care and its fiduciary duty by violating the AMA Code of Medical Ethics 1.3.10 and the Hippocratic Oath, because its policy is retaliatory and "promotes the self-interest of physicians over that of patients."[5]

Physicians have both a legal and ethical obligation to attend to their patients' needs. Physicians licensed in Illinois, for example, are specifically prohibited from abandoning their patients.[6] Furthermore, the American Medical Association's Council on Ethical and Judicial

Affairs mandates that "once having undertaken a case, the physician should not neglect the patient."[7]

The relationship between a physician and a patient, once established, continues until it is ended by the mutual consent of the parties, the patient's dismissal of the physician, the physician's withdrawal from the case, or the fact that the physician's services are no longer required. A physician who decides to withdraw his or her services must provide the patient with reasonable notice so that the services of another physician can be obtained. Premature termination of treatment is often the subject of a legal action for abandonment, the unilateral termination of a physician–patient relationship by the physician without notice to the patient. The following elements must be established in order for a patient to recover damages for abandonment:

- Medical care was unreasonably discontinued.
- The discontinuance of medical care was against the patient's will. Termination of the physician–patient relationship must have been brought about by a unilateral act of the physician. There can be no issue of abandonment if the relationship is terminated by mutual consent or by dismissal of the physician by the patient.
- The physician failed to arrange for care by another physician. Refusal by a physician to enter into a physician–patient relationship by failing to respond to a call or render treatment is not considered a case of abandonment. A plaintiff will not recover for damages unless he or she can show that a physician–patient relationship had been established.
- Foresight indicated that discontinuance might result in physical harm.
- The patient as a result of the physician's abandonment suffered actual harm.

Physicians must, as provided in the Hippocratic oath and codes of ethics, make care decisions for the benefit of their patients and not for their hurt or for any wrong. Terminating a physician–patient relationship must be done within legal guidelines, otherwise the physician can be held liable for abandonment. As noted next, compassion, trust, justice, and respect for patient privacy are all ethical principles and values that are intertwined with law.

COMPASSION

Compassion is a moral value hoped for in all caregivers. Those who truly possess it will have a more rewarding career and at the end of life be able to say, "I have not only lived, but I have lived for something, it was worthwhile, I had a reason for living and a reason for leaving. I led a purpose-fulfilled life." The following news clipping succinctly illustrates how one physician's experience when faced with a dying patient can spring forth compassion and a time for reflection.

Suddenly, unexpectedly, he grabs my shirt.

"Don't let me die!" he says, spraying me with blood.
He turns with effort, his yellow eyes searing into mine.

• • •

Hours later, my pager beeps again. It's the head nurse once more, summoning me back to "pronounce him dead."

• • •

"The family is waiting to see you," she says, as if I should've known.

• • •

The woman I take to be the deceased's mother reaches into a purse on the floor and unfurls a rumpled handkerchief. She buries her face in it. *Memento mori*, the ancient Romans said. Remember that you will die. This scene will be a permanent meditation throughout the rest of my career.

Richard E. Cytowic, Washingtonian, *March 2014*

Not all physicians possess the degree of compassion noted in the news clipping. The following *reality check* describes the world of Mrs. Smith who during an interview stated that she found in over 15 years of being passed from physician to physician only 4 of 26 physicians (15.83%) that she would describe as compassionate and empathetic to her as the pain racked her body from the top of her head to the soles of her feet.

Physician Lacks Compassion

Mrs. Smith arranged for an appointment to see Dr. Mean, a rheumatologist, who was a specialist in her particular disease process, systemic scleroderma. After scheduling her appointment, Mrs. Smith was asked to have her medical records faxed to Mean's office before her scheduled appointment on March 27. Two days before her scheduled appointment with Mean, Mrs. Smith called Mean's office to confirm that her records had arrived. She was told at that time that she was on Mean's calendar for March 23, not March 27. She had missed her appointment. Mrs. Smith had waited 2 months for this date, and her illness had gotten progressively worse. Mrs. Smith, desperate for help, pleaded with the scheduler to reschedule her as soon as possible. The scheduler explained to Mrs. Smith that Mean was a busy physician and that she could not schedule a new appointment until April 27, a month later.

Discussion

1. Describe how Dr. Mean violated the professional code of ethics for a physician.
2. Discuss what role a hospital ethics committee could play in addressing Dr. Mean's insensitivity to Mrs. Smith's needs? Explain your answer.

It is not only important for the physician to show compassion, but also the office staff that works with patients from the time they walk in the office door until the time they leave, as the following *reality check* illustrates.

Staff Affects Physician Practice Image

Mark was waiting to be seen by his physician in a multispecialty physician office practice. As Mark was waiting to see his physician, he observed a woman, most likely in her late 70s, limping into the office. She had a large leg brace that ran from her thigh to the calf of her leg. She struggled to push her husband in a wheelchair into the office. She carefully parked the wheelchair and approached the check-in counter. She apologized for being late for her appointment as she was late getting out of another physician's office. The patient was told, "You are late for your appointment. The office has a 15-minute late arrival rule. You will have to reschedule your appointment." She apologized for being late but said that she did tell the office staff she would be late. She was then told, "You can wait, and I will try to squeeze you into the schedule, but I don't know how long you will have to wait." The lady said, "I don't want to bother anyone. I will reschedule my appointment." She was directed around the corner to another desk to reschedule her appointment. Mark got up out of his chair, walked over to the scheduler, and said, "I don't believe this. Her husband is sitting in a wheelchair, and she is having difficulty walking. She can have my appointment, and I can reschedule." The lady suddenly turned to Mark and gave him a big hug. The scheduler asked, "Who is your physician?" Mark told her, and she said, "I am sorry, but this lady has a different physician." The lady, now a bit teary eyed, continued to make her appointment.

Discussion

1. Describe the ethical issues involved in this observation.
2. Consider and discuss how this event could have had a more pleasant outcome.

TRUST

Patients trust their physicians to provide them the necessary medical information to assist them in making the right treatment choices. The use of risky and unproven procedures that a patient's injury can result in a lawsuit. However, a physician will not be held liable for exercising his or her judgment in applying a course of treatment supported by a reputable and respected body of medical experts even if another body of expert medical opinion would favor a different course of treatment.

Surgeons and Medical Center Breach Trust

A young woman went to a medical center for removal of a benign fibroid tumor in her uterus, an outpatient procedure. By the end of the day, she was dead.

> The surgery was performed by two doctors—one on probation—who used equipment they were neither familiar with nor authorized to use, the Health Department said. In a highly unusual violation, the agency said, a salesman from Johnson & Johnson, which made the piece of equipment used in the surgery, operated its controls while the doctors performed their procedure on the woman. And the patient was never given the chance to consent to the use of the equipment or the presence of the salesman, the agency said.[8]

The actions of the surgeons and medical center in this case clearly place the spotlight on trust and the ability of health care organizations to competently monitor their professional staff. The community of patients across the nation trust that the physicians appointed and credentialed by hospitals are closely monitored and privileged strictly according to their proven capabilities. This trust must not falter.

Failure to Read Nurses' Notes

On October 17, the medical record indicated that Todd's sternotomy wound and the mid-lower left leg incision were reddened and his temperature was 99.6 degrees F. Dr. Sauls did not commonly read the nurses' notes but instead preferred to rely on his own observations of the patient. In his October 18 notes, he indicated that there was no drainage. The nurses' notes, however, show that there was drainage at the chest tube site. In contrast to the medical records showing that Todd had a temperature of 101.2 degrees F, Dr. Sauls noted that the patient was afebrile (normal, without fever).

On October 19, Dr. Sauls noted that Todd's wounds were improving, and he did not have a fever. Nurses' notes indicated redness at the surgical wounds and a temperature of 100 degrees F. No white blood count had been ordered. Again on October 20, the nurses' notes indicated redness at the site of the wound and a temperature of 100.8 degrees F. No wound culture had yet been ordered. Dr. Kamil, one of Todd's treating physicians, noted that Todd's nutritional status needed to be seriously confronted and suggested that Dr. Sauls consider supplemental feeding. Despite this, no follow-up to his recommendation appeared and the record is void of any action by Dr. Sauls to obtain a nutritional consult.

Todd was transferred to the intensive care unit on October 21 because he was gravely ill with profoundly depressed ventricular function. The following day the nurses' notes described the chest tube site as draining foul-smelling bloody purulence. The patient's temperature was recorded to have reached 100.6 degrees F. This was the first time that Dr. Sauls had the test tube site cultured. On October 23, the culture report from the laboratory indicated a staph infection, and Todd was started on antibiotics for treatment of the infection.

On October 25, at the request of family, Todd was transferred to St. Luke's Hospital. At St. Luke's, Dr. Leatherman, an internist and invasive cardiologist, treated Todd. Dr. Zeluff, an infectious disease specialist, examined Todd's surgical wounds and prescribed antibiotic treatment. On his admission to St. Luke's, every one of Todd's surgical wounds was infected. Despite the care given at St. Luke's, Todd died on November 2, 1988. The family brought a malpractice suit against the surgeon. The District Court entered judgment on a jury verdict for the defendant, and the plaintiff appealed, claiming the surgeon breached his duty of care owed to the patient by failing to (1) aggressively treat the surgical wound infections, (2) read the nurses' observations of infections, and (3) provide adequate nourishment, allowing the patient's body weight to waste away rapidly.

Dr. Sauls committed medical malpractice when he breached the standard of care he owed to Todd. Todd was effectively ineligible for a heart transplant, which was his only chance of survival because of the infections and malnourishment caused by Dr. Sauls's negligent care. Sauls's testimony convinced the Louisiana Court of Appeals that he failed to treat the surgical wound infections aggressively, that he chose not to take advantage of the nurses' observations of infection, and that he allowed Todd's body weight to waste away, knowing that extreme vigilance was required because of Todd's already severely impaired heart.

In cases in which a patient has died, the plaintiff need not demonstrate that the patient would have survived if properly treated. Rather, he need only prove that the patient had a chance of survival and that his chance of survival was lost as a result of the defendant/physician's negligence. The defendant/physician's conduct must increase the risk of a patient's harm to the extent of being a substantial factor in causing the result, but need not be the only cause. Dr. Sauls's medical malpractice exacerbated an already critical condition and deprived Mr. Todd of a chance of survival.

Todd trusted Dr. Sauls to do the right thing. Instead he failed to follow Todd's care closely enough to identify his declining health as a result of an infection—that was clearly indicated in the nurses' notes.

Failure to Refer for Consultation

1 in 4 Cancer Cases Missed: GPs Send Away Alarming Number of Patients, Delaying Vital Treatment

Tens of thousands of patients are initially told that their symptoms are "nothing to worry about" or advised to take painkillers or antibiotics for months.

They have to make repeated trips to their doctor before being given a correct diagnosis, the report concludes. Britain has one of the lowest cancer survival rates in Europe despite billions being invested in treatment over the last decade.

Experts blame late diagnosis for the alarmingly high death rates and say many tumors are spotted only when it is too late for successful treatment.

Sophie Borland and David Wilkes, Daily Mail, *March 1, 2011*[9]

When a practitioner determines or should have determined that a patient's ailment is beyond his or her scope of knowledge, technical skill or ability, or capacity to treat with a likelihood of reasonable success, he or she is under a duty to disclose such determination to the patient. The patient should be advised of the necessity of other or different treatments.

A physician has a duty to consult and/or refer a patient whom he or she knows or should know needs referral to a physician familiar with and clinically capable of treating the patient's particular ailments. Whether the failure to refer constitutes negligence depends on whether referral is demanded by accepted standards of practice. To recover damages, the plaintiff must show that the physician deviated from the standard of care and that the failure to refer resulted in injury.

The California Court of Appeals found that expert testimony is not necessary where good medical practice would require a general physician to suggest a specialist's consultation.[10] The court ruled that because specialists were called in after the patient's condition grew worse, it is reasonable to assume that they could have been called in sooner. The jury was instructed by the court that a general practitioner has a duty to seek consultation by a specialist if a reasonably prudent general practitioner would do so under similar circumstances.

A physician is in a position of trust, and it is his or her duty to act in good faith. If a preferred treatment in a given situation is outside a physician's field of expertise, it is his or her duty to advise the patient. Failure to do so could constitute a breach of duty. Today, with the rapid methods of transportation and easy means of communication, the duty of a physician is not fulfilled merely by using the means at hand in a particular area of practice.

Falsification of Records

The intentional alteration, falsification, or destruction of medical records to avoid liability for one's medical negligence is generally sufficient to show actual malice, and punitive damages may be awarded whether or not the act of altering, falsifying, or destroying records directly causes compensable harm. The evidence in *Dimora v. Cleveland Clinic Foundation*[11] had shown that the patient had fallen and broken five or six ribs; nevertheless, on examination, the physician noted in the progress notes that the patient was smiling and laughing pleasantly, exhibiting no pain on deep palpation of the area. Other testimony indicated that she was in pain and crying. This discrepancy between the written progress notes and the testimony of the witnesses who observed the patient was sufficient to raise a question of fact as to the possible falsification of documents by the physician to minimize the nature of the incident and the injury of the patient because of the possible negligence of the hospital personnel. The testimony of the witnesses, if believed, would have been sufficient to show that the physician falsified the record or intentionally reported the incident inaccurately in order to avoid liability for the negligent care of the patient.

Tampering with records sends the wrong signal to jurors and can shatter one's credibility. Altered records can create a presumption of negligence. The court in *Matter of Jascalevich*[12] held that "a physician's duty to a patient cannot but encompass his affirmative obligation to maintain the integrity, accuracy, truth, and reliability of the patient's medical record. His obligation in this regard is no less compelling than his duties respecting diagnosis and treatment of the patient because the medical community must, of necessity be able to rely on those records in the continuing care of that patient. The rendering of good care must not be jeopardized or prejudiced by false, misleading, or inaccurate entries in the patient's medical record. A deliberate falsification by a physician of a patient's medical record in order to protect one's own personal interests at the expense of the patient's is regarded as gross malpractice endangering the health or life of his patient.[13] The physician's oath to first do no harm was violated in this case.

Post-Cath Note Written Prior to Procedure

Dr. Benjamin, a physician consultant, noted that a cardiologist had documented a postprocedure catheterization note before the procedure was completed. The physician consultant discussed with the cardiologist the inappropriate record entry and had a peer-to-peer discussion to help the surgeon understand the ramifications of his actions. The organization was most grateful for the way the physician surveyor managed the situation as it made their job much easier in addressing the issue with the surgeon, whose nonadherence to hospital and medical staff policy the organization had difficulty trying to handle over the past year. They were pleased with the process.

Discussion

1. Who should have handled the discipline issues with the physician? Explain your answer. Consider in forming your answer: The surveyor had 3 days to survey the hospital to determine its compliance with accreditation standards and now the surveyor is involved in a counseling session taking valuable time out of his duties.
2. How should the hospital have dealt with the cardiologist?

JUSTICE

Does the value of life diminish with age? Do you see me? Do you hear me? Am I less valuable because I am older? We are all created equal in God's sight. But then, when it comes to supply and demand, everything we thought we learned about ethics is put to the test. Who gets the new lung when there is a limited supply? Are there criteria for determining what the right thing to do is? If so who decided what the criteria should be? The questions as to justice and the distribution of scare resources are numerous and the answers are not easily sorted out, as noted in the following *reality check*.

Care Based on Age

I was undergoing some minor revisions to a surgical procedure that I had 5 years earlier. I distinctly remember the surgeon speaking to one of his assistants during the surgery, as he wielded a scalpel in his hand, "I definitely take more time with younger patients, especially children, than older patients." As I lie there on a small surgical table, I thought what do I say? I could've smacked him for being so rude. What an uncomfortable situation for me to be in, knowing that the surgeon had already made an incision under a local anesthetic. He spoke as though I wasn't there. I thought I better just act as though I had not heard him. Afterwards I thought that was a stupid thought. It wasn't like he was whispering. He was actually somewhat loud as though I was under a general anesthetic. If a friend told me that this happened to him, I would most likely have found it hard to believe. A surgeon should always do his best, regardless of the patient's age. But then maybe I am living in La La land.

Anonymous

Discussion

1. Discuss what, if anything, the patient should have said to the surgeon. Consider when framing your answer the patient is thinking to himself, "Unfortunately I have to come back to have the stitches taken out."
2. Describe what action you would take, if any, as a board member. Assume you had been sitting outside the treatment room and you had overheard the surgeon's remarks. Further assume you were a friend of the patient and had dropped in the surgeon's office to pick him up to take him home.

RESPECT FOR PRIVACY

Respect for the privacy of medical information is a central feature of the physician–patient relationship. Under the Hippocratic Oath and modern principles of medical ethics derived from it, physicians are ethically bound to maintain patient confidences.

The physician–patient privilege imposes on a physician an obligation to maintain the confidentiality of each patient's communications. This obligation applies to all health care professionals. An exception to the rule of confidentiality of patient communications is the implied right to make necessary information available to others involved in the patient's care. Information received by a physician in a confidential capacity relating to a patient's health should not be disclosed without the patient's consent. Disclosure may be made under compelling circumstances (e.g., suspected child abuse) to a person with a legitimate interest in the patient's health.

The Code of Medical Ethics requires that patient information remain confidential and that physicians who violate that confidentiality be reported to the appropriate regulatory body as provided for in federal and state statutes and regulations. Section 6530 (23) of the New York State Education Law, for example, defines professional misconduct as the "revealing of personally identifiable facts, data or information obtained in a professional capacity without the consent of the patient." The State of New York Department of Health has set forth a penalty of censure, reprimand, suspension of license, revocation of license, annulment of license, limitation on further license, or fine for a person found guilty of professional misconduct (Public Health Law A4 230-a), which includes revealing patient information without consent or failing to maintain accurate information. The Department of Health is responsible for maintaining the standards and ethics of the profession and for enforcing those standards. In addition, the Principles of Medical Ethics of the American Medical Association states that physicians, including physicians employed by industry, have an ethical and legal duty to protect patient confidentiality.[14]

PHYSICIAN NEGLIGENCE

This section provides an overview of common medical mistakes. The reader should keep in mind when reading this section that "ethical values and legal principles are usually closely related, but ethical obligations typically exceed legal duties . . . The fact that a physician charged with allegedly illegal conduct is acquitted or exonerated in civil or criminal proceedings does not necessarily mean that the physician acted ethically."[15]

TWO SCHOOLS OF THOUGHT

Under the *two-schools-of-thought doctrine* a physician is not be liable for medical malpractice if he or she follows a course of treatment supported by reputable, respected, and reasonable medical experts. The doctrine is applicable only in medical malpractice cases in which there is more than one method of accepted treatment for a patient's disease or injury. A physician's treatment that results in a patient's injury does not constitute negligence merely because it was unsuccessful in a particular case. A physician cannot be required to guarantee the results of treatment. The mere fact that an adverse result may occur following treatment is not in and of itself evidence of professional negligence.

Patient Assessments

Patient assessments involve the systematic collection and analysis of patient–specific data necessary to determine patient care and treatment plans. The patient's plan of care is only as good as assessments conducted by the practitioners of the various disciplines (e.g., physicians, nurses, dietitians, physical therapists).

The physician's assessment involves an evaluation of the patient's history, symptoms, and physical examination results. It must be conducted within 24 hours of a patient's admission to the hospital. The findings of the clinical examination are used to determine the patient's plan of care. The assessment is the process by which a doctor investigates the patient's state of health, looking for signs of trauma and disease. It sets the stage for accurately diagnosing the patient's medical problems. A cursory and negligent assessment can lead to a misdiagnosis of the patient's health problems and/or care needs and, consequently, to poor care.

Failure to Respond to Emergency Call

Physicians on call for a specific service in an emergency department are expected to respond to requests for emergency assistance when such is requested. Failure to respond can result in a successful lawsuit should a patient suffer injury as a result of a physician's refusal to fulfill that known duty. Such decisions are both legally and morally wrong.

Family Medical History

When reviewing a patient's family history, the physician must not be indifferent or dismissive of the patient's complaints and thoughts as to the possible cause of his or her illness. Such was the case in the following news clipping.

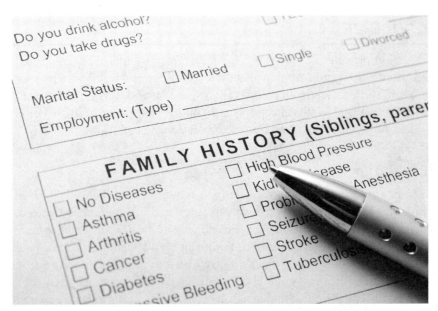

FIGURE 10-1 Family History (© Aleksandar Grozdanovski/Shutterstock, Inc.)

Bonded by Blood

A brother's history provides a clue to a woman's frightening and dangerous symptoms

Stein, who lives in Arlington, said she kept telling doctors and nurses about an odd coincidence involving her oldest brother—one she increasingly believed was relevant to her medical problems—but no one seemed to pay much attention.

"They were all sort of scratching their heads about what might be wrong, and I was getting so frustrated . . . ."

At her brother's suggestion, Stein said, she kept telling doctors about his CVID diagnosis, but no one seemed to follow up. "They'd say, 'Yeah that's interesting.'"

Sandra G. Boodman, The Washington Post, *February 25, 2014*

Patient Medical History

It is questionable in some cases as to whether a physician actually completes the process of obtaining a patient's medical history when the physician simply draws a diagonal line from the top right to the bottom left of the form and writes through the line "unremarkable" as noted in the following *reality check*.

Questionable Medical History Conducted

Smith was admitted to Community Hospital for surgery. Community Hospital medical staff bylaws require that a history and physical (H&P) exam be completed prior to patients' undergoing surgery. Smith's attending physician did not complete the H&P form. He simply drew a diagonal line from the top right to the bottom left of the H&P, indicating that the patient had no history of or current disease processes.

The patient's nurse, per hospital policy, completed a nursing assessment. The nurse documented on the patient admission assessment form that the patient had a history of transient ischemic attacks, diabetes, and hypothyroidism.

The anesthesiologist did not perform an anesthesia assessment before surgery. General anesthesia was administered without knowing the patient's previous experiences, if any, with anesthesia.

Failure of the attending physician to complete an appropriate H&P examination and the anesthesiologist's failure to perform a preanesthesia assessment placed the patient's life and health at risk. The physician did not complete the H&P. He merely went through the motions of completing a H&P examination because it was mandated that the patient have an H&P in his medical record prior to surgery.

Ethical and Legal Issues

1. Discuss the ethical issues and principles violated in this case.
2. What are the potential legal issues of concern in this case?
3. Discuss what actions the organization should consider to improve the quality of H&P documentation.

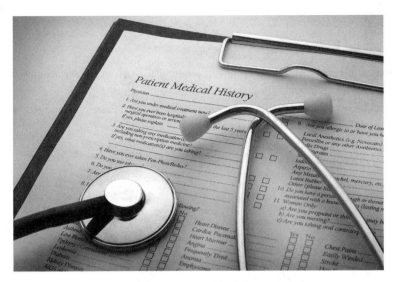

FIGURE 10-2 Patient Medical History (© Maksym Dykha/Shutterstock, Inc.)

Failure to obtain an adequate patient history and physical examination violates the standard of care owed to the patient. In *Foley v. Bishop Clarkson Memorial Hospital*,[16] Mr. Foley sued the hospital for the death of his wife. During her pregnancy, the patient was under the care of a private physician. She gave birth in the hospital on August 20, 1964, and died the following day. During July and August, her physician had treated her for a sore throat. Several days after her death, one of her children was treated in the hospital for a strep throat infection. There was no evidence in the hospital record that the patient had complained about a sore throat while in the hospital. The hospital rules required that an H&P had to be written promptly (within 24 hours of admission). No history had been taken, although the patient had been examined several times in regard to the progress of her labor. The trial judge directed a verdict in favor of the hospital. On appeal, the appellate court held that the case should have been submitted to the jury for determination. A jury might reasonably have inferred that if the patient's condition had been treated properly, the infection could have been combated successfully and her life saved. It also might have been reasonably inferred that if an H&P had been taken promptly when she was admitted to the hospital the throat condition would have been discovered and hospital personnel alerted to watch for possible complications of the nature that later developed. Quite possibly, this attention also would have helped in diagnosing the patient's condition, especially if it had been apparent that she had been exposed to a strep throat infection. The court held that a hospital must guard not only against known physical and mental conditions of patients, but also against conditions that reasonable care should have uncovered.

PATIENT DIAGNOSIS

Patient diagnosis refers to the process of identifying a possible disease or disease process, thus providing the physician with treatment options. Screens, assessments, reassessments, and the results of medical diagnostic testing such as electroencephalography (EEG),

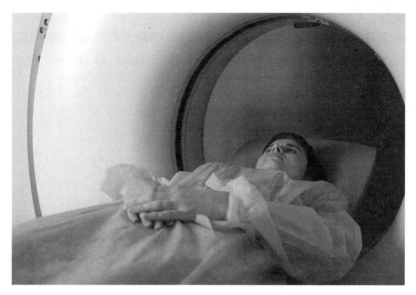

FIGURE 10-3 Patient Diagnostic Imaging Study (© bikeriderlondon/Shutterstock, Inc.)

electrocardiography (ECG), imaging, and laboratory findings are some of the tools of medicine that assists providers (e.g., physicians, osteopaths, dentists, podiatrists, nurse practitioners, physician's assistants) in diagnosing the possible causes of a patient's symptoms and medical problems from which a treatment plan is developed. The cases presented here describe some of the lawsuits that have occurred due to misdiagnoses and failure to properly treat the patient based on the results of diagnostic testing.

As Hands-On Doctoring Fades Away, Patients Lose

"In most hospitals today, the average amount of time a busy intern spends with a patient is four minutes," said Brendan Reilly, who until recently was the executive vice chair of medicine at New York Presbyterian Hospital. No longer are tests ordered based on the results of a careful physical exam and history, Reilly said, but the "technological tests become the primary source of information on the patient. It's backwards now," and the process is driving up health-care costs posed by sometimes unnecessary, risky procedures.

Sandra G. Boodman, The Washington Post, *May 20, 2014*

Even with all the diagnostic tools available to physicians, if they order the tests and fail to review or interpret them in conjunction with a patient's physical complaints and medical history, they are of little or no value. Tests results from imaging studies and laboratory results are useless if they are merely filed away after a cursory review as to their importance in arriving at an accurate diagnosis and appropriate treatment plan.

Concern Is Growing That the Elderly Get Too Many Medical Tests

Increasingly, questions are being raised about the over testing of older patients, part of a growing skepticism about the widespread practice of routine screening for cancer and other ailments of people in their 70s, 80s, and even 90s. Critics say there is little evidence of benefit—and considerable risk—from common tests for colon, breast, and prostate cancer, particularly for those with serious problems such as heart disease or dementia that are more likely to kill them.

• • •

Telling someone that screening is no longer necessary can be dicey, as California family physician Pamela Davis discovered when she advised her robust 86-year-old mother to stop getting mammograms and routine colon tests.

Her mother was incensed.

Sandra G. Boodman, Kaiser Health News, *September 12, 2011*

Discussion

1. There are some whose age is well hidden beneath their skin. As care and treatment options become safer (e.g., robotic surgery), should age alone be the sole criterion for determining the extent of medical care one should receive?
2. Do one's rights to care and treatment diminish with age?
3. Regardless of age, who should decide whether a particular diagnostic test or treatment is warranted?

Misdiagnosis

Her Doctor Dismissed the Lump in Her Breast

Many express anger at the practice where I had my breast exams. A few people even suggested that I look into legal action.

I choose not to walk down that political path, though. Sure, sometimes I allow the thought to creep into my head. What if it had been caught earlier? Would it still be in my lymph nodes? Would my prognosis be better? As soon as they pop up, I try to kick these thoughts to the curb. I will never know the answers, and blaming someone won't change my current reality. I choose to focus my energy on a path toward healing, not fault.

Kathryn Petrides, The Washington Post, *May 14, 2014*

Misdiagnosis is the most frequently cited injury event in malpractice suits against physicians. Although diagnosis is a medical art and not an exact science, early detection can be critical to a patient's recovery. Misdiagnosis may involve the diagnosis and treatment of a disease different from that which the patient actually suffers or the diagnosis and treatment of a disease that the patient does not have. Misdiagnosis in and of itself will not necessarily impose liability on a physician, unless deviation from the accepted standard of care and injury can be established.

My Physician Would Not Listen

I was left undiagnosed for over a year and a half. I had to endure extended chemotherapy for a stage III cancer because my GP would not listen to my concerns at first and then again 1.5 years later when the cancer had spread throughout my body to my lungs causing a nasty cough. I should've taken him to the GMC [Britain's General Medical Council] at the time but was more interested in getting better first! I made a diary all about it, just google my name; it's easy to find. I'm very grateful to be alive but it has left me broke, nothing or no one can fix that.

Tim Stollery

Fractured Skull, Not Intoxication

In *Ramberg v. Morgan*,[17] a police department physician at the scene of an accident examined an unconscious man who had been struck by an automobile. The physician concluded that the patient's insensibility was a result of alcohol intoxication, not the accident, and ordered the police to remove him to jail instead of the hospital. The man, to the physician's knowledge, remained semiconscious for several days and finally was taken from the cell to the hospital at the insistence of his family. The patient subsequently died, and the autopsy revealed massive skull fractures. The court found that any physician should reasonably anticipate the presence of head injuries when a car strikes a person. Failure to refer an accident victim to another physician or a hospital was actionable neglect of the physician's duty.

Although the presence of a physician does not ensure the correctness of the diagnosis or treatment, a patient is entitled to such thorough and careful examination as his or her condition and attending circumstances permit, with such diligence and methods of diagnosis as usually are approved and practiced by medical people of ordinary or average learning, judgment, and skill in the community or similar localities.

PATIENT TREATMENT

This section focuses on negligence cases that relate to medical treatment and various legal and ethical issues that health care professionals encounter when treating patients. *Patient treatment* is the attempt to restore the patient to health following a diagnosis. It is the application of various remedies and medical techniques, including the use of medications for the purpose of treating an illness or trauma. Treatment can be *active*, directed immediately to the cure of the disease or injury; *causal*, directed against the cause of a disease; *conservative*, designed to avoid radical medical therapeutic measures or operative procedures; *expectant*, directed toward relief of untoward symptoms but leaving cure of the disease to natural forces; *palliative*, designed to relieve pain and distress with no attempt to cure; *preventive/prophylactic*,

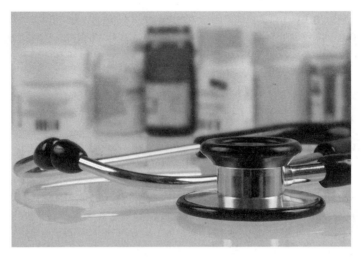

FIGURE 10-4   Patient Medications (© piotr_pabijan/Shutterstock, Inc.)

aimed at the prevention of disease and illness; *specific*, targeted specifically at the disease being treated; *supportive*, directed mainly to sustaining the strength of the patient; or *symptomatic*, meant to relieve symptoms without effecting a cure (i.e., intended to address the symptoms of an illness but not its underlying cause, as in scleroderma, lupus, or multiple sclerosis, for example).[18]

Medical practice guidelines are evidence-based best practices that are developed to assist physicians in the diagnosis and treatment of their patients. It should be remembered that best practices are not iron-clad rules. Skillful medical judgment demands that the physician determine how to use best practices and interpret the information.

Online Medical Treatment Advisor is a treatment program that uses medical specialists to accurately select the best and newest treatment for each patient, based on the individual patient's characteristics. Online Medical Treatment Advisor assesses each patient's symptoms with a knowledge base created by 1,500 specialist physicians. Online Medical Treatment Advisor includes treatments for 1,200 diseases.[19]

Autonomy and Informed Consent

Patients have a right to make their own treatment choices. When there are two or more medically acceptable treatment alternatives, a competent patient has the right to choose which option he or she wants after being informed of the risks, benefits, and alternatives of each option. The physician has a legal, ethical, and moral duty to respect a patient's *autonomy* and to provide only authorized medical treatment. It is inappropriate for physicians to pursue a treatment alternative other than the one to which their patient has given consent. Unless the patient consents to the physician's recommended treatment approach, the physician may not proceed with that approach even if the physician personally believes the recommended approach to be in the patient's best interests.[20]

The doctrine of *informed consent* is a theory of professional liability independent from malpractice. A physician's duty is to disclose known and existing dangers associated with a proposed course of treatment. The patient in *Leggett v. Kumar*[21] was awarded $675,000 for pain and disfigurement resulting from a mastectomy procedure. The physician in this case failed to advise the patient of treatment alternatives. He also failed to perform the surgery properly.

It is the physician's role to provide the necessary medical facts and the patient's role to make a subjective decision concerning treatment based on his or her understanding of those facts. Before subjecting a patient to a course of treatment, the physician has a duty to disclose information that will enable the patient to evaluate options and the risks attendant to a specific procedure. A failure to disclose any known and existing risks of a proposed treatment when such risks might affect a patient's decision to forgo treatment constitutes a prima facie violation of a physician's duty to disclose. If a patient can establish that a physician withheld information concerning the inherent and potential hazards of a proposed treatment, consent is abrogated. Consent for a medical procedure may be withdrawn at any time before the act consented to is accomplished.

With thousands of brand-name and generic drugs in use, it is no surprise that drug errors are one of the leading causes of patient injuries. Physicians should encourage the limited and judicious use of all medications and should document periodically the reason for their continuation. They should be alert to any contraindications and incompatibilities among prescription and over-the-counter drugs, and herbal supplements. Medication errors are often due to: administration of the wrong medication to the wrong patient; of the wrong dosage; at the wrong site; by the wrong route; or a combination of the aforementioned errors.

Medications

The Board of Regents in *Moyo v. Ambach*[22] determined that a physician had prescribed methaqualone fraudulently and with gross negligence to 20 patients. The Board of Regents found that the physician did not prescribe methaqualone in good faith or for sound medical reasons. His abuse in prescribing controlled substances constituted the fraudulent practice of medicine. Expert testimony established that it was common knowledge in the medical community that methaqualone was a widely abused and addictive drug. Methaqualone should not have been used for insomnia without first trying other means of treatment. On appeal, the court found that there was sufficient evidence to support the board's finding.

Damages were awarded in *Argus v. Scheppegrell*[23] for the wrongful death of a teenage patient with a preexisting drug addiction. It was determined that the physician had wrongfully supplied the patient with prescriptions for controlled substances in excessive amounts, with the result that the patient's preexisting drug addiction had worsened, causing her death from a drug overdose. The Louisiana Court of Appeal held that the suffering of the patient caused by drug addiction and deterioration of her mental and physical condition warranted an award of $175,000. Damages of $120,000 were to be awarded for the wrongful death claims of the parents, who not only suffered during their daughter's drug addiction caused by the physician's wrongfully supplying the prescription, but who also were forced to endure the torment of their daughter's slow death in the hospital.

Surgery

As noted in the following news clipping, surgical instruments inadvertently left in patients are reported by hospitals accredited by the Joint Commission. The various states also require the reporting of surgical errors, such as wrong patient, wrong surgery, and wrong site.

Joint Commission Alert: Preventing Retained Surgical Items

The Joint Commission today issued a Sentinel Event Alert urging hospitals and ambulatory surgery centers to take a new look at how to avoid mistakenly leaving items such as sponges, towels and instruments in a patient's body after surgery.

Known in medical terminology as the unintended retention of foreign objects (URFOs) or retained surgical items (RSIs), this is a serious patient safety issue that can cause death or harm patients physically and emotionally. The Joint Commission has received more than 770 voluntary reports of URFOs in the past seven years.

Elizabeth Eaken Zhani, The Joint Commission, *October 17, 2013*[24]

Wrong-site surgical mistakes have multiple causes, including draping the wrong surgical site, marking the wrong surgical site, and failing to mark the surgical site as required by hospital policy.

The Pain of Wrong-Site Surgery

Hospitals find it hard to protect patients from wrong-site surgery

"It's disheartening that we haven't moved the needle on this," said Peter Pronovost, a prominent safety expert and medical director of the John Hopkins Center for Innovation in Quality Patient Care. "I think we made national policy with a relatively superficial understanding of the problem." Pronovost suggests that doctors' lip service to the rules, which he calls "ritualized compliance," may be a key factor. Studies of wrong-site errors have consistently revealed a failure by physicians to participate in a timeout.

Sandra G. Boodman, Kaiser Health News, *June 20, 2011*[25]

Pregnant Woman Dies After Horrifying Medical Mixup

(Newser)—As far as medical mix-ups go, it's a horrifying one. In October 2011, a 32-year-old woman underwent an operation at Queen's Hospital outside of London; Maria De Jesus was suffering from appendicitis and needed to have her appendix removed. Instead, her right ovary was taken out, and De Jesus, who was 21 weeks pregnant with her fourth child at the time, ended up dying roughly three weeks later. The case is now in front of a medical tribunal, which is weighing the medical fates of the two doctors involved . . . .

Newser, Yahoo Shine, *April 17, 2014*[26]

Aggravation of Patient's Condition

Aggravation of a preexisting condition through negligence can result in a physician being liable for malpractice. If the original injury is aggravated by treatment or the failure to treat, liability can be imposed for injuries suffered as a result of the aggravation of the patient's condition.

Patient Infections

Physicians are increasingly at risk for lawsuits related to hospital-acquired infections (HAIs). According to the CDC over 700,000 HAIs occur each year in acute care hospital settings.[27] The serious nature of surgical site infections are all too common occurrences requiring intensive and costly care, as is illustrated in **Figure 10-5**. Both physicians and hospitals are at a greater risk of lawsuits when there are failures to implement and enforce recognized infection control practices, policies, and procedures.

The District Court of Appeals of Florida held in *Gill v. Hartford Accident & Indemnity Co.*[28] that the physician who performed surgery on a patient in the same room as the plaintiff should have known that the infection the patient had was highly contagious. The failure of the physician to undertake steps to prevent the spread of the infection to the plaintiff and his failure to warn the plaintiff led the court to find that hospital authorities and the plaintiff's physician caused an unreasonable increase in the risk of injury. As a result, the plaintiff suffered injuries causally related to the negligence of the defendant. The court held that the plaintiff's complaint does state a cause of action and alleges a duty and a breach of that duty.

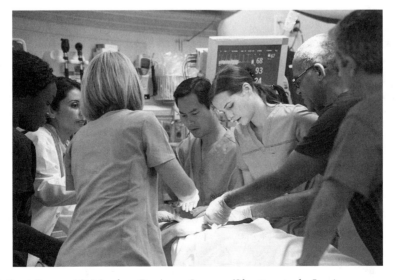

FIGURE 10-5 Patient Room (© Monkey Business Images/Shutterstock, Inc.)

Pain Management

Pain

I have been with Angie, my wife, on many of her appointments. One such appointment I vividly remember was at the university hospital pain center, described by some as one of the top medical centers in the country. Here, after several residents poked her, they left the room. They later returned with their supervising attending physician. He stood over my Angie as she lay on the examination table. Looking down at her, he said, "We treat bone pain here." Angie replied, "You advertise yourself as a pain-management center. I don't understand." The attending physician replied, "Anything we do for you would be very risky and most likely will not work." Angie described a new implantable device being used at Duke University Medical Center. The attending responded, "We never heard of that; however, we can suggest other procedures, but they do have associated risks." The attending then proceeded to describe the procedures to Angie. Both Angie and I thought, "This is a major teaching hospital? Why won't the physicians suggest looking into Duke's procedure as to the potential risks and benefits for Angie?" The attending suggested, "Why don't you think about the procedures we have discussed. Just schedule a new appointment before you leave."

Spouse

Discussion

1. Should the physicians have conducted research to determine if the Duke device might be helpful to Angie? Explain your answer.
2. What would you do, if you were Angie?

PHYSICIAN–PATIENT RELATIONSHIP

The physician–patient relationship entails special obligations for the physician to provide care to his or her patient. The physician's primary commitment must always be the patient's welfare and best interests, whether the physician is preventing or treating illness or helping the patient to cope with illness, disability, and death. It has long been recognized that the health and welfare of the patient depends on a collaborative effort between the physician and the patient. The physician must support the dignity of all patients and respect their uniqueness. The following guidelines serve to improve physician–patient relationships and help decrease the likelihood of malpractice suits:

- *Provide personalized treatment.* A patient is more inclined to sue an impersonal physician than one with whom he or she has developed a good relationship.
- *Conduct a thorough assessment*/history and physical examination that includes a review of all body systems.

- *Do not be dismissive* as to the patient's thoughts as to the cause of his or her ailments.
- *Develop a problems list* and comprehensive treatment plan that addresses the patient's problems.
- *Provide sufficient time* and care to each patient. Take the time to explain treatment plans and follow-up care to the patient, his or her family, and other professionals who are caring for your patient.
- *Request consultations* when indicated and refer if necessary.
- *Closely monitor* the patient's progress and, as necessary, make adjustments to the treatment plan as the patient's condition warrants.
- *Maintain timely*, legible, complete, and accurate records. Do not make erasures.
- *Do not guarantee* treatment outcome.
- *Provide for cross-coverage* during days off.
- *Do not overextend* your practice.
- *Avoid prescribing* over the telephone.
- *Do not become careless* because you know the patient. Seek the advice of counsel should you suspect the possibility of a malpractice claim.

CHAPTER REVIEW

1. The medical profession has long subscribed to a body of ethical statements developed primarily for the benefit of the patient.
   - *Hippocratic Oath* dates back to 400 BC.
   - Modified version of the *Hippocratic Oath* has been used by such medical schools as Johns Hopkins, Baylor College of Medicine, Tufts University School of Medicine.
   - American Medical Association code of ethical conduct for physicians.
2. Law and ethics interweave in patient care.
   - Hippocratic Oath and AMA Code of Ethics were violated when the physicians in *Scripps Clinic v. Superior Ct.* terminated a patient's care before ensuring the patient had continuing medical care.
   - Compassion, trust, justice, and respect for patient privacy are all ethical principles and values that are intertwined with law.
3. Physician negligence often involves one or more of the following:
   - Patient assessments
   - Medical diagnosis
   - Treatment

TEST YOUR UNDERSTANDING

TERMINOLOGY

autonomy	medical treatment	patient diagnosis
Hippocratic oath	misdiagnosis	patient treatment
informed consent	nonmaleficence	two-schools-of-thought
medical diagnosis	patient assessment	doctrine

REVIEW QUESTIONS

1. Describe how the *Hippocratic Oath* and modern codes of medical ethics apply to the practice of medicine.

2. Explain how the law and ethics intertwine in patient care.

3. Describe common medical errors relative to physician practice involving assessment, diagnosis, and treatment.

4. Discuss common guidelines that would be helpful in improving the physician–patient relationships.

NOTES

1. Hippocrates, written 400 BC, Translated by Francis Adams.
2. http://guides.library.jhu.edu/content.php?pid=23699&sid=190964.
3. http://www.ama-assn.org/ama/pub/physician-resources/medical-ethics/code-medical-ethics/principles-medical-ethics.page.
4. *Scripps Clinic v. Superior Ct.,* 134 Cal. Rptr. 2d 101 (2003).
5. *Id.*
6. *Bloomington Urological Associates v. Scaglia,* 686 N.E.2d 389 (1997).
7. American Medical Association Code of Medical Ethics: Current Opinions with Annotations, 8.11 (1996).
8. Jennifer Steinhauer, "Fatal Surgery Leads to Fine for Hospital," *The New York Times,* November 6, 1998. http://www.nytimes.com/1998/11/06/nyregion/fatal-surgery-leads-to-fine-for-hospital.html.
9. Sophie Borland and David Wilkes, "1 in 4 cancer cases missed: GPs send away alarming number of patients, delaying vital treatment," *MailOnline,* March 1, 2001; http://www.dailymail.co.uk/health/article-1361269/1-4-cancer-cases-missed-GPs-delaying-vital-treatment.html.
10. *Valentine v. Kaiser Found. Hosps.,* 15 Cal. Rptr. 26 (Cal. Ct. App. 1961) (dictum).
11. 683 N.E.2d 1175 (Ohio App. 1996).
12. 442 A.2d 635 (N.J. Super. Ct. 1982).
13. *Id.* at 644–45.
14. *Horn v. New York Times,* 100 N.Y.2d 85 (2003).
15. AMA, "Opinion 1.02 - The Relation of Law and Ethics," http://www.ama-assn.org/ama/pub/physician-resources/medical-ethics/code-medical-ethics/opinion102.page?
16. 173 N.W.2d 881 (Neb. 1970).
17. 218 N.W.2d 492 (Iowa 1928).
18. http://www.medical-dictionary.thefreedictionary.com/treatment.
19. http://www.ccspublishing.com/online_medical_treatment.htm.
20. See *Bankert v. United States,* 937 F. Supp. 1169, 1173 (D. Md. 1996).
21. 570 N.E.2d 1249 (Ill. App. Ct. 1991).
22. 23 N.Y.S.2d 645 (N.Y. App. Div. 1988).
23. 489 So. 2d 392 (La. Ct. App. 1986).
24. http://www.jointcommission.org/joint_commission_alert_preventing_retained_surgical_items/
25. Sandra G. Boodman, "Effort to end surgeries on wrong patient or body part falters," Kaiser Health News, June 20, 2011; http://www.kaiserhealthnews.org/Stories/2011/June/21/wrongsite-surgery-errors.aspx
26. https://shine.yahoo.com/parenting/pregnant-woman-dies-horrifying-medical-mixup-200700512.html.
27. Magill SS et al. Multistate Point-Prevalence Survey of Health Care-Associated Infections. *N Engl J Med* 2014;370:1198–1208.
28. 337 So. 2d 420 (Fla. Dist. Ct. App. 1976).

EMPLOYEE RIGHTS AND RESPONSIBILITIES

LEARNING OBJECTIVES

Upon completion of this chapter, the reader will be able to:

- Describe and understand the rights of employees.
- Describe the responsibilities of employees in the workplace.
- Discuss what professionals can do to improve professional relationships.

INTRODUCTION

This chapter provides an overview of the rights and responsibilities of employees, as well as independent contractors (e.g., physicians) in the health care work setting, many of which are expressed in state and federal laws. Applicable laws include employment practices, such as wages, hours, working conditions, union activity, and providing a safe work environment. This chapter demonstrates that balancing the rights and responsibilities of employees and their employer is not always an easy task. As is often said in the performance improvement process, it is not enough to do the right thing; it is doing the right thing well. As discussed next, with every right, there comes a corresponding duty equal to the right enjoyed.

EMPLOYEE RIGHTS

Man never fastened one end of a chain around the neck of his brother that God did not fasten the other end round the neck of the oppressor.

−ALPHONSE DE LAMARTINE (1790–1869)

This section introduces the reader to employee rights from both a legal and moral standpoint. "The Department of Labor (DOL) administers and enforces more than 180 federal laws. These mandates and the regulations that implement them cover many workplace activities for about 10 million employers and 125 million workers."[1]

FAIR TREATMENT AND EMPLOYMENT AT WILL

The common-law "employment-at-will" doctrine provides that employment is at the will of either the employer or the employee. The employer or employee may terminate employment for any or no reason, unless there is a contractual agreement in place that specifies the terms and duration of employment. Historically, termination of employees for any reason was widely accepted; however, contemporary thinking does not support this concept.

> An at-will prerogative without limits could be suffered only in anarchy, and there not for long; it certainly cannot be suffered in a society such as ours without weakening the bond of counter-balancing rights and obligations that holds such societies together.
>
> −Sides v. Duke Hospital[2]

Employment at will does not abrogate employee rights. Employees have faced discrimination involving age, race, creed, color, gender, wages, benefits, wrongful termination, as well as a host of other common labor issues. A variety of federal and state laws protect employee rights to be treated fairly in the workplace. The following listing describes but a few of the rights of employees in the workplace.

In recent years, the rule that employment for an indefinite term is terminable by the employer whenever and for whatever cause he chooses without incurring liability has been the subject of considerable scholarly debate and judicial and legislative modification. Consequently, there has been a growing trend toward a restricted application of the at-will employment rule whereby the right of an employer to discharge an at-will employee without cause is limited by either public policy considerations or an implied covenant of good faith and fair dealing.[3]

In *Sides v. Duke Hospital,* the North Carolina Court of Appeals found it to be an:[4]

> obvious and indisputable fact that in a civilized state where reciprocal legal rights and duties abound, the words "at will" can never mean "without limit or qualification,"

as so much of the discussion and the briefs of the defendants imply; for in such a state the rights of each person are necessarily and inherently limited by the rights of others and the interests of the public. An at-will prerogative without limits could be suffered only in an anarchy, and there not for long; it certainly cannot be suffered in a society such as ours without weakening the bond of counter-balancing rights and obligations that holds such societies together. . . .

If we are to have law, those who so act against the public interest must be held accountable for the harm inflicted thereby; to accord them civil immunity would incongruously reward their lawlessness at the unjust expense of their innocent victims.

The concept of the employment-at-will doctrine is embroiled in a combination of legislative enactments and judicial decisions. Some states, such as New York, have a tendency to be more employer oriented, whereas others, such as California, emerge as being much more forward thinking and in harmony with the constitutional rights of the employee.

The employment-at-will common law doctrine is not truly applicable in today's society and many courts have recognized this fact. In the last century, the common law developed in a laissez-faire climate that encouraged industrial growth and improved the right of an employer to control his own business, including the right to fire without cause an employee at will. . . . The twentieth century has witnessed significant changes in socioeconomic values that have led to reassessment of the common law rule. Businesses have evolved from small- and medium-size firms to gigantic corporations in which ownership is separate from management. Formerly there was a clear delineation between employers, who frequently were owners of their own businesses, and employees. The employer in the old sense has been replaced by a superior in the corporate hierarchy who is himself an employee.[5]

Some courts and legislative enactments have overturned the view that employers have total discretion to terminate workers who are not otherwise protected by collective bargaining agreements or civil service regulations. Montana legislation grants every employee the right to sue the employer for wrongful discharge. The mere fact that an employment contract is terminable at will does not give the employer an absolute right to terminate it in all cases. The Montana wrongful discharge statute of 1989 provides that a discharge is wrongful only if:

(1) it was in retaliation for the employee's refusal to violate public policy or for reporting a violation of public policy;

(2) the discharge was not for good cause and the employee had completed the employer's probationary period of employment; or

(3) the employer violated the express provisions of its own written personnel policy.[6]

Accordingly, "the evolving legal doctrines surrounding the breach of the duty of good faith and fair dealing still have primary importance."[7]

Fairness—When 6 + 1 = 9

Bill had nine evaluations during seven consulting assignments. One corporation submitted one original evaluation and two copies of the same evaluation. Policy requires that each corporation submit one evaluation for each consultant at the end of a consulting project. Unfortunately for Bill, the same evaluation by the same person was submitted three times. It was negative in 2 of 20 ratings. This skewed Bill's overall performance average in two categories to an overall score of "meets expectations." Bill—being a perfectionist—had "exceeds expectations" in all of the categories over the past 10 years. Bill believed that the data were flawed, and he approached Vinnie, his supervisor, to discuss his concerns. Vinnie brushed off Bill's concerns and said, "Everything would average out in the end. Don't worry about it."

Bill later learned that Vinnie was responsible for assuring the accuracy of aggregate data in the organization. Bill thought, "If the performance data are flawed, how can I trust any other data that Vinnie presents at corporate meetings?"

Bill decided to e-mail his concerns to Vinnie about the inaccurate aggregation of data in his evaluations. He made the analogy that, if he had seven algebra exams and in six he scored 100 and in one he scored 70, the aggregate data would be flawed if the score of 70 had been averaged into his total score three times. Bill was sure Vinnie would understand this analogy. Not so. Vinnie said to Bill, "We have already had this discussion. I don't want to hear about it again."

Discussion

1. Should Bill pursue his concerns, or should he accept the performance downgrade that has resulted from the use of flawed data? Discuss your answer.
2. Was Vinnie unreasonable in his thinking—"I've made up my mind, don't confuse me with the facts?"

Public Policy Exceptions

The public policy exception to the employment-at-will doctrine provides that employees may not be terminated for reasons that are contrary to public policy. Public policy originates with legislative enactments that prohibit, for example, the discharge of employees on the basis of handicap, age, race, color, religion, gender, national origin, pregnancy, filing of safety violation complaints with various agencies (e.g., the Occupational Safety and Health Administration), or union membership. Any attempt to limit, segregate, or classify employees in any way that would deprive any individual of employment opportunities on these bases is contrary to public policy.

Public policy also can arise as a result of judicial decisions that address those issues not covered by statutes, rules, and regulations. "[I]t can be said that public policy concerns what is right and just and what affects the citizens of the state collectively. It is to be found in the state's constitution and statutes and, when they are silent, in its judicial decisions."[8]

Public policy favors the exposure of crime, and the cooperation of citizens possessing knowledge thereof is essential to effective implementation of that policy. Persons acting in good faith, who have probable cause to believe crimes have been committed, should not be deterred from reporting them by fear of a lawsuit by those accused.[9]

In those instances in which state and federal laws are silent, not all courts concur with the use of judicial decisions as a means for determining public policy. A California court, for example, determined that a public policy exception to the at-will employment doctrine must be based on constitutional or statutory provisions rather than judicial policy making.[10]

FREEDOM FROM DISCRIMINATION

Employees have a right to be considered for a job without discrimination based on their skills and qualifications for the jobs for which they are applying. The job applicant must not be discriminated against, for example on the basis of race, age, creed, or color.

> The U.S. Equal Employment Opportunity Commission (EEOC) is responsible for enforcing federal laws that make it illegal to discriminate against a job applicant or an employee because of the person's race, color, religion, sex (including pregnancy), national origin, age (40 or older), disability or genetic information. It is also illegal to discriminate against a person because the person complained about discrimination, filed a charge of discrimination, or participated in an employment discrimination investigation or lawsuit. [11]

EQUAL PAY FOR EQUAL WORK

The Equal Pay Act (EPA) of 1963 is essentially an amendment to the Federal Labor Standards Act that was passed to address wage disparities based on gender. The EPA prohibits gender discrimination in the payment of wages for women and men performing substantially equal work in the same establishment. Under the EPA, a lawsuit may be filed by the Equal Employment Opportunity Commission (EEOC) or by individuals on their own behalf. If a complainant is paid full back wages under EEOC supervision or if the EEOC takes legal action first, a private suit may not be filed.

The EPA is applicable wherever the minimum wage law is applicable and is enforced by the EEOC. The EPA requires that employees who perform equal work receive equal pay. There are situations in which wages may be unequal as long as they are based on factors other than gender, such as in the case of a formalized seniority system or a system that objectively measures earnings by the quantity or quality of production.

REFUSE TO PARTICIPATE IN CARE

Caregivers have a right to refuse to participate in certain aspects of patient care and treatment. This can occur when there is conflict with one's cultural, ethical, and/or religious beliefs, such as the administration of blood or blood products, participation in elective abortions, and end-of-life issues such as disconnecting a respirator. In the attempt to honor staff rights, a patient's health must not be compromised. Questionable requests not to participate in certain aspects of a patient's care should be referred to an organization's legal counsel and/or the ethics committee for review and consultative advice.

Refusal to Participate in Elective Abortions Upheld

Caregivers have a right to refuse to participate in abortions and can abstain from involvement in abortions as a matter of conscience, religious beliefs, or moral conviction. In a Missouri case, *Doe v. Poelker,*[12] the city was ordered to obtain the services of physicians and personnel who had no moral objections to participating in abortions. The city also was required to pay the plaintiff's attorneys' fees because of the wanton disregard of the indigent woman's rights and the continuation of a policy to disregard and/or circumvent the U.S. Supreme Court's rulings on abortion.

Refusal to Participate in Therapeutic Abortion Insubordinate

In the attempt to honor staff rights, a patient's health must not be compromised. The New York Supreme Court, Appellate Division in *Larson v. Albany Medical Center*[13] held that although a nurse has the right to refuse to participate in an elective termination of pregnancy on grounds of freedom from religious discrimination in employment, the case before the court did not involve an elective procedure. The mother was in need of emergency care and the nurses were asked by their nursing supervisor to assist in an "emergency" evacuation of a dead fetus. The nurses launched an argument about elective abortions and the court ruled their action as insubordinate behavior.

Pharmacists Refusal to Fill Prescriptions

Some pharmacists' religious beliefs prohibit abortion or the use of birth control. They believe that dispensing such medications to others is an infringement on their freedom of religion. There are others who believe that pharmacists have an obligation to fill all prescriptions and that refusing to fill them violates the patients' freedom of conscience. The First Amendment protects individual free exercise of religion. The question here, "Does requiring pharmacists to fill prescriptions conflict with religious beliefs and violate their rights under the First Amendment?" Some say yes, because people whose religious beliefs prohibit birth control or abortion cannot freely exercise their religion if they are forced to dispense these medications. Others say no, because the patients' need to obtain their medication outweighs the pharmacists' rights.[14]

> Some states have subsequently proposed legislation and passed laws designed to allow doctors and other direct providers of health care to refuse to perform or assist in an abortion, and hospitals to refuse to allow abortion on their premises. Now, the issue is expanding as pharmacists are refusing to fill emergency contraception and contraception prescriptions.[15]

As each state often has different rulings on this issue, the reader should review applicable statutes in his or her state.

QUESTION PATIENT CARE

A caregiver has the right to question the care being rendered to a patient by another caregiver if there is reason to believe that the care is likely to be detrimental to the well-being of the patient. If for example, a caregiver believes that a particular order appears to be questionable, the caregiver has the responsibility to seek verification from the prescribing physician. If the prescribing physician believes the order to be correct and the caregiver still questions the order, the concern must be relayed to the employee's supervisor for verification and further follow-up if necessary.

CASE: PAVING HER WAY TO HEAVEN

The nurse-plaintiff in *Kirk v. Mercy Hosp. Tri-County*[16] was employed as a charge nurse with supervisory duties. A short time after one of her patients had been admitted to the hospital, the nurse diagnosed that the patient was suffering from toxic shock syndrome. The nurse believed that the physician would order antibiotics. After a period of time had passed without having received those orders from the physician, she discussed the patient's situation with the director of nursing. The nurse was told by the director to document what had happened. She was told to report the facts and stay out of the matter.

The nurse discussed the patient's condition and lack of orders with the chief of staff. Although the chief of staff took appropriate steps to treat the patient, the patient died. A member of the patient's family had told the nursing director that the nurse-plaintiff offered to obtain the medical records. The nursing director was later told that the nurse-plaintiff had told the family member that the physician was "paving [the patient's] way to heaven." The director terminated the plaintiff.

After her termination, the nurse received a service letter from the hospital that directed her to refrain from making any further false statements about the hospital and its staff.

The trial court entered a summary judgment for the defendant, stating that there were no triable issues of fact, and there was no public policy exception to the nurse's at-will termination. The nurse appealed.

The Missouri Court of Appeals held that the Nursing Practice Act provided a clear mandate of public policy that the nurses had a duty to provide the best possible care to patients. Public policy clearly mandates that a nurse has an obligation to serve the best interests of patients; therefore, if the plaintiff refused to follow her supervisor's orders to stay out of a case where the patient was dying from a lack of proper medical treatment, there would be no grounds for her discharge under the public policy exception to the employment-at-will doctrine.

Pursuant to the Nursing Practice Act, the plaintiff risked discipline if she ignored improper treatment of the patient. Her persistence in attempting to get the proper treatment for the patient was her absolute duty. The hospital could not lawfully require that she stay out of a case that would have obvious injurious consequences to the patient. Public policy, as defined in case law, holds that no one can lawfully do that which tends to be injurious to the public or against the public good.

Ethical and Legal Issues

1. Describe the ethical and legal issues in this case.
2. Did the hospital violate the rights and responsibilities of the nurse? Explain your answer.
3. Would the nurse's professional code of ethics support her actions in this case? Explain your answer.

SUGGEST CHANGING PHYSICIAN

There are circumstances in which a caregiver has a right to suggest that a patient or patient's family change to a different, more responsive physician. For example, in one case a patient began losing weight and having hallucinations. A nurse documented the patient's difficulties and attempted on several occasions to call the patient's physician. The physician failed to return the nurse's calls. When the patient's condition deteriorated further, the family contacted the nurse. After the nurse told the patient's family about her concerns, a member of the patient's family asked her what they should do. The nurse advised that she would reconsider their "choice of physicians." The nurse was subsequently terminated because she had advised the patient's family to consider changing physicians.

The nurse brought a lawsuit for wrongful discharge in violation of public policy. The language in the Nursing Practice Act of North Carolina and regulations of the Board of Nursing describe the practice of nursing as assessing a patient's health, which entails a responsibility to communicate, counsel, and provide accurate guidance to clients and their families. The nurse's comments that resulted in her termination were made in fulfillment of these responsibilities.

The North Carolina Court of Appeals held that the nurse stated a claim for wrongful discharge in violation of public policy. The nurse's termination for fulfilling her responsibilities as a practicing nurse violated state public policy and was a factual question for jury determination. Although there may be a right to terminate at-will employment for no reason or for an arbitrary or irrational reason, there can be no right to terminate such employment for an unlawful reason or purpose that contravenes public policy.[17]

FREEDOM FROM SEXUAL HARASSMENT

Employees have a right to be free from *sexual harassment*. Sexual harassment can be verbal or physical, and it includes a request for a sexual favor, sexual advances made as a condition of employment and unreasonably interfering with an employee's work performance, and creating an intimidating or offensive working environment. In 1980, the EEOC issued landmark sexual harassment guidelines that prohibit unwelcome sexual advances or requests that are made as a condition of employment. The guidelines also prohibit conduct that creates a hostile work environment. The U.S. Supreme Court held that a hostile work environment refers not only to conduct that is psychologically injurious but also to conduct that is perceived as abusive.

TREATMENT WITH DIGNITY AND RESPECT

One's dignity may be assaulted, vandalized, and cruelly mocked, but it cannot be taken away unless it is surrendered.

—AUTHOR UNKNOWN

Each employee has the right to be treated with dignity and respect and in a fair and consistent manner by the employer. Employers have a responsibility to respond to employee complaints and concerns regarding their rights to be treated with dignity and respect.

O.R. Becomes an Abusive Environment

Dr. D is the director of surgery at Union Medical Center. He has long been recognized for his disruptive behavior and outbursts of anger in the OR. Carol, the VP of nursing, makes an appointment to speak with you (Daniel, the new CEO) about the abusive disposition and mood swings of Dr. D in the OR.

"Daniel, Dr. D has a history of name-calling and berating Roberta, the O.R. manager in the presence of her staff. He fails to follow hospital policy and threatens that he is going to get her fired. Roberta has repeatedly spoken to Dr. D. several times for his failure to follow presurgical hand-washing technique. His postsurgical infection rate is the highest in the OR. We have spoken to the Infection Control Committee several times about this. They keep telling me that they will talk to him and yet nothing seems to change. Sometimes I think they are afraid of him. The staff is fearful of Dr. D and they have been reluctant to come forward with their concerns. I am new to the hospital and had hoped that we could resolve this without your intervention. However, we do need your help. Dr. D is recalcitrant and will not change. Roberta is a hard-working and conscientious supervisor. Today, Dr. D. again told Roberta that he was going to get her fired before the week was out. You know, she is an extremely conscientious nurse with patients being her first priority and is well liked by her coworkers. I went in Roberta's office earlier today and found her crying. She said she has put up with Dr. D. for 5 years and just cannot take his abusive outbursts any longer and has decided to resign her position and leave."

Daniel responds, "Carol, we are both new to this hospital and such abusiveness by any physician to any staff member will not be tolerated. I plan to speak to Roberta myself and follow up with the surgeon and if necessary, the medical board."

Discussion

1. If you were Daniel, how would you address this problem?
2. What procedures should be in place to handle disciplinary issues of this nature?
3. Would you talk to Roberta? What would you say?

FREEDOM FROM INTIMIDATION

Employees have a right to be free from intimidation by angry individuals and veiled threats by managers in the workplace. Employees have a right to be protected from the abuse of others whether they are managers, coworkers, or independent contractors such as physicians.

Hospitals Crack Down on Tirades by Angry Doctors

At a critical point in a complex abdominal operation, a surgeon was handed a device that didn't work because it had been loaded incorrectly . . . the surgeon slammed it down, accidentally breaking the technician's finger. . . .

> The 2011 incident illuminates a long-festering problem that many hospitals have been reluctant to address: disruptive and often angry behavior by doctors. Experts estimate that 3 to 5 percent of physicians engage in such behavior, berating nurses who call them in the middle of the night about a patient . . . demeaning co-workers they consider incompetent or cutting off patients who ask a lot of questions.
>
> *Sandra G. Boodman*, The Huffington Post, *March 5, 2013*

There is a tendency for those in power to abuse that power through threats, abuse, intimidation, and retaliatory discharge, all of which are cause for legal action. Employees who become the targets of a vindictive supervisor often have difficulty proving a bad-faith motive. In an effort to reduce the probability of wrongful discharge, some states, such as Connecticut,[18] Maine,[19] Michigan,[20] and Montana,[21] have enacted legislation that protects employees from terminations found to be arbitrary and capricious. The Montana Supreme Court upheld state legislation that protects workers against arbitrary discharge, while limiting the damages they can win.

> The National Labor Relations Act and other labor legislation illustrate the governmental policy of preventing employers from using the right of discharge as a means of oppression. . . . Consistent with this policy, many states have recognized the need to protect employees who are not parties to a collective bargaining agreement or other contract from abusive practices by the employer . . .

Recently those states have recognized a common law cause of action for employees at will who were discharged for reasons that were in some way "wrongful." The courts in those jurisdictions have taken various approaches: some recognizing the action in tort, some in contract.[22]

Dismissal of an employee shortly after a request for a grievance hearing regarding a salary discrepancy with another employee can raise an issue of liability for retaliatory discharge. The physician in *Jones v. Westside-Urban Health Center*[23] was found to have established a prima facie case of retaliatory discharge in which the record indicated that he had been fired from the hospital 5 days after his request for a grievance hearing on an alleged salary discrepancy.

Man of Integrity

How we want to be remembered by all throughout our career.

June 1978: Congratulations and good wishes on your appointment as administrator. This is a great responsibility but you are young and capable and it should be an interesting challenge. Most people of all stations working in the hospital are behind you and you certainly have the backing of the medical staff. This is a very good start. We will work 100% with you so please feel that you have our sincere backing. Once again, congratulations, good luck and good management.

—Bob

July 1978: Following our conversation yesterday, and for whatever it's worth, I'd just like to tell you that I think you're doing a terrific job! I like your administrative style and feel comfortable already. I'm very happy to be working with you. Have a good day!

—Yvonne

September 1998: Good luck in all your endeavors. It was my good fortune to be associated with you. People who are people-oriented should do well in any career path they choose. Happiness and good health.

—Natalie

November 2008: Daniel, before we talk about anything else, I want to first of all thank you for your approach to our staff. I want you to know I was happy to have had the pleasure to work with you. You had a wonderful way to put people at ease and glean information from them. You were able to determine from your questions the quality of care we offer here at Hennepin. When I think of the book, 'If Disney ran your hospital' and the fact that you went over and beyond what the book teaches ... I saw that in you. I have a report somewhere here on my desk as to staff feedback and how well you related to them ... You should see it. I am off to a meeting right now but I will share it with you.

—Jeanette

PRIVACY AND CONFIDENTIALITY

Employees have a right to privacy and confidentiality, such as information that the employer may become aware of as to an employee's health status. Modern technology enables employers to monitor their employees' activities through their computer site visits, e-mails, voicemail, and video monitoring (video monitoring is not permissible in bathrooms and locker rooms). Such monitoring is generally unregulated, and unless an organization's policy specifically states otherwise, the employer may listen, watch, and read an employee's workplace communications. Such information must be used wisely and discreetly without malice.

Employee rights often ride a fine line as related to privacy. As the following *reality check* illustrates, it is sometimes difficult to know where to draw the line between corporate integrity and employee rights.

Your Mail Has Been Intercepted

The XYZ Corporation has decided to open all mail sent to employees who work in the field. A memorandum was sent to the field staff saying, "Sorry, your mail will be either opened or returned to the sender if it is delivered to your workplace. If the sender is from a health care organization, it will be opened to determine if its contents relate to XYZ's business. If the mail is from any other person or place, it will be returned unopened to the sender. This action is necessary from a cost-savings standpoint. XYZ cannot afford to forward the on-average 60 pieces of mail that it receives each month addressed to field staff." What happens to opened mail that is not XYZ's business remains a mystery. What is it that drives an organization to make such decisions? Is it fear of competition, paranoia, distrust, or some other mysterious issue? The answer remains elusive.

Although it is legal for an organization to open all mail before sorting and delivering it, employees should be told that they should have no expectation of privacy and that they should not have anything personal sent to work that they don't want others to see. Managers should not be allowed to open an employee's mail indiscriminately, because the invasion of privacy will undermine employee morale. Policy should prohibit managers from opening employees' personal mail without good reason.[24]

Discussion

1. Discuss under what circumstances an organization should open an employee's mail.
2. Discuss any legal and ethical concerns (e.g., right to privacy).
3. Describe what should happen to the mail of an employee that is opened and is not intended for the organization? What if that information is confidential in nature and is shared with others?
4. Is forwarding 60 envelopes a month to employees who work at remote sites in 50 states 5 days a week asking too much of an accrediting corporation that charges over $45,000 for a 5-day review of a hospital's compliance with accreditation standards? Discuss your answer as to the impact such a policy can have on employee morale.

Trust Is Pivotal to Success

Without trust, privacy and confidentiality become meaningless. The most vital resource in a health care organization is the staff. The CEO must assign responsibilities to both line and staff employees on the basis of capability. The CEO must recognize the differences and needs of each individual, develop their strengths, and provide guidance in times of weakness. Like a conductor in a symphony orchestra, the CEO must produce organizational harmony among the staff. The CEO sets the tone for building trust in the organization. Therefore, it is imperative that he or she be attuned to the needs of those in the front line, those employees who conduct the day-to-day business of the organization and support its mission.

Jack, the newly appointed CEO of XYZ, has been working for 2 years in his position. Staff members have criticized his physical absence and his once-a-year appearance at employee luncheons. Except for the occasional memorandum drafted by other staff members, many employees at XYZ have become discouraged and distrustful of the top-tier vice presidents who were appointed by Jack to conduct business for XYZ. Employees are beginning to leave, and business is going elsewhere.

Discussion

1. Discuss why the CEO must earn the respect and trust of his or her staff. Discuss why:
   a. Without trust, one cannot lead.
   b. Being heard and not seen is not leadership.
2. What should Jack do to build trust in the organization?

Right to Family Medical Leave

Employees have a right to take a medical leave of absence under the *Family and Medical Leave Act of 1993 (FMLA),* which was enacted to grant temporary medical leave to employees under certain circumstances. The act provides that covered employers must grant an eligible employee up to a total of 12 work weeks of unpaid leave during any 12-month period for one or more of the following reasons: the birth and care of an employee's child; placement of an adopted or foster child with the employee; for the care of an immediate family member (spouse, child, or parent) with a serious health condition; or inability to work because of a serious health condition. It is illegal to terminate health insurance coverage for an employee on FMLA leave. Following an FMLA leave, the employee's job—or an equivalent job with equivalent pay, benefits, and other terms and conditions of employment—must be restored.

Whistleblowing

Employees have both a right and responsibility to report unethical conduct. *Whistleblowing* has been defined as an act of someone "who, believing that the public interest overrides the interest of the organization he serves, publicly blows the whistle if the organization is involved in corrupt, illegal, fraudulent, or harmful activity."[25] As noted in the following news clippings, the number of whistleblowing cases and settlements has resulted in major payouts by health care corporations.

Drug Firm to Pay $2.2 Billion in Fraud Settlement

Johnson & Johnson will pay $2.2 billion to resolve civil and criminal allegations involving the marketing of off-label, unapproved uses for three prescription drugs, Justice Department officials announced Monday.

• • •

Monday's settlement also will result in a significant payout for whistleblowers in three states—Pennsylvania, Massachusetts and California—who officials said will receive nearly $168 million of the government's take.

Brady Dennis with Sari Horwitz, The Washington Post, *November 5, 2013*

Physician Whistle-Blowers Can Sue Hospitals Without Delay, Appeals Court Rules

Judges say a law enables California doctors to take immediate legal action against health centers suspected of retaliation.

A 2007 amendment to California's whistle-blower protection law allows physicians lodging complaints about hospitals to sue the facilities for retaliating against them without the doctors first having to exhaust lengthy administrative remedies, a federal appeals court has ruled.

The ruling encourages more doctors to speak up about patient care concerns in health facilities, said Long X. Do, legal counsel for the California Medical Assn. The CMA wrote a friend-of-the-court brief in support of the doctor who is the plaintiff in the case.

Alicia Gallegos, American Medical News, *September 3, 2012*

Whistleblower Lawsuit Alleges Florida Hospital Filed Millions in False Claims

A whistleblower lawsuit based on insider information from a former Florida Hospital Orlando billing employee and a staff physician alleges that seven Adventist Health hospitals in Central Florida have overbilled the federal government for tens of millions of dollars in false or padded medical claims.

The suit claims Florida Hospital used improper coding for more than a decade to overbill Medicare, Medicaid and Tricare, all federal government payors. In addition, it alleges, the hospital commonly overbilled for a drug used, for example, in MRI scans and billed for computer analyses that were never performed.

Marni Jameson, Orlando Sentinel, *August 8, 2012*

According to the public policy exception, an employer may not rely on the employment-at-will doctrine as a basis for escaping liability for discharging an employee because of the doing of, or the refusing to do a wrongful act. Moreover, statutes in several jurisdictions protect an employee from an employer's retaliation for engaging in certain types of protected activities, such as whistleblowing.[26]

Health care organizations often describe their whistleblower policy in their compliance manuals. Compliance officers are responsible for providing information to employees regarding the organization's compliance program. The policies provide reporting procedures that ensure anonymity for employees through, for example, the use of phone hotlines answered by third parties not affiliated with the organization. Organizations must not retaliate against employees for disclosing activities that he or she reasonably believes is in violation of public policy, such as, fraudulent billing practices.

OSHA's Whistleblower Protection program, for example, enforces the whistleblower provisions of more than twenty whistleblower statutes protecting employees who report violations of various workplace safety, airline, commercial motor carrier, consumer product, environmental, financial reform, food safety, health insurance reform, motor vehicle safety, nuclear, pipeline, public transportation agency, railroad, maritime, and securities laws. Rights afforded by these whistleblower acts include, but are not limited to, worker participation in safety and health activities, reporting a work related injury, illness or fatality, or reporting a violation of the statutes.[27]

Although demotion, intimidation, reassignment, reduction in work hours, constructive discharge and so on are prohibited by law, there are often long-term negative affects on one's lifestyle, as noted in the following news clipping.

The Price Whistle-Blowers Pay for Secrets

"It's a life-changing experience," said John R. Phillips, founder of the law firm Phillips & Cohen and the man credited with devising the amendments that strengthened the government antifraud law, the False Claims Act, in 1986. "If you look at the field of whistle-blowers, you see a high degree of bankruptcies. You may find yourself unemployable. Home foreclosures, divorce, suicide and depression all go with this territory."

Paul Sullivan, The New York Times, *September 21, 2012*

SAFE ENVIRONMENT

Employees have a right to work in a safe environment, thus requiring the employer to provide appropriate safety conditions that includes providing the appropriate equipment (e.g., ventilation systems as required throughout the hospital, gowns, gloves, goggles) and signage posted as required in hazardous areas (e.g., isolation rooms for protection of both the employee and patient, hazardous medical gas storage areas).

UNEMPLOYMENT COMPENSATION

Employees have a right to unemployment compensation as well as worker's compensation for injuries resulting from the employees work environment. The Division of Unemployment Insurance is committed to providing high-quality, accurate, courteous, and dependable service to claimants and employers in a secure and confidential environment that demands accountability, integrity, and fairness.

EMPLOYEE RESPONSIBILITIES

I believe that every right implies a responsibility; every opportunity, an obligation; every possession, a duty.

–JOHN D. ROCKEFELLER, JR.

Employees are expected to adhere to their codes of professional ethics and to comply with their job-related duties and responsibilities as defined in their job description and the organization's policies and procedures. Rights and responsibilities run parallel to one another. With every right, there is a corresponding duty, for example, although there is a right to expect respect from others, there is a corresponding duty and responsibility to respect the rights of others. The following sections describe a few of the many responsibilities required of health care employees.

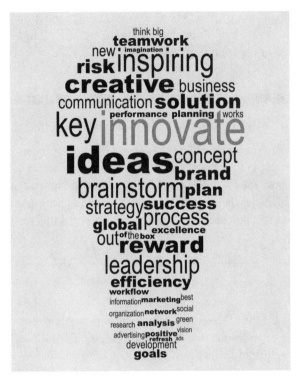

FIGURE 11-1   Working Together (© Archiwiz/Shutterstock, Inc.)

SHOW COMPASSION

How far you go in life depends on you being tender with the young, compassionate with the aged, sympathetic with the striving and tolerant of the weak and strong. Because someday in your life you will have been all of these.

—GEORGE WASHINGTON CARVER

The ability to show strength of character through compassion leads this list of employee responsibilities. Caregivers hold in their hands the gift to be instruments of God in the healing process. It is the compassionate caregiver who guides the patient as he or she struggles through illness, pain, and suffering. It is the compassionate caregiver who provides hope when there appears to be no hope.

Compassion for the Patient and Caregiver

Recently I started to show a health care worker a short video of a man who most likely weighed over 500 pounds. As a popular singer, he performed his last concert and maybe his last song; the caregiver noticed in the video that there was an oxygen tank beside his wheelchair with tubing leading from the tank into his nostrils. The caregiver abruptly turned away from the computer screen and ranted about how heavy people are so exasperating to work with. The caregiver proceeded to criticize the man saying that he was responsible for his own obesity, making it difficult for caregivers to lift and move. The singer had acknowledged in his public life that he knew he was addicted to food, which led to his early death. His message before singing a heartbreaking song was the purpose of showing the video. The message now goes further than this: the needs of the patient must be met with compassion and the provider must provide the caregiver with sufficient assistance to move such patients in order to prevent the caregiver from also becoming a patient.

Discussion

1. Discuss the various ethical issues affecting patients, caregivers, and hospitals.
2. Describe what actions you could take to make this a win-win scenario for the patients, caregivers and health care facilities.

COMPLY WITH STATE AND FEDERAL REGULATIONS

The governing body and its agents are responsible for compliance with federal, state, and local rules and regulations regarding the operation of the organization. Depending on the scope of the wrong committed and the intent of the governing body, failure to comply with the requirements of regulatory bodies can subject board members and/or their agents to civil liability and, in some instances, to criminal prosecution.

COMPLY WITH HOSPITAL POLICY

Employees are required by an organization's policies and procedures. The following *reality check* illustrates what can happen when there is a failure to comply with hospital policy.

My Surgical Journey

I was prepped for surgery and transported to the Operating Suite where I was placed in a corridor with multiple other patients on stretchers lined up against one side of the hallway waiting to be transported to their assigned OR room. I noticed various types of medical equipment lined up on the opposite side of the hallway. I am probably being a little too kind in my description of what I observed. I should say it was more like an obstacle course. The medical equipment was strewn not so neatly against the corridor wall. It was disturbing to see the equipment placed varying distances from the wall making it difficult for staff to navigate between patient stretchers and medical equipment. I thought to myself as a volunteer fireman and carpenter by trade, how would you ever transport me out of here in the event, for example, of an anesthesia gas explosion. But then my scheduled surgery was my priority at that moment.

After about 20 minutes lying on a stretcher in the OR corridor, in what seemed like a lifetime, I was slowly moved down the hallway by a transporter attempting to avoid hitting other stretchers and medical equipment on my way towards OR # 1, which had been designated for cardiac surgery patients.

As I was lying face up looking at the corridor ceiling, I noticed when passing one set of fluorescent lights that there were several flies and what appeared to be a roach lying on the bottom of the plastic cover protecting the florescent lights from breakage. I thought to myself, "Well at least they appear to be dead."

During my journey down the corridor I noticed physicians and nurses washing their hands at sinks prepping themselves for surgery. There was a sign above the sinks describing hand-washing techniques that staff must follow prior to participating in any surgical procedure. As I watched them scrubbing their hands I noticed one staff member who walked up to the sink and, by my observation, appeared not to have followed the hospital's hand-washing policy. I overheard a staff member comment as he walked away, "Oh he thinks he is King Tut. He never follows protocol. I would love to see how much bacteria we would find growing on a petri dish if we cultured his hands."

As the transporter moved me down the corridor, he abruptly stopped for a moment to allow surgical equipment being moved from OR #6 into the hallway and down the corridor. I noticed the equipment was placed in a position that partially blocked the fire exit. At that moment the exit door was opened by another staff member entering the OR suite and I observed medical equipment that appeared to be stored on the exit stairwell landing. Not that I know much about hospitals but it did seem odd that someone could enter the OR suite from a stairwell.

Finally by the time I arrived in OR #1, designated for open-heart surgery, the staff prepared to transfer me from my stretcher to the surgical table. I was a bit groggy from preanesthesia sedation but was awake during the transfer and noticed several tears in the surgical table mattress pad exposing the foam, which was protruding from the pad. A staff member noticed my observation and quickly finished covering the mattress pad with an OR sheet just prior to me being transferred onto the table. The tears appeared to measure 6 to 8 inches in length. I thought to myself, "What patients laid on this mattress pad before me and what body fluids seeped inside the mattress. Oh yes of course, how long was this mattress collecting body fluids from other patients and what might be growing inside it." Looking up at the ceiling, I thought, "Wow, those air vents appear to be covered with black and green mold."

Just prior to undergoing surgery I overheard one of the surgeons say, "I sure wish the hospital would get rid of those rusty lockers in the dressing room. And those showers should be used for showers and not as a storage area for clean surgical gowns and sterile gloves in cardboard boxes stored on the floor over shower drains. Where do they expect us to shower?" A surgical assistant replied, "Yes, you're right. Even if there was nothing stored in the shower, there are no showerheads or knobs to turn them on. It defeats the purpose of maintaining sterile technique in the OR if you have to travel from the employee showers on the ground floor to the OR on the fourth floor. And those chairs we sit on in the men's locker room should really be reupholstered. They are a mess and the foam is coming out of them." That was the last thing I remembered until after surgery.

My recovery from surgery was longer then I expected because I had developed a surgical site staph infection. By the time I got out of the hospital I felt like I had been through a train wreck. After discussing my experiences in the OR suite with some friends and family, they encouraged me to discuss my concerns with the hospital. I said, "You're right and I want the best care possible rendered at our community hospital." Not knowing who to talk to first, I decided to provide my surgical journey observations to the hospital's patient advocate in hopes that the issues in the OR suite would be addressed and the quality of care improved.

Discussion

1. Identify the ethical, and legal issues in this case.
2. Describe what your plan of action would be to prevent the recurrence of the issues identified. Include in your plan what hospital departments should be addressed in your plan.
3. If you were asked to write a response to the patient's complaints, how would it read?
4. This patient, a carpenter and volunteer fireman, identified his observations based on his skills and life experiences. Describe how he might have described his journey through the OR suite if he had a different set of skills, education, and training.

It is noteworthy that the observations of the carpenter or any other individual are limited by what they observe. As a surveyor of an accrediting body one would look for an approved disaster plan to provide for adequate space, staff, supplies, equipment, blood products, and transportation to handle mass casualties; expired medications; a universal protocol to help prevent wrong site wrong patient surgery; verification that professionals are credentialed and licensed, as appropriate, to perform the scheduled surgery; proper sterilization of surgical equipment and instruments; temperatures and humidity appropriately controlled; test tubes for cultures displaying expiration dates that have not expired; anesthesia gases and oxygen containers properly secured and stored; medical equipment properly maintained as required by the manufacturer; and the list goes on. In order to provide a safer environment, OR leadership should engage in walk-around inspections that would include, for example, the OR supervisor, infection control nurse, housekeeping, and engineering staff. For documentation and follow-up purposes, a checklist of surgical suite hazards should be required during inspections. Surgical suite inspection lists should be based on professional guidelines and feedback from staff and other hospital committee meetings. In order not to reinvent the wheel, examples of OR checklists can be easily found by conducting a web search.

COMPLY WITH JOB DESCRIPTIONS

Employees have a responsibility to comply with the responsibilities outlined in their job descriptions. Failure to do so can be hazardous to patient safety as well as lead to termination of the employee who fails to perform the duties required in a professional and acceptable manner.

HONOR PATIENT WISHES

Caregivers have a responsibility to honor a patient's right to participate in decisions regarding his or her care, including the right to formulate advance directives and have those directives honored.

MAINTAIN CONFIDENTIALITY

The duty of employees and staff to maintain confidentiality encompasses both verbal and written communications. This requirement also applies to consultants, contracted individuals, students, and volunteers. Information about a patient, regardless of the method in which it is acquired, is confidential and should not be disclosed without the patient's permission. Those who come into possession of the most intimate personal information about patients have both a legal and an ethical duty not to reveal confidential communications. The legal duty arises because the law recognizes a right to privacy. To protect this right, there is a corresponding duty to obey. The ethical duty is broader and applies at all times.

Health care professionals who have access to medical records have a legal, ethical, and moral obligation to protect the confidentiality of the information in the records. The communications between a physician and his or her patient and the information generated during the course of the patient's illness are generally accorded the protection of confidentiality. Medical records, with proper authorization, may be used for the purposes of research, statistical evaluation, and education.

Compliance Officer and Confidentiality

The employee who decides to place confidence and trust in a corporate compliance officer must understand the following points, among others, prior to filing a complaint against any organizational practice, individual, and/or department within or entity owned by the organization:

- The compliance officer is hired by and is responsible to the corporation by which he or she is hired.
- Compliance officers often report directly to the organization's corporate counsel and/or chief executive officer and/or board of directors/trustees.
- The compliance officer is expected to abide by the laws of the land and follow the code(s) of ethics applicable to compliance officers in general and any ethical principles or codes of ethics that apply to his or her profession. For example, a compliance officer who is a lawyer is expected to adhere to those professional code(s) of ethics that apply to lawyers from both a professional and state licensing standpoint. Failure to do so can result in professional discipline and sanctions against the compliance officer.
- Compliance officers are expected to maintain confidentiality of the names of employees who file complaints.
- Organizations often have compliance hotlines to protect the identity of employees who file complaints.

The compliance officer has a difficult balancing act in maintaining the confidentiality of employees, working for the organization, adhering to standards of ethical conduct, and abiding by applicable federal and state laws. This is no easy task, as Phil was about to learn.

Phil, having exhausted all other appeals, called Beth, the compliance officer, to speak with her about a decision that the human resources department had made that he believed was out of compliance with the Federal Equal Pay Act. The office assistant, Mary, stated, "Beth will not be in the office until next week." Phil then scheduled a telephone conference with Beth for the following week. He asked Mary, "Will my telephone conference with Beth remain confidential?" Mary said, "Most certainly. Our office is here for you. Everything in our office remains confidential."

The following week Phil called Beth to discuss his concern that certain professionals were performing the same work as he was and were getting paid more. He described the specifics of his concern. Beth asked, "Is it OK for me to reveal your name to human resources so that I can obtain the necessary records that I would need from them to see if you are being paid equally to others for the same work?" Phil agreed to Beth's request.

During his discussion with Beth, Phil asked that his conversations with her remain confidential. Beth responded, "If you wanted confidentiality, then you should have asked for it before speaking to me."

Discussion

1. What lessons could employees learn from Phil's experience?
2. If you were Phil, discuss how you would handle compliance issues in the future.

ADHERE TO SAFE PRACTICES

Caregivers have a responsibility to adhere to safe practices in order to minimize patient injuries. This responsibility requires employees to adhere to national patient safety goals (e.g., comply with the Centers for Disease Control and Prevention (CDC) hand-washing guidelines, patient identification, verification of operative site), the purpose of which is to protect the health of the patient.

Failure to Comply with Hand Hygiene Guidelines

Smith was a healthy young lady until suddenly she experienced neck pain and needed surgery. She was admitted to a postsurgical care unit at a major teaching hospital. Upon entering her assigned four-bedded room, she and her husband observed a bloody suction bottle hanging from a wall at the head of her assigned bed. The bed rails were rusting with dried body fluids from previous patients. They were uneasy about having a surgical procedure performed but they decided the physician's skills were more important then an unclean room. The morning following surgery, a physician entered the room with three residents and examined each of four postsurgical patients. The first patient examined was a post surgical amputee, who was later diagnosed with a staph infection. Mrs. Smith was the fourth patient to be examined in the room. Even though each of the patients' wounds had been examined and dressings changed, the physicians failed to change their gloves between patients. Following examination of Mrs. Smith, they proceeded to remove their gloves and tossed them in Mrs. Smith's bedside wastebasket. All four patients contracted a staff infection. History repeated itself. CDC hygiene recommendations, though adopted by the hospital, were not followed, to the patients' detriment.

Discussion

1. Discuss the principles of ethics violated in this case.
2. Describe what values were violated and what action the hospital should take to reduce the likelihood of similar occurrences in the future.

The CDC has estimated that "nosocomial [hospital-acquired] bloodstream infections are a leading cause of death in the United States. If we assume a nosocomial infection rate of 5%, of which 10% are bloodstream infections, and an attributable mortality rate of 15%, bloodstream infections would represent the eighth leading cause of death in the United States."[28] It is believed that such infections have resulted in as many as 100,000 deaths and billions of dollars in additional health care costs. These numbers do not reflect nonhospital-acquired infections that have occurred in physicians' offices. The serious nature of these numbers validate the importance of complying with sterile techniques through recommended hand washing and maintaining a sterile environment for patients.

ADHERE TO PROFESSIONAL STANDARDS

Caregivers have a responsibility to maintain a professional attitude in the performance of their work. The operation of a hospital requires the coordination of a wide variety of disciplines and departments, each with different responsibilities that depend on each other. Thus, staff cooperation and communication are essential for ensuring professionalism in the provision of high-quality patient care.

Unprofessional conduct, incompatibility, and lack of cooperation in a hospital are appropriate considerations for discharging an employee or denying staff privileges. The ability to work with others is a reasonably definite standard proscribing the conduct on which discharge or other adverse action is based. Today's health care environment has become increasingly complex. The operation of a hospital requires the coordination of numerous employees and departments, each with different responsibilities that build and depend on each other. Thus, staff cooperation and communication are essential to ensuring a high quality of patient care. Disruptive behavior in the workplace can affect the morale and teamwork of the staff, as well as cause actual harm to patients. A hospital's evaluation of an employee or physician's attitude and ability to work with others is not unduly vague and is directly related to the goal of good patient care.[29]

MAINTAIN PROFESSIONAL RELATIONSHIPS

Employees are responsible for maintaining an appropriate professional relationship with patients, families, coworkers, and others who come into contact with the organization (e.g., consultants).

Shoot the Consultant

Justin, a new consultant, was assigned to review an organization's human resources department and provide recommendations on how to improve processes and systems. As Justin was new to the job, Mel, a more seasoned consultant, was assigned to work with him. Justin was working on a preliminary report to be presented to the organization later that day. Judy, the organization's coordinator assigned to work with Justin, was asked to provide additional information on its staffing process. Justin believed that the organization's staffing processes were well done. Mel, whispering in Justin's ear, out of Judy's eyesight, said,

"I disagree. These processes are not what we would expect to see in place, but then, this is your assignment. I am just here to evaluate you." Justin understood his message. Justin described to Judy his concerns about human resources staffing processes as Mel stood in the back of the room watching their interaction. Judy turned to Mel and said, "Don't you think Justin is wrong?" Mel quickly replied, "I am just an observer." Judy left the room as Justin completed his report.

Later that afternoon Justin presented his report to the organization's leadership. Justin made his suggestions for improvement. After his report, the CEO asked whether there were any questions regarding Justin's report. Mel was sitting to the immediate left of Justin, and Judy was to the left of Mel. Judy, leaning over to look at Justin, pointing at him, said, "I could just shoot him." After a few moments of silence, followed by a few goodbyes, Justin handed his report to the CEO. He, along with Mel, got up to leave the room. Judy, ignoring Justin, shook Mel's hand and hugged him goodbye as she looked at Justin with contempt.

Discussion

1. Assuming that Mel adequately explained his recommendations, discuss what other actions, if any, Justin might have taken to defuse Judy's discontent.
2. What action should the CEO take regarding Judy's apparent disrespect? Explain your answer.

Sexual Harassment

Employers have a responsibility to maintain a workplace that is free of sexual harassment. This not an easy task to achieve. Forms of sexual harassment include a request for sexual favors, demeaning comments, sexually explicit jokes, pinching and fondling of a coworker, sexually explicit jokes sent through e-mails, and so on. Health care professionals must not breach their legal and ethical obligations through sexual harassment or illicit relationships with employees and/or patients. Engagement of health professionals in such affairs, even if the affairs are consensual, is morally wrong. Sexual harassment cases are often litigated in both civil and criminal arenas. Health care professionals finding themselves in such unprofessional relationships should seek help for themselves as well as refer their patients to other appropriate professionals. Besides being subject to civil and criminal litigation, health care professionals also are subject to having their licenses revoked for sexual improprieties.

Organizations should take action to prevent claims of sexual improprieties by training supervisory personnel to recognize and correct questionable behavior before it becomes a problem. Policy and procedures regarding sexual harassment should be included in an organization's orientation programs. The following cases illustrate the pervasiveness of sexual improprieties by professionals in a variety of settings.

Nurse's Relationship with Patient

A nurse's sexual relations with a patient can give rise to disciplinary action resulting in the nurse's loss of license. In *Heinecke v. Department of Commerce,*[30] a male nurse lost his license after having a sexual relationship with a patient, even though she was no longer a patient at the hospital where they met. The fact that the nurse resigned from the hospital and was living with the patient was not a sufficient defense to support such behavior.

Physician's Inappropriate House Call

A hospital technologist in *Copithorne v. Framingham Union Hospital*[31] alleged that a staff physician raped her during the course of a house call. The technologist's claim against the hospital had been summarily dismissed for lack of proximate causation. On appeal, the dismissal was found to be improper when the record indicated that the hospital had received notice of allegations that the physician had assaulted patients on and off the hospital's premises. The hospital had instructed the physician to have another individual present when visiting female patients and had instructed nurses to "keep an eye on him." The physician's sexual assault was foreseeable. There was evidentiary support for the proposition that failure to withdraw the physician's privileges had caused the rape when the technologist asserted that it was the physician's good reputation in the hospital that had led her to seek his services.

Avoid Relationships with a Patient's Spouse

The sexual relationship that a psychiatrist had with the spouse of a patient was found to be improper in *Richard v. Larry*.[32] California Civil Code Section 43.5, abolishing causes of action for alienation of affection, criminal conversation, and seduction of a patient over the age of consent, did not bar damages for emotional distress caused by the alleged professional negligence of the psychiatrist who had sexual relations with the plaintiff's wife. The psychiatrist owed a special duty to use due care for his patient's health. The statute was not intended to lower the standard of care that psychiatrists owed their patients. Besides an action against the psychiatrist, allegations that the psychiatrist was an agent of the hospital stated a cause of action against the hospital.

The Bureau of Professional Medical Conduct had charged the petitioner in *Goldberg v. De Buono*,[33] a licensed physician and psychiatrist, with moral unfitness, gross negligence and incompetence, negligence on more than one occasion, and incompetence by reason of his alleged sexual relationship with a patient. After a hearing, a hearing committee of the State Board for Professional Medical Conduct sustained the specifications of moral unfitness, gross negligence, and negligence, and the committee recommended revocation of the petitioner's license. The New York Supreme Court, Appellate Division, rejected the petitioner's assertion that the committee erred in crediting the testimony of Patient A and her daughter. Issues of credibility, even as to witnesses with psychiatric illnesses, are exclusively for the administrative fact-finder to determine. The petitioner conceded his sexual relationship with Patient A, but contended that the physician–patient relationship had been terminated at the time the sexual relationship occurred. Inasmuch as the respondent's medical expert testified that the relationship was not terminated and the petitioner's relationship with Patient A constituted a serious deviation from accepted standards of practice, the court was satisfied that the committee's determination was supported by substantial evidence.

REPORT UNETHICAL BEHAVIOR

Caregivers have both a right and responsibility to report impaired, incompetent, and unethical colleagues in accordance with the legal requirements of each state. Unethical behavior includes conduct that threatens patient care or welfare, behavior that violates state licensing provisions, and conduct that violates criminal statutes.

PROTECT PATIENTS FROM HARM

Caregivers have an ethical and legal responsibility to protect patients from harm. The rules of ethics applicable to nurses, for example, specifically recognize a nurse's obligation to safeguard not only patients' health but their safety as well. These are not duties invented by courts of equity but rather tenets of ethical responsibility issued by the profession itself.

REPORT PATIENT ABUSE

Caregivers have both a right and responsibility to report patient abuse. Statutes protect employees against retaliation by employers for reporting patient abuse. An employer may not, therefore, discharge an employee for fulfilling this societal obligation.

WORK WITH TEAM SPIRIT

Employees have a responsibility to work together as team in the delivery of high-quality patient care, as noted, for example, in the following *reality check*.

Teamwork Requires Community Input

Dr. White, the medical director of Anytown hospital's cancer center, had been working on a plan for a new cancer center for the community. Dr. White was particularly concerned with seeking input from community leaders as to their ideas for developing a model comprehensive treatment program for patients. After several visits to various well-respected programs in California, New York, and Texas at his own expense, he was certain he wanted to match and if possible surpass the excellence he found at these centers. Knowing that the administration had other projects in mind, his feeling was that there is room for more than one capital program at a time.

Bill, the director of a major corporation, recently visited the cancer center where his close friend Dr. White discussed his preliminary plans with him. Bill was impressed and joking laughed, "You have my vote. Count me in for a million dollars." Dr. White held back his tears saying, "You are serious, aren't you?" Bill replied, "Yes I am. That is, on one condition." Dr. White replied, "I am listening." Bill continued, "There must be serious-minded community involvement, including cancer patients. Not token input, but valued community participation." Dr. White continued, "We are on the same page."

Bill, before leaving, said to Dr. White, "I am truly excited to be part of your dream to answer such a spiritual calling in the plans you shared with me today."

Discussion

1. Discuss the importance of involving community input when developing and reviewing new and existing care programs.
2. Consider and discuss what training you might provide community members interested in the planning process.

MAINTAIN PROFESSIONAL COMPETENCIES

It is expected that each professional have current understanding of one's area of specialization and practice. Education has value and is a legal necessity in order to be in conformity with the national standard of care of one's profession. Every professional is responsible to be current in his or her knowledge and skills. This comes by reading professional literature, attending continuing education programs, and mentoring.

U.S. Cancer-Care Delivery is "in Crisis": Report

NEW YORK (Reuters)—Cancer treatment has grown so complex, many U.S. doctors can't keep up with new information and are offering incorrect treatment, failing to explain options and leaving patients to coordinate their own care, according to a report released on Tuesday by the Institute of Medicine, part of the National Academy of Sciences.

• • •

Treating the disease, which can require precisely matching a tumor's molecular characteristics to a drug, has become so complicated that many physicians lack "core competencies in caring for patients with cancer," the report concludes.

Sharon Begley, Reuters, *September 10, 2013*[34]

This news clipping succinctly describes the educational crisis brought about by the massive delivery of new drugs being brought to market and research being conducted that requires more emphasis on translational medicine, as well as the need for computer-assisted diagnosis and treatment as a tool for caregivers in delivering highquality patient care. Search the National Institute of Medicine's website at http://iom.edu for the full report, *Delivering High-Quality Cancer Care: Charting a New Course for a System in Crisis.*

For the reader, student and practitioner, the educational process is just beginning with the awarding of a diploma, degree, and license or certification to practice in one's area of training. There is no short cut in the learning process; however.

Show me a good caregiver and I will show you a person who not only provides good care but also provides it well and seeks ways to make it even better by improving his or her own competencies.

—GP

HELPFUL ADVICE

The following listing provides some helpful advice to caregivers for building a spirit of teamwork and improving the quality of patient care.

- Build consensus when solving problems.
- Do not blame others for your mistakes.
- Do not say the physician is not here when he or she is.

- Do not say the physician will soon be here when he or she has already left the building.
- Do not say that this will not hurt, when you know it will.
- Do not say that you are busy when you are not.
- Take responsibility for caring and communicating.
- Include the patient in the decision-making process.
- Take the time to explain to patients the risks, the benefits, and alternatives to each course of treatment.
- Show respect and sensitivity to the patient's needs.
- Listen to what the patient is saying without interruption.
- Do not make fun of a patient's decision-making capacity. Patients are human and have the frailties that all must someday endure.
- Prohibit others from demeaning and criticizing a patient's wishes because of his or her frail condition.
- Remember that your feelings and those of family may be different from those of the patient. It is, however, the patient who faces the consequences of his or her decisions. You are, therefore, responsible for considering the patient's wishes sacred and protecting the patient from those who would disregard them.

THE CAREGIVER'S PLEDGE

- I will be compassionate.
- I will not neglect my duties and responsibilities.
- I will read instructions and follow protocols.
- I will seek verification of questionable orders.
- I will report concerns for patient safety (e.g., staffing concerns).
- I will not assume responsibilities beyond my capabilities.
- I will call for help when a patient's medical needs suddenly change.
- I will continuously improve my skills and participate in continuing education opportunities.

CHAPTER REVIEW

1. Staff rights include:
   - Fair treatment and employment at will
   - Freedom from discrimination
   - Equal pay for equal work
   - Refusal to participate in patient care
   - Questioning of patient care
   - Suggesting a change of physician
   - Freedom from sexual harassment
   - Treatment with dignity and respect
   - Freedom from intimidation
   - Privacy and confidentiality
   - Family medical leave
   - Whistleblowing
   - Safe environment
   - Unemployment compensation

2. Staff responsibilities include:
   - Show compassion
   - Honor a patient's autonomy
   - Comply with state and federal regulations
   - Comply with hospital policy
   - Comply with job descriptions
   - Honor patient wishes
   - Maintain confidentiality
   - Adhere to safe practices
   - Adhere to professional standards
   - Maintaining professional relationships
   - Report unethical behavior
   - Protect patients from harm
   - Report patient abuse
   - Work with a team spirit
   - Maintain professional competencies
3. Helpful advice to caregivers for maintaining a spirit of teamwork.

TEST YOUR UNDERSTANDING

TERMINOLOGY

employment at will   sexual harassment
Family and Medical Leave Act of 1993   whistleblowing

REVIEW QUESTIONS

1. Describe the rights of employees.

2. Describe under what circumstances an employee has a right to refuse to participate in a patient's procedure.

3. Does a nurse have a right to question the care being rendered to a patient? Explain your answer.

4. Is the employment-at-will concept appropriate in today's society?

5. Describe the responsibilities of employees as described in this chapter.

6. Describe what caregivers can do to build a spirit of teamwork and improve the quality of patient care.

NOTES

1. http://www.dol.gov/opa/aboutdol/lawsprog.htm#workerscomp.
2. 328 S.E.2d 818 (N.C. Ct. App. 1985).
3. 44 A.L.R. 4th 1136 (1986).
4. *Sides v. Duke Hosp.,* 328 S.E.2d 818 (N.C. Ct. App. 1985).
5. *Pierce v. Ortho Pharm. Corp.,* 417 A.2d 505, 509 (N.J. 1980).
6. MONT. CODE ANN. § 39-2-904 (1989).
7. Montana Employment Law and the 1987 Wrongful Discharge From Employment Act: A New Order Begins, LeRoy H. Schramm, 125 Montana Law Review, Vol. 51 (1990).
8. *Palmateer v. International Harvester Co.,* 421 N.E.2d 876, 878 (Ill. 1981).
9. *Joiner v. Benton Community Bank,* 411 N.E.2d 229, 231 (Ill. 1980).
10. *Gantt v. Sentry Ins.,* 824 P.2d 680, 687–688 (Cal. 1992).
11. http://www.eeoc.gov/eeoc/index.cfm.
12. 515 F.2d 541 (8th Cir. 1975).
13. 676 N.Y.S. 2d 293 (N.Y. App., 1998).
14. National Constitutional Center, "Laws Protecting Pharmacist's Refusal," http://www.constitutioncenter.org/education/ForEducators/DiscussionStarters/PharmacistConscienceLaws.shtml.
15. http://www.ncsl.org/issues-research/health/pharmacist-conscience-clauses-laws-and-information.aspx.
16. 851 S.W.2d 617 (Mo. Ct. App. 1993).
17. *Deerman v. Beverly Cal. Corp.,* 518 S.E.2d 804 (N.C. App. 1999).
18. Conn. Gen. Stat. Ann. A4 31–51m(a) (West 1987).
19. Me. Rev. Stat. Ann. 26, A4A4 831–840 (West 1987).
20. Mich. Comp. Laws Ann. A4A4 15.361–369 (West 1981).
21. Mont. Code Ann. A4 39-2-901 (1987).
22. *Pierce v. Ortho Pharm. Corp.,* 417 A.2d 505, 509 (N.J. 1980).
23. 760 F. Supp. 1575 (D.C. Ga. 1991).
24. Alexander Hamilton Institute, "Mail policy considerations: Maintaining the right to open employee mail," BusinessManagement Daily, November 9, 2001; http://www.legalworkplace.com/maintaining-right-open-employee-mail-pla.aspx.
25. Whistleblowing: The Report of the Conference of Professional Responsibility 6 (1972); see also Annotation, 99 A.L.R. Fed. 778.
26. Annotation, 99 A.L.R. Fed. 775.
27. http://www.whistleblowers.gov.
28. Richard P. Wenzel and Michael B. Edmond, "The impact of hospital-acquired bloodstream infections," *Emerg Infect Dis* [Internet serial], March/April 2001; http://wwwnc.cdc.gov/eid/article/7/2/70-0174.htm.
29. *Freilich v. Upper Chesapeake Health, Inc.,* 313 F.3d 205 (2002).
30. 810 P.2d 459 (Utah 1991).
31. 520 N.E.2d 139 (Mass. 1988).
32. 243 Cal. Rptr. 807 (Cal. Ct. App. 1988).
33. 711 N.Y.S.2d 81 (N.Y. App. Div. 2000).
34. http://uk.reuters.com/article/2013/09/10/us-usa-health-cancer-idUKBRE9891EI20130910?feedType=RSS&feedName=healthNews.

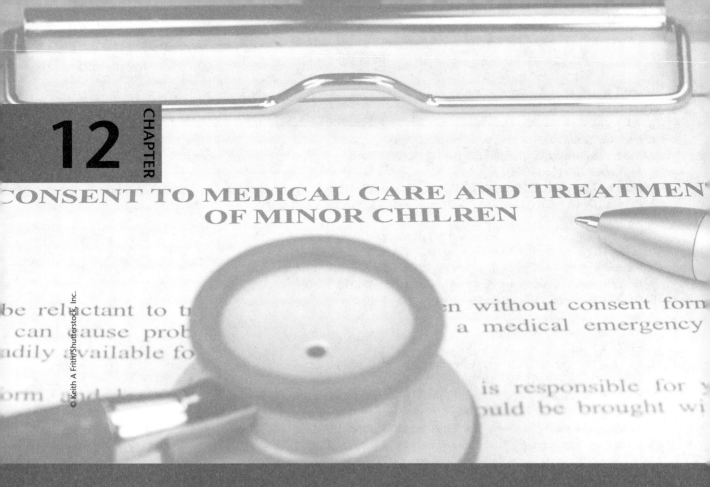

12 CHAPTER

CONSENT TO MEDICAL CARE AND TREATMENT OF MINOR CHILREN

PATIENT CONSENT

LEARNING OBJECTIVES

Upon completion of this chapter, the reader will be able to:

- Discuss informed consent and how it applies the patient's right to self-determination.
- Describe how various codes of professional ethics address a patient's right to informed consent and self-determination.
- Explain and give examples of verbal, written, and implied consent.
- Describe under what circumstances statutory consent can be inferred.
- Describe how caregivers can determine a patient's capacity to consent and what action should be taken if the patient is unable to consent to recommended care choices.
- Describe what factors the courts could take into consideration when determining the adequacy of consent.
- Explain why a patient has a right to refuse treatment.
- Understand the importance of state interests when a parent refuses life saving treatment for a child.

INTRODUCTION

. . . no right is held more sacred, or is more carefully guarded, by the common law, than the right of every individual to the possession and control of his own person.

−UNION PACIFIC RY. CO. V. BOTSFORD[1]

Consent is the voluntary agreement by a person who possesses sufficient mental capacity to make an intelligent choice to allow something proposed by another to be performed on himself or herself. Consent changes touching that otherwise would be nonconsensual to touching that is consensual. Consent can be either express or implied.

Express consent can take the form of either a verbal agreement or can be accomplished through the execution of a written document authorizing medical care. *Implied consent* is determined by some act of silence, which raises a presumption that consent has been authorized.

Consent must be obtained from the patient or from a person authorized to consent on the patient's behalf before any medical procedure can be performed. Every individual has a right to refuse to authorize a touching. This chapter reviews many of the issues surrounding consent in the health care setting.

INFORMED CONSENT

Informed consent is a legal concept that provides that a patient has a right to know the potential risks, benefits, and alternatives of a proposed procedure. The right to be free of unwanted medical treatment has long been recognized in this country. An "individual's right to make decisions vitally affecting his private life according to his own conscience . . . is difficult to overstate . . . because it is, without exaggeration, the very bedrock on which this country was founded."[2]

The right to control the integrity of one's own body spawned the doctrine of informed consent.[3] The United States Supreme Court has held that a competent adult patient has the right to decline any and all forms of medical intervention, including lifesaving or life-prolonging treatment.[4]

Informed consent is predicated on the duty of the physician to disclose to the patient sufficient information to enable the patient to evaluate a proposed medical or surgical procedure before submitting to it. Informed consent requires that a patient have a full understanding of that to which he or she has consented. An authorization from a patient who does not understand to what he or she is consenting is not effective consent.

Unreported Robot Surgery Injuries Open New Questions for FDA

When Sheena Wilson, 45, underwent robotic surgery for a hysterectomy in May, she didn't know the Intuitive Surgical Inc. system used by her doctor was previously tied to a variety of injuries for the same procedure.

> Her rectum was badly burned in the operation, said Wilson, a mother of two from Parlin, New Jersey. Now she is on long-term disability, fearful of losing her job and facing a third corrective surgery, she said in a telephone interview.
>
> "If I had known there were other people who had injuries, I would never have done this surgery," said Wilson, who has filed suit against Intuitive and her doctor. "Whatever they have in place is not working."
>
> *Robert Langreth*, Bloomberg, *December 30, 2013*[5]

Hospitals generally do not have an independent duty to obtain informed consent or to warn patients of the risks of a procedure to be performed by a physician who is not an agent of the hospital. It is the treating physician who has the education, expertise, skill, and training necessary to treat a patient and determine what information a patient should have in order to give informed consent.

CODES OF ETHICS

The first American Medical Association Code of Medical Ethics was written in 1847. Section I of the 1998–1999 edition, titled "Fundamental Elements of the Patient–Physician Relationship," provides "the patient has the right to receive information from physicians and to discuss the benefits, risks, and costs of appropriate treatment alternatives." Because the American Medical Association is an organization composed of experts in the field of medicine, its code of ethics and the duties of physicians prescribed therein should be understood to reflect the standard of care of the profession on the issue of informed consent. Social policy does not accept the "paternalistic" view that the physician may remain silent because divulgence might prompt the patient to forgo needed therapy.

The American Dental Association Code of Ethics also reflects the standard of care for the dental profession. Part III, Section 1, of the American Dental Association Code of Ethics, titled "Principle: Patient Autonomy," provides "the dentist has a duty to respect the patient's rights to self-determination and confidentiality," and Section 1A provides that "the dentist should inform the patient of the proposed treatment, and any reasonable alternatives, in a manner that allows the patient to become involved in treatment decisions." These American Medical Association and American Dental Association ethical standards embrace the doctrine of informed consent.

The American Nurses Association code of ethics for nurses provides in part in Provision 1.4 the following as to a patient's right to self-determination:

> . . . Patients have the moral and legal right to determine what will be done with their own person; to be giving accurate, complete, and understandable information in a manner that facilitates that facilitates an informed judgment; to be assisted with weighing the benefits, burdens, and available options in their treatment, including the choice of no treatment; to accept, refuse, or terminate treatment without deceit, undue influence, duress, coercion, or penalty; and to be given necessary support throughout the decision-making and treatment process.[6]

PROOF OF CONSENT

Consent can be verbal, written, or implied. The law requires verbal or written consent for the intentional touching that involves medical or surgical procedures. Consent can also be implied in emergency situations.

Oral consent is as binding as written consent. There is no legal requirement that a patient's consent be in writing; however, oral consent is more difficult to corroborate.

Written consent provides visible proof of a patient's wishes. Because the function of a written consent form is to preserve evidence of informed consent, the nature of the treatment, the risks, benefits, and consequences involved should be incorporated into the consent form. States have taken the view that consent, to be effective, must be "informed consent." An informed consent form should include the following elements:

* The nature of the patient's illness or injury
* The name of the proposed procedure or treatment
* The purpose of the proposed treatment
* The risks and probable consequences of the proposed treatment
* The probability that the proposed treatment will be successful
* Any alternative methods of treatment along with their associated risks and benefits
* The risks and prognosis if no treatment is rendered
* An indication that the patient understands the nature of any proposed treatment, the alternatives, the risks involved, and the probable consequences of the proposed treatment
* The signatures of the patient, physician, and witnesses
* The date the consent is signed

Health care professionals have an important role in the realm of informed consent. They can be instrumental in averting major lawsuits by being observant as to a patient's doubts, changes of mind or confusion, or misunderstandings expressed by a patient regarding any proposed procedures he or she is about to undergo.

Implied consent can be assumed when immediate treatment is required to preserve the life of a patient or to prevent an impairment of the patient's health and it is impossible to obtain the consent of the patient or representative legally authorized to consent for him or her, an emergency exists, and consent is implied. This privilege to proceed in emergencies without consent is accorded to physicians because inaction at this time may cause greater injury to the patient and would be contrary to good medical practice; however, if possible, consultation should be undertaken before a procedure is commenced, and every effort must be made to document the medical need for proceeding with treatment without consent. The patient's record should clearly indicate the nature of the threat to life or health, its immediacy, and its magnitude.

Unconscious patients are presumed under law to approve treatment that appears to be necessary. It is assumed that such patients would have consented if they were conscious and competent; however, if a patient expressly refuses to consent to certain treatment, such treatment may not be instituted after the patient becomes unconscious. Similarly, conscious patients suffering from emergency conditions retain the right to refuse consent. If a procedure is necessary to protect one's life or health, every effort must be made to document the medical necessity for proceeding with medical treatment without consent. It must be shown that the emergency situation constituted an immediate threat to life or health.

In *Luka v. Lowrie*,[7] involving a 15-year-old boy whose left foot had been run over and crushed by a train, consultation by the treating physician with other physicians was an important factor in determining the outcome of the case. On the boy's arrival at the hospital, the defending physician and four house surgeons decided that it was necessary to amputate the foot. The court said that it was inconceivable that had they been present, the parents would have refused consent in the face of a determination by five physicians that amputation would save the boy's life. Thus, despite testimony at the trial that the amputation may not have been necessary, professional consultation before the operation supported the assertion that a genuine emergency existed and could have implied consent.

Consent also can be implied in nonemergency situations. For example, a patient may voluntarily submit to a procedure, implying consent, without any explicitly spoken or written expression of consent. In the Massachusetts case of *O'Brien v. Cunard Steam Ship Co.*,[8] a ship's passenger who joined a line of people receiving injections was held to have implied his consent to a vaccination. The rationale for this decision is that individuals who observe a line of people and who notice that injections are being administered to those at the head of the line should expect that if they join and remain in the line they will receive an injection. The plaintiff entered the line voluntarily. The plaintiff had opportunity to see what was taking place at the head of the line and could have exited the line but chose not to do so. The jury appropriately determined this to be consent to the injection. The *O'Brien* case contains all of the elements necessary to imply consent to a voluntary act: The procedure was a simple vaccination. The proceedings were visible at all times, and the plaintiff was free to withdraw up to the instant of the injection.

Whether a patient's consent can be implied is frequently asked when the condition of a patient requires some deviation from an agreed-on procedure. If a patient expressly prohibits a specific medical or surgical procedure, consent to the procedure cannot be implied. The same consent rule applies if a patient expressly prohibits a particular extension of a procedure even though the patient voluntarily submitted to the original procedure.

STATUTORY CONSENT

The age of consent is the minimum age at which a person is considered to be legally competent to consent to medical care. Many states have adopted legislation concerning emergency care. An emergency in most states eliminates the need for consent. When a patient is clinically unable to give consent to a lifesaving emergency treatment, the law implies consent on the presumption that a reasonable person would consent to lifesaving medical intervention; this is defined as *statutory consent*. When an emergency situation does arise, there may be little opportunity to contact the attending physician, much less a consultant. The patient's records, therefore, must be complete with respect to the description of the patient's illness and condition, the attempts made to contact the physician as well as relatives, and the emergency measures taken and procedures performed. If time does not permit a court order to be obtained, a second medical opinion, when practicable, is advisable.

CASE: PATIENT EMERGENCY—FAVOR PRESERVING LIFE

Any glimmer of uncertainty as to a patient's desires in an emergency situation should be resolved "in favor of preserving life." The patient in *Matter of Hughes*[9] signed a standard blank hospital form titled "Refusal to Permit Blood Transfusion." There was no indication on the form that the consequences of her refusal had been explained to her in the context of the elective surgical procedure she was about to undergo. The form should have contained an unequivocal statement that under any and all circumstances blood is not to be used and an acknowledgment that the consequences of the refusal were fully explained. The form should fully release the physician, all medical personnel, and the hospital from liability should complications arise from the failure to administer blood, thereby resolving any doubt as to the physician's responsibility to his patient. If Hughes had refused to sign such a form, her physician could then have decided whether to continue with Hughes's treatment or to aid her in finding a physician who would carry out her wishes.

The court emphasized that this case arose in the context of elective surgery. This was not an emergency situation where the physician and patient did not have time to discuss fully the potential risks, benefits, and alternatives of the planned surgery and the conflict arising over the patient's religious beliefs. Patients have an obligation to make medical preferences known to the treating physician, including the course to follow if life-threatening complications should arise. This protects the patient's right to freedom of religion and self-determination. In addition, it is helpful to the hospital when faced with the dilemma of trying to preserve life whenever possible and honoring the patient's wishes to forgo life-sustaining treatment.

Ethical and Legal Issues

1. Describe the relevant ethical principles violated in this case.
2. Describe the relevant legal issues in this case. What actions could the parties to this lawsuit have taken beforehand to prevent this case from becoming a legal issue?

CAPACITY TO CONSENT

A patient is considered competent to make medical decisions regarding his or her care unless a court determines otherwise. Generally speaking, medical personnel make the determination of a patient's decision-making capacity. The clinical assessment of decision-making capacity should include the patient's ability to understand the risks, benefits, and alternatives of a proposed test or procedure; evaluate the information provided by the physician; express his or her treatment options/plan; and voluntarily make decisions regarding his or her treatment plan without undue influence by family, friends, or medical personnel.

If a patient is unable to make decisions by reason of age or incapacity, a patient appointed decision maker may "substitute his or her judgment" on behalf of the patient. Before declaring an individual incapacitated, the attending physician must find with a reasonable degree of medical certainty that the patient lacks capacity. A notation should be placed in the patient's medical record describing the cause, nature, extent, and probable duration of incapacity.

Before withholding or withdrawing life-sustaining treatment, a second physician must confirm the incapacity determination and make an appropriate entry on the medical record before honoring any new decisions by a health care agent.

CASE: LACK OF CONSENT AND PATIENT DEATH

Four siblings, in *Riser v. American Medical Int'l, Inc.,*[10] brought a medical malpractice action against Dr. Lang, a physician who performed a femoral arteriogram on their 69-year-old mother, who died due to the procedure.

Riser had been admitted to Hospital A experiencing impaired circulation in her lower arms and hands. She had multiple medical diagnoses, including diabetes mellitus, end-stage renal failure, and arteriosclerosis. Her physician, Dr. Sottiurai, ordered bilateral arteriograms to determine the cause of the patient's impaired circulation. Hospital A could not accommodate Sottiurai's request, and Riser was transferred to Dr. Lang, a radiologist at Hospital B. Lang performed a femoral arteriogram rather than the bilateral brachial arteriogram ordered by Sottiurai. The procedure seemed to go well, and the patient was prepared for transfer back to the hospital; however, shortly after the ambulance departed the hospital, the patient suffered a seizure in the ambulance and was returned to Hospital B. Riser's condition deteriorated, and she died 11 days later. The plaintiffs claimed in their lawsuit that Riser was a poor risk for the procedure. The district court ruled for the plaintiffs, awarding damages in the amount of $50,000 for Riser's pain and suffering and $100,000 to each of Riser's children. Lang appealed.

The Louisiana Court of Appeal held that Lang failed to obtain consent from the patient. Riser was under the impression that she was about to undergo a brachial arteriogram, not a femoral arteriogram. Two consent forms were signed; neither form authorized the performance of a femoral arteriogram. O'Neil, one of Riser's daughters, claimed that her mother said, following the arteriogram, "Why did you let them do that to me?"[11]

Ethical and Legal Issues

1. Describe how the physician violated his professional duty to the patient.
2. Should the hospital have intervened and prevented the femoral arteriogram? Explain your answer.

ADEQUACY OF CONSENT

A physician should provide as much information about treatment options as is necessary based on a patient's personal understanding of the physician's explanation of the risks of treatment and the probable consequences of the treatment. The needs of each patient can vary depending on age, maturity, and mental status.

Some courts have recognized that the condition of the patient may be taken into account to determine whether the patient has received sufficient information to give consent. The individual responsible for obtaining consent must weigh the importance of giving full disclosure to the patient against the likelihood that such disclosure will seriously and adversely affect the condition of the patient.

When questions do arise as to whether adequate consent has been given, some courts take into consideration the information that is ordinarily provided by other physicians. A physician must reveal to his or her patient information just as a skilled practitioner of good standing would provide under similar circumstances. A physician must disclose to the patient the potential of death, serious harm, and other complications associated with a proposed procedure.

Failure to Inform—Alternative Procedures

The operation you get often depends on where you live. One patient underwent a mastectomy only to learn that a less destructive alternative procedure was available in a region near her home. The procedure, a lumpectomy, has the same survival rate as a mastectomy. The patient claims that the surgeon never informed her about the alternative.

Discussion

1. Describe the ethical and legal issues involved in failing to discuss alternative treatments with a patient.
2. Should a physician describe every possible alternative treatment procedure with his or her patient? Explain your answer.

COMPETENT PATIENT

A competent adult patient's wishes concerning his or her person may not be disregarded. The court in *In re Melideo*[12] held that every human being of adult years has a right to determine what shall be done with his or her own body and cannot be subjected to medical treatment without his or her consent. When there is no compelling state interest that justifies overriding an adult patient's decision, that decision should be respected. State interests include preserving life, preventing suicide, safeguarding the integrity of the medical profession, and protecting innocent third parties.

SPOUSE

The patient in *Greynolds v. Kurman*[13] suffered a transient ischemic attack, a sudden loss of neurological function caused by vascular impairment to the brain. He was taken to an emergency department. Because of the patient's prior medical history, which included transient ischemic attacks, he was at high risk for a stroke. After receiving the results of noninvasive tests, Dr. Rafecas, a consulting physician, ordered a cerebral angiogram. Dr. Kurman performed the angiogram, and the patient suffered a stroke during the procedure that left him severely disabled.

The patient and his wife filed a medical malpractice action against Rafecas and Kurman, asserting that Rafecas had negligently recommended the procedure and that Kurman had performed the procedure without obtaining informed consent. The court of appeals held that the evidence was sufficient to support a judgment in favor of the patient and his wife.

The jury needed to determine that the risks involved in the cerebral angiogram were not disclosed, that the risks involved in the procedure materialized and caused the stroke, and that a reasonable person in the position of the patient would have decided against having the angiogram had the risks associated with the procedure been disclosed. The jury concluded that the patient did not consent to the angiogram because he "was not . . . capable of comprehending the consent form" and further noted that Kurman should have sought consent from the next of kin, specifically the spouse. Given the evidence of the patient's condition when he signed the consent forms, his past medical history, and his increased risk of suffering complications during an angiogram, the court found that evidence supported a finding of lack of informed consent.

PARENTAL CONSENT

Parents generally have the right to authorize medical care for minor children, generally under the age of 18. Consent laws for minors often vary from state to sate and should be referenced as necessary. Children who are emancipated have a right to make their own medical care decisions. Although parents may have a right to refuse medical care in certain instances, such refusal is reportable by the caregiver to the state if such refusal can result in harm to the child.

CASE: PARENTS REFUSE TREATMENT

When parents in *In re Guardianship of L.S.*[14] refused to consent to medically necessary care for their minor child based on their religious convictions, the trial court appointed the hospital as a temporary guardian to make decisions to provide medically necessary, lifesaving treatment for the child. The evidence presented to the trial court in the form of an affidavit from a hospital physician stated that the parents were refusing medically necessary blood transfusions, that the child would require blood transfusions to survive, and that the child was unable to respond to this risk. The trial court reasonably concluded from this information that the child was at risk of substantial and immediate physical harm. The trial court's decision to appoint a temporary guardian was based on the child's best interest and protected the state's interest in the welfare of children within the state.

In the midst of an emergency, the district court was confronted with the task of balancing the competing interests of the child, the parents, the hospital, and the state. Throughout the proceedings, the district court took numerous steps to protect the interests of the child and the parents, including requiring notice and a hearing within 24 hours after the original order, allowing the parents time to obtain counsel before reaching a final determination.

"Substantive due process guarantees that no person shall be deprived of life, liberty, or property for arbitrary reasons." The due process clause of the Fourteenth Amendment protects those liberty interests that are deemed fundamental and are "deeply rooted in this Nation's history and tradition." Certain family privacy rights, including the parent–child relationship, have therefore been recognized as fundamental rights. The Nevada Supreme Court adopted a "reasonableness test" to address family privacy cases involving "competing interests within the family."

Although a parent has a fundamental liberty interest in the "care, custody, and management" of his or her child, that interest is not absolute. "The state also has an interest in the welfare of children and may limit parental authority," even permanently depriving parents of their children; therefore, although the parents have a parental interest in the care of their son, both the state and L.S. have an interest in preserving the child's life. As L.S. is unable to make decisions for himself, the state's interest is heightened. The parents' liberty interest in practicing their religion must also give way to the child's welfare. Hence, the district court found that the parents' refusal to consent to treatment put L.S.'s life at substantial risk. Additionally, the state has an interest in protecting "the ethical integrity of the medical profession" and in allowing hospitals the full opportunity to care for patients under their control, especially when medical science is available to save that patient's life.

Here, the child's interest in self-preservation and the state's interests in protecting the welfare of children and the integrity of medical care outweigh the parents' interests in the care, custody, and management of their children, as well as their religious freedom. The combined weight of the interests of the child and the state are great and therefore mandate interference with parental rights.

The Supreme Court of Nevada affirmed the order of the district court appointing Valley Hospital as temporary guardian.

CONSENT BY MINORS

Parental consent is not required when a minor is married or otherwise emancipated. Most states have enacted statutes making it valid for married and emancipated minors to provide effective consent. Several courts have held the consent of a minor to be sufficient authorization for treatment in certain situations. In any specific case, a court's determination that the consent of a minor is effective and that parental consent is unnecessary will depend on such factors as the minor's age, maturity, mental status, and emancipation and the procedure involved, as well as public policy considerations.

The courts have held, as a general proposition, that the consent of a minor to medical or surgical treatment is ineffective and that the physician must secure the consent of the minor's parent or someone standing in loco parentis; otherwise, he or she will risk liability. Although parental consent should be obtained before treating a minor, treatment should not be delayed to the detriment of the child. The various states have laws allowing children to be treated without consent in order to protect the minor (e.g., provision of emergency care, protect the minor from child abuse, abortion, treat venereal diseases) and safeguard the public health of the community (e.g., communicable and venereal diseases).

INCOMPETENT PATIENTS

The attending physician, who is in the best position to determine if a patient is incompetent, should become familiar with his or her state's definition of legal incompetence. In any case in which a physician doubts a patient's capacity to consent, the consent of the legal guardian or next of kin should be obtained. If there are no relatives to consult, application should be made for a court order that would allow the procedure. It may be the duty of the court to assume responsibility of guardianship for a patient who is non compos mentis. The most frequently cited conditions indicative of incompetence are mental illness, mental retardation, senility, physical incapacity, and chronic alcohol or drug abuse.

A person who is mentally incompetent cannot legally consent to medical or surgical treatment; therefore, consent of the patient's legal guardian must be obtained. When no legal guardian is available, a court that handles such matters must be petitioned to permit treatment.

Subject to applicable statutory provisions, when a physician doubts a patient's capacity to consent, even though the patient has not been judged legally incompetent, the consent of the nearest relative should be obtained. If a patient is conscious and mentally capable of giving consent for treatment, the consent of a relative without the consent of the competent patient would not protect the physician from liability.

Guardian

Consent of the patient ordinarily is required before treatment. When a patient is either physically unable or legally incompetent to consent and no emergency exists, consent must be obtained from a person who is empowered to consent on the patient's behalf. A guardian is an individual who by law is invested with the power and charged with the duty of taking care of a patient by protecting the patient's rights and managing the patient's estate. *Guardianship* is often necessary in those instances in which a patient is incapable of managing or administering his or her private affairs because of physical and/or mental disabilities or because he or she is under the age of majority.

Temporary Guardian

The courts can grant temporary guardianship if it is determined necessary for the well being of the patient.

Case: Physician and Administrator File for Temporary Guardianship

The court in *In re Estate of Dorone* granted temporary guardianship.[15] In this case, the physician and administrator petitioned the court on two occasions for authority to administer blood. A 22-year-old male patient brought to the Hospital Center by helicopter after an automobile accident was diagnosed as suffering from an acute subdural hematoma with a brain contusion.

It was determined that the patient would die unless he underwent a cranial operation. The operation required the administration of blood, to which the parents would not consent because of their religious beliefs. After a hearing by telephone, the court of common pleas appointed the hospital's administrator as temporary guardian, authorizing him to consent to the performance of blood transfusions during emergency surgery. A more formal hearing did not take place because of the emergency situation that existed. Surgery was required a second time to remove a blood clot, and the court once again granted the administrator authority to authorize administration of blood. The superior court affirmed the orders, and the parents appealed. The Pennsylvania Supreme Court held that the judge's failure to obtain direct testimony from the patient's parents and others concerning the patient's religious beliefs were not in error when death was likely to result from withholding blood. The judge's decisions granting guardianship and the authority to consent to the administration of blood were considered absolutely necessary in the light of the facts of this case. Nothing less than a fully conscious contemporary decision by the patient himself would have been sufficient to override the evidence of medical necessity.

Ethical and Legal Issues

1. Should a hospital act to save a patient's life if he or she has not given written consent to a procedure?
2. What types of monetary awards should the court give the plaintiff, if any? Why?

RIGHT TO REFUSE TREATMENT

The individual's right to make decisions vitally affecting his private life according to his own conscience . . . is difficult to overstate . . . because it is, without exaggeration, the very bedrock on which this country was founded.

—*Wons v. Public Health Trust*[16]

Adult patients who are conscious and mentally competent have the right to refuse medical care to the extent permitted by law, even when the best medical opinion deems it essential to life. A patient's right to make decisions regarding his own health care is addressed in the Patient Self-Determination Act of 1990.[17] The act provides that each person has a right under state law (whether statutory or as recognized by the courts of the state) to make decisions concerning his or her medical care, including the right to accept or refuse medical or surgical treatment.

A competent patient's refusal to consent to a medical or surgical procedure must be adhered to, whether the refusal is grounded in lack of confidence in the physician, fear of the procedure, doubt as to the value of a particular procedure, or mere whim. The U.S. Supreme Court stated that the "notion of bodily integrity has been embodied in the requirement that informed consent is generally required for medical treatment" and the "logical corollary of the doctrine of informed consent is that the patient generally possesses the right not to consent, that is, to refuse treatment."[18] The common-law doctrine of informed consent is viewed as generally encompassing the right of a competent individual to refuse medical treatment.

The question of liability for performing a medical or surgical procedure without consent is separate and distinct from any question of negligence or malpractice in performing a procedure. Liability can be imposed for a nonconsensual touching of a patient, even if the procedure improved the patient's health.

The courts perform a balancing test to determine whether or not to override a competent adult's decision to refuse medical treatment. The courts balance state interests, such as preservation of life, protection of third parties, prevention of suicide, and the integrity of the medical profession, against a patient's rights of bodily integrity and religious freedom. The most frequently used state right to intervene in a patient's decision-making process is for the protection of third parties. In *In re Fetus Brown*,[19] the state of Illinois asserted that its interest in the well-being of a viable fetus outweighed the patient's right to refuse medical treatment. The state argued that a balancing test should be used to weigh state interests against patient rights. The appellate court held that it could not impose a legal obligation on a pregnant woman to consent to an invasive medical procedure for the benefit of her viable fetus.

Adult patients who are conscious and mentally competent have the right to refuse medical care to the extent permitted by law even when the best medical opinion deems it essential to life. Such a refusal must be honored whether it is grounded in religious belief or straightforward objection to the procedure. Every person has the legal right to refuse to permit a touching of his or her body. Failure to respect this right can result in a legal action for assault and battery. If a patient refuses consent, every effort should be made to explain the importance of the procedure. Coercion through threat, duress, or intimidation must be avoided.

A hospital generally has no common-law right or obligation to thrust unwanted medical care on a patient who, having been sufficiently informed of the consequences, competently and clearly declines such care. A patient's common-law right of bodily self-determination is entitled to respect and protection. Before a patient leaves a health care facility against medical advice, every attempt should be made to have a release form completed (**Figure 12-1**) and included in the patient's permanent record.

All reasonable steps should be taken to (1) inform the patient of the benefits and risks of treatment and (2) secure the patient's written informed consent to refuse examination and treatment. If the patient refuses to sign the "refusal to consent form," documentation of a patient's refusal of care should be placed in the patient's medical record.

REFUSAL OF CARE BASED ON RELIGIOUS BELIEFS

As part of their religious beliefs, Jehovah's Witnesses generally have refused the administration of blood, even in emergency situations. Case law over the past several decades has developed to a point where any person, regardless of religious beliefs, has the right to refuse medical treatment.

CASE: A MOTHER'S RIGHT, A CHILD'S DEATH

Harrell, a Jehovah's Witness, was 6 months pregnant when physicians discovered a life-threatening blood condition that could rapidly deteriorate, placing both her life and the life of the fetus in jeopardy. Because of her religious beliefs, Harrell objected to a blood transfusion. After an emergency hearing during which the Harrells could not summon an attorney, the court ruled that a blood transfusion could be given to Harrell if it was necessary to save the life of the fetus and that after the child was born a blood transfusion could be given to the child if necessary to save the child's life. The Harrells appealed. The child was delivered by Caesarean section and died 2 days later. No blood transfusion was given to Harrell or to the child. As a result, the hospital and the state claimed that the *appeal* of the trial court's order was moot. Because of the hospital's serious misunderstanding about its standing to bring

Hospital _____

Address _____

Phone _____

Refusal of Care and Treatment
(Leave Against Medical Advice)

The patient meets all of the following criteria:

1. The patient is over the age of 18 years of age.

2. The patient exhibits no evidence of:

_____ Altered level of consciousness

_____ Alcohol or drug ingestion that would impair judgment

3. The patient understands the nature of his or her medical condition, including the risks, benefits, and of alternative treatments, as well as, the consequences of refusing care treatment alternatives.

Acknowledgement of Information (initial each of the following lines)

_____ I have been advised that medical care on my behalf is necessary, and that refusal of care and assistance could be hazardous to my health, and under certain circumstances, including disability or death.

_____ I acknowledge that I may have a medical problem which may require additional medical attention, and that NDSP or an ambulance is available to transport me to the hospital. Instead, I elect to seek alternative medical care and/or refuse further evaluation, treatment and/or transport.

Release of Liability (initial on line)

_____ By signing this form, I am releasing _____ (name of hospital or healthcare facility) of any liability or medical claims resulting from my decision to refuse care against medical advice.

_____ I have read and understand the Acknowledgement ofInformation and Release of Liability.

_____ If I change my mind, or my condition changes, I will call 911 in an emergency and request that I be taken to the _____ Hospital emergency room or call my private doctor, for follow-up care as appropriate.

Signature _____   Date _____

Witness Information

Signature: _____   Name Printed: _____   Date: _____

Signature: _____   Name Printed: _____   Date: _____

FIGURE 12-1   Refusal of Care and Treatment

such proceedings, the Florida District Court of Appeal addressed the issue as capable of repetition yet evading review.

The Florida constitution guarantees that a competent person has the constitutional right to choose or refuse medical treatment, and that right extends to all relevant decisions concerning one's health. The state has a duty to ensure that a person's wishes regarding medical treatment are respected. That obligation serves to protect the rights of the individual from intrusion by the state unless the state has a compelling interest great enough to override this constitutional right (e.g., protection of innocent third parties).

Harrell argued that the hospital should not have intervened in her private decision to refuse a blood transfusion. She claimed that the state had never been a party in this action, had not asserted any interest, and that the hospital had no authority to assume the state's responsibilities.

The Florida District Court of Appeal concluded that a health care provider must not be forced into the position of having to argue against the wishes of the facility's own patient. Patients do not lose their right to make decisions affecting their lives when they enter a health care facility. A health care provider's function is to provide medical treatment in accordance with the patient's wishes and best interests, not supervene the wishes of a competent adult. A health care provider must comply with the wishes of a patient to refuse medical treatment unless ordered to do otherwise by a court of competent jurisdiction. A health care provider cannot act on behalf of the state to assert state interests. When a health care provider, acting in good faith, follows the wishes of a competent and informed patient to refuse medical treatment, the health care provider is acting appropriately and cannot be subjected to civil or criminal liability. [20]

Ethical and Legal Issues

1. Is the Florida District Court of Appeal's conclusion binding in all states?
2. Do you think the hospital made the correct decisions in this case? Discuss your answer.

CASE: MOTHER REFUSES BLOOD, SPOUSE DISAGREES

What would you do if a patient, a Jehovah's Witness, signs a consent form refusing a blood transfusion and her husband, who is not a Jehovah's Witness, consents to a blood transfusion to save his wife's life?

The plaintiff, Bonita Perkins, in *Perkins v. Lavin*,[21] was a Jehovah's Witness. She gave birth to a baby at the defendant's hospital. After going home, she began hemorrhaging and returned to the hospital. She specifically informed the defendant's employees that she was not to be provided any blood or blood derivatives, and she signed a form to that effect:[22]

> I request that no blood or blood derivatives be administered to [plaintiff] during this hospitalization, notwithstanding that such treatment may be deemed necessary in the opinion of the attending physician or his assistants to preserve life or promote recovery. I release the attending physician, his assistants, the hospital, and its personnel from any responsibility whatever for any untoward results due to my refusal to permit the use of blood or its derivatives.

Because of the plaintiff's condition, it became necessary to perform an emergency dilation and curettage. She continued to bleed and her condition deteriorated dramatically. Her blood count dropped, necessitating administration of blood products as a lifesaving measure. Her husband, who was not a Jehovah's Witness, consented to a blood transfusion, which was administered. The plaintiff recovered and filed an action against the defendant for assault and battery. The plaintiff's claim as to assault and battery was sustained.

The plaintiff specifically informed the defendant that she would consider a blood transfusion an offensive contact. Although both parties have noted that the plaintiff's husband provided his consent for the transfusion, the defendant has not argued that his consent was sufficient to overcome plaintiff's direction that she was not to receive a transfusion. The plaintiff submitted sufficient evidence to the trial court to establish that there was, at least, a genuine issue as to whether the defendant intentionally invaded her right to be free from offensive contact. Because of the plaintiff's recognition that the defendant acted to save her life, a jury may find that she is entitled to only nominal damages.

Ethical and Legal Issues

1. Should the court be the ultimate decision maker when there is a dispute over whether or not a lifesaving measure should be administered to a nonconsenting patient?
2. Should a parent have the right to refuse a lifesaving treatment (e.g., transfusion) for a minor? Explain.

CASE: MOTHER REFUSES TREATMENT, SPOUSE AGREES

Vega, a Jehovah's Witness, executed a release requesting that no blood be administered to her during her hospitalization. Vega's husband also signed the release. She delivered a healthy baby. After the delivery, Vega bled heavily. Her obstetrician, Dr. Sood, recommended a dilation and curettage (D&C) to stop the bleeding. Although Vega agreed to permit Sood to perform the D&C, she refused to allow a blood transfusion. Before undergoing the procedure, she signed a second release refusing any transfusions and releasing the hospital from liability. Despite the D&C, Vega continued to hemorrhage.

Because Sood and the other physicians involved in Vega's care believed that it was essential that she receive blood in order to survive, the hospital requested that the court issue an injunction that would permit the hospital to administer blood transfusions. The trial court convened an emergency hearing at the hospital and appointed Vega's husband as her guardian. At the hearing testimony, Vega's husband testified that, on the basis of his religious beliefs as a Jehovah's Witness, he continued to support his wife's decision to refuse transfusions and believed that she would take the same position if she were able to participate in the hearing.

The court, relying on the state's interests in preserving life and protecting innocent third parties, granted the hospital's request for an injunction permitting it to administer blood transfusions. Vega was given blood transfusions. She recovered and was discharged from the hospital.

Vega sued, arguing that if her refusal of blood transfusions interfered with certain state interests, it should be the state itself, not a private hospital, that asserts state's interests. The hospital responded that because it was charged with Vega's care it had a direct stake in the outcome of the controversy and was a proper party to bring the action.

The hospital had a legitimate interest in receiving official guidance in resolving the "ethical dilemma" it faced: whether to practice medicine by trying to save a patient's life despite that patient's refusal to consent to treatment or to practice medicine in accordance with the patient's wishes and likely watch the patient die, knowing nonetheless that it had the power to save her life. The hospital had conflicting interests and was in the role not of opposing its patient but of a party seeking the court's guidance in determining its obligations under the circumstances.

Vega claimed that the state's interest in the welfare of her child is not sufficiently compelling as to outweigh her interest in refusing blood transfusions. Vega maintained that the trial court's injunction, issued at the behest of the hospital, violated her common-law right of self-determination, her federal constitutional right to bodily self-determination, her federal constitutional right to free exercise of religion, and her state constitutional right of religious liberty. The court concluded that, under the circumstances of this case, the issuance of the injunction, followed by the administration of blood transfusions, violated Vega's common-law right of bodily self-determination.

Although the hospital's interests are sufficient to confer standing in this case, they are not sufficient to take priority over Vega's common law right to bodily integrity, even when the assertion of that right threatens her own life. The hospital had no common-law right or obligation to thrust unwanted medical care on a patient who, having been sufficiently informed of the consequences, competently and clearly declined that care. The hospital's interests were sufficiently protected by Vega's informed choice, and neither it nor the trial court was entitled to override that choice. Vega's common-law right of bodily self-determination was entitled to respect and protection.[23]

Ethical and Legal Issues

1. What would you do if a patient refused a blood transfusion and the spouse agreed with her decision, knowing that a blood transfusion may be necessary to save her life?
2. Should a hospital challenge a patient's refusal of lifesaving blood transfusions?

Competent adolescents have the right to deny treatment according to Skagit County Superior Court Judge John Meyer when he had to decide if a 14-year-old patient with leukemia had the right to refuse a blood transfusion. The patient, Dennis Lindberg, a Jehovah's Witness had denied the transfusion based on his religious beliefs.

Ethics experts and Jehovah's Witness officials said such a court case is unusual these days. Most cases involving transfusions stem from surgical cases, and current policy at Children's is to inform parents that while the hospital will do everything it can to avoid transfusions, it will not let a child die for want of blood, said Dr. Doug Diekema, an ethics consultant there.[24]

Are Teens Old Enough for Life/Death Decisions?

When Skagit County Superior Court Judge John Meyer came to work he expected to be hearing a few small matters.

Instead, he made a decision in a case that he said has "perhaps more profound interest and implication than any matter I have ever heard on the bench."

Meyer decided Wednesday to allow 14-year-old Dennis Lindberg of Mount Vernon to refuse blood transfusions—based on his religious beliefs.

It's a case that brings into sharp relief the tensions in laws and ethics over whether adolescents should be able to make such serious health-care decisions for themselves.

Janet I. Tu, The Seattle Times, *November 30, 2007*

Judge John Meyer's decision should by no means be applied as a standard for all similar cases involving a minor patient's right to refuse treatment. The courts of various jurisdictions may have reached a different decision than that of Judge Meyer of the Skagit County Superior Court. In future cases of this sort, no court can use a customized cookie cutter approach to stamp out decisions because every case is composed of a different set of facts and circumstances to which the law must be applied. It seems to be an oxymoron to prohibit minors from obtaining treatment for most medical conditions without first obtaining parental consent on the one hand and on the other hand allowing the minor to deny lifesaving treatment. It is unclear how the courts will respond to the same or similar cases as they arise in other jurisdictions.

Interestingly, Dr. James L. Bernat wrote an article titled "Ask the Neurologist: What If Your Patient Refuses Blood Transfusions Due to Religious Beliefs? in *Neurology Today*, a publication of the American Academy of Neurology:

> One memorable experience in which I performed an ethics consultation on a minor patient whose Jehovah's Witness parents refused consent for blood transfusion yielded an unexpected outcome. After the bioethics committee requested and obtained a court order mandating treatment, rather than being angry or resentful with us for superseding their parental authority through the judiciary, the parents were relieved that their child would survive. It became clear to us in retrospect that they felt compelled to refuse blood transfusions on behalf of their child for them to remain true to their religious beliefs.[25]

CHAPTER REVIEW

1. *Consent*
   * Voluntary agreement by a person who possesses sufficient mental capacity to make an intelligent choice to allow something proposed by another to be performed on himself or herself.

- Forms of consent
  - *Express*
    - Verbal
    - Written
  - *Implied*
    - Presumption that consent has been authorized
2. *Informed consent*
   - Legal concept that provides that a patient has a right to know
     - Risks
     - Benefits
     - Alternatives of a proposed procedure
   - Informed consent is predicated on the duty of the physician to disclose to the patient sufficient information to enable the patient to evaluate a proposed medical or surgical procedure before submitting to it.
3. *Statutory consent*
   - Age of consent
   - Emergency consent
     - Generally presumed when immediate action is required to prevent death or permanent impairment of a patient's health
     - Documentation justifying the need for treatment
4. Capacity to consent
   - Individuals incompetent to give consent
   - No relatives or other parties from whom consent can be obtained
     - Application should be made for a court order that would allow a needed procedure.
5. Adequacy of consent
   - Requires that that consent be informed consent.
     - Varies depending on age, maturity, and mental status.
   - Competent patient
   - Spouse
   - Parental consent
   - Consent by minors
   - Incompetent patients
   - Guardian
6. Right to refuse treatment
   - Often based on religious beliefs.
   - Complexities occur when the consent for a minor's treatment is involved.
     - Generally because states interests are at issue, as in the case of a minor.
   - Patients refusing care should be requested to sign a release form.
     - Documentation should be placed in the patient's medical record as to their refusal of treatment.

TEST YOUR UNDERSTANDING

TERMINOLOGY

consent	implied consent	statutory consent
express consent	informed consent	written consent
guardianship	oral consent	

REVIEW QUESTIONS

1. Discuss informed consent and how it applies the patient's right to self-determination.

2. Describe what information the patient should be provided prior to consenting to a recommended treatment.

3. Describe how various codes of professional ethics address a patient's right to informed consent and self-determination.

4. Explain and give examples of verbal, written, and implied consent.

5. Describe the purpose of statutory consent.

6. Describe under what circumstances statutory consent to treatment can be inferred.

7. Discuss why is it important to assess a patient's decision-making capacity.

8. Describe what factors the courts could take into consideration when determining the adequacy of consent.

9. Can a patient give consent and then withdraw it? Discuss your answer.

10. Explain why a patient has a right to refuse treatment.

NOTES

1. 141 U.S. 250, 251 (1891).
2. Wons v. Public Health Trust, 500 So. 2d 679, 687 (Fla. Dist. Ct. App. 1987), aff'd 541 So. 2d 96 (Fla. 1989).
3. In re Duran, 769 A.2d 497 (Pa. 2001).
4. Cruzan v. Director, Missouri Dep't of Health, 497 U.S. 261 (1990).
5. http://mobile.bloomberg.com/news/2013-12-30/unreported-robot-surgery-injuries-open-questions-for-fda.html
6. http://www.nursingworld.org/MainMenuCategories/EthicsStandards/CodeofEthicsforNurses/Code-of-Ethics.pdf.
7. 136 N.W. 1106 (Mich. 1912).
8. 28 N.E. 266 (Mass. 1891).
9. 611 A.2d 1148 (N.J. Super Ct. 1992).
10. 620 So. 2d 372 (La. Ct. App. 1993).

11. Id. at 380.
12. 390 N.Y.S.2d 523 (N.Y. Sup. Ct. 1976).
13. 632 N.E.2d 946 (Ohio Ct. App. 1993).
14. No. 38242 (Nev. 2004).
15. 534 A.2d 452 (Pa. 1987).
16. 500 So. 2d 679, 687 (Fla. Dist. Ct. App. 1987), aff'd 541 So. 2d 96 (Fla. 1989).
17. Public Law 101-508, November 5, 1990, sections 4206 and 4751 of the Omnibus Budget Reconciliation Act.
18. Cruzan v. Director, Missouri Dep't of Health, 497 U.S. 261, 269 (1990).
19. 689 N.E.2d 397 (Ill. App. Ct. 1997).
20. Harrell v. St. Mary's Hosp., Inc., 678 So. 2d 455 (Fla. Dist. Ct. App. 1996).
21. 648 N.E.2d 839 (Ohio App. 9 Dist. 1994).
22. Id. at 840.
23. Stamford Hosp. v. Vega, 674 A.2d 821 (Conn. Super. Ct. 1996).
24. *Carol M. Ostrom*, The Seattle Times, *November 29, 2007.* http://seattletimes.com/html/health/2004041765_transfusion29m.html.
25. *Neurology Today*, Vol. 11, Issue 10, May 19, 2011 pp. 27-8, 30-12.

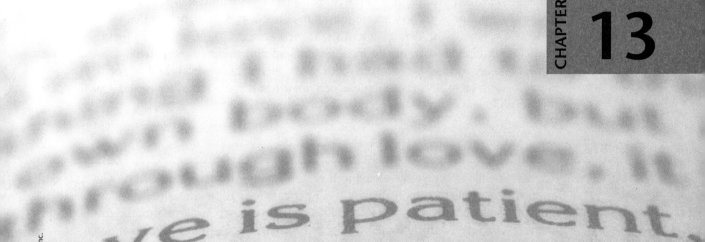

CHAPTER 13

PATIENT ABUSE

LEARNING OBJECTIVES

Upon completion of this chapter, the reader will be able to:

- Understand the pervasiveness of abuse
- Identify the signs of abuse
- Describe the reporting requirements for abuse

INTRODUCTION

Love and knowledge led upwards to the heavens, but always pity brought me back to earth; cries of pain reverberated in my heart of children in famine, of victims tortured, and of old people left helpless. I long to alleviate the evil, but I cannot, and I too suffer. This has been my life; I found it worth living.

—BERTRAND RUSSELL (ADAPTED)

Patient abuse refers to the mistreatment or neglect of individuals in the health care setting. Abuse often occurs to those who are most vulnerable and dependent on others for care (e.g., patients diagnosed with dementia and Alzheimer's disease, those who are physically weak). Abuse is not limited to an institutional setting and may occur in the patient's home. Abuse can take many forms—physical, psychological, medical, financial, and so forth. It is not always easy to identify because injuries can often be attributed to other causes. This chapter reviews child and senior abuse in a variety of settings.

CHILD ABUSE

An abused child is generally defined as a person younger than 18 years of age whose parent or other person legally responsible for his or her care inflicts, or allows to be inflicted, on that child physical injury by nonaccidental means that causes or creates a substantial risk of death, serious or protracted disfigurement, protracted impairment of physical or emotional health, or protracted loss or impairment of the function of any bodily organ; commits, or allows to be committed, a sex offense against that child; and/or allows, permits, or encourages the child to engage in an act considered unlawful. An abused child is one who may have suffered intentional serious mental, emotional, sexual, and/or physical injury inflicted by a parent or other person responsible for the child's care. The United States Code defines a *child abuse crime* as "a crime committed under any law of a State that involves the physical or mental injury, sexual abuse or exploitation, negligent treatment, or maltreatment of a child by any person."[1] Some states extend the definition to include a child suffering from starvation. Other states include moral neglect in the definition of abuse. Others mention immoral associations; endangering a child's morals; and the location of a child in a disreputable place or in association with vagrant, vicious, or immoral persons.

Child abuse continues to be of serious concern throughout the nation as noted by Joo Yeun Chang, the associate commissioner of the Children's Bureau, Department of Health and Human Services, in a report titled *Child Maltreatment 2012*.

- From 2008 to 2012, overall rates of victimization declined by 3.3%, from 9.5 to 9.2 per 1,000 children in the population. This results in an estimated 30,000 fewer victims in 2012 (686,000) compared with 2008 (716,000).
- Since 2008, overall rates of children who received a [Child Protective Services] CPS response increased by 4.7%, from 40.8 to 42.7 per 1,000 children in the population. This results in an estimated 107,000 additional children who received a CPS response in 2012 (3,184,000) compared to 2008 (3,077,000).
- Nationally, four-fifths (78.3%) of victims were neglected, 18.3% were physically abused, 9.3% were sexually abused, and 8.5% were psychologically maltreated.[2]

It is estimated that 1,640 children died of abuse and neglect at a rate of 2.20 children per 100,000 children in 2012.[3] The full document describing child maltreatment in 2012 is available from the Children's Bureau website at http://www.acf.hhs.gov/programs/cb/ research-data- technology/statistics-research/child-maltreatment. The Children's Bureau in the Administration on Children, Youth and Families, the Administration for Children and Families within the U.S. Department of Health and Human Services (HHS), addresses this important issue in many ways. As noted in the following news clipping, the horrors of child abuse continue seemingly unabated.

Mother gets 99 years for beating, gluing daughter: Has the US had it with bad parents?

Elizabeth Escalona, a 23-year-old mother of five, was sentenced to 99 years in prison after severely beating her daughter and gluing the girl's hands to a wall. The sentence is one sign that society—and the courts—are taking child abuse more seriously.

A 99-year prison sentence for a 23-year-old Dallas mother who admitted she had acted like a "monster" when gluing her daughter's hands and beating her into a coma last year suggests that society and the courts are taking a harsher view of neglectful, abusive, and violent parents, experts say.

Patrik Jonsson, The Christian Science Monitor, *October 13, 2012*

REPORTING ABUSE

The U.S. Code describes a state's reporting requirements for child abuse as follows:

> In each State, an authorized criminal justice agency of the State shall report child abuse crime information to, or index child abuse crime information in, the national criminal history background check system. A criminal justice agency may satisfy the requirement of this subsection by reporting or indexing all felony and serious misdemeanor arrests and dispositions.[4]

Child abuse statutes have been enacted by the states to protect abused children and provide civil immunity for those making or participating in good-faith reports of suspected child abuse. Most states also provide immunity from criminal liability. The New York State Social Services Law provides that "[a]ny person, official, or institution participating in good faith in the making of a report, the taking of photographs, or the removal or keeping of a child pursuant to this title shall have immunity from any liability, civil or criminal, that might otherwise result by reason of such actions."[5] Even in states that do not provide immunity, it is unlikely that anyone making a good-faith report of suspected child abuse would be subject to criminal liability. State laws generally specify what persons are required to report suspected child abuse that comes before them in their official capacities. In some states, failure to report a case of suspected child abuse carries criminal penalties as well as civil liability for the damages resulting from such failure.[6]

Child Abuse Fears Must Be Reported by Doctors, But Some Cases Pose Dilemmas

. . . As she turned her head on the way out the door, I noticed minor swelling around her eye. When I asked about it, she said, without hesitation, "Oh, my father hit me." Like all pediatricians, I am mandated by law to report any concern of child abuse . . .

Day after day, she begged me to rescind the report . . .

This spring, I received a message from her. She'd be home from college in the summer, she wrote. Could she shadow me at work as she explored a possible career in health care?

Her e-mail gave me hope.

Ilana Sherer, The Washington Post, *August 15, 2011*

Most states protect the persons required to report cases of child abuse. In a few states, certain identified individuals who are not required to report instances of child abuse, but who do so, are protected. Child abuse laws may or may not provide penalties for failure to report. Those in the health care setting who are required to report or cause a report to be made when they have reasonable cause to suspect that a child has been abused include the following: administrators, physicians, interns, registered nurses, chiropractors, social service workers, psychologists, dentists, osteopaths, optometrists, podiatrists, mental health professionals, and volunteers in residential facilities.

DETECTING ABUSE

What constitutes an abused child is difficult to determine because it is often impossible to ascertain whether a child was injured intentionally or accidentally. An individual who reports child abuse should be aware of the physical and behavioral indicators of abuse and maltreatment that appear to be part of a pattern (e.g., bruises, burns, broken bones). In reviewing the indicators of abuse and maltreatment, the reporter does not have to be absolutely certain that abuse or maltreatment exists before reporting. Rather, abuse and maltreatment should be reported whenever they are suspected, based on the existence of the signs of abuse and maltreatment and in light of the reporter's training and experience. Behavioral indicators include, but are not limited to, substantially diminished psychological or intellectual functioning, failure to thrive, no control of aggression, self-destructive impulses, decreased ability to think and reason, acting out and misbehavior, or habitual truancy. Such impairment must be clearly attributable to the unwillingness or inability of the person responsible for the child's care to exercise a minimum degree of care toward the child.

GOOD-FAITH REPORTING

Any report of suspected child abuse must be made with a good-faith belief that the facts reported are true. The definition of good faith as used in a child abuse statute may vary from state to state; however, when a health care practitioner's medical evaluation indicates reasonable cause to believe a child's injuries were not accidental and when the health care practitioner is not acting from his or her desire to harass, injure, or embarrass the child's parents, making the report will not result in liability.

Statutes generally require that when a person covered by a statute is attending a child and suspects child abuse, the staff member must report such concerns. Typical statutes provide that an oral report be made immediately, followed by a written report.

The criminal and civil risks for health care professionals lie not in *good-faith reporting* of suspected incidents of child abuse but in failing to report such incidents. Most states have legislated a variety of civil and criminal penalties for failure to report suspected child abuse incidents. New York, for example, provides:[7]

1. Any person, official, or institution required by this title to report a case of suspected child abuse or maltreatment who willfully fails to do so shall be guilty of a Class A misdemeanor.

2. Any person, official, or institution required by this title to report a case of suspected child abuse or maltreatment who knowingly and willfully fails to do so shall be civilly liable for the damages proximately caused by such failure.

IMMUNITY AND GOOD-FAITH REPORTING

A minor child and his mother brought an action for damages against physicians for failing to diagnose disease and filing erroneous child abuse reports in *Awkerman v. Tri-County Orthopedic Group*.[8] The Wayne County Circuit Court granted the physicians' motions for partial summary judgment, and the plaintiffs appealed. The Michigan Court of Appeals held that the child abuse reporting statute provides immunity to persons who file child abuse reports in good faith even if the reports were filed because of negligent diagnosis of the cause of the child's frequent bone fractures, which was eventually diagnosed as osteogenesis imperfecta. The court of appeals also held that damages for shame and humiliation were not recoverable pursuant to Michigan statute. Immunity from liability did not extend to damages for malpractice that may have resulted from the failure to diagnose the child's disease as long as all the elements of negligence were present.

Child Abuse Can Be Elusive

Child abuse is not always obvious to the caregiver and can unfortunately go undetected to the detriment of the child. I learned this early on in my training. I was a first-year resident at General Medical Center and was on tour in the hospital's pediatric unit with Peggy, the unit charge nurse. As we walked down the corridor I noticed a young child in room 106 in a full leg cast, which had been placed in traction. I asked Peggy what had happened to the patient. Peggy said, "Oh that's Gracie. Poor thing. She broke her femur tripping over a toy in her home." I thought to myself that was a major injury for tripping over a toy. I questioned Peggy further and she told me that she knew where I was leading by my questions and said, "Oh you can be assured that Gracie had not been abused. She has the sweetest mother and father. Although they are divorced one of her parents is here everyday. I even questioned the mother and she assures me it was an accident."

I had an uneasy feeling about the mother's story and decided to visit the radiology department to review Gracie's X-rays with the radiologist on duty. I walked into the imaging reading room where I found three radiologists reviewing various imaging studies. I introduced myself as a first-year resident to Dr. Patrick Williams, the medical director of radiology. I asked Dr. Williams, "Do you have time to review Gracie's X-rays with me." The radiologist replied, "No problem. What is Gracie's last name." I told him and he pulled up Gracie's X-rays electronically on a computer screen. As soon as he pulled up the X-rays he said, "Oh yes, Gracie has a compound fracture of the femur." He was very patient as he thoroughly reviewed with me Gracie's case. He pointed out the compound fracture of the femur with the computer cursor. I asked him, "Do you think the injury could have occurred from Gracie tripping over a toy at home on a plush carpet." He replied, "That would be highly unlikely." He called over one of his partners and said, "Does this patient's injury look like she tripped over a toy." Looking at me he said, "Is this what you were told you?" I said, "Well, yes, I was." He looked at me and said, "I have been reading imaging studies for over 20 years. It is highly unlikely that Gracie's compound fracture of her left femur is the result of her tripping over a toy." The third radiologist in the room commented, "Definitely not caused by a slip on a toy."

Following my review with the radiologists, I called Peggy and asked if she had time to review Gracie's medical record with me after lunch. Peggy replied, "Sure thing, I will see you after lunch."

After lunch I went to the pediatric unit. Upon arriving on the unit Peggy and Caroline, a hospital social service worker, greeted me. Caroline said, "I contacted child welfare in the county in which Gracie resides. They informed me that Gracie was an active child abuse case, which they have been following for the past 6 months. They thanked me for the information and will be in the hospital late this afternoon to follow up."

Discussion

1. Discuss what lessons the caregiver can learn from the resident's observations and persistence in learning more about the cause of Gracie's injury.
2. Assume you are the hospital's director of inservice education, explain what steps you might take to reeducate staff as how to identify and report suspicions of child abuse.

SENIOR ABUSE

People at their weakest are often treated the worst.

—NINA SANTUCCI

Senior abuse is the harmful treatment of older people and includes abandonment; emotional, financial (e.g., theft or misuse of a senior individual's money or property by a person in a position of trust), verbal, mental, sexual, or physical abuse; corporal punishment; and involuntary restraint and seclusion. Neglect is the failure to provide the care necessary to prevent physical harm (e.g., the failure of staff to turn a patient periodically to prevent pressure sores) or mental anguish.

The American Psychological Association estimates that "4 million older Americans are victims of physical, psychological or other forms of abuse and neglect."[9]

Those statistics may not tell the whole story. For every case of elder abuse and neglect reported to authorities, experts estimate as many as 23 cases go undetected. The quality of life of older individuals who experience abuse is severely jeopardized, as they often experience worsened functional and financial status and progressive dependency, poor self-rated health, feelings of helplessness and loneliness and increased psychological distress. Research also suggests that older people who have been abused tend to die earlier than those who have not been abused, even in the absence of chronic conditions or life-threatening disease.[10]

A *USA Today* review of 2 years of inspection records (between 2000 and 2002) for more than 5,300 assisted-living facilities in seven states found that what should be havens for senior persons may in reality be exposing them to deadly risks. The study indicates that medication errors and poor staff training resulted in many of the injuries identified.[11]

The Centers for Medicare & Medicaid Services (CMS) is the federal agency responsible for reviewing the effectiveness of state surveys. CMS evaluates the performance of state surveyors by conducting federal surveys in which federal surveyors resurvey a nursing facility recently inspected by state surveyors. The results of the two surveys are compared as to the deficiencies identified between the two surveys.[12]

Federal comparative surveys can find two types of understatement: (1) missed deficiencies, which can occur when a state surveyor fails to cite a deficiency altogether, or (2) cases where state surveyors cite deficiencies at too low a level. In May 2008, we reported that a substantial proportion of federal comparative surveys conducted from fiscal years 2002 through 2007 identified missed deficiencies that either had the potential to or did result in harm, death, or serious injury to nursing home residents.[13]

There is no shortage of case stories as to the abuse of patients in nursing facilities. Both print and broadcast news are replete with stories of elder abuse. On Long Island nine nursing home employees were charged following investigation of a resident's death. "As CBS 2's Jennifer McLogan reported, of the nine employees charged, seven of them were arrested in connection with the October 2012 death of 72-year-old patient Aurelia Rios. Licensed professional Kethlie Joseph is charged with criminally negligent homicide and *administrator* David Fielding is accused of an alleged cover-up.[14]

On January 10, 2014 in an editorial titled *A Welcome Emphasis On Elder Abuse* the *News Tribune* writes, "Examples of elder abuse in the headlines range from baffling to horrifying: from the lonely old widower conned out of his life savings by a pretty young woman to the invalid grandmother found restrained to her bed, covered in bedsores and filth."[15] There is an endless stream of headlines and news stories as to how widespread and pervasive senior abuse is, as the following examples show:

- The California Attorney General has estimated that 200,000 elderly Californians are abused each year.[16]

- Financial Abuse Cost Elderly Billions[17]
- Like many Americans, Mary Kantorowski has been ordered to leave her home, but it's not a bank telling her to get out—it's her own son.[18]
- Jasmine Kassim, now serving 75 months in prison for bilking five seniors out of more than $1 million dollars.[19]
- Judge Timothy Lamb in addressing two defendants said, "In short, by your offending you have let down your colleagues, you have damaged patient trust and you have undermined the quality of care for the elderly and vulnerable at Whipps Cross (University Hospital)."[20]

REPORTING SENIOR ABUSE

Most states have enacted statutes mandating the reporting of senior abuse. In general, senior abuse is less likely to be reported than child abuse. Physical and emotional neglect, as well as verbal and financial abuse, are perceived as the most prevalent forms of senior abuse. Seniors often fail to report incidents of abuse because they fear retaliation and not being believed. Threats of placement in a nursing home or shame that a family member is involved often prevent senior citizens from seeking help.

Kansas statute 39-1402, for example, requires reporting of abuse, neglect or exploitation of its residents. The statute obligates the following persons to report elder abuse.

> (a) Any person who is licensed to practice any branch of the healing arts, a licensed psychologist, a licensed master level psychologist, a licensed clinical psychotherapist, a chief administrative officer of a medical care facility, an adult care home administrator or operator, a licensed social worker, a licensed professional nurse, a licensed practical nurse, a licensed marriage and family therapist, a licensed clinical marriage and family therapist, licensed professional counselor, licensed clinical professional counselor, registered alcohol and drug abuse counselor, a teacher, a bank trust officer and any other officers of financial institutions, a legal representative or a governmental assistance provider who has reasonable cause to believe that a resident is being or has been abused, neglected or exploited, or is in a condition which is the result of such abuse, neglect or exploitation or is in need of protective services, shall report immediately such information or cause a report of such information to be made in any reasonable manner to the department on aging . . .[21]

Kansas Governor Sam Brownback signed into law H.B. 2504 that imposes strict penalties against those who commit elder abuse. "Attorney General Derek Schmidt says elderly residents will have new protections against fraud and financial abuse under a new state law . . . The law is aimed at protecting people 70 and older who are victims of financial abuse. People convicted of large-scale abuse could be sentenced to more than 40 years in prison."[22]

Signs of Abuse

Hidden Camera

Gale . . . wasn't prepared for the rough treatment and cruel taunts she says her ailing mother suffered at the nursing home. She cried as a nurse's aide chastised her mother for failing to straighten her arthritic-stricken legs. And she watched in disbelief as an assistant jerked her mother off her rubber bed pad and pushed her into the bed's metal rails. All of these images were caught . . . by a "granny cam"—a camera hidden in her mother's room.

Deborah Sharp, USA Today, *September 14, 1999*

Signs of senior abuse or neglect of a senior include the following:

- Physical Abuse
  - bruises, black eyes, welts, lacerations, and rope marks;
  - bone fractures, broken bones, and skull fractures;
  - open wounds, cuts, punctures, untreated injuries in various stages of healing;
  - sprains, dislocations, and internal injuries/bleeding;
  - broken eyeglasses/frames, physical signs of being subjected to punishment, and signs of being restrained;
  - laboratory findings of medication overdose or under utilization of prescribed drugs;
  - an elder's report of being hit, slapped, kicked, or mistreated;
  - an elder's sudden change in behavior; and
  - the caregiver's refusal to allow visitors to see an elder alone.
- Sexual Abuse
  - bruises around the breasts or genital area;
  - unexplained venereal disease or genital infections;
  - unexplained vaginal or anal bleeding;
  - torn, stained, or bloody underclothing; and
  - elder's report of being sexually assaulted or raped.
- Emotional or Psychological Abuse
  - being emotionally upset or agitated;
  - being extremely withdrawn and noncommunicative or nonresponsive;
  - unusual behavior usually attributed to dementia (e.g., sucking, biting, rocking); and
  - an elder's report of being verbally or emotionally mistreated.
- Neglect
  - dehydration, malnutrition, untreated bed sores, and poor personal hygiene;
  - unattended or untreated health problems;
  - hazardous or unsafe living condition/arrangements (e.g., improper wiring, no heat, or no running water);
  - unsanitary and unclean living conditions (e.g., dirt, fleas, lice on person, soiled bedding, fecal/urine smell, inadequate clothing); and
  - an elder's report of being mistreated.

- Abandonment
  - the desertion of an elder at a hospital, a nursing facility, or other similar institution;
  - the desertion of an elder at a shopping center or other public location; and
  - an elder's own report of being abandoned.
- Financial or Material Exploitation
  - sudden changes in bank account or banking practice, including an unexplained withdrawal of large sums of money by a person accompanying the elder;
  - the inclusion of additional names on an elder's bank signature card;
  - unauthorized withdrawal of the elder's funds using the elder's ATM card;
  - abrupt changes in a will or other financial documents;
  - unexplained disappearance of funds or valuable possessions;
  - substandard care being provided or bills unpaid despite the availability of adequate financial resources;
  - discovery of an elder's signature being forged for financial transactions or for the titles of his/her possessions;
  - sudden appearance of previously uninvolved relatives claiming their rights to an elder's affairs and possessions;
  - unexplained sudden transfer of assets to a family member or someone outside the family;
  - the provision of services that are not necessary; and
  - an elder's report of financial exploitation.
- Self-Neglect
  - dehydration, malnutrition, untreated or improperly attended medical conditions, and poor personal hygiene;
  - hazardous or unsafe living conditions/arrangements (e.g., improper wiring, no indoor plumbing, no heat, no running water);
  - unsanitary or unclean living quarters (e.g., animal/insect infestation, no functioning toilet, fecal/urine smell);
  - inappropriate and/or inadequate clothing, lack of the necessary medical aids (e.g., eyeglasses, hearing aids, dentures); and
  - grossly inadequate housing or homelessness.[23]

DOCUMENTATION

Caregivers who suspect abuse are expected to report their findings. Symptoms and conditions of suspected abuse should be defined clearly and objectively. The abuse of senior individuals is not a localized or isolated problem. Unfortunately, it permeates our society. *Behind Closed Doors,* a landmark book on family violence, stated that the first national study of violence in American homes estimated that one in two homes was the scene of family violence at least once a year.[24]

> We have always known that America is a violent society. . . . What is new and surprising is that the American family and the American home are perhaps as much or more violent than any other single institution or setting (with the exception of the military, and only then in the time of war). Americans run the greatest risk of assault, physical injury and even murder in their own homes by members of their own families.[25]

It is difficult to determine the extent of senior abuse because the abused are reluctant to admit that their children or loved ones have assaulted them. Unfortunately, the abuse of senior persons remains hidden from the public, and the findings of the 1990 report are as current today as when they were first published in 1990 when the Senate Select Committee on Aging reported the following:[26]

- Senior abuse is less likely to be reported than child abuse.
- Physical violence, including negligence, and financial abuse appear to be the most common forms of abuse, followed by abrogation of basic constitutional rights and psychological abuse.
- Most instances of senior abuse are recurring events rather than one-time occurrences.
- Victims are often 75 years of age or senior, and women are more likely to be abused than men.
- Senior people are often ashamed to admit that their children or loved ones abuse them, or they may fear reprisals if they complain.
- Many middle-aged family members, finally ready to enjoy time to themselves, are resentful of a frail and dependent senior parent.
- Finally, the majority of the abusers are relatives.

The plaintiffs in *In re Estate of Smith v. O'Halloran*[27] instituted a lawsuit in an effort to improve deplorable conditions in many nursing homes. The court concluded that:[28]

> The evidentiary record . . . supports a general finding that all is not well in the nation's nursing homes and that the enormous expenditures of public funds and the earnest efforts of public officials and public employees have not produced an equivalent return in benefits. That failure of expectations has produced frustration and anger among those who are aware of the realities of life in some nursing homes, which provide so little service that they could be characterized as orphanages for the aged.

Surveyors of health care organizations should look for signs of patient abuse by watching for the following:

- Physician's order for restraints
- Time-limited orders
- The number of patients that are physically restrained
- The types of restraints being used
- Whether or not the restraints are applied correctly
- How often restrained patients are observed by the staff
- Signs of overmedication
- Signs of mental and physical abuse of patients
- Signs of harassment, humiliation, or threats from staff or patients
- Whether patients are comfortable with the staff
- The numbers of patients with bruises or other injuries
- Evidence of patient neglect or patients left in urine or feces without cleaning

CASE: WANTON NEGLECT OF RESIDENTS

The defendant in *State v. Cunningham,*[29] the owner and administrator of a residential care facility, housed 30 to 37 mentally ill, mentally retarded, and senior residents. The Iowa Department of Inspections and Appeals conducted various surveys at the defendant's facility between October 1989 and May 1990. All of the surveys except for one resulted in a $50 daily fine assessed against the defendant for violations of the regulations.

On August 16, 1990, a grand jury filed an indictment charging the defendant with several counts of wanton neglect of a resident in violation of Iowa Code section 726.7 (1989), which provides, "A person commits wanton neglect of a resident of a health care facility when the person knowingly acts in a manner likely to be injurious to the physical, mental, or moral welfare of a resident of a health care facility. . . . Wanton neglect of a resident of a health care facility is a serious misdemeanor."

The district court held that the defendant had knowledge of the dangerous conditions that existed in the health care facility but willfully and consciously refused to provide or to exercise adequate supervision to remedy or attempt to remedy the dangerous conditions. The residents were exposed to physical dangers and unhealthy and unsanitary physical conditions and were grossly deprived of much-needed medical care and personal attention. The conditions were likely to and did cause injury to the physical and mental well-being of the facility's residents. The defendant was found guilty on five counts of wanton neglect. The district court sentenced the defendant to 1 year in jail for each of the five counts, to run concurrently. The district court suspended all but 2 days of the defendant's sentence and ordered him to pay $200 for each count, plus a surcharge and costs, and to perform community service. A motion for a new trial was denied, and the defendant appealed.

The Iowa Court of Appeals held that there was substantial evidence to support a finding that the defendant was responsible for not properly maintaining the nursing facility, which led to prosecution for wanton neglect of the facility's residents. The defendant was found guilty of knowingly acting in a manner likely to be injurious to the physical or mental welfare of the facility's residents by creating, directing, or maintaining hazardous conditions and unsafe practices; fire hazards and circumstances impeded safety from fire. The facility was not properly maintained (e.g., findings included broken glass in patients' rooms, excessive hot water in faucets, dried feces on public bathroom walls and grab bars, insufficient towels and linens, cockroaches and worms in the food preparation area, no soap available in the kitchen, at one point only one bar of soap and one container of shampoo found in the entire facility). Dietary facilities were unsanitary and inadequate to meet the dietary needs of the residents. There were inadequate staffing patterns and supervision in the facility, and improper dosages of medications were administered to the residents.[30]

The defendant argued that he did not "create" the unsafe conditions at the facility. The court of appeals disagreed. The statute does not require that the defendant create the conditions at the facility to sustain a conviction. The defendant was the administrator of the facility and responsible for the conditions that existed.

Ethical and Legal Issues

1. Do you agree with the court's finding? Discuss your answer.
2. Discuss how both ethics and the law are intertwined in this case.

CASE: ABUSE OF RESIDENTS

The operator of a nursing facility appealed an order by the Department of Public Welfare revoking his license because of resident abuse in *Nepa v. Commonwealth Department of Public Welfare.*[31] Substantial evidence supported the department's finding. Three former employees testified that the nursing facility operator had abused residents in the following incidents:[32]

He unbuckled the belt of one of the residents, causing his pants to drop, and then grabbed a second resident, forcing them to kiss. (Petitioner's excuse for this behavior was to shame the resident because of his masturbating in public.)

On two occasions he forced a resident to remove toilet paper from a commode after she had urinated and defecated in it. (Denying that there was fecal matter in the commode, the petitioner made the excuse that this would stop the resident from filling the commode with toilet paper.)

He verbally abused a resident who was experiencing difficulty in breathing and accused him of faking as he attempted to feed him liquids.

The nursing facility operator claimed that the findings of fact were not based on substantial evidence and that even if they were the incidents did not amount to abuse under the code. The defendant attempted to discredit the witnesses with allegations from a resident and another employee that one of his former employees got into bed with a resident and that another had taken a picture of a male resident while in the shower and had placed a baby bottle and a humiliating sign around the neck of another resident. The court was not impressed. Although these incidents, if true, were reprehensible, they were collateral matters that had no bearing on the witnesses' reputation for truthfulness and therefore could not be used for impeachment purposes. The court held that there was substantial evidence supporting the department's decision and that the activities committed by the operator were sufficient to support revocation of his license:[33]

> We believe Petitioner's treatment of these residents as found by the hearing examiner to be truly disturbing. These residents were elderly and/or mentally incapacitated and wholly dependent on Petitioner while residing in his home. As residents, they are entitled to maintain their dignity and be cared for with respect, concern, and compassion.
>
> Petitioner testified that he did not have adequate training to deal with the patients he received who suffered from mental problems. Petitioner's lack of training in this area is absolutely no excuse for the reprehensible manner in which he treated various residents. Accordingly, DPW's order revoking Petitioner's license to operate a personal care home is affirmed.

Ethical and Legal Issues

1. Do the facts of this case support the court's finding? Discuss your answer.
2. Discuss why senior citizens are often reluctant to report abuse.

CASE: ABUSIVE SEARCH

A nurse in *People v. Coe*[34] was charged with a willful violation of the public health law in connection with an allegedly abusive search of an 86-year-old resident at a geriatric center and with the falsification of business records in the first degree. The resident, Mr. Gersh, had heart disease and difficulty in expressing himself verbally. Another resident claimed that two $5 bills were missing. Nurse Coe assumed that Gersh had taken them because he had been known to take things in the past. The nurse proceeded to search Gersh, who resisted. A security guard was summoned, and another search was undertaken. When Gersh again resisted, the security guard slammed a chair down in front of him and pinned his arms while the defendant nurse searched his pockets, failing to retrieve the two $5 bills. Five minutes later, Gersh collapsed in a chair gasping for air. Coe administered cardiopulmonary resuscitation but was unsuccessful, and Gersh died.

Coe was charged with violation of the New York Penal Law for falsifying records because of the defendant's "omission" of the facts relating to the search of Gersh. These facts were considered relevant and should have been included in the nurse's notes regarding this incident. "The first sentence states, 'Observed resident was extremely confused and talks incoherently. Suddenly became unresponsive . . .' This statement is simply false. It could only be true if some reference to the search and the loud noise was included."[35] A motion was made to dismiss the indictment at the end of the trial.

The court held that the search became an act of physical abuse and mistreatment, that the evidence was sufficient to warrant a finding of guilt on both charges, and that the fact that searches took place frequently did not excuse an otherwise illegal procedure:[36]

> It may well be that this incident reached the attention of the criminal justice system only because, in the end, a man had died. In those instances which are equally violative of residents' rights and equally contrary to standards of common decency but which do not result in visible harm to a patient, the acts are nevertheless illegal and subject to prosecution. A criminal act is not legitimized by the fact that others have, with impunity, engaged in that act.

Ethical and Legal Issues

1. With the number of senior abuse cases occurring so frequently, discuss why society waits for extreme violence to occur before preventative actions are taken.
2. Having studied ethics and the moral breakdown that appears to have occurred in society, what steps do you believe can be taken to reverse the trend of violence faced by our seniors?

CASE: FORCIBLE ADMINISTRATION OF MEDICATIONS

The medical employee in *In re Axelrod*[37] sought review of a determination by the commissioner of health that she was guilty of resident abuse. Evidence showed that the employee, after a resident refused medication, "held the patient's chin and poured the medication down her throat."[38] There was no indication or convincing evidence that an emergency existed that would have required the forced administration of the medication. The court held that substantial evidence supported the commissioner's finding that the employee had been guilty of resident abuse.

Ethical and Legal Issues

1. Discuss the ethical and legal ramifications of this case.
2. What sentence should the employee receive? Why?
3. What message should the court be sending to other potential abusers of patients?

INTIMIDATION OF ABUSIVE RESIDENT/DISCIPLINARY OVERKILL

A difficult and abusive 80-year-old resident of a veteran's home in *Beasley v. State Personnel Board*[39] slapped the face of an aide who was assisting him. The resident, referring to his inability to have sex, said that he might as well have his penis cut off. The aide, Beasley, stated that she said to the resident if he did not behave, then she might accommodate him. A nursing supervisor who passed by at that moment noted that a nursing assistant and a hospital aide who were standing nearby laughed and did nothing to intervene. Beasley was fired and the other two employees were suspended for 10 days. After the state board upheld the punishments, the three employees went by mandate to the superior court, where Beasley's dismissal was ruled too severe. The trial court found that action against the nursing assistant and hospital aide, although harsh, was within discretion.

On appeal, the court held that Beasley's comments did not constitute misconduct, and the veterans' home nursing assistant and hospital aide did not commit actionable conduct by "sort of laughing." When this incident was viewed in its context and in light of the whole record, it did not support the state personnel board's finding that Beasley's attitude toward patients was poor.

CASE: DEFICIENT CARE

In *Montgomery Health Care Facility v. Ballard*,[40] three nurses testified that the facility was understaffed. "One nurse testified that she asked her supervisor for more help but that she did not get it."[41] A nursing home resident, Mrs. Stovall, expired as the result of multiple infected bedsores. The estate of the patient brought a malpractice action against the nursing home. First American Health Care, Inc., is the parent corporation of the Montgomery Health Care Facility, a nursing home. The trial court entered a judgment on a jury verdict against the home, and an appeal was taken. The Alabama Supreme Court held that reports compiled by the Alabama Department of Public Health concerning deficiencies found in the nursing home were admissible as evidence. Evidence showed that the care given to the deceased was deficient in the same ways as noted in the survey and complaint reports, which indicated that deficiencies in the home included:[42]

> Inadequate documentation of treatment given for decubitus ulcers; 23 patients found with decubitus ulcers, 10 of whom developed those ulcers in the facility; dressings on the sores were not changed as ordered; nursing progress notes did not describe

patients' ongoing conditions, particularly with respect to descriptions of decubitus ulcers; ineffective policies and procedures with respect to sterile dressing supplies; lack of nursing assessments; incomplete patient care plans; inadequate documentation of doctor's visits, orders, or progress notes; am care not consistently documented; inadequate documentation of turning of patients; incomplete "activities of daily living" sheets; "range of motion" exercises not documented; patients found wet and soiled with dried fecal matter; lack of bowel and bladder retaining programs; [and] incomplete documentation of ordered force fluids.

From a corporate standpoint, the parent corporation of the nursing facility could be held liable for the nursing facility's negligence, where the parent company controlled or retained the right to control the day-to-day operations of the home. The defendants had argued that the punitive damage award of $2 million against the home was greater than what was necessary to meet society's goal of punishing them. The Alabama Supreme Court, however, found the award not to be excessive. "The trial court also found that because of the large number of nursing home residents vulnerable to the type of neglect found in Mrs. Stovall's case, the verdict would further the goal of discouraging others from similar conduct in the future."[43]

Ethical and Legal Issues

1. Could any legislation be enacted or policies, procedures, rules, and regulations be implemented as proactive measures to prevent this type of widespread abuse? Describe your answer.
2. Do you agree with the court that the award will discourage others from similar behavior? Explain.

LOOK CLOSER, SEE ME

Donna Fannin read the poem "Look Closer, See ME" to every nursing assistant class she ever taught. This wonderful poem was found among the meager belongings of an 89-year-old nursing home patient in Scotland following her death. It has been widely published since then. It is a reminder to us all that our bodies and relationships continue to change, and someday many of us will experience what she has felt.[44]

Look Closer, See ME

What do you see, Nurses?/ What do you see?/ What are you thinking?/ When you're looking at me?

A crabbit old woman,/ Not very wise,/ Uncertain of habit/ With faraway eyes? Who dribbles her food/ And makes no reply/ When you say in a loud voice,/ "I do wish you'd try!"

Who seems not to notice/ The things that you do,/ And forever is losing/

A stocking or shoe? Who, resisting or not,/ Lets you do as you will,/ With bathing and feeding,/The long day to fill.

Is that what you're thinking?/ Is that what you see?/ Then open your eyes, Nurse,/ You're not looking at ME. I'll tell you who I am/ As I sit here so still/ As I do at your bidding/ As I eat at your will.

I'm a small child of ten,/ With a Mother and Father,/ Brothers and sisters/ Who love one another. A young girl of sixteen,/ With wings on her feet,/ Dreaming that soon,/ A lover she'll meet.

A bride soon at twenty,/ My heart gives a leap./ Remembering the vows/ We have promised to keep. At twenty-five now,/ I have young of my own,/ Who need me to guide them,/And a secure happy home.

A woman of thirty/ My young they grow fast,/ Bound to each other/ With ties that should last. At forty, my young sons/ Have grown and have gone,/ But my man's beside me/To see I don't mourn.

At fifty, once more/ Babies play round my knee,/ Again we know children,/ My husband and me. Dark days are upon me,/ My husband is dead./ I look to the future/ And shudder with dread.

For my young are all rearing/ Young of their own,/ And I think of the years/And the love I have known.

I'm an old woman now,/ And nature is cruel,/ 'Tis her jest to make old age/ Look like a fool. The body, it crumbles,/ Grace and vigor depart/ There is now a stone,/ Where I once had a heart.

But inside this old carcass,/ A young girl still dwells,/ And now and again,/ My battered heart swells. I remember the joys,/ I remember the pain,/ And I'm living and loving/ All over again.

I think of the years,/ All too few, gone too fast,/ And accept the stark fact/ That nothing can last. So, open your eyes, people,/ Open and see,/ Not a crabbit old woman,/ Look closer, See ME.

CHAPTER REVIEW

1. Patient Abuse
   - Mistreatment or neglect of individuals who are under the care of a health care organization.
   - Abuse is not limited to an institutional setting and may occur in an individual's home as well as in an institution.
   - Signs of abuse include:
     ○ Physical (e.g., sexual), psychological, medical, financial
     ○ Difficult to identify because injuries can be attributed to other causes
2. Child Abuse
   - Defined as a child under the age of 18 one who has suffered intentional serious mental, emotional, sexual, and/or physical injury inflicted by a parent or other person responsible for the child's care.

- Reporting child abuse.
  - All states have enacted various child abuse statutes to provide civil immunity for those making or participating in good-faith reports of suspected child abuse.
- Detecting child abuse.
  - Individual who report child abuse should be aware of the physical and behavioral indicators of abuse and maltreatment that appear to be part of a pattern (e.g., bruises, burns, broken bones).
  - Caregivers must report the suspicion of child abuse with good faith motives.
  - Caregivers are immune from liability for good faith reporting.

3. Senior Abuse
   - Seniors often fail to report incidents of abuse because they fear retaliation and not being believed.
   - Most states have enacted statutes mandating the reporting of senior abuse.
   - Signs of Elder Abuse:
     - Unexplained or unexpected death; broken bones; sudden and unexpected emotional outbursts, agitation, or withdrawal; bruises, welts, discoloration, or burns; absence of hair; dehydration and malnourishment without an illness-related cause; hesitation to talk openly; implausible stories; and unusual or inappropriate bank account activity.
   - Reporting elder abuse
     - Caregivers who suspect abuse are expected to report their findings. Symptoms and conditions of suspected abuse should be defined clearly and objectively.
     - Signs of abuse should be accurately and thoroughly documented.
   - Senior abuse is less likely to be reported than child abuse.
   - Cases of elder abuse include:
     - Neglect
     - Physical abuse
     - Abusive search
     - Forcible administration of medications
     - Intimidation
     - Deficient care

4. *Look Closer, See ME*
   - A poem close to many hearts and interpreted "don't see through the patient, see the patient you are treating."

TEST YOUR UNDERSTANDING

TERMINOLOGY

child abuse crime	patient abuse
good faith reporting	senior abuse

REVIEW QUESTIONS

1. What is patient abuse?

2. Discuss common signs of abuse for both children and seniors.

3. Describe what should a caregiver do when he or she suspects another unrelated person, caregiver or family member has been abusing a patient.

4. Discuss the importance of accurate and complete documentation of suspected abuse.

5. Describe what good-faith reporting means.

6. Discuss why patients are often reluctant to complain about their abusers and caregivers.

7. When a health care provider reports abuse, should the accuser's identity be revealed to the accused? Explain your answer.

8. Should caregivers be disciplined for reporting abuse if it proves to be false? Explain your answer.

9. Discuss the patient poem "Look Closer, See Me."

NOTES

1. Title 42 U.S. Code, Chapter 67 § 5119c (3).
2. http://www.acf.hhs.gov/sites/default/files/cb/cm2012.pdf
3. http://www.acf.hhs.gov/sites/default/files/cb/cm2012.pdf#page=11.
4. Title 42 U.S. Code, Chapter 67, Subchapter VI § 5119 (a).
5. N.Y. Soc. Serv. Law A4 419 (McKinney 1992).
6. N.Y. Soc. Serv. Law A4 420 (McKinney 1992).
7. N.Y. Soc. Serv. Law A4 420 (McKinney 1992).
8. 373 N.W.2d 204 (Mich. Ct. App. 1985).
9. http://www.apa.org/pi/aging/resources/guides/elder-abuse.aspx.
10. *Id.*
11. "Havens for elderly may expose them to deadly risks," *USA Today*, May 25, 2004, at 1.
12. http://www.gao.gov/new.items/d10434r.pdf.
13. *Id.*
14. *CBS New York/AP, February 11, 2014.* http://newyork.cbslocal.com/2014/02/11/9-arrested-in-l-i-nursing-home-probe-following-patients-death/.
15. http://www.thenewstribune.com/2014/01/10/2986582/a-welcome-emphasis-on-elder-abuse.html
16. Arthur Meirson, Prosecuting Elder Abuse: Setting the Gold Standard in the Golden State, 60 HASTINGS L.J. 431, 434 (2008).

17. http://www.nbcnews.com/id/41992299/ns/business-consumer_news/t/financial-abuse-costs-elderly-billions/#.U1eogcYgvG4.

18. http://www.newser.com/tag/18247/1/elder-abuse.html.

19. http://www.lawyersandsettlements.com/articles/financial-elder-abuse/interview-financial-elder-abuse-19203.html#.U1fuLcYgvG4.

20. *Suzannah Hills*, MailOnline, *August 23, 2013*. http://www.dailymail.co.uk/news/article-2400887/Jailed-Whipps-Cross-Hospital-carers-physically-verbally-abused-patients.html.

21. http://kansasstatutes.lesterama.org/Chapter_39/Article_14/.

22. *Greg Palmer*, WIBW.com, *April 22, 2014. The Associated Press*, The Kansas City Star, *April 22*. http://www.wibw.com/home/headlines/Kansas-Elder-Abuse-Measure-Becomes-Law-256157141.html.

23. http://ncea.aoa.gov/FAQ/Type_Abuse/#abandonment.

24. Richard J. Gelles, Murray A. Strauss, & Suzanne K. Steinmetz, *Behind Closed Doors: Violence in the American Family,* Anchor Press/Doubleday: Garden City, NY (1980).

25. *Id.*

26. Senate Subcommittee on Health and Long-Term Care, supra note 53.

27. 557 F. Supp. 289 (D. Colo. 1983).

28. *Id.* at 293.

29. *State v. Cunningham,* 493 N.W.2d 884 (Iowa Ct. App. 1992).

30. *Id.* at 887–888.

31. 551 A.2d 354 (Pa. Commw. Ct. 1988).

32. *Id.* at 355.

33. *Id.* at 357.

34. 501 N.Y.S.2d 997 (N.Y. Sup. Ct. 1986).

35. *Id.* at 1001.

36. *Id.*

37. 560 N.Y.S.2d 573 (N.Y. App. Div. 1990).

38. *Id.*

39. 178 Cal. Rptr. 564 (Cal. Ct. App. 1981).

40. 565 So. 2d 221, 224 (Ala. 1990).

41. *Id.* at 224.

42. *Id.* at 223–224.

43. *Id.* at 226.

44. Donna Fannin, "Your Granny's Nurses: Look Closer, See ME," Gather.com, May 16, 2006; http://www.gather.com/viewArticle.action?articleId=281474976752728.

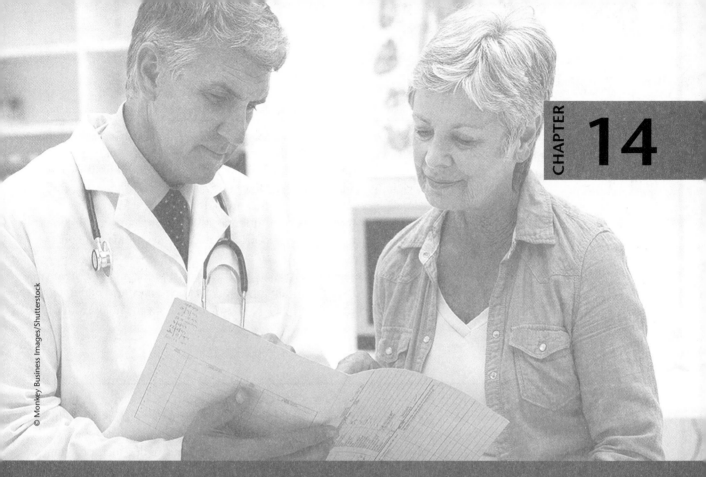

© Monkey Business Images/Shutterstock

PATIENT RIGHTS AND RESPONSIBILITIES

Freedom makes a huge requirement of every human being. With freedom comes responsibility.

–ELEANOR ROOSEVELT

LEARNING OBJECTIVES

Upon completion of this chapter, the reader will be able to:

- Describe and understand patient rights
- Describe and understand patient responsibilities
- Explain how rights and responsibilities are tethered together and are not mutually exclusive but equally important

INTRODUCTION

This chapter provides an overview of the rights and responsibilities of patients. Every person possesses certain rights guaranteed by the Constitution and its amendments, including freedom of speech, religion, and the right not to be discriminated against on the basis of race, creed, color, or national origin. In addition, citizens have a variety of rights and responsibilities as provided for in federal, state, and local laws that are not in conflict with the Constitution. The Supreme Court has interpreted the Constitution as also guaranteeing certain other rights not expressly mentioned, such as the right to privacy and self-determination and the right to accept or reject medical treatment.

A professional relationship between the physician and the patient is essential for the provision of proper medical care. Both staff and patients should be aware of and understand not only their own rights and responsibilities but also the rights and responsibilities of one another.

PATIENT RIGHTS

Patients of the various states have certain rights and protections guaranteed by state and federal laws and regulations. Patients have a right to receive a clear explanation of tests, diagnoses, prescribed medications, prognosis, and treatment options.[1] Most federal, state, and local programs specifically require, as a condition for receiving funds under such programs, an affirmative statement on the part of the organization that it will not discriminate. For example, the Medicare and Medicaid programs specifically require affirmative assurances by health care organizations prohibiting discrimination.

The continuing trend of consumer awareness, coupled with increased governmental regulations, makes it advisable for caregivers to understand the scope of patient rights. The Patient Self-Determination Act of 1990 (PSDA)[2] describes the rights of patients to make their own health care decisions. Health care organizations may no longer passively permit patients to exercise their rights but must educate patients as to their rights. The PSDA provides that each individual has a right under state law (whether statutory or as recognized by the courts of the state) to make decisions concerning his or her medical care, including the right to accept or refuse medical or surgical treatment and the right to formulate advance directives.

Patient rights may be classified as either legal, those emanating from law, or human statements of desirable ethical principles such as the right to be treated with dignity and respect. The rights of patients discussed here do not exist in a vacuum without limitations. They are tethered to moral obligations and responsibilities that have their roots in the law, ethics, moral principles, and religious values. To kill another human being, for example, is wrong and punishment will follow if the life of another is taken.

RIGHT TO KNOW ONE'S RIGHTS

Patients have a right at the time of admission to be provided in writing a copy of his or her rights and responsibilities. The patient's rights and responsibilities are documented in a statement most often referred to as *The Patient's Bill of Rights*. Access to a copy of a patient rights and responsibilities should be available to the general public when so requested. A limited random sample of three hospitals in two states revealed that staff members were often reluctant and suspicious as to why a copy of the patient's bill of rights was being requested. All three hospitals would not provide a copy on site. One hospital after a second visit reluctantly provided a copy via e-mail.

Health Insurance Portability and Accountability Act

Patients have a right to receive a "Notice of Privacy Standards," a requirement under the *Health Insurance Portability and Accountability Act* (45 CFR 164.520).

> The HIPAA Privacy Rule gives individuals a fundamental new right to be informed of the privacy practices of their health plans and of most of their health care providers, as well as to be informed of their privacy rights with respect to their personal health information. Health plans and covered health care providers are required to develop and distribute a notice that provides a clear explanation of these rights and practices. The notice is intended to focus individuals on privacy issues and concerns, and to prompt them to have discussions with their health plans and health care providers and exercise their rights.[3]

The issues of confidentiality and privacy have both ethical and legal implications. Caregivers must safeguard each patient's right to privacy and the right to have information pertaining to his or her care kept confidential.

Disclosures Permitted

Patient information (e.g., diagnoses, anesthesia history, surgical and other invasive procedures, drug allergies, medication usage, lab test results, and imaging studies) may be disclosed to other providers who may be caring for the patient to provide safe health care treatment. The following list describes some of the ways a health care provider may disclose medical information about a patient without his or her written consent.

- Disclosure of information to third-party payers so the providers of care bill for services rendered
- Disclosure of information necessary to render care and treatment
- Disclosure of information as may be required by a law enforcement agency
- Disclosure of information as may be required to avert a serious threat to public health or safety
- Disclosure of information as required by military command authorities for their medical records
- Disclosure of information to worker's compensation or similar programs for processing of claims
- Disclosure of information in response to a subpoena for a legal proceeding
- Disclosure of information to a coroner or medical examiner for purposes of identification

Limitations on Disclosures

Some of the individual rights a patient has regarding disclosure of access to his or her medical information are as follows:

- Right to request restrictions or limitations regarding information used or disclosed about one's treatment.
- Right to an accounting of nonstandard disclosures: The patient has a right to request a list of the disclosures made of information released regarding his or her care.
- Right to amend: If a patient believes that medical information regarding his or her care is incorrect or incomplete, he or she has a right to request that the information be corrected.
- Right to inspect and copy medical information that may be used to make decisions about one's care.
- Right to file a complaint with the provider, or the Secretary of the Department of Health and Human Services in Washington, DC, if a patient believes his or her privacy rights have been violated.
- Right to a paper copy of a notice pertaining to patients.
- Right to know of restrictions on rights. Any restrictions on a patient's visitors, mail, telephone, or other communications must be evaluated for their therapeutic effectiveness and fully explained to and agreed upon by the patient or patient representative.

Explanation of One's Rights

Patients have a right to receive an explanation of their rights and responsibilities. The rights of patients must be respected at all times. Each patient is an individual with unique health care needs. The patient has a right to make decisions regarding his or her medical care, including the decision to discontinue treatment, to the extent permitted by law.

RIGHT TO ASK QUESTIONS

The patient has a right to ask questions and caregivers have a responsibility to listen. Caregivers must not become dismissive or trivialize the importance of a patient's opinion as to the cause of his or her medical complaints and ailments. Although a patient may be anxious, the questions asked should not be disregarded.

Attributed to Socrates, the classical Greek philosopher, is the *socratic method of teaching and learning* by asking and answering questions. Patients have the right ask questions regarding their care from entry to the hospital through the time of departure. Questions regarding care should include, for example, "I saw blood in my IV tubing. Is this okay? Is it infiltrating?" or "My wound dressing seems wet. Is this okay? Should the dressing be changed?" Patients should not hesitate to ask for:

- clarification of a caregiver's instructions
- interpretation of a caregiver's handwriting
- instructions for medication usage (e.g., frequency, dosing, drug–drug or drug–food interactions, contraindications, side effects)

- clarification of a physician's diet orders
- explanation of treatment plan
- a copy of the organization's handwashing policy
- a description of the hospital's procedures to prevent wrong-site surgery
- consultations and second opinions
- accurate and complete discharge instructions
- verification that their advance directives are on file (e.g., living will)
- confirmation that contact information for the patient's surrogate decision maker is on file in the event the patient becomes incapacitated and cannot make health care decisions

This listing is but a sampling of the many questions that patients have a right to ask during the course of their care in any health care setting.

As the information regarding patient care increases at an alarming rate, the more important it is for the patient to become more informed by asking questions. Dr. Ranit Mishori explains in *Don't Let a Hospital Make You Sick*, "The problem is not that we have an epidemic of negligent doctors. Rather, it's that the health-care system has grown so complicated that there is a greater chance than ever of things falling through the cracks. Another problem is that hospitals produce massive amounts of data, including lab and X-ray reports, medication lists, doctors' orders, and dietary restrictions. It is easier than ever for critical communications to get lost, and hospitals often don't have thorough backup systems."[4]

Sandra G. Boudman, a reporter for the Washington Post writes in an article *Bonded by Blood*, "Doctors talk to doctors happily," she said, "it's sometimes hard to get them to listen to patients." She hoped that such a conversation might lead to an answer that could help spring her from the hospital or at least enable doctors to investigate—or to rule out—a potential disease and get to the bottom of her medical problem.[5]

Accreditation Standards and Patient Right to Ask Questions

Hillary was the lead consultant assigned to speak at a state-sponsored conference. The purpose of the conference was to review new accreditation standards designed to encourage patients to ask questions about their care. They were scheduled to be effective on January 1. Hillary scheduled four consultants to speak with her on a variety of topics. Rebecca, one of the more junior of the consultants, addressed the right of patients to ask questions. She spoke about the newly designed program that would require health care providers to encourage patients to *speak up and ask questions* about any concerns they may have regarding their care. Following her presentation, Rebecca asked for questions from the audience. One participant said, "I really don't understand the need for this standard. Patients don't seem to have a problem complaining." Rebecca began to flounder as she attempted to continue answering the questions of what was to be a generally disgruntled person. Hillary listened intently but said nothing.

Jerome, a more experienced consultant, raised his hand. After being recognized by Rebecca, he responded, "Many patients are not afraid to ask questions and complain when they believe things are not going right. These often are ambulatory patients who can leave a particular provider if they become dissatisfied. Other, more seriously ill inpatients may fear some sort of retaliation if they complain. This is often the case in long-term care facilities." A caregiver in the audience strongly disagreed. Jerome said, "I realize this is not the case with all patients. This fear can often arise, however, with an elderly person or extremely ill individual who is too weak and feels vulnerable and fearful of offending the caregiver, believing that his or her care could be less than desirable if he or she asks too many questions or complains. Seniors have sometimes been abused at home or under the care of third parties and are often not willing to risk confrontation."

Figuring a picture is worth 1,000 words, Jerome had asked for an overhead projector and proceeded to show some newspaper clippings illustrating why some patients have developed a fear to ask questions. After the session was over, the audience member who had raised the issue approached Jerome and said, "Not all caregivers are like the ones you displayed!" Jerome said, "I agree. I tried to illustrate for you why some patients are fearful." Jerome thought to himself that this caregiver was too combative to continue the discussion.

Discussion

1. Do you agree with Jerome's attempt to help Rebecca by responding to the concern of the contentious caregiver?
2. What approach would you have taken in responding to a persistent quarrelsome caregiver? Explain your answer.

My Question Disregarded

As I was lying on a minor surgery table waiting for my physician to arrive in the treatment room I noticed a Joint Commission sign lying sideways in the corner of the room on a countertop. The title on the sign read "Speak Up." Although it was lying behind several other documents and pieces of medical equipment, I recognized the title on the sign. Its purpose is to encourage patients to ask questions they have about their care. The sign is also a reminder to the physician to ask patients if they have any questions about their care.

As I was thinking about the difficulty in reading the sign, a physician came into the room with a woman in a white uniform. I didn't recognize her nor did I recognize him, as it was a group practice. There were no introductions, I felt like I was just part of an assembly line. The physician sat on a swivel chair directly behind me and said, "You haven't been here in 3 years." I commented that it had not seemed that long. He then asked the young woman to inject the site on my chest to numb it for a biopsy. I decided to test out the sign and "Speak Up."

I asked her smiling, tongue in cheek, as to what her credentials were to administer the injection. She seemed annoyed that I asked the question and did not answer me and proceeded with the injection. I was sort of embarrassed having asked the question. To break the silence, I pointed out the Joint Commission "Speak-Up" sign in the corner of the room. The physician said, "Oh, that. That is Dr. R's sign." I thought to myself, I would think it would apply to everyone in the office. Needless to say, they did not introduce themselves.

The physician seemed to conduct a somewhat cursory exam, after which he completed the biopsy. He then left the room saying to the unknown woman to give me instructions. She walked to the exit door, turned around and verbally gave me her rapid fire instructions and left the room before I could ask her a question. My mouth was actually halfway open to ask a question. I could not get a word out of my mouth. Actually as I reflect back I thought it was a bit comical with me sitting there in the room with my mouth half open starting to ask a question as the door closed.

Patient

Discussion

1. Identify the ethical issues in this case.
2. What action should the patient take, if any, to notify the director of the practice of your experience? Note: The physician advertised in a local magazine that her practice is *Joint Commission* accredited.

Right to Examination and Treatment

Patients have a right to expect the physician will conduct an appropriate history and physical examination based on the patient's presenting complaints. The assessment is the process by which a physician investigates the patient's state of health, looking for signs of trauma and disease. It sets the stage for accurately diagnosing the patient's medical problems that leads to an agreed-upon treatment plan. A cursory assessment can lead to a misdiagnosis and inappropriate treatment plan. As reported by Karen Asp in *Shape Magazine*, "Is Your Dr. Missing the Mark?": "It took almost my whole life to get the right diagnosis because no one person had asked me enough questions."[6]

Primary care physicians often refer complex patients, such as those with autoimmune diseases with multiple systems failure, to specialists when their disease processes become too complex for them to treat. Unfortunately, challenging patients are often passed on a seemingly endless discouraging journey from specialist to specialist. The patient can often feel as though he or she is on a merry-go-round answering the same routine questions by consulting physicians, residents, and medical students, as noted in the following *reality check*. Medical students are often ill equipped to conduct an adequate history and physical on patients with multiple diagnoses. Patients trapped in the referral merry-go-round often become discouraged only to find that they often know more about their disease processes than many of the caregivers to whom they have been referred for help as noted in the letter to the patient's physician.

The Merry-Go-Round—Letter to My Doctor

When I went to your office, it was with great hopes that someone was finally going to piece together all of the bizarre symptoms I have been experiencing over the past several months and get to the cause of my pain. I was quite frankly shocked by how I was treated as a patient—especially one experiencing a health crisis.

A medical student, who wrote my history and current health problems on the pages of a small "yellow sticky pad," examined me. You were not in the room when he examined me, and then I saw you for approximately 10 minutes.

You took the card of my New York doctor and said you were going to call him, and then you said you would call me regarding what you thought the next steps should be.

I called you on Friday because my local doctor said that you had not called, and I was told you were on vacation. I asked that you call me. You never did. I called you yesterday again, but you did not answer, nor did you return my call.

On Monday, I received a letter—from a medical student, I assume. Although I empathize with the demands on your time, I have never seen a handwritten letter, which I received, informing me of test results I provided to you prior to my appointment with you. You never mentioned the liver enzyme elevations or my February test done in New York. Moreover, no mention was made regarding any plan to help me alleviate immediate problems.

Doctor, I am not a complainer or a person with a low pain tolerance. Since moving here, I've had fainting episodes, severe chest pain and pressure, leg and arm pain and stiffness, congestion on the left side when the pain kicks in, and by 3 p.m. I have to go home and lie down because I'm so weak and tired. I cannot continue to exist like this. It is not normal.

If you're too busy and don't want to take me as a patient, you will not offend me. Frankly, I need attention now to get these things resolved. Testing my cholesterol in a month will not address the problem. I've been treated for that for 3 years.

Please call or write to me so I can get another doctor if I have to.

Patient

[The physician never responded.]

Discussion

1. The physician never responded to the patient's letter of desperation. Discuss what you would suggest the patient should do.
2. Describe the legal and ethical and issues that appear in the correspondence.
3. As the patient continues on her merry-go-round, discuss what you would advise her to do.

Right to Emergency Care

Emergency care is well recognized as a patient right. Although regulations and court decisions recognize the right to emergency care; disparaging remarks have been made by some caregivers who resent treating patients they consider nonurgent or emergent in their care needs, as noted in the *reality check*.

Your Dad Needlessly Raises the Costs of Health Care

My dad lived in a small country town in southwest Pennsylvania. While visiting with him I noticed that he was having some difficulty breathing.

He had been a heavy smoker most of his life. In addition, he was exposed to the secondary smoke from a country bar that would seep through our floorboards from two stories below. Because of the severity of his breathing difficulty, I convinced him to go to the hospital emergency department. It was a Sunday, and it was his only option.

After undergoing a physical examination, a variety of blood tests, and chest X-rays, the emergency department physician came out to greet me and took the liberty to say, "Well, your dad is okay. There is nothing wrong with him. It is people like your dad that raise the costs of health care. They run to the emergency department with every little problem." Needless to say, I was shocked but relieved that Dad was okay. I said nothing to the physician out of respect for my dad, but I hope the physician is reading these words today.

Unfortunately, relief was short lived. Dad received a call the following day. He was asked to follow up with his family physician because the radiologist noted a shadow on his chest X-ray. Dad called me in New York and asked what I thought. I attempted to reassure him but, knowing his history of smoking, I keep silent as the sadness invaded my body.

Dad was diagnosed with lung cancer. Although dad refused chemotherapy, he did agree to radiation treatments. Mom relayed to me how his big event of the week was when he returned home from his treatments he would say, "Those cookies they gave me were actually pretty good." Yes, there are a lot of compassionate people who work in the hospital, but there are a few that give it a bad name.

Administrator

Take Time to Educate

I had to make an emergency room visit a couple weeks ago. While I was there for heart problems, I was told that they believed I had a blood clot and decided to order some imaging studies.

Next thing I know, a male nurse came to my room with discharge papers, telling me. "They couldn't find a blood clot." I was relieved to hear that I did not have a blood clot but was disturbed that a doctor never took the time to talk to me or share that information with me. I also noticed on my discharge papers that I had a potassium deficiency. I asked the nurse about it and she said, "Oh, don't worry. It's no big deal. Eat a banana. They are full of potassium."

I saw my cardiologist a few days later because my condition was worsening, and when I told him about my experience in the emergency room, he was very upset that no one bothered to contact him about that I, his cardiology patient was in the emergency room.

I guess I'm okay . . . I am on potassium supplements now and have to have follow-up with periodic blood work this to check my potassium levels. My heart rate has not changed much, but the EKG and Holter monitor were negative.

Patient

Discussion

1. What would be your expectations of the nurse and physician if you were the patient?
2. Do you believe this to be a typical encounter in an emergency department? Explain your answer.

RIGHT TO ADMISSION

Whether a person is entitled to admission to a particular hospital depends on the statute establishing that hospital. Governmental hospitals, for example, are by definition creatures of some unit of government; their primary responsibility is to provide service to the population within the jurisdiction of that unit. Military hospitals, for example, have been established to care for those persons who are active members of the military. Veteran hospitals were established to care for veterans. Although the public in general has no legal right of admission, government hospitals and their employees owe a duty to extend reasonable care to those who present themselves for assistance and are in need of immediate attention. With respect to such persons, governmental hospitals are subject to the same rules that apply to private hospitals, as noted in the following case.

CASE: STROKE PATIENT REFUSED TREATMENT

For example, the patient–plaintiff in *Stoick v. Caro Community Hospital*[7] brought a medical malpractice action against a government physician alleging the physician determined that she was having a stroke and required hospitalization but refused to hospitalize her. The plaintiff's daughter-in-law called the defendant, Caro Family Physicians, P.C., where the patient had a 1:30 p.m. appointment. She was told to take the patient to the hospital. On arriving at the hospital, there was no physician available to see the patient, and a nurse directed her to Dr. Loo's clinic in the hospital. On examination, Loo noted right-sided facial paralysis, weakness, dizziness, and an inability to talk. He told the patient that she was having a stroke and that immediate hospitalization was necessary. Loo refused to admit her because of a hospital policy that only the patient's family physician or treating physician could admit her. The plaintiff went to see her physician, Dr. Quines, who instructed her to go to the hospital immediately.

He did not accompany her to the hospital. At the hospital, she waited approximately 1 hour before another physician from the Caro Family Physicians arrived and admitted her. Loo claimed that he did not diagnose the patient as having a stroke and that there was no bad faith on his part.

The court of appeals reversed, holding that the plaintiff did plead sufficient facts constituting bad faith on the part of Loo. His failure to admit or otherwise treat the patient was a ministerial act for which governmental immunity does not apply and might be found by a jury to constitute negligence.

Ethical and Legal Issues

1. Discuss the legal and ethical issues in this case.
2. If you were the chief executive officer, discuss what action would you take to prevent similar occurrences in the emergency department.

RIGHT TO HAVE SPECIAL NEEDS ADDRESSED

Patients who have language barriers or hearing or vision impairments have a right to special help to have their needs addressed in order to ensure proper care. Many health care organizations maintain a list of employees with various language competencies and sign language skills in order to provide patients with high-quality care.

EXECUTE ADVANCE DIRECTIVES

Patients have a right to execute advance directives. A patient who becomes incapacitated or unable to make decisions on his or her behalf has a right to appoint a surrogate decision maker to make decisions on his or her behalf. Each patient at the time of admission should be queried to determine if they have executed advance directives and if a designated decision maker has been identified. Patients who have formerly executed advance directives should file a copy with the hospital and primary care physician.

RIGHT TO KNOW CAREGIVERS

Patients have a right to know the names and positions of the caregivers who will care for them while in the hospital. Patients should know who is treating them by name, discipline, role, and responsibility in their care plan. Caregivers should identify themselves to patients by name and discipline.

RIGHT TO TRUST CAREGIVERS

Patients have a right to trust the caregivers who provide their care. Forty-three year-old William McCormack found that where trust should be at its peak cannot always be presumed. When he had his appendix removed in 2013 and the hospital bill was settled, he at least could feel at ease knowing his appendix was removed in time and that was one less medical problem he would have to concern himself with in the future. That unfortunately was mistaken trust in this case. The pathology report showed the appendix had not been removed and no one informed him that he still had an appendix. Specimens sent to pathology for microscopic examination must be labeled as to the tissue being sent for review by a pathologist. This is in accordance with national standards and hospital practice. What happened here was a failure to follow up and let the patient know that tissue had been removed but it was not his appendix.[8]

Eighteen-month-old Josie King suffered third-degree burns after she had crawled into a hot bath at home. She was taken to a hospital where she died of dehydration despite the mother's concern that Josie was dehydrated.

What Josie King's Story Should Teach Us

She died despite the fact that her mother raised her concerns with hospital staff about Josie being denied liquids and being administered narcotics as she watched her daughter deteriorate.

• • •

While reading about little Josie's story, a familiar feeling came over me: frustration. Despite more information being available to the public than ever, we are still encouraged to trust medical personnel with little question. Josie's story underscores a reality that we are too often encouraged to forget: doctors and nurses are just human and make mistakes.

Maria Andreu, nj.com, *September 21, 2009*[9]

Misdiagnosed: What to Do When Your Doctor Doesn't Know What You Can Do

Knowing how and why diagnoses are missed might help you steer your own doctor in the right direction. Here are some steps you can follow.

• Keep detailed records
• Come prepared to ask the right questions
• Be assertive
• Be honest
• Explore new avenues
• Trust your gut
• In the absence of a diagnosis, treat your symptoms

Mary A. Fischer, AARP Newsletter, *July/August 2011*

RIGHT TO ACCESS A PATIENT ADVOCATE

Most organizations have adopted policies and procedures to address patient complaints. A patient advocate generally addresses patient concerns. Access to a patient advocate is often described in patient handbooks. Patient advocacy services should be available to both patients and families. Many states have mandated by legislation the establishment of ombudsman and patient advocacy programs. In fulfilling their commitments and obligations to patients, health care executives function as moral advocates and models. Being a model means that decisions and actions will reflect personal integrity and ethical leadership that others will seek to emulate.[10] Patient advocacy by all caregivers should be considered a routine responsibility. Caregivers are closest to observing the care being rendered to the patient and are more aware of when things are not going right. Intervention earlier in a patient's care is more important than watching a bad scenario in a patient's care unfold.

RIGHT TO CHAPLAINCY SERVICES

Today I will take the time to be happy and will leave my footprints and my presence in the hearts of others.

–AUTHOR UNKNOWN

Patients have a right to chaplaincy services. The purpose of a pastoral care program is to affirm the valuable role of spiritual care as an integral part of a patient's healing process. Accordingly, the program will make available to patients and their families spiritual support while they are in the hospital, in accordance with their wishes. The hospital supports the role of the clergy and pastoral care volunteers as important members of the healing team.

A multifaith chapel as well as televised services are available in many hospitals. Some hospitals provide spiritual devotions and reflections that are broadcast daily. Music and meditation are often provided as an adjunct for pain management and stress reduction at the bedside.

Chaplains are often available as a first call option for ethics consultations. The hospital chaplain coordinates liaison between patient and area clergy. Consultations with the patient care team contribute to the holistic care of patients, family, and staff through assessment, pastoral conversation, and other interventions. Caregivers often refer patients to a chaplain for:

- patients/families/caregivers who are experiencing life-changing events
- patients who lack effective social, psychological, or spiritual support
- patients who have complicated personal relationships
- patients who express spiritual or religious concerns
- patients who are in a remorseful state of mind
- patients who express hopelessness, worthlessness, anger, or depression
- patients who receive news of life-threatening conditions
- families at times of death of the patient

Hospital pastoral care departments should provide a patient information brochure at the time of admission that describes the services offered. For example, an introductory statement to such a brochure could be worded to include:

- When a loved one is hospitalized—or when you require hospitalization yourself—it is perfectly normal to feel anxious, worried, and sometimes overwhelmed.
- We know how you feel. At times like this, it's good to have a helping hand. The hospital's pastoral care department is here to help you cope with the emotional struggle associated with hospitalization.
- No matter what your religious affiliation, a representative of the pastoral care department is always available to offer spiritual and emotional support.
- Someone will lend an ear and offer comforting words. He or she will help you draw on your spiritual strength in these times of need.

Services offered by a chaplaincy program should:

- offer pastoral support to patients and their families at time of crisis, which may include prayer, scripture reading, and counseling
- provide for enhanced communications between patients, their families, and hospital personnel
- be available to clinical staff by providing counseling and support during or after emotional emergency situations
- provide appropriate referrals to the social service department, the local clergy, and community agencies as needed

RIGHT TO ETHICS CONSULTATION

Patient's rights in many hospitals allow for patients and/or families to access an ethics committee for consultation when faced with challenging treatment decisions that involve ethical dilemmas. Dilemmas often arise when two or more choices often have some degree of a negative outcome. Conflict can arise when there is a difference of opinion between families and care providers, or when the family is unsure about what course of treatment is best for the patient. Ethics committee consultation can provide an objective perspective. Ethics committees are consultative in nature. Recommendations of an ethics committee should not be considered as binding. Ethics consultations are helpful when, for example, when making end-of-life decisions.

RIGHT TO CHOOSE TREATMENT

Patients have the right to choose the medical care they wish to receive. They have a right to know their treatment options and to accept or refuse care. As medical technology becomes more advanced, care decisions become more complicated to make. Should I have the surgery? Do I want to be maintained on a respirator? Frequently, these decisions involve not only medical questions, but moral and ethical dilemmas as well. What has the greater value, the length of life or the quality of life? What is the right choice? Although patients have a right to make their own care and treatment decisions, they often face conflicting religious and moral values in their decision-making process. Often, it is difficult to make a choice when two roads may seem equally desirable.

RIGHT TO INFORMED CONSENT

Patients have a right to receive a full explanation of treatment options in order to make an informed decision prior to consenting to a proposed procedure or treatment. This information should include the risks, benefits, and alternatives of each procedure or treatment option. The right to receive information from the physician includes information about the illness, the suggested course of treatment, and the prospects of recovery in terms that can be understood.

RIGHT TO REFUSE TREATMENT

The responsibility of the physician is to objectively balance the risks and benefits of each treatment option. This balancing act can lead to a dilemma where the physician's recommended procedure differs from the procedure the patient is willing to accept. Pressing a patient to undergo an unwanted procedure is a form of paternalism that could represent a failure to respect the patient's right of self-determination.

RIGHT TO TIMELY RESPONSE TO CARE NEEDS

Patients have a right to have their care needs addressed within a reasonable time frame. Delay in responding to patient needs can place a patient's life at risk.

RIGHT TO RECEIVE QUALITY CARE

Health care professionals are expected to monitor the quality of each patient's care beginning with the history and physical, followed by the development of the treatment plan, and ultimately the delivery of care to the patient. The patient has a right to expect that the quality of care rendered will be based on best practices recognized by the medical profession.

RIGHT TO COMPASSIONATE CARE

I would suggest if you don't see me, don't come to see me.

—DANIEL

Patients have a right to receive considerate and compassionate care from caregivers. There appears to be less time for compassion in the practice of medicine than at the turn of the 20th century. Providers of care seem to have taken the assembly-line approach to patient care with little thought as to the need to help alleviate their fears. Dr. Robert E. Rakel, Department of Family Medicine at Baylor College of Medicine in Houston, wrote in the *Journal of the American Board of Family Practice*, "It has been said that more mistakes in medicine are made by those who do not care than by those who do not know."[11]

> The caring function of family medicine emphasizes our personalized approach to health care and our commitment to understanding the patient as a person, respecting the person as an individual, and showing compassion for his or her discomfort. Compassion, from the word *patior*, literally means "to suffer with," to share in another's distress and to be moved to give relief. Compassion reflects the physician's willingness to share the patient's anguish and to attempt to understand what the sickness means to that person.[12]

It seems with the progress of medicine there has at the same time been a decline in compassion for the patient. Patients fill out numerous forms prior to their visit to the physician's office and yet the caregiver often fails to read the information the patient has provided, as noted in the following *reality check*.

Compassionate Care

During the past 5 years, I have filled out numerous standardized forms that ask questions that have been repeatedly asked by a wide variety of physician specialists and other caregivers. I've been told that my most recent specialist had great credentials. He came highly recommended. I grew more hopeful as I drove to his office during the early morning rush hour in a metropolitan city. I would finally meet someone who cared and understood my disease processes. As I walked into his office, I noted that my medical chart was lying on the desk in front of him. The sight of it on his desk comforted me, thinking that he had actually read my answers. His staff had said he wanted the chart several weeks prior to my appointment because he needed time to familiarize himself with my case. I soon realized several minutes into the conversation that he had not reviewed my medical chart. The forms that I had so painstakingly completed, hoping for an answer to my illness, had not been read. He inquired as to what medications I was taking. My husband accompanied me that day and noticed that the list of medications was laid in front of him; he didn't hesitate to point that out to the physician. The doctor asked questions within a predetermined range—one was, "What is your pain on a scale of 1 to 10?" How do I answer that? I am off your scale. I cannot remember not being in pain for the past 5 years. I sometimes wonder what it must have been like to be pain free. I don't know that feeling anymore. Hello, is anyone out there?

Eventually, I was admitted to the hospital for the first time. My nerve endings felt frayed, my stomach churned, my worries were multiplying, and my thoughts turned to, "Is it time to get more bad news?" I was extremely ill. The waiting area in the admissions office was uncomfortable and uninviting. Privacy was minimal and soft music was nonexistent. I wondered what was going to happen to me.

Things got worse when I was finally admitted to a room. I was in an unfamiliar room with drab, nondescript walls, and I was dependent upon people who barely had the time to dispense medications. The physicians and other staff members were rushing about, engaged in their everyday tasks. No one seemed to have time for me.

Confusion set in, and the fear of being in a strange place triggered fear. Unfamiliar people looked at me, touched me, and asked me the same questions over and over again. The questioning seemed never ending. I wondered, "Do these people ever talk to each other?" The surroundings were sterile and unfriendly, adding to my uneasy feelings.

Why can't health care facilities be more compassionate and patient friendly? Why must I worry about complaining and fear retribution? Provisions should be made for a serene environment with calming colors and carefully chosen people to gently ease answers from a frightened patient. More attention is needed in making a patient's room a calm and inviting place, which would help to soothe and carry the patient through troubling times.

Patient

Discussion

1. In what way did the physician show a lack of concern for the patient's needs?
2. Describe how hospitals can provide a compassionate and comforting environment for patients.

Ms. Ying Tai Choi's daughter, Ching Cheung, described how a hospice nurse failed to stay and care for her 85-year-old mother during the last hour of her life. The hospice had promised to be there for Cheung's mother and to provide the care she needed as she passed from this life to the next. They were not there. The nurse left Choi and her daughter during the last hour of need.

Terminal Neglect for Hospice Patients?

Ying Tai Choi lay on a hospital bed arranged in the living room of her daughter's house. A pulse oximeter pinged intermittent warning about her mother's oxygen levels. She heaved for breath sometimes and panted at others. Sounds of gurgling and congestion came from her throat. The skin behind her fingernails was turning dark.

"She is leaving soon," the hospital nurse told Choi's daughter.

Then the nurse left the house and drove away . . . .

• • •

"Everyone later said they are 'sorry,'" Cheung said. "But what is 'sorry'? That is just another word."

David A. Fahrenthold, The Washington Post, *May 4, 2014*

Reading this news clipping, one quickly realizes that not much has changed over the years. This is unfortunately the real world in which we live. The article is so descriptive of how humanity fails itself over and over again. It was as timely in the 20th century as it is now in the 21st century. Although compassion is not so easily taught to an adult as it is to a child, the struggle and the need to bring life to the study of ethics and the law are clearly borne out in this article.

RIGHT TO RESPECT

The right to respect is a common right enjoyed by patients, families, and caregivers. Respect is more than a two-way street. It is not just about what is right for you and me but requires respect of all persons.

Right to Pain Management

I am locked in a prison of pain, where doctors hold the key. Why can't they think beyond the box and develop a cure for me?

—Nina Santucci

Pain is the body's way of alerting the patient that something is not quite right. *Pain management* is the process whereby caregivers work with the patient to determine the cause of pain and develop a pain control treatment plan. The process involves educating the patient as to the importance of pain management in the healing process. With current treatments, pain can often be prevented or at least be better controlled.

Patients have a right to have a pain assessment and management of any pain identified. A *pain rating scale* is a visual tool often used to help patients describe their pain level. It helps the caregiver know how well treatment is working and whether change in the treatment plan is necessary. The pain assessment scale is a tool often used because of its ease of use in performing a task. Just as important as the severity of pain are its locations and type (e.g., burning sensation, throbbing, dull, stabbing, numbing, sharp, shooting). A diagram of the body should be used so the patient can more easily identify the various locations of his or her pain. The severity of pain can be described to the physician to assist in diagnosing and treating the patient. All patients have a right to:

- A pain control treatment plan developed with the caregiver
- Alternative and/or complementary strategies included in the pain management plan that might help improve the efficacy of traditional treatment options (e.g., pain medications), for example, acupuncture, imagery, meditation, reiki (ancient Japanese touch therapy)
- Inclusion of family and caregivers in the decision-making process
- An explanation of the medications, anesthesia, or other treatments planned
- An explanation of the risks, benefits, and alternatives (e.g., acupuncture) to suggested treatment(s)
- Request changes in treatment if pain persists
- Refuse pain treatment(s) recommended
- Receive pain medication in a timely manner

Right to Privacy and Confidentiality

Patients have a right to expect that information regarding their care and treatment will be kept confidential. Confidentiality requires that the caregiver safeguard a patient's confidences within the constraints of law. Caregivers must be careful not to discuss any aspect of a patient's case with others not involved in the case. Written permission must be obtained before a patient's medical record can be made available to anyone not associated with the patient's care.

A lack of patient privacy was discovered when hospital records were discovered online. "The breach at Stanford Hospital in Palo Alto, Calif., exposed the names and diagnoses of 20,000 patients who visited the hospital's emergency department between March 1, 2009, and Aug. 31, 2009 are affected."[13] in another instance on the heels of its first Health Insurance

Portability and Accountability Act (HIPAA) privacy rule, "the Department of Health and Human Services (HHS) has doled out a $1 million fine against Massachusetts General Hospital for a data breach involving 192 patients being treated for infectious diseases."[14]

UCLA Workers Snooped in Spears Medical Records

UCLA Medical Center is taking steps to fire at least 13 employees and has suspended at least six others for snooping in the confidential medical records of pop star Britney Spears during her recent hospitalization in its psychiatric unit, a person familiar with the matter said Friday.

• • •

"Each member of our workforce, which includes our physicians, faculty, employees, volunteers and students, is responsible to ensure that medical information is only accessed as required for treatment, for facilitating payment of a claim or for supporting our health care operations," chief compliance and privacy officer Carole A. Klove wrote in an e-mail to all employees.

Charles Ornstein, Los Angeles Times, *March 15, 2008*

The limitations of space and financial restraints make it difficult to continuously preserve a patient's right to privacy in many hospital settings (e.g., emergency departments). Even so, health care organizations have a responsibility to provide for a reasonable amount of privacy for patients.

Phlebotomist Discloses Patient Information at Public Tavern

The phlebotomist, in *Bagent v. Blessing Care Corp.,*[15] revealed the results of a patient's pregnancy test to the patient's sister at a public tavern. Although the hospital attempted to have the case dismissed for the phlebotomist's breach of confidentiality, invasion of privacy, and the negligent infliction of emotional distress, the appeals court determined that there were triable issues of fact precluding dismissal of the case. It was asserted that the phlebotomist had been trained to maintain the confidentiality of patient information and that she knew that she had violated the patient's rights.

Right to Know Hospital's Adverse Events

The Florida Supreme Court in the cases *Florida Hospital Waterman, Inc., etc. v. Teresa M. Buster, et al.* and *Notami Hospital of Florida, Inc., etc. v. Evelyn Bowen, et al.*[16] ruled that hospitals under Amendment 7 (approved by the voters on November 2, 2004, and codified as Article X, Section 25 of the Florida Constitution) must reveal their records of past acts of malpractice that have been performed at the hospital. In Florida, patients now have a right to know about, ask for, and/or receive records about adverse medical incidents that have occured at the hospital.

Amendment 7 to the Florida Constitution reads in part:

Section 25. Patients' right to know about adverse medical incidents.

(a) Patients have a right to have access to any records made or received in the course of business by a health care facility or provider relating to any adverse medical incident.

(b) In providing such access, the identity of patients involved in the incidents shall not be disclosed, and any privacy restrictions imposed by federal law shall be maintained.

RIGHT TO DISCHARGE

Patients have a right to be discharged and not be detained in a health care setting merely because of an inability to pay for services rendered. An unauthorized detention of this nature could subject the offending organization to charges of false imprisonment. Although patients have a right not to be held against their will, there are circumstances in which reasonable detainment can be justified (e.g., a minor may be released only to a parent or authorized guardian).

Discharge Orders

When discharging a patient, a physician should issue and sign all discharge orders. If there is no need for immediate care, the patient should be advised to seek follow-up care with his or her family physician.

CASE: RELEASE FROM HOSPITAL CONTRAINDICATED

The patient–plaintiff in *Somoza v. St. Vincent's Hospital*[17] was admitted to the hospital during the 29th week of her pregnancy. Dr. Gutwein, a resident, was caring for the patient. The results of a sonogram were abnormal, and the radiologist recommended a follow-up sonogram. Despite the abnormal sonogram and various findings on the physical examinations, Dr. Svesko decided to release the plaintiff because her pain had subsided. Dr, Gutwein signed an order discharging the patient from the hospital. Four days later, the patient returned to the hospital suffering severe pain and soon thereafter delivered twin girls diagnosed as suffering from cerebral palsy. The patient became a plaintiff bringing a medical malpractice action against the hospital and Dr. Svesko arising out of the premature birth of the twins. The defendants filed a motion for summary judgment, which was denied and the defendants appealed.

The New York State Supreme Court, Appellate Division, held that there were material issues of fact as to whether the mother's symptoms exhibited during her physical assessment contraindicated her release from the hospital. Dr. Sherman, an expert witness for the plaintiff testified that the plaintiff's discharge was "a departure from good and accepted medical practice. The resident clearly had an obligation to examine even a private patient in the face of a changing cervix and not just to discharge her pursuant to some attending physician's order."[18] A hospital whose staff carries out a physician's order may be held responsible where the hospital staff knows, or should know, that the orders are clearly contraindicated by normal practice.

Ethical and Legal Issues

1. Discuss how both the hospital and caregivers failed both legally and ethically in caring for the patient.
2. Discuss how you would work with caregivers in general to prevent similar incidents from occurring in the future.

RIGHT TO TRANSFER

Patients have a right to be transferred when the admitting hospital is unable to address a patient's care needs. This is required when a hospital does not, for example, have a neurosurgeon on staff when such is required for a serious head injury. For this reason, it is imperative that hospitals execute transfer agreements for services they do not offer with other health care organizations.

Transfer agreements help ensure the smooth transfer of a patient from one facility to another when such is determined appropriate by the attending physician(s). Generally speaking, a transfer agreement is a written document that sets forth the terms and conditions under which a patient may be transferred from a facility unable to treat a patient's particular ailment to a facility that can provide the kind of care crucial to the patient's recovery.

Transfer agreements should be written in compliance with and reflect the provisions of the many federal and state laws, regulations, and standards affecting health care organizations. The parties to a transfer agreement should be particularly aware of applicable federal and state regulations.

Patients also have a right to choose a receiving facility, whenever possible. The Medicaid patient in *Macleod v. Miller*[19] was entitled to an injunction preventing his involuntary transfer from a nursing home. The patient had not been accorded a pretransfer hearing, as was required by applicable regulations. In addition, it was determined that the trauma of transfer might result in irreparable harm to the patient. The appeals court remanded the case to the trial court with directions to enter an order prohibiting the defendants from transferring the plaintiff pending exhaustion of his administrative remedies.

RIGHT TO ACCESS MEDICAL RECORDS

The courts have taken the view that patients have a legally enforceable interest in the information contained in their medical records and therefore have a right to access their records. Some states have enacted legislation permitting patients access to their records. Patients may generally have access to review and/or obtain copies of their records, X-rays, and laboratory and diagnostic tests. Access to information includes that maintained or possessed by a health care organization and/or a health care practitioner who has treated or is treating a patient. Organizations and physicians can withhold records if it is determined that the information could reasonably be expected to cause substantial and identifiable harm to the patient (e.g., for patients in psychiatric facilities, institutions for the mentally disabled, alcohol and drug treatment programs).

RIGHT TO ACCESS LAB REPORTS

The Department of Health and Human Services (HHS) released a statement on February 3, 2014 that strengthens the right of patients to access their lab test reports.

> As part of an ongoing effort to empower patients to be informed partners with their health care providers, the Department of Health and Human Services (HHS) has taken action to give patients or a person designated by the patient a means of direct access to the patient's completed laboratory test reports.
>
> "The right to access personal health information is a cornerstone of the Health Insurance Portability and Accountability Act (HIPAA) Privacy Rule," said Secretary Kathleen Sebelius. "Information like lab results can empower patients to track their health progress, make decisions with their health care professionals, and adhere to important treatment plans."[20]

Some hospitals have been made it easier for patients to access their lab results by either hard copy or through electronic access to their lab results.

Hospital Peer-Review Materials Discoverable: Patient's Right to Know

Florida voters, in November 2004, adopted the "Patients' Right to Know About Adverse Medical Incidents" amendment to Florida's constitution ("Amendment 7"). In a medical malpractice action in which the plaintiffs sought the production of documents relating to the investigation of the decedent's death and any medical incidents of negligence, neglect, or default of any health care provider who rendered services to the decedent, the trial court properly held that the Patient's Right to Know Amendment to the state constitution was self-executing and allowed for the discovery during the course of litigation. The patient should have been provided with information and documents that emanate from the self-policing processes of health care providers; however, the court's retroactive application of the amendment was found to be improper.[21]

RIGHT TO KNOW THIRD-PARTY CARE RELATIONSHIPS

Patients have a right to know the hospital's relationships with outside parties that may influence their care and treatment. These relationships may be with educational institutions, insurers, and other caregivers.

RIGHT TO KNOW HOSPITAL CHARGES

Patients have a right to transparency when requesting information about hospital emergency room, outpatient, and inpatient treatment charges. The North Carolina Senate is considering a bill titled the Health Care Cost Reduction and Transparency Act to be effective, which is intended to allow patients to compare treatment costs among different providers. Hospitals and ambulatory surgical facilities would be required to annually provide financial information for their 50 most common episodes of care to the North Carolina Health Information Exchange (Exchange), which allows free public access to its most current information. The Act is intended to allow patients to compare treatment costs among different providers.[22] As noted in the *reality check*, hospital charges are necessarily transparent.

Hospital Charges Not So Transparent

I traveled to Florida for a continuing education program on patient care in my specialty. I unfortunately forgot my asthma inhaler. When I got off the plane after landing and not knowing where to go, as I was new to the area and it was late evening, I decided to go to a local hospital emergency department for a prescription. I was in no distress but was concerned that I had forgotten my inhaler. I unfortunately made the mistake of believing that an emergency room was an appropriate place to go for help and advice when traveling. I sat in a hallway, had my temperature and blood pressure taken, and inhaled some albuterol. My visit from beginning to end was about 20 minutes.

Upon returning home, I received an emergency room bill in excess of $3,000, so now I was distressed. Although I have an insurance policy, there is a $2,000 deductible that I was responsible to pay. I decided to request more detail on my bill. After a less than pleasant experience with the billing department I decided also to request a copy of my medical record. For a hospital that claimed transparency on its website, it took me 6 weeks and several annoying phone conversations with hospital staff to obtain the billing information and a copy of what turned out to be an 18-page barely readable computerized medical record that listed yes and no answers to questions I was never specifically asked. I couldn't believe it and said to my husband, "Wow, the bill says $27.00 for the medication and I have to pay $2,973 to inhale it."

In summary, I discovered there was no transparency the hospital publicized on its website. Transparency is an overused platitude that has little meaning. For me, I totally understand the U.S. citizen's frustration with the health care system.

Anonymous

PATIENT RESPONSIBILITIES

Patients' Responsibilities—Avoiding Putting Others at Risk

At one extreme, we see and hear news reports about a tuberculosis patient who travels the world, potentially infecting someone else, or about a person with AIDS who passes on his disease intentionally.

• • •

In the United States, we have an obligation not to harm others either through intentional or unintentional means. It's our responsibility to act in such a way that we keep others from being infected or injured. In some cases, there are laws that speak to this responsibility, warranting eventual arrest or a lawsuit. In others, it's simply common sense or even the golden rule.

Trisha Torrey, About.com Guide, *April 8, 2010*

Patients have responsibilities as well as rights. One cannot exist without the other in an orderly society. Various patient responsibilities are described next.

MAINTAIN A HEALTHY LIFESTYLE

Living a health lifestyle involves both a right and a responsibility. Each person must take responsibility for living well through exercise, diet, stress control, and maintaining positive social relationships, which will be rewarded with a richer and fuller life that should better prepare people for whatever health obstacles the future may hold. Recognizing what is right and what is wrong for one's health is not enough, it must me recognized and practiced.

KEEP APPOINTMENTS

Patients have a responsibility to promptly notify caregivers whenever they are unable to keep a scheduled appointment. Failure to notify caregivers of a cancellation means longer delays for other patients who may be finding it difficult to schedule appointments with physicians.

MAINTAIN CURRENT MEDICATION RECORDS

Patients have a responsibility to maintain a current accurate record of their medications, including dosages, route of administration, and frequency. Drug allergies should be included on the list. Medication records should be reviewed periodically to be sure the listing is current. A copy should be provided to treating physicians and treating facility.

PROVIDE FULL AND HONEST DISCLOSURE OF MEDICAL HISTORY

Provide full disclosure of all information relevant to one's medical condition, medical complaints, symptoms, location and severity of pain, previous pain control concerns, past illnesses, treatments, surgical or other invasive procedures, hospitalizations, medications, and allergies. Information provided must be accurate, timely, and complete. Selectively in the information provided to the physician or hospital for whatever the reason can lead caregivers down the wrong path when treating the patient. The court of appeal in *Fall v. White*[23] affirmed the superior court's ruling that the patient had a duty to provide the physician with accurate and complete information and to follow the physician's instructions for further care or tests.

Why Would My Patient Not Tell Me the Truth?

Several months ago I nearly collided with one of my patients at the subway entrance. She was so busy lighting a cigarette that she didn't even notice me. I, on the other hand, was shocked to see her mid-drag. A mere two days earlier she had been sitting in my office telling me how she hadn't smoked in more than six months.

. . . in a survey of pregnant women, urine tests for tobacco byproducts revealed that 34 percent of women who said they didn't smoke actually did.

Daphne Miller, The Washington Post, *March 15, 2011*

REPORT UNEXPECTED CHANGES IN HEALTH STATUS

Relay to caregivers unexpected changes in your health status. Make it known whether you clearly understand the plan of care. Ask questions to seek clarification of concerns when in doubt about the plan of care.

CASE: RIGHTS AND RESPONSIBILITIES CONFLICT

Several months after having stomach surgery, Vicki Marsingill, in *Marsingill v. O'Malley*, 58 P.3d 495 (2002), called her surgeon, Dr. O'Malley, complaining of abdominal pain and nausea. O'Malley advised Marsingill to go to the emergency room and offered to meet her there, but Marsingill said she felt better and declined to go.

O'Malley left it up to Marsingill whether to seek emergency room treatment. O'Malley informed Marsingill that the doctors in the emergency room would probably take X-rays and insert a nasogastric tube to relieve the pressure in her stomach. After hearing that she would likely need to have a nasogastric tube inserted if she went to the emergency room, Marsingill ended the call, telling O'Malley that she was feeling better.

Later that night, Marsingill's husband found her unconscious on the bathroom floor. Paramedics rushed her to the hospital, where an emergency operation later revealed that she had experienced an intestinal blockage, but by then the obstruction had caused Marsingill to go into shock. She suffered brain damage and partial paralysis.

Marsingill sued O'Malley, claiming that he lacked the skill and knowledge to advise her properly and that the information he gave her over the telephone did not allow her to make an intelligent treatment decision.

Section 8.08 of the AMA Code of Medical Ethics addresses the duty of disclosure, providing, "The patient's right of self-decision can be effectively exercised only if the patient possesses enough information to enable an intelligent choice." Marsingill's experts maintained that O'Malley had violated Section 8.08 by failing to give her enough information to make an intelligent choice about whether to seek emergency room treatment. O'Malley acknowledged that Section 8.08 applied to his conduct—that he did have an obligation to give Marsingill enough information so that she could make an intelligent choice as to whether she should go to the emergency room.

Marsingill's proposed instruction by the judge to the jury would have required the jury to decide the sufficiency of O'Malley's communications from the standpoint of a reasonable patient in Marsingill's position. The trial court rejected the proposed "reasonable patient" instruction.

O'Malley acquiesced in Marsingill's decision not to go to the emergency room. In the context of a preexisting patient–physician relationship involving postoperative care, a physician's recommendation to do nothing in the face of threatening symptoms is the equivalent of a treatment recommendation and should be accompanied by a duty of disclosure.

A physician's acquiescence in a patient's decision not to seek treatment in the same circumstances should likewise be regarded as equivalent to a treatment recommendation subject to the same duty.

The superior court deprived Marsingill of her right to have the jury decide the issue directly from the standpoint of a reasonable patient, and the case was remanded for a new trial on Marsingill's claim for breach of the duty to provide sufficient information to allow her to make an intelligent treatment choice.

The appellate court ruled that the jury should have been instructed to use the reasonable patient standard to determine whether O'Malley gave Marsingill sufficient information about her condition and treatment choices. On remand, the jury must be instructed to decide the claim from the standpoint of a reasonable patient.

There will always be an endless number of "what-if" scenarios. In the end, this question remains: What should one do, knowing that whatever decision is made there will always be some doubt as to whether the decision made was the right one? Armed with the knowledge in this book, the reader will be a more effective caregiver and better able to make critical health care decisions.

Ethical and Legal Issues

1. Explain the court's reasoning for remanding this case back to the trial court.
2. Discuss how you would assess the failure of both the patient and physician as to their rights and responsibilities in this case.

ADHERE TO THE AGREED-UPON TREATMENT PLAN

Be sure to follow the treatment plan recommended. Accept responsibility for the consequences of failing to adhere to the caregiver's instructions. Refrain from self-administration of medications not prescribed by the physician, as well as those you may have brought to the hospital with you. Be considerate of the rights of others (e.g., noise control, no-smoking rules, respect for the rights and property of others).

WHEN IN DOUBT, SEEK A SECOND OPINION

When in doubt, seek a second opinion. Participate in marking the site of a surgical or other invasive procedure. Communicate to staff your care preferences, including that you have selected as a decision maker in the event you become incapacitated and unable to make decisions for yourself.

STAY INFORMED

Understand caregiver instructions. Consider the following case where a patient had been sedated during the performance of a colonoscopy at an endoscopy center. He decided to drive himself home against medical advice. Claims against the clinic and a nurse were dismissed with respect to fatal injuries that the patient received during a one-car collision. The trial court correctly ruled that the nurse had no duty to prevent the patient from leaving its premises once she repeatedly warned the patient not to drive. The nurse was justified in relying upon the patient's false representations that he had a friend available to drive him home. She was not required to keep the patient in a gown in the recovery room once she learned the truth, and she was not required to use other options to prevent him from driving, such as putting him in a taxicab, putting him in a hotel, calling the police, admitting him to the hospital, personally driving him home, taking his keys away from him, or physically restraining him. The center and the nurse owed no legal duty to the patient to do more than warn him that he should not drive. The center is not an insurer of the patients' safety. The patient acted recklessly in ignoring the advice he was given and suffered the consequences. The circuit court correctly found no duty to ensure that no patient drives after the procedure.[24]

Ask Questions

The necessity and responsibility to ask questions cannot be overstated. A knowledgeable patient is a good patient. If you are unsure of a caregiver's instructions, be sure to seek clarification and a written copy of the proposed treatment plan. Ask questions and seek clarification when in doubt about the plan of care. Patients have a responsibility to ask questions and understand explanations. Such questions include: "What is this medication for?" "What diet am I on?" "Since you are going to change my dressing, did you wash your hands?"

Accurately Describe Symptoms

Accurately describe the location and severity of pain.

Advisory Commission Describes Patient Responsibilities

A 1997 report to the president by the Advisory Commission on Consumer Protection and Quality in the Health Care Industry clearly describes patient responsibilities:

> In a health care system that protects consumers' rights, it is reasonable to expect and encourage consumers to assume reasonable responsibilities. Greater individual involvement by consumers in their care increases the likelihood of achieving the best outcomes and helps support a quality improvement, cost-conscious environment. Such responsibilities include:

- Take responsibility for maximizing healthy habits, such as exercising, not smoking, and eating a healthy diet.
- Become involved in specific health care decisions.
- Work collaboratively with health care providers in developing and carrying out agreed upon treatment plans.
- Disclose relevant information and clearly communicate wants and needs.
- Use the health plan's internal complaint and appeal processes to address concerns that may arise.
- Avoid knowingly spreading disease.
- Recognize the reality of risks and limits of the science of medical care and the human fallibility of the health care professional.
- Be aware of a health care provider's obligation to be reasonably efficient and equitable in providing care to other patients and the community.
- Become knowledgeable about his or her health plan coverage and health plan options (when available) including all covered benefits, limitations and exclusions, rules regarding use of network providers, coverage and referral rules, appropriate

processes to secure additional information, and the process to appeal coverage decisions.

- Show respect for other patients and health workers.
- Make a good-faith effort to meet financial obligations.
- Abide by administrative and operational procedures of health plans, health care providers, and government health benefit programs.
- Report wrongdoing and fraud to appropriate resources or legal authorities.[25]

CHAPTER REVIEW

1. Patients' rights include the right to be informed of their rights and responsibilities at the time of admission, emergency care, admission, have special needs addressed, execute advance directives, know caregivers, trust caregivers, access a patient advocate, chaplaincy services, ethics consultation, choose treatment, informed consent, refuse treatment, timely response to care needs, receive quality care, compassionate care, respect, pain management, privacy and confidentiality, know hospital's adverse events, discharge, transfer, access medical records, know third-party care relationships, and know hospital charges.

2. Patient Responsibilities
   - Maintain a healthy lifestyle.
   - Keep appointments.
   - Maintain current medication records.
   - Provide full and honest disclosure of medical history.
   - Report unexpected changes in health status.
   - Adhere to the agreed-upon treatment plan.
   - When in doubt, seek a second opinion.
   - Stay informed.
   - Ask questions.
   - Accurately describe symptoms.
   - Pain control.

3. Rights and responsibilities converge when each person acknowledges and practices a healthy lifestyle.

TEST YOUR UNDERSTANDING

TERMINOLOGY

Health Insurance Portability and Accountability Act	pain management	socratic method of teaching and learning
pain	pain rating scale	
	Patient's Bill of Rights	

REVIEW QUESTIONS

1. Discuss the various rights of patients discussed in this chapter.

2. Discuss the various responsibilities of patients discussed in this chapter.

3. Describe why a patient's responsibilities are as important as his or her rights.

4. Explain the importance of patient rights and responsibilities from both an ethical and legal point of view.

5. Discuss the importance of living a healthy lifestyle.

6. Describe patient responsibilities as reported in the 1997 report to the president by the Advisory Commission on Consumer Protection and Quality in the Health Care Industry

NOTES

1. Your Rights as a Hospital Patient in New York State, State of New York, Department of Health.

2. 42 U.S.C. 1395cc(a)(1).

3. http://www.hhs.gov/ocr/privacy/hipaa/understanding/coveredentities/notice.html.

4. *Dr. Ranit Mishori*, Parade, *February 8, 2009.*

5. *Sandra G. Boudman*, The Washington Post, *February 25, 2014.*

6. *Karen Asp*, Shape Magazine, *March 2013.*

7. 449 N.E.2d 628 (Ind. Ct. App. 1983).

8. *Richard Liebson*, The Journal News, *April 10, 2014,* http://www.lohud.com/story/news/local/westchester /2014/04/09/bronxville-man-sues-hospital-doc-appendix-mulligan/7514765/.

9. Maria Andreu, "What Josie King's story should teach us," nj.com, September 21, 2009; http://www.nj.com/ parenting/maria_andreu/index.ssf/2009/09/what_josie_kings_story_should.html.

10. http://www.ache.org/ABT_ACHE/code.cfm.

11. Robert E. Rakel, MD, *Compassion and the Art of Family Medicine: From Osler to Oprah.* J Am Board Fam Med. 2000;13(6). http://www.medscape.com/viewarticle/405817_2.

12. *Id.*

13. Ryan Jaslow, "Patient Privacy in Spotlight after Hospital Records Spotted Online," *CBS News*, September 9, 2011.

14. http://www.infosecurity-magazine.com/view/16228/mass-general-takes-1-million-hit-for-losing-193-patient- records/.

15. 844 N.E.2d 649 (Ill. App. 2006).

16. Supreme Court of Florida, No. SC06-912 (March 6, 2008).

17. 596 N.Y.S.2d 789 (N.Y. App. Div. 1993).

18. *Id.* at 791.

19. 612 P.2d 1158 (Colo. Ct. App. 1980).

20. http://www.hhs.gov/news/press/2014pres/02/20140203a.html.

21. Florida Hosp. Waterman, Inc. v. Buster, 932 So.2d 344 (Fla. App. 2006).

22. http://www.ncga.state.nc.us/Sessions/2013/Bills/Senate/HTML/S473v3.html.

23. 449 N.E.2d 628 (Ind. Ct. App. 1983).

24. *Young v. Gastro-IntestinalCenter, Inc., No. 04-595 (Ark.* 2005).

25. President's Advisory Commission on Consumer Protection and Quality in the Health Care Industry. "Chapter 8: Consumer Bill of Rights and Responsibilities," in *Consumer Responsibilities*, (July 17, 1998). http://www .hcqualitycommission.gov/cborr/chap8.html (accessed October 12, 2010).

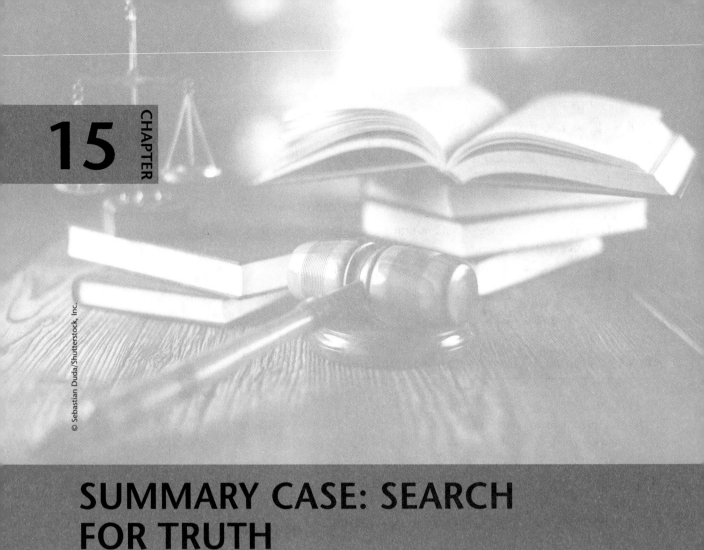

SUMMARY CASE: SEARCH FOR TRUTH

"There is nothing," says Plato, "so delightful as the hearing or the speaking of truth"—for this reason there is no conversation so agreeable as that of the man of integrity, who hears without any intention to betray, and speaks without any intention to deceive.

—THOMAS SHERLOCK

LEARNING OBJECTIVES

Upon completion of this chapter, the reader will be able to:

- Understand that in each encounter with another person there is the spoken word that may not always clearly describe the intent of the message.

- Understand how values are intertwined in the communication process and how they can be instrumental in changing the course of one's journey through life.

To laugh often and love much; to win the respect of intelligent persons and the affection of children; to earn the approbation of honest citizens and endure the betrayal of false friends; to appreciate beauty; to find the best in others; to give of one's self; to leave the world a bit better, whether by a healthy child, a garden patch or a redeemed social condition; to have played and laughed with enthusiasm and sung with exultation; to know even one life has breathed easier because you have lived—this is to have succeeded.

—Bessie Anderson Stanley

The Pillars of Moral Strength list many of the virtues and values that make up each individual's moral character. What sets each individual apart from one another? In the final analysis, it is the degree and worth a person assigns to each virtue and value and the price he or she is willing to pay to be the person he or she wants to be. Believing requires practicing what you believe. If we do not possess the courage to do what is right, all other virtues begin to crumble and our lives become empty. The virtues and values listed on the pillars of moral strength are not merely words but they do define who we are.

Each person must evaluate for himself who he is, what values and moral strengths are important. When responding to the discussion questions following the closet drama in this chapter, apply the virtues and values presented in the Pillars of Moral Strength.

The closet drama that follows is designed to provide the reader with a better understanding of communications, human conflict, and the real world of working relationships. This drama is intriguing in that it arises out of the complex and diversified affairs of humanity.

My words fly up, my thoughts remain below: Words without thoughts never to heaven go.

—William Shakespeare

Communication is the exchange of thoughts, messages, or information through speech, signals, writing, or behavior. It is the art and technique of using words effectively to impart information or ideas. The process of communication includes both verbal and nonverbal messages. Communication requires a sender, a message, and an intended recipient, the receiver.

Communications can be transmitted verbally through words, which are the tools of thought. The more words you thoroughly understand, the more effectively you can articulate your thoughts and ideas to other people. The sender of information can also transmit a message through body language, posture, gestures, facial expressions, and eye contact. Clothing styles, hairstyles, and tone of voice are forms of nonverbal communication. *Nonverbal communication* has been called the silent language and plays a key role in the day-to-day communications process. During face-to-face communication, body language and the tone of one's voice play a significant role, and they may have greater impact on the listener than the intended content of the spoken words.

Both managers and employees tend to perceive each new experience as reinforcing preconceived notions and biases and, at the same time, screen out those things that do not strengthen their ideas or individual conceptions of the real world. There is a tendency to make value judgments from one's own perspective and to evaluate all new knowledge according to its positive or negative impact on preconceived beliefs.

The sender's personal filters and the receiver's personal filters may vary based on different religious beliefs, regional traditions, cultures, gender, race, and more, which may

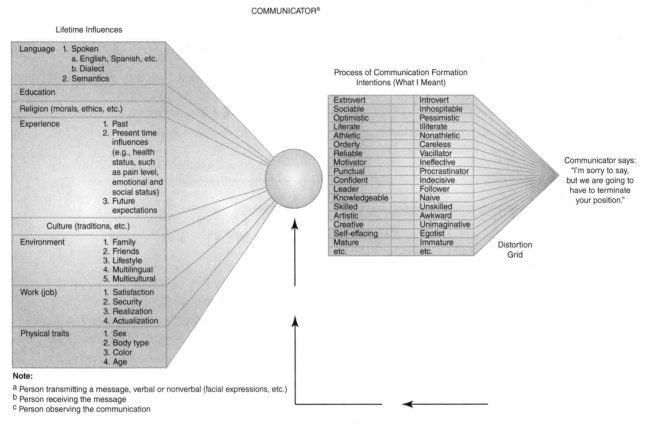

FIGURE 15-1 Process of Communications

alter the intended meaning of the message. Barriers to effective communication include the *noise interferences*: (1) environmental (e.g., disruption of communication by a barking dog); (2) physiological impairment (e.g., deafness, blindness, pain); (3) semantic (e.g., "coke" could refer to coal, cocaine, or a beverage); (4) syntactical (e.g., mistakes in grammar); (5) organizational (e.g., corporate policies on grievance procedures that differ from the employee handbooks); (6) cultural (e.g., stereotyping the followers of a particular religion because of extremists); and (7) psychological (e.g., stress, fear, anger, or sadness that may cause someone to lose focus in the moment and thus distort effective communications). A person's personal beliefs, lack of motivation, personality conflicts, and resistance to change often prevent the parties to a conversation from effectively communicating with one another. For communication between two people to be effective, each person must recognize and seek to overcome barriers that prevent it. It should be remembered that with each new person added to a conversation, the barriers to effective communications becomes more complex.

The chart in **Figure 15-1** is helpful in understanding the communications process that unfolds in the following case drama. Health care professionals, regardless of their field of training without a doubt will face similar issues during their career. This drama ends with a variety of thought-provoking questions.

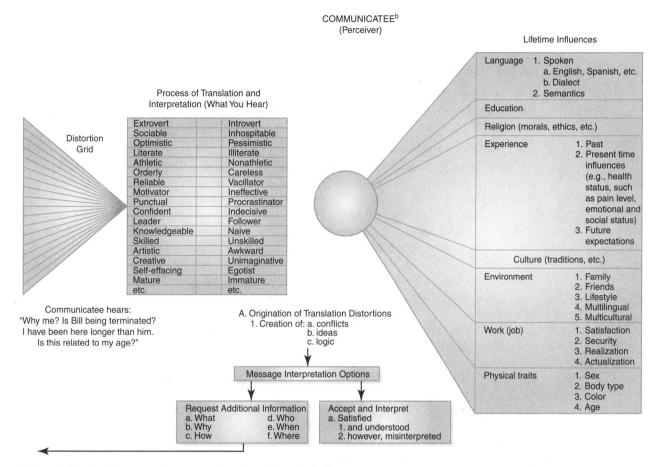

FIGURE 15-1 Process of Communications (*Continued*)

Case: Code of Silence

Characters

Mr. Daniel Marcus: Administrative reviewer

Magistrate: Hearing officer

Counselor Hadrian: Counsel representing Mr. Marcus

Mr. Damon Antonio: Nurse reviewer

Counselor Luke: Counsel representing the defendants

Dr. Machiavelli: Physician reviewer

Ms. Ophelia Cicero: Athens Health Center guide

Ms. Margaret Galeria: Nurse trainee

Dr. Caesar: Patient's physician

Mr. Bruce Verus: Mr. Marcus's manager

Ms. Carol Titus: Mr. Verus's manager

Settings

Rome: Mr. Marcus's hometown

Health Review Council: An entity responsible for evaluating the quality of care in health centers from Rome to Athens.

Courtroom of the Chief Magistrate: Site of the hearing in Athens

Athens Health Center: A local medical facility in Athens that Mr. Marcus was assigned to review

Pelopidas Street Inn: Hotel where the reviewers lodged

Daniel Marcus worked for the Health Review Council, whose mission is to review the quality of patient care in health care settings from Maine to California and Alaska to Puerto Rico. He traveled much of the time, writing, consulting, educating, and reviewing the quality of care rendered to patients. His travels took him to hundreds of health centers in villages and cities. In order to have some semblance of family life, he stayed at various inns during his travels. He sacrificed family life to serve a call and a mission to help improve the quality of patient care by encouraging each health center to set higher standards and to practice state-of-the-art medicine—to fly with eagles. Daniel encouraged caregivers to dare to dream, to become possibility optimists and not impossibility pessimists.

Daniel collected numerous practices from the centers he visited, sharing them throughout his travels. He spent 15 years traveling, reviewing patient care centers, and organizing the information that he had gathered solely to share that information with his colleagues, the Health Review Council leadership as well as the health centers he visited. He encouraged the brightest and best to freely share best practices for improving the health of the people. He challenged many not to merely collect and sell health care information but to provide it freely to all health care centers. Even the Health Review Council eventually recognized from Daniel's work that best practices should be freely shared with health care organizations that ultimately served to improve the quality of patient care.

As politics began to change in Rome and Athens with the appointment of new and inexperienced members to the Health Review Council, Daniel watched as leadership turned back the clock by implementing decisions long abandoned by the previous leadership. He struggled in making a decision to leave his position where he was certain he made an enduring difference. Daniel, however, decided to pursue his passion for writing. He describes here the defining moments that led him at the end of the day to give notice to the Health Review Council of his decision to leave, a fortuitous decision for him. Those defining moments that led to Daniel's ultimate decision to leave his employment with the Health Review Council followed a long and mysterious flow of events that were revealed during a hearing before the chief magistrate in Athens, where the drama begins and ends.

Events of Sunday, October 2

[Counselor Hadrian prepares to question Mr. Antonio regarding his October 2 arrival at the Pelopidas Street Inn in Athens.]

Magistrate: Counselor Hadrian, you may proceed with your questioning.

Counselor Hadrian: Magistrate, for the record, this complaint was filed on behalf of Mr. Marcus, who was abruptly removed, without provocation, from his review of the Athens Health Center on Pelopidas Street in Athens.

Magistrate: Counselor Hadrian, you may proceed.

Counselor Hadrian: I would like to call Mr. Antonio to the stand.

Magistrate: So granted.

[Counselor Hadrian calls Mr. Antonio to the witness stand.]

Counselor Hadrian: Could you please state your full name?

Mr. Antonio: Mr. Damon Antonio.

Counselor Hadrian: Who is your employer?

Mr. Antonio: The Health Review Council.

Counselor Hadrian: Where is the council located?

Mr. Antonio: In Washington, DC.

Counselor Hadrian: Could you tell the magistrate what your position is with the council?

Mr. Antonio: I am a nurse reviewer.

Counselor Hadrian: Could you describe what you do as a nurse reviewer for the council?

Mr. Antonio: I review health centers' quality of care provided to the citizens of Rome to Athens.

Counselor Hadrian: Mr. Antonio, could you describe for the magistrate what can happen to a center if it should fail to meet care standards?

Mr. Antonio: It can lose its Medicaid and Medicare reimbursement funding.

Counselor Hadrian: Do you review centers in a particular region of the United States?

Mr. Antonio: No, I am not assigned to any particular region of the country.

Counselor Hadrian: How long have you been reviewing health centers with the Health Review Council?

Mr. Antonio: Approximately 7 years.

Counselor Hadrian: Are you aware of how many years Mr. Marcus had worked for the Health Review Council?

Counselor Luke: Objection.

Magistrate: I will allow the question if he knows the answer.

[The magistrate looks at Mr. Antonio.]

Magistrate: You may answer the question if you know the answer, Mr. Antonio.

Mr. Antonio: Over 16 years.

Counselor Hadrian: Prior to October 2, had you ever worked with Dr. Machiavelli?

Mr. Antonio: Yes, the previous week.

Counselor Hadrian: Do you know how long Dr. Machiavelli had worked for the Health Review Council at that time?

Counselor Luke: Objection.

Magistrate: Again, I will allow the question if he knows the answer.

[The magistrate looks at Mr. Antonio.]

Magistrate: You may answer the question if you know the answer, Mr. Antonio.

Mr. Antonio: A year and a half.

Counselor Hadrian: Who was assigned as team leader during that review?

Mr. Antonio: I was.

Counselor Hadrian: Did there come a time when you were assigned to review health care services in Athens?

Mr. Antonio: Yes.

Counselor Hadrian: Do you know who was assigned to lead that team?

Mr. Antonio: Yes, it was Dr. Machiavelli.

Counselor Hadrian: Based on length of service, do you believe it was logical to appoint Dr. Machiavelli as team leader?

Mr. Antonio: Well, it didn't make sense. I thought it was strange.

Counselor Luke: Objection, Magistrate. He can't speak to that decision.

Magistrate: Objection sustained. That will be stricken from the record. Counselor Hadrian, you may call a witness who can address that issue at a later time. You may proceed with your questioning.

Counselor Hadrian: Do you recall the dates of that review?

Mr. Antonio: No.

Counselor Hadrian: Would an itinerary from that trip refresh your recollection?

Mr. Antonio: Yes.

Counselor Hadrian: Magistrate, I would like to approach Mr. Antonio with what has been labeled Exhibit A, the October assignment sheet for Mr. Marcus.

Magistrate: You may proceed.

[Counselor Hadrian hands Exhibit A to Mr. Antonio.]

Counselor Hadrian: Do you recognize this document?

Mr. Antonio: Yes.

Counselor Hadrian: What do you recognize Exhibit A to be?

Mr. Antonio: The October assignment sheet for Mr. Marcus.

Counselor Hadrian: Looking at Exhibit A, is it a fair and accurate representation of the health center to which you were assigned to work?

Mr. Antonio: Yes.

Counselor Hadrian: Does this refresh your recollection as to your work assignment?

Mr. Antonio: Yes, it does.

Counselor Hadrian: What were the dates of your assignment in Athens?

Mr. Antonio: October 3 through 7.

Counselor Hadrian: What health center were you assigned to review?

Mr. Antonio: Athens Health Center on Pelopidas Street.

Counselor Hadrian: Does Mr. Marcus's itinerary reflect which health reviewers were assigned to review the Athens Health Center on Pelopidas Street?

Mr. Antonio: Yes.

Counselor Hadrian: Could you read the names and titles of those health reviewers listed on the assignment sheet?

Mr. Antonio: Yes, Mr. Daniel Marcus, administrator reviewer. Dr. Machiavelli, physician reviewer. Mr. Damon Antonio, nurse reviewer. Ms. Margaret Galeria, nurse review trainee.

Counselor Hadrian: Were the individuals listed on Mr. Marcus's assignment sheet present during the week that you reviewed patient care at the Athens Health Center?

Mr. Antonio: Yes, they were.

Counselor Hadrian: Can you tell the magistrate where you stayed in Athens?

Mr. Antonio: Yes, the Pelopidas Street Inn.

Counselor Hadrian: Is that on the same street as the Athens Health Center?

Mr. Antonio: Yes, it is.

Counselor Hadrian: When did you arrive at the inn?

Mr. Antonio: On Sunday, October 2.

Counselor Hadrian: Do you recall what time of day you arrived?

Mr. Antonio: I don't recall the time. I know it was in the afternoon.

Counselor Hadrian: Was it two o'clock or three o'clock?

Counselor Luke: I object, Mr. Antonio has already answered this question. He doesn't know what time he arrived.

Magistrate: Objection sustained.

Counselor Hadrian: Upon your arrival at the inn, did you observe Mr. Marcus in the lobby area?

Mr. Antonio: Yes, I did. I had just gotten off an elevator and he was sitting at a table.

Counselor Hadrian: What was he doing at the table?

Mr. Antonio: He was having a late lunch as I recall.

Counselor Hadrian: Did you have a conversation with him?

Mr. Antonio: Yes, I walked past the registration desk to greet him.

Counselor Hadrian: Do you recall that conversation?

Mr. Antonio: Yes.

Counselor Hadrian: Could you describe your conversation with Mr. Marcus?

Mr. Antonio: I said, "Daniel, I haven't seen you in a long time. How are you doing?"

Counselor Hadrian: And what, if anything, was his response?

Mr. Antonio: He said he was doing well and asked how I was.

Counselor Hadrian: Was there any further conversation?

Mr. Antonio: Yes. I asked about how his wife was doing.

Counselor Hadrian: Why did you ask about his wife?

Mr. Antonio: She had some medical problems.

Counselor Hadrian: And what was his response?

Mr. Antonio: As I recall, he said she was doing fine.

Counselor Hadrian: Did there come a time during your conversation with Mr. Marcus when you asked him if he knew or had ever reviewed health centers with Dr. Machiavelli?

Mr. Antonio: Yes, I asked him if he knew or ever worked with Dr. Machiavelli.

Counselor Hadrian: Had you ever worked with Mr. Marcus before?

Mr. Antonio: Yes.

Counselor Hadrian: Did you enjoy working with Mr. Marcus?

Counselor Luke: I object to the question, Your Honor. I see no relevance for asking this question.

[The magistrate hesitates for a moment.]

Gossip May Put an Evil Eye on People

"Gossip changes the way we view people, but it also changes the way we literally see a person," said Lisa Barrett, . . . a psychology professor at Northeastern University, in an interview. "Gossip reaches all the way down into our visual system."

Christian Torres, The Washington Post, *June 6, 2011*

Magistrate: Counselor Hadrian?

Counselor Hadrian: Your Honor, I will establish the relevance of that question as I continue my questioning.

Magistrate: I will allow the question. Mr. Antonio, you may respond.

Mr. Antonio: Yes, I enjoyed working with him.

Counselor Hadrian: What, if anything else, did you say?

Mr. Antonio: I don't recall.

Counselor Hadrian: Let me refresh your recollection. Do you recall saying that Dr. Machiavelli was a physician health reviewer?

Mr. Antonio: Yes, I did say that.

Counselor Hadrian: Do you recall saying Dr. Machiavelli was a retired admiral?

Mr. Antonio: Yes, I did say that.

Counselor Hadrian: Were you ever in the military?

Mr. Antonio: Yes, I was. Well, actually I am now in the air force reserves.

Counselor Hadrian: And what was you rank?

Mr. Antonio: I was a captain in the air force. Actually I still am. I am in the reserves.

Counselor Hadrian: Since you were rushing to check in, why was this information so important?

Mr. Antonio: Well, I was trying to establish if Mr. Marcus knew Dr. Machiavelli.

Counselor Hadrian: What was Mr. Marcus's response?

Mr. Antonio: Excuse me, what is the question?

Counselor Hadrian: What was Mr. Marcus's response to your question as to whether or not he knew Dr. Machiavelli?

Mr. Antonio: He said that he did not know him.

Counselor Hadrian: Did he say anything else?

Mr. Antonio: Yes, he asked me why I had asked that question.

Counselor Hadrian: Did you answer his question?

Mr. Antonio: No.

Counselor Hadrian: And why did you not answer his question?

Mr. Antonio: I told him that I had just worked with Dr. Machiavelli the previous week and that I would like to know his impression of him at the end of the Athens Health Center review.

Counselor Hadrian: What role did you play in your previous health center review with Dr. Machiavelli?

Mr. Antonio: I was the team leader in charge of the overall review.

Counselor Hadrian: You stated that you had just worked with Dr. Machiavelli, is that correct?

Mr. Antonio: Yes.

Counselor Hadrian: And you are referring to the week prior to the Athens Health Center review?

Mr. Antonio: Yes.

Counselor Hadrian: Was there any other conversation that you recall from this brief encounter with Mr. Marcus?

Mr. Antonio: No, not to my recollection.

Counselor Hadrian: So your conversation was somewhat short, is that correct?

Mr. Antonio: Yes, it was.

Counselor Hadrian: So was it less than, or more than, 5 minutes in length?

Counselor Luke: I object, Your Honor. That question has already been answered.

Magistrate: I will allow the question. You may answer the question, Mr. Antonio.

Mr. Antonio: Less than 5 minutes.

Counselor Hadrian: Was it less than 4 minutes?

Counselor Luke: Again, I object, Your Honor. Mr. Antonio has already answered that question.

Magistrate: Objection sustained.

Counselor Hadrian: So, Mr. Antonio. We have established that you spoke to Mr. Marcus for less than 5 minutes. You asked how he and his wife were, and then you asked Mr. Marcus if he would give you his impression of Dr. Machiavelli at the end of the Athens Health Center review. Is that correct?

Mr. Antonio: Yes.

Counselor Hadrian: Why was your conversation so short, especially since you had not seen Mr. Marcus in such a long time?

Counselor Luke: I object, Your Honor; that question has already been answered.

Magistrate: Objection overruled. I will allow the witness to answer.

Mr. Antonio: I was just checking into the hotel. I wanted to get my things to my room.

Counselor Hadrian: So you were happy to see that Marcus was on the review?

Mr. Antonio: Yes.

Counselor Hadrian: And why was that?

Mr. Antonio: I had worked with him before. He has always been pleasant to work with, and I enjoyed his professional stature, wisdom, and sense of humor.

Counselor Hadrian: Did you meet up with Mr. Marcus later that day to discuss old times, anything?

Mr. Antonio: No, I did not.

Counselor Hadrian: So you had not seen Mr. Marcus in some time, you always enjoyed reviewing with him, and you did not meet with him later in the day. Yet, your third question was to ascertain his impression of Dr. Machiavelli at the end of the review. Is that correct?

Mr. Antonio: Yes, I guess, about the third question.

Counselor Hadrian: Did you have any other questions at that time?

Mr. Antonio: No, I just told him I had to check in.

Counselor Hadrian: What was so important about asking that specific question that you were willing to wait 5 days for an answer?

Counselor Luke: I object, Your Honor. That question has already been answered.

Magistrate: I will allow the question. You may answer the question, Mr. Antonio.

Mr. Antonio: Well, I felt he had sort of a military style of reviewing. It seemed as though he thought he had some sort of right to be in charge of the previous week's survey.

Counselor Hadrian: But he was not the team leader. Is that correct?

Mr. Antonio: That is correct.

Counselor Hadrian: You were the team leader. Correct?

Mr. Antonio: Yes, and I think he resented that.

Counselor Hadrian: And why do you believe he resented that?

Mr. Antonio: Partially because I was at a lower rank and in a different branch of the military. Also, I was thinking that he was having difficulty in adapting to civilian life.

Counselor Hadrian: So on the week we are talking about here, Dr. Machiavelli is now the team leader? Is that correct?

Mr. Antonio: Yes.

Counselor Hadrian: So were you concerned about Dr. Machiavelli being in charge?

Mr. Antonio: Yes, sort of.

Counselor Hadrian: So Mr. Marcus was a friend?

Mr. Antonio: Yes.

Counselor Hadrian: A good friend.

Counselor Luke: Magistrate, I object. The question has been asked and answered.

Magistrate: I will allow the question. Counselor Hadrian, you may proceed.

Counselor Hadrian: So you considered Marcus a trusted colleague with whom you enjoyed working.

Mr. Antonio: Yes, I did.

Counselor Hadrian: And, to your knowledge, he thought the same of you?

Mr. Antonio: Yes.

Counselor Hadrian: Yet you foresaw there might be problems on this review?

Counselor Luke: Magistrate, I object to the form of the question.

Magistrate: Your objection is overruled! Counselor Hadrian, you may proceed with your questioning.

Counselor Hadrian: Mr. Antonio, you stated that you and Mr. Marcus had a good working relationship, yet you failed to warn your friend of a possible problem ahead during this review. Is that correct?

Counselor Luke: Magistrate, I object.

Magistrate: I will allow the question.

Mr. Antonio: Could you repeat the question?

Counselor Hadrian: In summary, did you hang your friend out to dry?

Counselor Luke: Magistrate, I object. Counselor Hadrian is badgering my client.

Magistrate: Objection sustained. Counselor Hadrian, do you wish to reword that question?

Counselor Hadrian: No. I have no further questions at this time but reserve the right to recall Mr. Antonio to the witness stand.

Magistrate: Granted. We will take a short recess.

Events of Wednesday Afternoon, October 5

[Counselor Hadrian questions Mr. Marcus regarding Day 3 of the Athens Health Center review.]

Counselor Hadrian: Before we proceed, could you please verify if the testimony previously provided by Mr. Antonio is, to your recollection, fair and accurate?

Mr. Marcus: Yes, it was.

Counselor Hadrian: Thank you. Could you please describe for the magistrate what occurred on the afternoon of Wednesday, October 5?

Mr. Marcus: Yes, I can. I would like to refer to my notes.

Counselor Hadrian: Magistrate, I would like to place into evidence the notes that Mr. Marcus is going to refer to as he describes what occurred on the afternoon of Wednesday, October 5.

Magistrate: You may proceed.

Counselor Hadrian: Mr. Marcus, how long have you been working for the Health Review Council?

Marcus: Approximately 15 years.

Counselor Hadrian: Could you please describe for the magistrate what occurred on the afternoon of Wednesday, October 5?

Mr. Marcus: Yes, I can. At approximately 12:50 p.m. Dr. Machiavelli asked what activity I had planned to review for the afternoon.

Counselor Hadrian: And what did you say?

Mr. Marcus: I said, since none of the reviewers asked for a complex medical case, I was planning to ask the health center's staff for such a case to review.

Counselor Hadrian: What, if anything else, did you say to Dr. Machiavelli at that time?

Mr. Marcus: I asked if that was okay with him.

Counselor Hadrian: And what did he say?

Mr. Marcus: He said, "That sounds like a good idea."

Counselor Hadrian: Then what happened?

Mr. Marcus: Ophelia Cicero, my Athens Health Center guide, opened the door to the room where I had just finished eating lunch with my colleagues. She entered the room and inquired if I had a particular case in mind that I would like to review.

Counselor Hadrian: And what did you say?

Mr. Marcus: I said yes and suggested a complex medical case.

Counselor Hadrian: What is the responsibility of the health center guide?

Mr. Marcus: That person is responsible for leading me to each patient care area where I plan to review a case. Ophelia also had a scribe with her who was assigned to take notes on all conversations.

Counselor Hadrian: So, Ms. Cicero located the type of case you requested?

Mr. Marcus: Yes, Ophelia said that she had such a case. She escorted me to the patient care unit where the patient had been admitted.

Counselor Hadrian: Did you review the patient's record?

Mr. Marcus: Yes, the charge nurse searched for the patient's record that I planned to review and brought it to me.

Counselor Hadrian: Is that part of the patient care review process?

Mr. Marcus: Yes, it is.

Counselor Hadrian: Then what happened?

Mr. Marcus: I was introduced to the staff nurse assigned to care for the patient.

Counselor Hadrian: Then what happened?

Mr. Marcus: The staff nurse reviewed the record with me.

Counselor Hadrian: What questions, if any, did you ask her?

Mr. Marcus: I asked her for some preliminary information about the patient, which included the patient's age and diagnosis.

Counselor Hadrian: How did the nurse respond?

Mr. Marcus: She answered my questions, providing me with the patient's admitting information and medical problems.

Counselor Hadrian: Did you ask any other questions?

Mr. Marcus: Yes. While reviewing the patient's lab results I noticed that some tests were out of normal range. I asked whether any of the patient's lab results helped to identify the patient's medical problems.

Counselor Hadrian: So that is part of the Health Review Council's expectations of you?

Mr. Marcus: Yes, it is.

Counselor Hadrian: What was the nurse's response?

Mr. Marcus: She said that she could not answer the question. A nurse manager in the room where I was reviewing the patient's record asked if I would like to speak to Dr. Caesar, the patient's physician.

Counselor Hadrian: What was your response?

Mr. Marcus: I said sure, provided he is available and not too busy caring for other patients.

Counselor Hadrian: Then what happened?

Mr. Marcus: Dr. Caesar was summoned. Upon entering the room, he stood inside the doorway, at which time I introduced myself. He appeared somewhat disturbed that he had been interrupted in his work.

Counselor Hadrian: In your opinion, why do you believe Dr. Caesar was disturbed?

Counselor Luke: Objection, Magistrate. I see no relevance to this question. It is mere speculation as to why the physician was disturbed.

Magistrate: I will allow the question. Mr. Marcus, you may proceed with your response.

Mr. Marcus: It is normal, in general, for physicians to be anxious when questioned by a reviewer from the Health Review Council. Reviewers are not always the highlight of a physician's or any other caregiver's day. To be questioned about a patient's care can be intimidating.

Counselor Hadrian: Then what happened?

Mr. Marcus: Well, he introduced himself and he asked what questions I had and what kind of physician I was.

Counselor Hadrian: What was your response?

Counselor Hadrian: I stated that I was not a physician and that I just had a few questions for him.

Counselor Hadrian: What questions did you ask?

Mr. Marcus: I asked Dr. Caesar if the patient's lab results revealed any other disease processes than what the patient was admitted for.

Counselor Hadrian: What was his response?

Mr. Marcus: He said that he was there only to treat the patient's immediate needs and not all of the patient's complex issues.

Counselor Hadrian: Then what happened?

Mr. Marcus: I let the remaining questions pass and asked if it would be okay if I visited with the patient.

Counselor Hadrian: What did he say?

Mr. Marcus: He said that would be fine and started to leave the room.

Counselor Hadrian: Then what happened?

Mr. Marcus: I asked Dr. Caesar if he would ask the patient if it would be okay for me to interview him.

Counselor Hadrian: And how did Dr. Caesar respond?

Mr. Marcus: He said, "That's not necessary."

Counselor Hadrian: Then what happened?

Mr. Marcus: He quickly left the conference room and walked down the hallway to the patient's room.

Counselor Hadrian: Did you follow Dr. Caesar down the hallway?

Mr. Marcus: Yes, I did. The scribe who recorded her observations of the review followed us.

Counselor Hadrian: Did you follow Dr. Caesar into the patient's room?

Mr. Marcus: No, I waited for him to return to the hallway.

Counselor Hadrian: Then what happened?

Mr. Marcus: Dr. Caesar returned and said, "I had to awaken the patient. He is willing to speak to you."

Counselor Hadrian: Then what happened?

Mr. Marcus: I entered the patient's room and walked toward the patient's bed. Dr. Caesar stood with his back to the wall facing the patient's bed. The scribe had also followed me into the room and stood by Dr. Caesar, taking notes.

Counselor Hadrian: Then what happened?

Mr. Marcus: Dr. Caesar asked me if I wanted him to leave. I said he was welcome to stay if he wished.

Counselor Hadrian: Did he remain in the room?

Mr. Marcus: Yes, and I began to introduce myself to the patient. As I began to introduce myself, the patient interrupted, "I know who you are." I asked, "How do you know?" He said with a smile, "My wife is a nurse. She works here. She told me you might be coming."

Counselor Hadrian: Then what happened?

Mr. Marcus: I said that I had only a few questions that I would like to ask him. He said okay. I asked about his care at Athens Health Center. He stated that he was receiving excellent care. After some discussion about his care, the patient repeated that he was getting very good care.

Counselor Hadrian: Then what happened?

Mr. Marcus: I thanked him for his time and for speaking to me. I began to leave the patient's room, but Dr. Caesar said he would like to say something.

Counselor Hadrian: And what did you reply?

Mr. Marcus: I said that would be fine.

Counselor Hadrian: What did Dr. Caesar say?

Mr. Marcus: He began to describe to the patient his disease process and described how he could die of his disease. I was shocked and bewildered by his comments. I looked at the patient, observing that he was traumatized and saddened.

Counselor Hadrian: Then what happened?

Mr. Marcus: I said, "You will be okay." I was not about to repeat Dr. Caesar's prognosis.

Counselor Hadrian: Why were you bewildered?

Mr. Marcus: The patient had been under Dr. Caesar's care in the hospital for 2 weeks. I could not think of a reason why Dr. Caesar would say that. The timing of that statement was inappropriate and added nothing to the interview but more stress for the patient.

Counselor Hadrian: Were you telling the patient that he would be okay clinically?

Mr. Marcus: No, I was not referring to his clinical condition but was responding to his emotional status at the time.

Counselor Hadrian: Then what happened?

Mr. Marcus: I thanked the patient again and left the room.

Counselor Hadrian: Then what happened?

Mr. Marcus: Dr. Caesar quickly followed me to the doorway, somewhat agitated, and said, "Don't you ever tell my patients they will be okay."

Counselor Hadrian: Please continue.

Mr. Marcus: A nurse asked if we could move the conversation down the hall, away from the patient's doorway, at which time Dr. Caesar asked me again, "What kind of physician are you?"

Counselor Hadrian: So he had asked you this question twice: "What kind of physician are you?"

Mr. Marcus: Yes, and I restated that I was not a physician. I attempted to calm him down, extended my hand, and thanked him for his time.

Counselor Hadrian: Did he shake your hand?

Mr. Marcus: Yes, he did. I think I caught him off guard when I extended my hand. I don't think he was expecting that.

Counselor Hadrian: Then what happened?

Mr. Marcus: He turned and walked away.

Counselor Hadrian: Were any nurses listening to you during the time you were in the hallway with Dr. Caesar?

Mr. Marcus: Yes, the scribe was taking notes, and the nurse manager was present. The nurse stated that this was unusual behavior by Dr. Caesar.

Counselor Hadrian: Then what happened?

Mr. Marcus: At that point, Ophelia had arrived and led me back up the hallway, with the scribe following closely behind. As we walked down the hall Ophelia asked what had happened, and I described the scene to her. Ophelia then asked the scribe, "Why didn't you intervene? I knew from the minute Dr. Caesar entered the chart review room he was going to be a problem. I should have stayed with you, Daniel. I would never have let him get away with that. But while you were reviewing the chart, I was called to another unit where he had had a problem with a staff nurse earlier in the day."

Counselor Hadrian: Did the scribe respond to Ms. Cicero?

Mr. Marcus: Yes, she said that she didn't think she needed to get involved.

Counselor Hadrian: Did the scribe say anything else to you?

Mr. Marcus: Yes, she later asked me if I thought she should have intervened.

Counselor Hadrian: And what did you say to her?

Mr. Marcus: I told her no and that if she intervened it might have inflamed the situation. She had to work at Athens Health Center after I left, and I didn't think she needed a poor working relationship with Dr. Caesar.

Counselor Hadrian: Do you now regret, in retrospect, her not intervening?

Counselor Luke: Magistrate, I strongly object. We are talking about what happened, not what Mr. Marcus wishes had occurred.

Magistrate: Objection sustained. Counselor Hadrian, do you have any further questions at this time?

Counselor Hadrian: Not at this time, but I will most likely recall Mr. Marcus to the witness stand.

Magistrate: I understand. We will take a short break at this time. Counselor Luke and Counselor Hadrian, I would like to see you in my chambers.

Events of Thursday Morning, October 6

The most striking contradiction of our civilization is the fundamental reverence for truth, which we profess and the thorough-going disregard for it, which we practice.

–Vilhjalmur Stefansson

[Magistrate hearing continues with Counselor Hadrian questioning Mr. Antonio.]

Counselor Hadrian: Did you know if Mr. Marcus had ever previously reviewed the Athens Health Center?

Mr. Antonio: To my knowledge, he had not.

Counselor Hadrian: Did Mr. Marcus ever say to you if he knew any employee on the staff of the Athens Health Center?

Mr. Antonio: No, he did not.

Counselor Hadrian: Did you and your colleagues brief the Athens Health Center's leadership each morning on your previous day's findings?

Mr. Antonio: Yes, we did.

Counselor Hadrian: What is the purpose of briefings?

Mr. Antonio: The reviewers describe to the health center's leadership the previous day's observations, possible written citations, as well as opportunities for improving patient care.

Counselor Hadrian: Do you recall the substance of Mr. Marcus's report on Thursday morning, which would be the beginning of the fourth day of your review of the Athens Health Center?

Mr. Antonio: I don't recall.

Counselor Hadrian: Do you recall if he was complimentary in his observations on the previous day's activities?

Mr. Antonio: I am sure he was, yes. But I don't recall the specifics. As with all the reviews that I worked on with Daniel, he was sensitive to recognizing the good things he observed. We all did that.

Counselor Hadrian: How much time is generally allotted to each health reviewer to present at the morning briefings?

Mr. Antonio: Generally 10 minutes.

Counselor Hadrian: Is that time set in stone?

Mr. Antonio: No, it is not.

Counselor Hadrian: Did the reviewers stick to the time allotted?

Mr. Antonio: No.

Counselor Hadrian: Did you stick to your time limit?

Mr. Antonio: Not always.

Counselor Hadrian: Did Dr. Machiavelli stick to his time limit?

Mr. Antonio: Not always. He had a habit of going off on tangents and criticized others for doing so.

Counselor Hadrian: So there were days that you stuck to your schedule and there were days that you did not. Is that correct?

Mr. Antonio: Yes, that is correct.

Counselor Hadrian: And why didn't you always stick to your time allotment?

Mr. Antonio: It depended on the number of observations I had.

Counselor Hadrian: Were there any other factors as to why a reviewer may have gone over his or her allotted time to present his or her report?

Mr. Antonio: Yes, it depended on how many times Dr. Machiavelli interrupted to add something in an attempt to clarify or relate a personal experience to emphasize what information a reviewer was relaying.

Counselor Hadrian: In your experience, have you ever observed a health reviewer say, "I pass" and say nothing more?

Mr. Antonio: No.

Counselor Hadrian: So reviewers generally have something to say?

Mr. Antonio: Yes, most health reviewers have something to say.

Counselor Hadrian: Do you recall Mr. Marcus reporting on a physician's disruptive behavior Thursday morning, October 6th?

Mr. Antonio: Yes, that I do remember.

Counselor Hadrian: Do you recall the physician's name?

Mr. Antonio: Yes, I do.

Counselor Hadrian: And what was his name?

Mr. Antonio: Dr. Caesar.

Counselor Hadrian: Could you summarize what Mr. Marcus reported? Question withdrawn. Mr. Antonio, can you describe what events occurred that ultimately resulted in Mr. Marcus reporting the disruptive behavior of Dr. Caesar to the hospital's leadership that morning.

Counselor Luke: Objection. Counsel has not established the physician was disruptive.

Magistrate: Objection sustained.

Counselor Hadrian: Let me reword that. Can you describe what Mr. Marcus reported at the Thursday morning leadership briefing?

Mr. Antonio: He reviewed with us what he observed during a review of a patient's care on Wednesday the 6th.

Counselor Hadrian: Is reviewing a patient's care part of the review process?

Mr. Antonio: Yes, it is.

Counselor Hadrian: So you would say that reviewing a patient's care is a fairly important aspect of the review process?

Mr. Antonio: Yes, very much so.

Counselor Hadrian: Would you say that Mr. Marcus was within his right to review the patient's case?

Mr. Antonio: Yes, that is the main purpose of our reviews. That's what we are trained to do.

Counselor Hadrian: Could you describe the kinds of activities that occur during a case review?

Mr. Antonio: Yes. The reviewer selects a case for review. Staff members who participate in the patient's care are interviewed. In complex medical cases the staff will often refer to the patient's medical record in order to more accurately respond to the reviewers questions. If the staff experiences difficulty in answering the questions, the patient's physician, if available, would be asked to help in answering the reviewers questions.

Counselor Hadrian: Do you recall if Mr. Marcus said during the Thursday morning briefing that the center's staff asked Dr. Caesar to review the patient's case with him?

Mr. Antonio: Yes, he did. He described Dr. Caesar's unprofessional conduct during the interview to both him and the patient.

Counselor Hadrian: In what way was Dr. Caesar unprofessional to Mr. Marcus?

Mr. Antonio: Following Mr. Marcus's interview with the patient, Dr. Caesar told him not to ever tell any of his patients that they would be okay.

Counselor Hadrian: In order to save time here, have you read the transcript of Mr. Marcus's testimony?

Mr. Antonio: Yes.

Counselor Hadrian: Is Mr. Marcus's description of what occurred on Wednesday afternoon in the patient's room a fair and accurate representation of what he reported on Thursday morning to the Athens Health Center leadership?

Mr. Antonio: Yes, it is accurate to my recollection.

Counselor Hadrian: When this incident began to unfold, do you recall who Mr. Marcus reported was in the patient's room with him?

Mr. Antonio: Yes, there was Mr. Marcus, Dr. Caesar, the patient, and the scribe.

Counselor Hadrian: Why did, if you know, Mr. Marcus report the incident with Dr. Caesar on Thursday morning?

Mr. Antonio: He was concerned this might be a pattern with Dr. Caesar, but he said perhaps he'd just had a bad day or been very busy. If there was a pattern of bad behavior in his record, it needed to be addressed.

Counselor Hadrian: Did you see Ms. Cicero, during the Wednesday morning briefing, lean toward Mr. Marcus and whisper something to him?

Mr. Antonio: Yes.

Counselor Hadrian: Did you ever learn what Ms. Cicero said?

Mr. Antonio. Yes, at Thursday's luncheon. Daniel told the nurse trainee and myself.

Counselor Hadrian: And what did he say?

Mr. Antonio: He said she whispered, "Good job. Your presentation was fair and well balanced."

Counselor Hadrian: And what did you think of her comments?

Mr. Antonio: I just told Daniel she was right.

Counselor Hadrian: Meaning?

Mr. Antonio: That Daniel was very diplomatic in his approach to a delicate matter. He really left it up to the Athens Health Center's leadership to determine how to handle the matter. He could have reported the incident to the Health Review Council but chose a more diplomatic route.

Counselor Hadrian: If Mr. Marcus had reported the incident to a council manager, what do you think the manager would have said to him?

Mr. Antonio: "Good job, Mr. Marcus. I am pleased that you presented this incident at the leadership meeting. This way it cannot be swept under a rug."

Counselor Hadrian: Interesting comment, Mr. Antonio. Do you think certain leaders in an organization would do such a thing?

Counselor Luke: Objection, Counselor Hadrian is asking an opinion about organizations in general.

Magistrate: Objection sustained. Counselor Hadrian, please stick to the facts of this case before me.

[Counselor Hadrian acknowledges the magistrate's admonition.]

Counselor Hadrian: Do you believe that one often gets an answer to a question by the way he or she words or asks a question?

Mr. Antonio: Yes, I do.

Counselor Hadrian: Do you believe that the tone in one's voice and the way a question is presented will influence the listener?

Mr. Antonio: Yes.

Counselor Hadrian: So the listener could draw the conclusion he or she wanted or thought was intended?

Mr. Antonio: Yes.

Counselor Hadrian: So if Dr. Machiavelli had reported Mr. Marcus's encounter with Dr. Caesar to the Health Review Council, the response he received from the council might have been different than if Mr. Marcus reported this incident, or let's say, even you?

Mr. Antonio: Yes, of course. I first of all saw no reason for Dr. Machiavelli to have, well, to be blunt, to have gotten involved and offered his two cents.

Counselor Hadrian: If you had reported Mr. Marcus's encounter with Dr. Caesar to the council, based on your previous reviews with Dr. Machiavelli, do you think you might have presented the incident differently than he would have?

[Mr. Antonio hesitates for a time that seems like forever, and the magistrate waits patiently for an answer.]

Mr. Antonio: Yes, I do. Everyone is different.

Counselor Hadrian: Do you recall if Mr. Marcus spent an inordinate amount of time reporting on his encounter with Dr. Caesar?

Mr. Antonio: No, he had a long report but presented it within a reasonable amount of time.

Counselor Hadrian: Do you think Dr. Machiavelli would agree with you?

Mr. Antonio: No.

Counselor Hadrian: And why is that?

Mr. Antonio: It was just an observation. Well, he did comment later that the morning briefings had to be shortened.

Counselor Hadrian: As the reviewers presented their reports that morning, were there ever interruptions by Dr. Machiavelli?

Mr. Antonio: Yes, he generally had a few of his own personal stories that he added to the conversation.

Counselor Hadrian: Had he interrupted your report and made further comments?

Mr. Antonio: Yes, on several occasions that morning.

Counselor Hadrian: Did he interrupt Mr. Marcus on Thursday morning?

Mr. Antonio: Not as I recall.

Counselor Hadrian: Do you recall Dr. Machiavelli being uneasy and fidgeting in his chair as Mr. Marcus presented his report?

[Mr. Antonio again hesitates. The magistrate appears uneasy and ready for a break.]

Magistrate: Mr. Antonio, could you please answer the question?

Mr. Antonio: Yes, I do recall that Dr. Machiavelli was uneasy, actually a bit rude in his facial expressions.

Counselor Hadrian: Where were you sitting at the time Mr. Marcus presented his report?

Mr. Antonio: I was sitting at the head of the table with Ms. Galeria and other members of the organization's leadership.

Counselor Hadrian: So you could actually see Dr. Machiavelli's facial expressions, let's say, in a face-to-face manner?

Mr. Antonio: That is correct.

Counselor Hadrian: Are you aware if anyone else in the Athens Health Center's leadership observed Dr. Machiavelli's mannerisms?

Mr. Antonio: Yes. The table was oval in shape and I could easily see that the leadership must have been wondering why Dr. Machiavelli seemed so disengaged with Mr. Marcus.

Counselor Hadrian: So you were actually sitting where the organization's leadership could observe Dr. Machiavelli's behavior?

Counselor Luke: Objection, this question has already been answered.

Magistrate: Objection overruled. Mr. Antonio, you may proceed with your answer.

Mr. Antonio: Yes, I was.

Counselor Hadrian: Did Ms. Galeria also note his behavior?

Mr. Antonio: Yes.

Counselor Hadrian: Are you aware as to whether or not Mr. Marcus was distracted by his behavior?

Mr. Antonio: I believe so, but I noticed he tried not to look at Dr. Machiavelli's body language. Actually, I'm sure it was distracting to him.

Counselor Hadrian: Did Mr. Marcus mention to you whether or not the Athens Health Center's leadership had noted Dr. Machiavelli's behavior?

Mr. Antonio: Yes, according to Daniel, Ophelia said, "Dr. Machiavelli appeared to be somewhat disengaged with you. He didn't do this with any of the other reviewers."

Counselor Hadrian: So Mr. Marcus pretty much felt the same way?

Mr. Antonio: Yes, he remarked that he had never met Dr. Machiavelli and could not understand his behavior.

Counselor Hadrian: Do you agree that Dr. Machiavelli's behavior was out of line in that setting?

Mr. Antonio: Yes, without question.

Counselor Hadrian: Magistrate, I have no further questions at this time.

Events of Thursday Luncheon, October 6

[After a short recess, Counselor Hadrian recalls Mr. Antonio to the witness stand.]

Counselor Hadrian: Returning to that afternoon luncheon on Thursday, where did you have lunch?

Mr. Antonio: In the Athens Health Center's library.

Counselor Hadrian: Did there come a time at lunch that Mr. Marcus again asked why you had asked him for his impression of Dr. Machiavelli at the end of the survey?

Mr. Antonio: Yes.

Counselor Hadrian: Was Dr. Machiavelli in the room when this conversation took place?

Mr. Antonio: No.

Counselor Hadrian: Do you know where he was?

Mr. Antonio: I am not sure. He had left the room. I think he went to speak to the CEO.

Counselor Hadrian: Did you answer Mr. Marcus's question?

Mr. Antonio: I told Daniel I did not want to get in the middle of this.

Counselor Hadrian: Mr. Antonio, reflecting back to Sunday in the Pelopidas Street Inn, don't you think you already placed yourself in the middle?

Counselor Luke: Objection.

Magistrate: I will allow the question. You can answer the question, Mr. Antonio.

Mr. Antonio: Well, uh, well, I didn't think this would happen.

Counselor Hadrian: What did you expect to happen? Dr. Machiavelli would give Marcus a hard time?

Mr. Antonio: Well, I didn't expect it to go this far.

Counselor Hadrian: Far? What do you mean?

Mr. Antonio: Well, Dr. Machiavelli had a bit of, uh, uh . . .

Counselor Hadrian: Uh, uh, what?

Mr. Antonio: I just didn't think Dr. Machiavelli would be so hard on Daniel.

Counselor Hadrian: I see. So, it sounds like he gave you some problems during a previous review?

[Mr. Antonio hesitates as the magistrate stares at him. Even the magistrate guards seem mesmerized by the hearing. Counselor Hadrian, getting impatient, asks the question again.]

Counselor Hadrian: Mr. Antonio, could you please answer the question?

Mr. Antonio: Could you please repeat the question?

Counselor Hadrian: Did you have a previous encounter with Dr. Machiavelli at a previous health center review?

Mr. Antonio: Well, yes, I did.

Counselor Hadrian: And you are referring to the health center review that took place the week prior to the one that was being conducted at the Athens Health Center?

Mr. Antonio: Yes, I am.

Counselor Hadrian: Were you happy or unhappy with Dr. Machiavelli's behavior at that review, that is, the review prior to the Athens review?

Mr. Antonio: I was not totally happy.

Counselor Hadrian: So, again, you chose to allow Marcus to walk into the minefield?

Counselor Luke: I object to this line of questioning.

Magistrate: Objection . . .

[Before the magistrate can say "sustained" or "overruled, " Counselor Hadrian breaks in . . .]

Counselor Hadrian: I withdraw my question.

Magistrate: Withdrawal noted. You may proceed.

Counselor Hadrian: And now that Dr. Machiavelli was in charge of the review at the Athens Health Center, you thought his style would match his name and that he might have met his match in Mr. Marcus. Is that right?

Counselor Luke: Objection, he is leading the witness.

Magistrate: Objection sustained.

Counselor Hadrian: What, if anything else, did Mr. Marcus say to you about you being placed in the middle of something?

Mr. Antonio: He just kept asking me, in the middle of what? He was trying to prod an answer out of me.

Counselor Hadrian: And you refused to give an answer. Is that correct?

Mr. Antonio: Yes.

Counselor Hadrian: Did he say anything else that you recall?

Mr. Antonio: Uh, no, uh, I mean I don't recall.

Counselor Hadrian: Did he refresh your memory?

Mr. Antonio: What do you mean?

Counselor Hadrian: Going back to your conversation with Mr. Marcus on the first day in the inn lobby, did he ask again at lunch on Thursday why you wanted to know what he thought of Dr. Machiavelli on the last day of the Athens review?

Mr. Antonio: Yes, he did.

Counselor Hadrian: And you replied you would tell him on Friday at the end of the Athens review. Is that correct?

Mr. Antonio: Yes.

Counselor Hadrian: So, previously, on the record, Mr. Marcus said he never met Dr. Machiavelli. Is that correct?

Mr. Antonio: Yes.

Counselor Hadrian: So you knew that there was something Mr. Marcus should know, but you sort of let him walk into the middle of a minefield and find out for himself. And you call yourself his friend. Is that correct?

Counselor Luke: Magistrate, I have already objected to this question!

Magistrate: I will allow the question. I believe I see where Counselor Hadrian is leading, and we need to hear it. You may answer the question, Mr. Antonio.

Mr. Antonio: Well, I wouldn't put it that way.

Counselor Hadrian: How would you put it?

Counselor Luke: I object.

Magistrate: Objection overruled. You may answer the question.

Mr. Antonio: I just did not want to get involved. I did not expect Dr. Machiavelli would be so rude to Marcus.

Counselor Hadrian: What else did Mr. Marcus say during that luncheon?

Mr. Antonio: He said Dr. Machiavelli was not responsive to him except that Dr. Machiavelli shifted around in his chair with inappropriate body language during the morning sessions when he presented his daily report to the Athens leadership. He said, "I don't even know him. Why is he doing that?"

Counselor Hadrian: Do you recall anything else that Mr. Marcus might have said regarding Machiavelli's body language?

Mr. Antonio: No.

Counselor Hadrian: Let me refresh your memory. Do you recall Mr. Marcus saying to you and Ms. Galeria that the Athens staff sensed that Dr. Machiavelli appeared to be disengaged with him the morning he made his reports and that Dr. Machiavelli did not do this with any of the other health reviewers?

Mr. Antonio: Yes, I believe I answered that before. I recall that.

Counselor Hadrian: Do you recall if anyone else was present in the room during this conversation?

Mr. Antonio: Yes, as you just said, Ms. Galeria, the nurse trainee.

Counselor Hadrian: Did she participate in this conversation?

Mr. Antonio: No.

Counselor Hadrian: Magistrate, I may wish to call Ms. Galeria to the witness stand at a later date.

Magistrate: Understood.

Counselor Hadrian: Before we proceed, do you recall if, earlier during the Thursday luncheon, Mr. Marcus gave you some sort of CD?

Mr. Antonio: Yes, he did.

Counselor Hadrian: In general, do you recall what was contained on that disc?

Mr. Antonio: Yes, Mr. Marcus had collected thousands of pages of best practices over the years that he shared with reviewers and the health centers he reviewed.

Counselor Hadrian: Could you describe for the magistrate why Mr. Marcus collected and distributed those practices?

Mr. Antonio: Yes, I think so. It was sort of a mission with him to share best practices so that health care organizations did not have to waste valuable time "reinventing the wheel." He believed that human resources should be used wisely, and if organizations were willing to share with one another, everyone benefited.

Counselor Hadrian: Are you aware of anyone else in your career that has embarked on such a project?

Mr. Antonio: No, I am not. Mr. Marcus is the only reviewer that I am aware of.

Counselor Hadrian: Since, as you well know, Mr. Marcus is no longer with the Health Review Council, has it come to your attention that the council is now sharing such or similar information freely, sort of borrowing the idea from Mr. Marcus?

Mr. Antonio: Yes, I am aware that this has occurred.

Counselor Hadrian: About this disc, did Mr. Marcus provide you with any specific instructions as to with whom it should or should not be shared?

Mr. Antonio: Yes.

Counselor Hadrian: What was his request?

Mr. Antonio: He requested that we use these disc files for personal reference. He asked that they not be shared with others at this time. He was in the process of editing them and wanted to share a copy with us.

Counselor Hadrian: Did you agree to his request?

Mr. Antonio: Yes, I did.

Counselor Hadrian: Are you aware that Ms. Galeria received a copy of the disc?

Mr. Antonio: Yes.

Counselor Hadrian: Did she agree to Mr. Marcus's request?

Mr. Antonio: Yes, she did. We both agreed.

Counselor Hadrian: Do you recall shortly after the Athens Health Center review that a member of the Health Review Council used certain files from that disc during a conference call with all of your colleagues in Rome to improve the quality of the conference call?

Mr. Antonio: Yes, I recall that; however, I did not provide a copy to anyone at the council.

Counselor Hadrian: Was Mr. Marcus credited with providing that information in any way?

Mr. Antonio: No, he was not.

Counselor Hadrian: Do you know who provided the disc to the leadership at the Health Review Council?

Mr. Antonio: No, I am not aware of how the council obtained a copy of the disc.

Counselor Hadrian: Did the information on this disc serve to improve your approach in conducting health center reviews?

Mr. Antonio: Yes, definitely.

Counselor Hadrian: Mr. Antonio, do you recall anything else that Mr. Marcus asked you at the Thursday lunch?

Mr. Antonio: No.

Counselor Hadrian: Let me refresh your memory. Did Mr. Marcus ask you again, and I quote: "Mr. Antonio, you asked for my impression of Dr. Machiavelli on Sunday, before I ever met him, and now you don't want to answer as to why you asked that question?"

Counselor Luke: I object; this question has been asked and answered many times over.

Counselor Hadrian: I am setting the background for my next question.

Magistrate: Objection overruled. Mr. Antonio, you may proceed.

Mr. Antonio: Yes, he did say that.

Counselor Hadrian: And how did you respond?

Mr. Antonio: I said I didn't want to get in the middle of it. I suggested that he sit down with Dr. Machiavelli and talk to him.

Counselor Hadrian: And what did Mr. Marcus say?

Mr. Antonio: He said, the middle of what? He said he'd tried on several occasions to speak to Dr. Machiavelli but he was nonresponsive.

Counselor Hadrian: Did Mr. Marcus relate to you his attempts at conversation with Dr. Machiavelli in an elevator at the Pelopidas Street Inn?

Mr. Antonio: Yes, he said that his last attempt to have a casual conversation with Dr. Machiavelli was on the elevator on Tuesday evening at the inn after that day's review.

Counselor Hadrian: And did Mr. Marcus describe how Dr. Machiavelli responded?

Mr. Antonio: He said that Dr. Machiavelli failed to respond and that he got off on a floor just below his, walked away, never said good night, never acknowledged that he, Mr. Marcus, was in the elevator. He said that Dr. Machiavelli just got off the elevator and walked away, with the elevator doors closing being him.

Counselor Hadrian: In other words, he ignored Mr. Marcus's attempt at any conversation?

Counselor Luke: Objection, Your Honor—he is leading the witness.

Magistrate: Objection sustained.

Counselor Hadrian: Does Dr. Machiavelli appear to have a hearing problem that you are aware of?

Mr. Antonio: Oh no, quite the opposite.

Counselor Hadrian: Could you describe the size of that elevator?

Counselor Luke: I object, Your Honor. I see no relevance to this line of questioning.

Magistrate: Let us see where this is going. Overruled. Mr. Antonio, you may answer the question.

Mr. Antonio: It was small. Six people, and it would have been crowded.

Counselor Hadrian: So, even if Dr. Machiavelli was hard of hearing, he most likely heard Mr. Marcus's comment.

Mr. Antonio: Yes.

Events of Thursday Late Afternoon, October 6

The withholding of truth is sometimes a worse deception than a direct misstatement. There is an idiom in truth which falsehood never can imitate.

—Lord Napier

[Counselor Hadrian recalls Mr. Antonio to the witness stand to testify regarding events of late afternoon on Thursday, October 6. Counselor Hadrian's first questions of Mr. Antonio at this time have to do with Mr. Marcus having just finished the fourth day of his 5-day review in Athens and returning to the conference room assigned by the Athens Health Center as home base for the health reviewers. Both the morning briefings with the Athens Health Center leadership and the afternoon debriefings with the reviewers were being held there. But as Mr. Marcus headed back to the conference room shortly before that evening's debriefing, he observed his colleagues Mr. Antonio and Ms. Galeria scurry past him, avoiding eye contact, as if they just wanted to get out of the Athens Health Center. Mr. Marcus thought that was strange, and he supposed that there must not be an afternoon debriefing after all.]

Counselor Hadrian: Mr. Antonio, following lunch on Thursday, did you again see Mr. Marcus before leaving the Athens Health Center?

Mr. Antonio: Yes.

Counselor Hadrian: And when was that?

Mr. Antonio: I saw him at the end of the day.

Counselor Hadrian: And where were you when you saw him?

Mr. Antonio: I was leaving the review for the day and was headed back to the inn.

Counselor Hadrian: And who was with you?

Mr. Antonio: Ms. Galeria.

Counselor Hadrian: Did you and Ms. Galeria leave separately from Mr. Marcus?

Mr. Antonio: Yes.

Counselor Hadrian: With whom did you leave at the end of the day to return to the Pelopidas Street Inn on Monday, Tuesday, and Wednesday?

Mr. Antonio: We all left together.

Counselor Hadrian: Who are "we"?

Mr. Antonio: The nurse trainee, Mr. Marcus, Dr. Machiavelli, and myself.

Counselor Hadrian: So you and Ms. Galeria left on Thursday without Marcus and Dr. Machiavelli?

Mr. Antonio: Yes.

Counselor Hadrian: And why was that?

Counselor Luke: Magistrate, I object. I fail to see any relevance to this question.

Magistrate: Overruled. You may answer the question.

Mr. Antonio: Dr. Machiavelli said he talked to Bruce and they planned a conference call with Daniel.

Marcus: Who is Bruce?

Mr. Antonio: Bruce Verus. He is Mr. Marcus's manager at the council office.

Counselor Hadrian: So you generally meet as a team at the end of each day to debrief and review the team's findings?

Mr. Antonio: Yes.

Counselor Hadrian: On Thursday, October 6, you did not have such a meeting?

Mr. Antonio: No.

Counselor Hadrian: So you walked past Mr. Marcus on Thursday with Ms. Galeria, and you saw Mr. Marcus coming toward the two of you. Is that correct?

Mr. Antonio: Yes.

Counselor Hadrian: So were you in the hallway when you spotted him, or someplace else?

Mr. Antonio: We were in an office area when we passed him in a small aisle between desks.

Counselor Hadrian: Did he ask where you were going?

Mr. Antonio: I don't recall.

Counselor Hadrian: So you never acknowledged that you saw him. Is that correct?

Mr. Antonio: Well, what could I say?

Counselor Hadrian: I am asking the questions. You are to answer them. Magistrate, could you please instruct the witness as to protocol.

Magistrate: Mr. Antonio, answer the questions. I don't want a cat-and-mouse game before me.

Mr. Antonio: I did not acknowledge him.

Counselor Hadrian: How far apart were you when you walked by him?

Mr. Antonio: A few feet.

Counselor Hadrian: Did you make eye contact with him?

Mr. Antonio: No, I did not.

Counselor Hadrian: So you knew that a confrontation was awaiting Mr. Marcus when he met up with Dr. Machiavelli?

Counselor Luke: Objection.

Magistrate: Overruled.

Counselor Hadrian: So you knew Mr. Marcus was about to be ambushed when he walked into the conference room.

Mr. Antonio: Uh—

Counselor Luke: Objection, Your Honor.

Magistrate: Objection sustained. Counselor Hadrian, please tone down your question a few notches.

Counselor Hadrian: Were you aware that Dr. Machiavelli was waiting for Mr. Marcus to return from his day's activities?

Mr. Antonio: Yes, I was.

Counselor Hadrian: And what else did you know?

Mr. Antonio: That Bruce maneuvered to have Mr. Marcus removed from the review.

Counselor Hadrian: Maneuvered?

Mr. Antonio: Oh, uh, I mean planned.

Counselor Hadrian: So you knew that your "friend" was going to be facing an early removal from the review. Is that correct?

Mr. Antonio: Yes, I did.

Counselor Hadrian: You considered Mr. Marcus your friend earlier in the week. Are you still friends?

Mr. Antonio: I assume so.

Counselor Hadrian: Do you think your assumption is accurate?

Counselor Luke: Objection, the question has been asked and answered.

Magistrate: Objection sustained.

Counselor Hadrian: So who held the higher rank, you or Dr. Machiavelli?

Mr. Antonio: Dr. Machiavelli.

Counselor Hadrian: Mr. Antonio, were you intimidated by Dr. Machiavelli because of his rank?

[Mr. Antonio was in fact intimidated, but he does not wish to reveal that to the magistrate.]

Mr. Antonio: No.

Counselor Hadrian: Let me reword that question. Because of Dr. Machiavelli's previous service as a admiral, do you believe you held back from responding to Marcus when he kept asking you why you wanted his opinion of Dr. Machiavelli? Did you feel like you were in the middle, like you were between a rock and a hard place?

Counselor Luke: Objection.

Magistrate: What is the basis for your objection?

Counselor Luke: Objection withdrawn.

Magistrate: Mr. Antonio, you may answer the question.

Mr. Antonio: Well, yes. He had a higher rank—substantially higher rank.

Counselor Hadrian: I have no more questions at this time.

Events of Thursday Evening, October 6

[Marcus is recalled to the witness stand.]

Counselor Hadrian: When you arrived back at the conference room, how did Dr. Machiavelli greet you?

Mr. Marcus: There was no greeting, really. He just said, "Follow me. We have to go to another room for a conference call with Bruce. We can't make a conference call from the phone in this room."

Counselor Hadrian: Then what happened?

Mr. Marcus: I asked, "What conference call?"

Counselor Hadrian: How did Dr. Machiavelli respond to your question?

Mr. Marcus: He disregarded the question.

Counselor Hadrian: Then what happened?

Mr. Marcus: We walked into a small conference room, probably 9 feet by 11 feet, that had a small, circular conference table with four chairs around it and a telephone in the middle.

Counselor Hadrian: Then what happened?

Mr. Marcus: Dr. Machiavelli placed a phone call to Bruce, who was sitting in his office waiting.

Counselor Hadrian: Who is Bruce?

Mr. Marcus: Bruce Verus. He is my supervisor at the council office.

Counselor Hadrian: You may continue.

Mr. Marcus: Bruce stated that he was removing me the from the Athens Health Center review until he conducted an investigation.

Counselor Hadrian: Did he ever explain to you what he was investigating?

Mr. Marcus: No, he did not. I asked if it had something to do with me reporting Dr. Caesar's behavior.

Counselor Hadrian: What was his response?

Mr. Marcus: He just reiterated that he had to conduct some sort of investigation. I assumed it had to do with my reporting Dr. Caesar at the Thursday morning briefing with the Athens leadership.

Counselor Hadrian: So he did not answer your question?

Mr. Marcus: No, he did not give an answer. Basically, he said he was my manager, end of story. I think he needed time to make up something from whole cloth.

Counselor Hadrian: What do you mean by "whole cloth"?

Mr. Marcus: He had to fabricate an answer; he did not have a clear answer ready. He had to come up with something.

Counselor Hadrian: Do you know if Mr. Verus was an officer in the military?

Mr. Marcus: Yes, he was.

Counselor Hadrian: What branch of the service was he in?

Mr. Marcus: He was in the army.

Counselor Hadrian: Did he have a higher rank than Dr. Machiavelli?

Mr. Marcus: No, he did not. He was a captain.

Counselor Hadrian: Did you ask any other questions as to why you were being removed from this review?

Mr. Marcus: Yes, I asked Bruce why I would be removed from a review at the end of the fourth day of a 5-day survey, especially in light of the fact that the fifth day was truly only a half-day of reviewing and one half-day having lunch and preparing the final report.

Counselor Hadrian: And what did he say?

Mr. Marcus: He said he is the supervisor and that it was his decision.

Counselor Hadrian: Did Mr. Verus describe how he was going to go about his investigation?

Mr. Marcus: He said that he wanted to talk to the CEO, but she had gone on vacation after the review. He said that, after her return from vacation, he would get back to me within 2 weeks.

Counselor Hadrian: Did Mr. Verus get back to you?

Mr. Marcus: No, he did not. As a matter of fact, I learned later from Ophelia that the CEO of the Athens Health Center had resigned her position as CEO. I assume that is one of the reasons she was said to be on vacation.

Counselor Hadrian: Do you doubt that Mr. Verus actually ever spoke to the CEO?

Mr. Marcus: Yes, I have my doubts. But then, I don't know. There is no written record of any discussion.

Counselor Hadrian: Did he tell you why he wanted to talk to the CEO?

Mr. Marcus: No, he did not.

Counselor Hadrian: How did you learn that the CEO resigned?

Mr. Marcus: Ophelia Cicero, my guide at the Athens Health Center, related this information to me after I had returned home.

Counselor Hadrian: Did Ms. Cicero contact you, or did you contact her?

Mr. Marcus: She e-mailed me on my corporate e-mail and asked that I call her. She said that she preferred not to communicate through e-mail.

Counselor Hadrian: Did she include a telephone number in the e-mail?

Mr. Marcus: Yes, she provided me with her direct line at the Athens Health Center, as well as her cell phone number.

Counselor Hadrian: Do you have any notes of that telephone conversation?

Mr. Marcus: Yes.

[Counselor Hadrian speaks to the magistrate.]

Counselor Hadrian: Magistrate, I would like to show these papers to the witness.

Magistrate: Request granted.

Counselor Hadrian: Do you recognize these papers?

Mr. Marcus: Yes.

Counselor Hadrian: What do you recognize them to be?

Mr. Marcus: These are the notes I took during the phone conversation I had with Ophelia.

Counselor Hadrian: Magistrate, I would like to have these notes marked as Exhibit B and have Marcus read them into the record.

[The following notes are read by Mr. Marcus and entered into the record.]

Notes by Ophelia

Marcus, first of all, I want to thank you. I want you to know it was a pleasure to work with you. You have a wonderful way of putting people at ease and of politely gleaning information from them. You were able to determine from your questions the quality of care we offer here at the Athens Health Center. When I think of the book If Disney Ran Your Hospital *and the fact that you went over and beyond in customer service . . . I saw that in you. I have a report somewhere here on my desk from staff feedback and how well you related to them—you should see it. I am off to a meeting right now, but I will share it with you later.*

Your presentation regarding Dr. Caesar was fair and well balanced during the Thursday morning session.

The team leader was less than polite to you. He was disengaged with you, but he did not act this way with the other health reviewers. Other staff members commented on this behavior.

On Friday morning I was told you would not be back. Dr. Machiavelli never mentioned a thing about you or why you were not there. Health reviewers were coming and going all week, so I don't think anyone thought anything about it. I was very disturbed about the whole thing.

If anybody asks me, you will get a good report.

A Mind Is a Terrible Thing to Change

A politician may be able to survive cavorting with prostitutes, sexting with coeds and comingling with interns, but heaven forbid he should change his mind—the transgression that trumps all compassion.

Or thinking.

After all, thinking can lead to that most dangerous territory for a politician—doubt—and, inevitably, the implication that dare not be expressed: "I could be wrong."

Kathleen Parker, The Washington Post, *June 12, 2011*

Events of December 27–29 Educational Conference

[Counselor Hadrian continues to question Mr. Marcus regarding his early dismissal from participating in the review at the Athens Health Center by Mr. Verus, who claimed he wanted to investigate Mr. Marcus's encounter with Dr. Caesar. This seems to be a typical shoot-the-messenger investigation.]

Counselor Hadrian: Did there come a time when you approached Mr. Verus and asked him for the results of his investigation?

Mr. Marcus: Yes, I did at noon on the first day of the annual training conference, December 27–29.

Counselor Hadrian: Up until that time, did you have any feedback from Mr. Verus as to the results of his investigation?

Mr. Marcus: No, I did not. That's why I decided to contact him at the conference.

Counselor Hadrian: Did you ever provide information as to what occurred at the Athens Health Center to Mr. Verus prior to the conference?

Mr. Marcus: Yes, I did.

Counselor Hadrian: In what form did you relate that information?

Mr. Marcus: I relayed the information in the form of several memoranda to Bruce on the date of my encounters with Dr. Caesar, Health Care Council reviewers, and Athens Health Center staff.

Counselor Hadrian: Could you explain to the magistrate why you wrote memoranda to Mr. Verus the day he removed you from the Athens Health Center review?

Mr. Marcus: I wanted to get across the facts of my experience with Dr. Caesar and not depend on recollection at a later date, which turned out to be *much* later. I simply did not wish to be accused of making up a story.

Counselor Hadrian: During the investigation, did you ever meet your accusers in the same room, in the presence of Mr. Verus or any other leadership member, to ask them questions?

Mr. Marcus: No.

Counselor Hadrian: How would you describe the investigation?

Mr. Marcus: It was somewhat amorphous.

Counselor Hadrian: So you would suggest that it was trumped up?

Counselor Luke: Objection, Counselor Hadrian is leading Mr. Marcus.

Magistrate: Objection sustained.

Counselor Hadrian: So when you saw Mr. Verus at the December educational conference, what was the essence of your conversation?

Mr. Marcus: I told Bruce that his mysterious investigation had gone on for several months and that I would like to know what was going on.

Counselor Hadrian: And what did he say?

Mr. Marcus: He said, "You're right, I should have gotten back to you sooner. Well, let's see—I've got a half-hour slot for you on the 29th at 3:00."

Counselor Hadrian: How did you respond?

Mr. Marcus: I asked for more time and an earlier meeting, but he said he was too busy and didn't have time for me.

Counselor Hadrian: So, repeat for the record, please. On what day of the conference was this that you spoke with Mr. Verus about wanting to meet with him concerning the investigation?

Mr. Marcus: It was on December 27, at noon, on the first day of the conference.

Counselor Hadrian: So you eventually did meet with Mr. Verus.

Mr. Marcus: Yes.

Counselor Hadrian: Where did he meet with you?

Mr. Marcus: He met me in a small conference room at the hotel.

Counselor Hadrian: Was he alone?

Mr. Marcus: No, his manager, Carol Titus, was also there.

Counselor Hadrian: Why was Ms. Titus there?

Mr. Marcus: I am not sure, other than to provide Bruce support. She added nothing to the discussion.

Counselor Hadrian: What happened at this half-hour meeting?

Mr. Marcus: Bruce provided me with a five-page document that he wanted me to sign. It appeared to have been hastily written during the conference.

Counselor Hadrian: So Mr. Verus gave you 30 minutes to sign a five-page document. Is that correct?

Mr. Marcus: Yes.

Counselor Hadrian (handing the document to Marcus): Is this the document he wanted you to read, digest, and sign in less than 30 minutes?

Mr. Marcus: Yes.

Counselor Hadrian: Magistrate, I would like to mark this document into evidence as Exhibit C.

Magistrate: So ordered.

Counselor Hadrian: Mr. Marcus, could you read the contents of Exhibit C?

Mr. Marcus: Yes.

[Marcus reads Exhibit C into the record.]

Counselor Hadrian: As you read from Exhibit C, you recommended that the hospital purchase a car wash to help pay for a dental clinic. What is that about?

Marcus: Some physicians, nurses, and myself were brainstorming ideas on how to prevent the pediatric dental clinic at the Athens Health Center from closing due to the lack of funds.

Counselor Hadrian: So these five pages sound as though someone was pulling snippets of communications out of context and placing his or her spin on the communications that you were having with staff at the hospital. Is that correct?

Counselor Luke: Objection, he is leading the witness.

Magistrate: I will allow the question. Mr. Marcus, you may answer the question.

Mr. Marcus: Yes, that is correct. He said that I had to sign the document before returning to work. I said, "This was supposed to have been a review of your investigation, but instead, I am handed a five-page document and told I have to sign it here and now."

Counselor Hadrian: Then what happened?

Mr. Marcus: I said, "I need more time to review what you have written here." He then asked how much time I needed, and I said 21 days to prepare a response.

Counselor Hadrian: Then what happened?

Mr. Marcus: I noticed that his supervisor, Ms. Titus, who had claimed she was there just to observe, shook her head "no" at Bruce. He then said to me, "Can you get back to me by Friday?"

Counselor Hadrian: Then what happened?

Mr. Marcus: I said it was already Wednesday afternoon and that I needed at least the weekend. He looked over at Ms. Titus again, and she gave him a reluctant nod okay.

Counselor Hadrian: The document also notes that you suggested holding a car wash. For clarification purposes, could you explain in more detail why you suggested a car wash?

Counselor Luke: Objection, this has nothing to do with this hearing.

Magistrate: Objection overruled. Since it was important enough to place in the five-page report, it is important enough to discuss. You may continue, Mr. Marcus.

Mr. Marcus: We were talking about fundraising in one of the Athens Health Center's clinics, as I recall. They were concerned that they might have to close it due to lack of funds, and we got into a discussion of how to save the clinic. I said that, in life, there is something everybody can do in order to fund health care projects. When I reviewed health centers, I would often say that all age groups and people from all walks of life have something to offer. For example, kids could organize car washes, nursing home patients could knit sweaters for selling in gift shops, and there are so many other things that people could do to raise funds. It was an example of what can be done when you're considering closing programs that benefit the community. The statement was taken out of context, and honestly, Dr. Machiavelli and friends didn't understand that.

Counselor Hadrian: I have no more questions for Mr. Marcus at this time. I would like to call Dr. Caesar to the witness stand.

Magistrate: We will take a 15-minute break. Counselors, I would like to speak with you in my chambers.

[**Following the break, the magistrate and counselors return to the hearing.**]

Magistrate: Counselor Hadrian, you may continue.

Counselor Hadrian: At some point, were you told that Mr. Marcus was reviewing a case of yours?

Dr. Caesar: Yes, I was.

Counselor Hadrian: Do you recall who told you?

Caesar: One of the staff nurses.

Counselor Hadrian: Were you invited by the nurse to attend the review?

Dr. Caesar. Yes, I was.

Counselor Hadrian: Did you go to the conference room?

Dr. Caesar: Yes, I did.

Counselor Hadrian: Did Mr. Marcus at any time introduce himself to you as a physician?

Dr. Caesar: No, he did not.

Counselor Hadrian: Did there come a time when Mr. Marcus asked about the care of one of your patients?

Dr. Caesar: Yes, he did.

Counselor Hadrian: Did you object to his questions?

Dr. Caesar: No, I did not.

Counselor Hadrian: Were you aware that such questions are part of the process of reviewing the quality of health care at the Athens Health Center?

Dr. Caesar: Yes, I was aware but not of the protocol as to how the reviewers could go about the process in only 5 days.

Counselor Hadrian: So are you more understanding now of what Mr. Marcus's role was in this process?

Dr. Caesar: Yes, I am.

Counselor Hadrian: Did there come a time when Mr. Marcus asked to speak to the patient?

Dr. Caesar: Yes.

Counselor Hadrian: So Mr. Marcus talked to your patient?

Dr. Caesar: Yes, he did.

Counselor Hadrian: What happened after he spoke to your patient?

Dr. Caesar: I asked if I could say something.

Counselor Hadrian: What did you say to the patient?

Dr. Caesar: I was blunt with the patient as to the serious nature of his prognosis.

Counselor Hadrian: How did the patient react?

Dr. Caesar: He started to break down.

Counselor Hadrian: Then what happened?

Dr. Caesar: Mr. Marcus told the patient that he would be okay.

Counselor Hadrian: Then what happened?

Dr. Caesar: I quickly followed Mr. Marcus out of the room, stopped him, and told him to never tell a patient of mine that he would be okay.

Counselor Hadrian: Did there come a time when the nurse asked that you and Mr. Marcus step away from the entrance to the patient's room?

Dr. Caesar: Yes, she did not want to upset the patient.

Counselor Hadrian: Why were you disturbed with Mr. Marcus?

Dr. Caesar: Well, I was upset that Mr. Marcus had said to my patient that he would be okay. But that was only because I thought he was speaking clinically about my patient.

Counselor Hadrian: So you now understand that Mr. Marcus was not speaking as to your clinical skills or competence?

Dr. Caesar: That is correct.

Counselor Hadrian: So his departing words were . . . ?

Dr. Caesar: He thanked me for my time.

Counselor Hadrian: Did he extend his hand and say thank you?

Dr. Caesar: Yes, he did.

Counselor Hadrian: Did the nurses ever explain to you that Mr. Marcus was not a physician?

Dr. Caesar: Yes, they explained that to me the following day. Honestly, I can't believe that this was taken to such an extreme. I thought it was over. I had no clue this was a continuing saga. I don't understand why no one ever spoke to me. After all, it was just the two of us that spoke to one another.

Counselor Hadrian: Let's back up a minute. Let me paraphrase here: you said that you were never aware that Mr. Marcus was being investigated because of this incident?

Dr. Caesar: I never knew there was an investigation. No one ever asked me any questions about our interactions, and I have since apologized to Mr. Marcus for my failure to recognize that he was not a physician and was merely getting a general picture of the patient's satisfaction with his care.

Counselor Hadrian: Are you aware that Mr. Marcus resigned his position as a result of this incident, because of the wall of silence surrounding this mystery investigation?

Dr. Caesar: No, I was never aware that there was an investigation. I thought our interaction was over the day I left that unit. No one ever spoke to me.

Counselor Hadrian: Did Mr. Marcus ever contact you regarding the incident?

Dr. Caesar: Yes, he did.

Counselor Hadrian: Did you ever receive an e-mail, Dr. Caesar?

Dr. Caesar: Yes, I did.

Counselor Hadrian: Were there several e-mails back and forth between you and Marcus?

Dr. Caesar: Yes, there were several e-mails.

Counselor Hadrian (handing copies of the e-mails to Dr. Caesar): Are these the e-mails that were exchanged between you and Mr. Marcus?

Dr. Caesar: Yes, they are.

Counselor Hadrian: Magistrate, I would like to mark these e-mails into evidence as Exhibits D, E, and F.

Magistrate: So ordered. You may proceed.

Counselor Hadrian: The e-mails by date and time are as follows:

EXHIBIT D December 19 (8:24 a.m.)

Dr. Caesar:

As you may or may not know, as a result of your treatment of me during my survey at your hospital, I never again worked for the Health Review Council. Isn't it sad how you found it necessary to be so rude to me? I hope each time you look in the mirror that you always remember that day. I was never anything but polite toward you and compassionate toward your patient. I hope that someday you will find the strength to apologize. And as I said, I was not a doctor and was not judging your clinical skills. Why you kept asking if I was a doctor was a mystery to me. Maybe you had me mixed up with the Joint Commission team leader, who was a physician. Even though I found you rude on that one occasion, I do wish you much success.

    Sincerely, Daniel Marcus

EXHIBIT E December 19 (10:15 a.m.)

Dear Mr. Marcus,

Thank you for contacting me. We have so many interactions in life, good and bad; although this case was obviously the latter, it is a rare opportunity to try to clear the air and, perhaps, for me to apologize. Based on what you wrote, that may not be possible, but I would like to try. If you would be willing to send me a phone number, I would like to talk to you about it. I will be watching my e-mail all day, and I offer to telephone you at any time you prefer.

    Even though it has been a year, I remember you, that day, and my patient's case very well. My patient struggled with a potentially life-threatening condition that had baffled many of my colleagues, and to add to it, he was the husband of a colleague of mine. At that time, we were uncertain if he would improve (the condition frequently leads to long-term disability and is associated with high mortality). The comment that I remember most clearly was to the effect of "Don't worry, you will be okay." I am paraphrasing, of course.

    That's a completely understandable and considerate thing to say to a sick person in the hospital. However, it would not be an appropriate comment coming from a physician (which I was told by a nurse on the floor that you were). That, along with your confident demeanor (an attribute) and your probing me with questions regarding different possible diagnoses (asked in a manner similar to my old attending physicians), increased my anxiety to the point that I assumed you were criticizing me as a physician. That's when I snapped at you not to tell my patients they would be okay. To be honest, I would snap at any medical student or resident who made a remark like yours, and it would be justified, but what I said to you was certainly not.

    Regardless of all that, I'm sorry, and if you would be so kind as to send a contact number, I will call you promptly.

    Take care, and like your comment to me, I do wish you the best,

    Dr. Caesar

EXHIBIT F December 19 (11:28 a.m.)

Dear Dr. Caesar,

I truly was happy to see your quick response. It was important for me to let you know that I was never for a moment judging your clinical skills. I have always taken pride in working well with physicians. When I left my hospital as administrator in _____, both my physicians and nurses wore black armbands wanting me to stay. I have read about your successful career and just wanted you to know a little more about me and that I was not a gotcha-type administrator reviewer. I have always been an out-of-the-box-type guy seeing the tough world in which physicians must practice.

I would be eager to speak with you on a happier note. My home number is ___-___-___. Again and again, I appreciate your nice comments.

Sincerely,

Daniel Marcus

Counselor Hadrian: So, Dr. Caesar, did there come a time that you called Mr. Marcus?

Dr. Caesar: Yes, the same day the e-mails were written.

Counselor Hadrian: Do you recall the substance of that conversation?

Dr. Caesar: Yes, I do.

Counselor Hadrian: Could you summarize it for the magistrate?

Dr. Caesar: Yes, I can. On the same day that Mr. Marcus and I corresponded through e-mails, I called Mr. Marcus and said, "You can have an interaction with someone for 10 minutes, and there are high stakes to be paid in those 10 minutes. I must tell you that 36 hours after you left, I never heard anything about our conversation regarding my patient. I am so sorry you went through all of this. Actually, we need people like you working in our medical societies. Our conversation just shows what can happen in a high-stakes environment. There are occasions, there are times, when I have interactions that are antithetical to why I went into medicine. If I learned anything in medicine, it is that life is short. Daniel, if you ever need a letter or anything else to clear this up, I will be happy to do anything I can." That is close to what I told him, and like I said, I just can't believe this has gone on for so long. No one ever talked to me. I can't for the life of me believe that a reviewer was removed from a survey from doing his job. You know, I teach ethics, and I find this behavior totally unethical.

Counselor Hadrian: During your telephone conversation, did you ever ask Mr. Marcus if he wanted you to send a letter on his behalf?

Dr. Caesar: Yes, I did.

Counselor Hadrian: How did Mr. Marcus respond to your suggestion?

Dr. Caesar: He said that it wasn't necessary, and he thanked me for the offer.

Counselor Hadrian: Thank you, Dr. Caesar. Thank you. Magistrate, I would like to summarize at this point.

Magistrate: You may proceed.

Counselor Hadrian: In summary, there was no investigation that included Mr. Marcus, or Ms. Cicero, or Dr. Caesar. The notes of the scribe were never forthcoming and were apparently misplaced or destroyed. The positive feedback about Mr. Marcus from the staff at the Athens Health Center to Ms. Cicero can no longer be located. There is no evidence of a written conversation between the CEO and Mr. Verus. The memo that was once offered to Mr. Marcus by Mr. Verus and was supposedly from the CEO was never provided. In fact, Ms. Titus claims that it never existed. The investigation, in my opinion, was completely fabricated, and a snowball started to roll downhill at the Health Review Council. The new leadership apparently was brought into an incident that they were not willing to understand. They relied on staff managers who wished that Marcus would just disappear. They had to cover themselves. They made an unfortunate decision cloaked in a "code of silence." The truth was made so convoluted by the old leadership that the new leadership had no clue what to do and could only rely on what was being regurgitated to them. It is unfortunate that the Health Review Council's leadership never admitted to their wrongdoing. *(Pause)* Magistrate, this is a case of "don't confuse me with facts." I have no more questions.

Magistrate: Counselor Luke, do you have any witnesses or documents to bring forth?

Counselor Luke: No, I do not.

Magistrate: Counselor Hadrian, you may sum up your thoughts.

Counselor Hadrian: In summary, I will be brief as to the Health Review Council's handling of this case. The council's practice of strict arbitrary rulings and secretive proceedings is unconscionable. An organization whose goal it is to help ensure the quality of health care throughout the nation has failed to ensure the rights of its own employees, in this case, Mr. Daniel Marcus. The council became confused and buried in its own morass of poor decision making. It lacked the ability to see the light of day. The council's attitude, *I have already made up my mind. Don't confuse me with the facts*, is appalling. It is an indictment as to the trustworthiness of this organization's leadership. I find in this case no good-faith attempt by the Health Review Council to clear Marcus's good name. It is a sad day when an organization fails to live up to its own ethical standards.

Magistrate: Having listened to the testimony as to what occurred during this review, I need no time for further consideration, for I have heard enough. I hereby strongly reprimand the leadership of the council for failing to ferret out the truth. Based on what I have heard, I do not believe the full truth will ever be heard, because they've dug themselves in so deeply that even they do not know what the truth is.*

 To seek for the truth, for the sake of knowing the truth, is one of the noblest objects a man can live for.

—WILLIAM RALPH INGE

Please refer to the Pillars of Moral Strength when answering the following discussion questions.

Discussion

1. Describe the ethical and legal issues in this closet drama as they relate to the various characters.
2. Describe the virtues and values in play.

---

*The playwright who wrote this closet drama remains anonymous and retains the rights of ownership of the information contained herein.

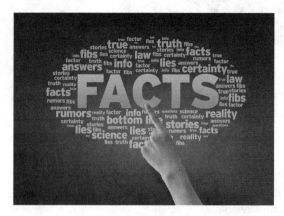

FIGURE 15-2   Facts Spawn Truth(© Bildagentur Zoonar GmbH/Shutterstock, Inc.)

3. Describe why you think there was a breakdown in communications between Dr. Caesar and Marcus.

4. In light of the fact that 70% of diagnoses are made as the result of lab tests, would you expect Marcus to inquire what the lab results had revealed about the patient's state of health?

5. Describe your overall impression of this case, and how you would have handled it if you were Marcus.

6. After considering yourself in the position of each character in this closet drama, describe which role you would have chosen to play. Explain your choice of character.

7. How would you describe the culture of the Health Review Council?

8. Using the communications process in **Figure 15-2**, how would you describe the values of each character in this case?

TEST YOUR UNDERSTANDING

Terminology

communication   noise interference   nonverbal communication

GLOSSARY

Abandonment: Unilateral severance by the physician of the professional relationship between himself or herself and the patient without reasonable notice at a time when the patient still needs continuing care.

Abortion: Premature termination of pregnancy at a time when the fetus is incapable of sustaining life independent of the mother.

Ad litem: A Latin term meaning "for the suit." A *guardian ad litem* is a person appointed by a court to defend a legal action on the part of a child or incapacitated person. A *guardian ad litem* is specifically appointed for the purposes of a suit.

Admissibility (of evidence): Refers to the issue of whether a court, applying the rules of evidence, is bound to receive or permit introduction of a particular piece of evidence.

Advance directives: Written instructions expressing one's health care wishes in the event that he or she becomes incapacitated and is unable to make such decisions.

Adverse drug reaction: An unusual or unexpected response to a normal dose of a medication; an injury caused by the use of a drug in the usual, acceptable fashion.

Affidavit: A voluntary statement of facts, or a voluntary declaration in writing of facts, that a person swears to be true before an official authorized to administer an oath.

Agent: An individual who has been designated by a legal document to make decisions on behalf of another individual; a substitute decision maker.

Americans with Disabilities Act (ADA): Federal act that bars employers from discriminating against disabled persons in hiring, promotion, or other provisions of employment.

Appellant: Party who appeals the decision of a lower court to a court of higher jurisdiction.

Appellee: Party against whom an appeal to a higher court is taken.

Artificial nutrition and hydration: Providing food and liquids, such as intravenous feedings, when a patient is unable to eat or drink.

Assault: Intentional act that is designed to make the victim fearful and produces reasonable apprehension of harm.

Attestation: Act of witnessing a document in writing.

Autonomy: Right of an individual to make his or her own independent decisions.

Battery: Intentional touching of one person by another without the consent of the person being touched.

Beneficence: Describes the principle of doing good, demonstrating kindness, and helping others.

Best evidence rule: Legal doctrine requiring that primary evidence of a fact (such as an original document) be introduced or that an acceptable explanation be given before a copy can be introduced or testimony given concerning the fact.

Borrowed servant doctrine: Refers to a situation in which an employee is temporarily placed under the control of someone other than his or her primary employer. It may involve a situation in which an employee is carrying out the specific instructions of a physician. The traditional example is that of a nurse employed by a hospital who is "borrowed" and under the control of the attending surgeon during a procedure in the operating room. The temporary employer of the borrowed servant can be held responsible for the negligent acts of the borrowed servant under the doctrine of *respondeat superior*. This rule is not easily applied, especially if the acts of the employee are for the furtherance of the objectives of the employer. The courts apply a narrow application if the employee is fulfilling the requirement of his or her position.

Captain-of-the-ship doctrine: A doctrine making the physician responsible for the negligent acts of other professionals because he or she had the right to control and oversee the totality of care provided to the patient.

Cardiopulmonary resuscitation: A lifesaving method used by caregivers to restore heartbeat and breathing.

Case citation: Describes where a court's opinion in a particular case can be located. It identifies the parties in the case, the text in which the case can be found, the court writing the opinion, and the year in which the case was decided. For example, the citation *Bouvia v. Superior Court (Glenchur)*, 225 Cal. Rptr. 297 (Ct. App. 1986), is described as follows:

- *Bouvia v. Superior Court (Glenchur)* identifies the basic parties involved in the lawsuit.
- 225 Cal. Rptr. 297 identifies the case as being reported in volume 225 of the California Reporter at page 297.
- Ct. App. 1986 identifies the case as being in the California Court of Appeals in 1986.

Case law: Aggregate of reported cases on a particular legal subject as formed by the decisions of those cases.

Certiorari: Writ that commands a lower court to certify proceedings for review by a higher court. This is the common method of obtaining review by the U.S. Supreme Court.

Charitable immunity: Legal doctrine that developed out of the English court system that held charitable institutions blameless for their negligent acts.

Civil law: Body of law that describes the private rights and responsibilities of individuals. The part of law that does not deal with crimes, it involves actions filed by one individual against another (e.g., actions in tort and contract).

Clinical privileges: On qualification, the diagnostic and therapeutic procedures that an institution allows a physician to perform on a specified patient population. Qualification includes a review of a physician's credentials, such as medical school diploma, state licensure, and residency training.

Closed-shop contract: Labor–management agreement that provides that only members of a particular union may be hired.

Common law: Body of principles that has evolved and continues to evolve and expand from court decisions. Many of the legal principles and rules applied by courts in the United States had their origins in English common law.

Comorbidities: Two or more coexisting medical conditions or disease processes that are additional to an initial diagnosis. [http://medical-dictionary.thefreedictionary.com/Comorbidities].

Complaint: The first pleading, in an alleged negligence action, filed in a court by the plaintiff's attorney. It is the first statement of a case by the plaintiff against the defendant and states a cause of action, notifying the defendant as to the basis for the suit.

Congressional Record: Document in which the proceedings of Congress are published. It is the first record of debate officially reported, printed, and published directly by the federal government. Publication of the *Congressional Record* began March 4, 1873.

Consent: *See Informed consent.*

Consequentialism: A moral theory that determines good or bad, right or wrong, based on good outcomes or consequences.

Contextualism: An ethical doctrine that considers the rightness or wrongness of an action, such as lying, to be based on the particular circumstances of a given situation. The implication is that lying is acceptable in one situation but not in another, even though the situation may be similar. In other words, it depends on the context within which something occurs.

Criminal negligence: Reckless disregard for the safety of others. It is the willful indifference to an injury that could follow an act.

Decision capacity: Having the mental capacity to make one's own decisions. Mental capacity refers to the ability to understand the risks, benefits, alternatives, and consequences of one's actions. Inferred in this interpretation is knowing the decision maker can reasonably distinguish right from wrong and good from bad.

Defamation: Injury of a person's reputation or character caused by the false statements of another made to a third person. Defamation includes both libel and slander.

Defendant: In a criminal case, the person accused of committing a crime. In a civil suit, the party against whom the suit is brought, demanding that he or she pay the other party legal relief.

Demurrer: Formal objection by one of the parties to a lawsuit that the evidence presented by the other party is insufficient to sustain an issue or case.

Deontological ethics: An ethical approach that focuses on duty rather than on the consequences, when determining the right conduct to be followed.

Deposition: A method of pretrial discovery that consists of statements of fact taken by a witness under oath in a question-and-answer format as it would be in a court of law with opportunity given to the adversary to be present for cross-examination. Such statements may be admitted into evidence if it is impossible for a witness to attend a trial in person.

Determinism: The view that nothing happens without a cause.

Directed verdict: When a trial judge decides that the evidence and/or law is clearly in favor of one party, the judge may direct the jury to return a verdict for the appropriate party. The conclusion of the judge must be so clear and obvious that reasonable minds could not arrive at a different conclusion.

Discharge summary: That part of a medical record that summarizes a patient's initial complaints, course of treatment, final diagnosis, and instructions for follow-up care.

Discovery: To ascertain that which was previously unknown through a pretrial investigation; it includes testimony and documents that may be under the exclusive control of the other party.

Dogmatic: The stubborn refusal to consider challenges to your own ethical point of view.

Do not resuscitate (DNR): Directive of a physician to withhold cardiopulmonary resuscitation in the event that a patient experiences cardiac arrest.

Durable power of attorney: Legal instrument enabling an individual to act on another's behalf. In the health care setting, a *durable power of attorney for health care* is the authority to make medical decisions for another.

Ethical conduct: Conducting oneself in a manner consistent with acceptable principles of right and wrong. Such conduct may relate to one's community, country, profession, and so on.

Ethical dilemma: A situation that forces a person to make a decision that involves breaking some ethical norm or contradicting some ethical value. It involves making a decision between two or more possible actions where any one of the actions can be justified as being the right decision, but, whatever action is taken, there always remains some doubt as to whether the correct course of action was chosen. The effect of an action may put others at risk, harm others, or violate the rights of others.

Ethicist: One who specializes in ethics.

Ethics: A set of principles of right and wrong conduct; a theory or system of moral values, of what is right and what is wrong. Ethics is a system of values that guides behavior in relationships among people in accordance with certain social roles.

Ethics committee: A committee created to deal with ethical problems and dilemmas in the delivery of patient care.

Euthanasia: A Greek word meaning "the good death." It is an act conducted for the purpose of causing the merciful death of a person who is suffering from an incurable condition, such as providing a patient with medications to hasten his or her death.

Evidence: Proof of a fact, which is legally presented in a manner prescribed by law, at trial.

Expert witness: Person who has special training, experience, skill, and knowledge in a relevant area and who is allowed to offer an opinion as testimony in court.

Futility: Having no useful result. Futility of treatment, as it relates to medical care, occurs when the physician recognizes that the effect of treatment will be of no benefit to the patient. Morally, the physician has a duty to inform the patient when there is little likelihood of success.

Good Samaritan laws: Laws designed to protect those who stop to render aid in an emergency. These laws generally provide immunity for specified persons from a civil suit arising out of care rendered at the scene of an emergency, provided that the one rendering assistance has not done so in a grossly negligent manner.

Grand jury: Jury called to determine whether there is sufficient evidence that a crime has been committed to justify bringing a case to trial.

Grievance: The process undertaken to resolve a labor–management dispute when there is an allegation by a union member that management has failed in some way to meet the terms of a labor agreement.

Guardian: Person appointed by a court to protect the interests of and make decisions for a person who is incapable of making his or her own decisions.

Health: According to the World Health Organization, "[a] state of complete physical, mental, and social well-being and not merely the absence of disease or infirmity."

Health Care Financing Administration (HCFA): Federal agency that coordinates the federal government's participation in the Medicare and Medicaid programs.

Health care proxy: Document that delegates the authority to make one's own health care decisions to another, known as the health care agent, when one has become incapacitated or is unable to make his or her own decisions.

Hearsay rule: Rule of evidence restricting the admissibility of evidence that is not the personal knowledge of the witness.

Holographic will: A will handwritten by the testator.

Home health agency: An agency that provides home health services. Home health care involves an array of services provided to patients in their homes or foster homes because of acute illness, exacerbation of chronic illness, and disability. Such services are therapeutic and/or preventative.

Home health care: Home health care is an alternative for those who fear leaving the secure environment of their home. Such care is available through home health agencies. These agencies provide a variety of services for the elderly living at home. Such services include part-time or intermittent nursing care; physical, occupational, and speech therapy; medical social services, home health aide services, and nutritional guidance; medical supplies other than drugs and biologicals prescribed by a physician; and the use of medical appliances.

Hospice care: Care provided for terminally ill persons, provided in a setting more economical than that of a hospital or nursing facility. Hospice care is often sought after a decision has been made to discontinue aggressive efforts to prolong life. A hospice program includes such characteristics as support services by training individuals, family involvement, and control of pain and discomfort.

Hydration: Intravenous addition of fluids to the circulatory system.

Immoral: Behavior that is in opposition to accepted societal, religious, cultural, and/or professional standards.

Incapacity: An individual's lack of ability to make decisions for himself or herself.

Incompetent: Individual determined by a court to be incapable of making rational decisions on his or her own behalf.